Basic pathophysiology

A CONCEPTUAL APPROACH

Basic pathophysiology

A CONCEPTUAL APPROACH

Maureen E. Groër, R.N., Ph.D.

Associate Professor, College of Nursing,
University of Tennessee at Knoxville,
Knoxville, Tennessee

Maureen E. Shekleton, R.N., B.S.N., M.S.N.

Formerly Assistant Professor of Nursing,
Lewis University, Lockport, Illinois

with a contribution by
Kenneth J. Kant, Ph.D.

Associate Professor, College of Nursing,
University of Tennessee at Knoxville,
Knoxville, Tennessee

with 423 illustrations

The C. V. Mosby Company

ST. LOUIS • TORONTO • LONDON   1979

The C. V. Mosby Company
11830 Westline Industrial Drive, St. Louis, Missouri 63141

Library of Congress Cataloging in Publication Data

Groër, Maureen E., 1944-
  Basic pathophysiology.

  Bibliography: p.
  Includes index.
  1. Physiology, Pathological. I. Shekleton,
Maureen E., joint author. II. Title.
RB113.G67 616.07   78-21170
ISBN 0-8016-1983-1

GW/CB/CB 9 8 7 6 5 4 3 2   02/B/219

TO OUR STUDENTS

past, present, and future

Preface

This textbook of basic pathophysiology has been written primarily for students in health-related fields. Students and practitioners of health care should find this approach to pathophysiology very meaningful. Concepts of pathophysiologic mechanisms have broad application to the areas of medicine, nursing, and allied health. All too often the student or practitioner has been faced with a need to understand disease mechanisms at a basic level in order to give intelligent and creative care. While many curricula offer courses in pathophysiology, a textbook that is both theoretic and conceptual has been lacking. The student in the past has been required to extensively review the physiologic, medical, pathologic, and nursing literature to gain information and ultimately to formulate concepts in pathophysiology. This textbook has organized the vast field of pathophysiologic knowledge, including the latest research results, into major *conceptual* areas. These concepts have been unified by the utilization of systems theory as it applies to living organisms. Disease as a loss of the steady state is continually emphasized. With this in mind therapeutic approaches are discussed as mechanisms that act to restore and maintain the steady state.

Each chapter in this book is preceded by a list of objectives. The student is encouraged to review these objectives carefully before beginning the study of the chapter. These objectives should later be used as an aid for the student in self-testing. Accomplishment of these objectives requires not only an increase in knowledge of specific disease states but also that the student form concepts and be able to use these concepts

to problem solve. The suggested readings at the end of each chapter are provided for those students who wish to further increase their knowledge of pathophysiology. This textbook is not a dictionary of diseases but rather a conceptual approach to disease mechanisms. Students wishing to learn the signs and symptoms of unusual disease conditions are therefore referred to textbooks of internal or clinical medicine.

Although each chapter is complete in itself, it is generally expected that cohesiveness is achieved by study of the entire book. It is only after study of the many mechanisms of disease in the various organ systems that the student will begin to appreciate the tremendous interaction of the systems in response to disease.

This textbook should also serve as a valuable reference for students enrolled in all core-curriculum, science-based courses. Although there are many excellent textbooks to support the medical, nursing, and allied health content, there are few textbooks that offer a conceptual, comprehensive, and scientific approach to disease in terms of pathophysiologic mechanisms. Thus, this textbook will be an adjunct to core textbooks and should prove very useful in both the study of theory and in practice. Furthermore, the use of systems theory throughout the book may serve to unify without squelching each individual's own style of health care delivery. Systems theory in general is broadly pertinent to health care and is often part of the conceptual framework of many nursing and other curricula. Students will appreciate its significance even more in the light of the content presentation of this textbook.

We wish to acknowledge Bernice Carroll for

her consultation on the illustrations and tables in this book.

We would like to express our deep appreciation to the following friends and colleagues who reviewed portions of the manuscript as it was being prepared. Their candid and helpful analyses were of great value, and we thank them for the time they spent.

Mary Ellen Banks, R.N., M.S.N.

Assistant Professor,
University of Tennessee College of Nursing,
Knoxville, Tennessee

Kathleen Canda, R.N., M.S.N.

Instructor of Nursing,
Lutheran Medical Center School of Nursing,
Cleveland, Ohio

Kathleen Conlon, R.N., M.S.N.

Assistant Professor,
University of Tennessee College of Nursing,
Knoxville, Tennessee

Juyne De Lessio, R.N., M.A.

Assistant Professor,
Lewis University College of Nursing,
Lockport, Illinois

Patricia Droppleman, R.N., M.S.N.

Assistant Professor,
University of Tennessee College of Nursing,
Knoxville, Tennessee

Judith Dulle, R.N., M.S.N.

Assistant Professor,
Lewis University College of Nursing,
Lockport, Illinois

Dale Goodfellow, R.N., M.S.N.

Associate Professor,
University of Tennessee College of Nursing,
Knoxville, Tennessee

Sylvia Hart, R.N., Ph.D.

Dean,
University of Tennessee College of Nursing,
Knoxville, Tennessee

Mary Lue Jolly, R.N., M.S.N.

Assistant Professor,
University of Tennessee College of Nursing,
Knoxville, Tennessee

Fortunata Kennedy, R.N., M.S.N.

Assistant Professor,
Lewis University College of Nursing,
Lockport, Illinois

Margaret Pierce, R.N., M.S.N.

Assistant Professor,
University of Tennessee College of Nursing,
Knoxville, Tennessee

Dennis Rio, Ph.D.

Associate Professor,
Lewis University,
Lockport, Illinois

The following students also assisted us in reviewing sections of the manuscript, giving us needed insight and perspective or assisting us in other ways: Sarah Carlson, Karen Wimberly, Michael Imbrogna, Theresa McNally, Jacqueline Pociek, Ann Perona, Karen Smith, Sandra Smith, and Mary Ann Todd.

We are also grateful to Linda Welch, who endured much inconvenience so cheerfully when faced with deadlines and rewrites. Judith Canning, Bess Ariens, and Lynne Boeing also assisted with some of the typing, and their help is greatly appreciated.

The excellent illustrations in this textbook were done by Jack Tandy. Pat Fallon, B.F.A., also did a number of illustrations. We wish to acknowledge both of them for their skill and hard work.

Lastly, we wish to thank our husbands and children for their tolerance and sacrifice that they showed throughout the writing of this book.

Maureen E. Groër
Maureen E. Shekleton

Contents

PART ONE

Health and disease: man as an open system

CHAPTER 1

The steady state and pathophysiology: adaptive and compensatory mechanisms of health and disease

Health and disease are extremely complex concepts and are interpreted in many different ways. Health is not only a physiologic parameter but a psychologic and cultural one as well. Furthermore, the idea that health or "wellness" is determined in large part by the individual complicates the precise defining of health and disease. Nevertheless, in terms of physiologic functioning it is possible to define normality and abnormality (pathophysiology) within certain limits and to measure certain phenomena that change with disease.

When the normal physiology of an organism is so disrupted that the function of the organism deteriorates and the organism becomes unstable and subject to further possible attacks on its function and very survival, pathophysiologic mechanisms are likely to arise, and disease results. There are, of course, a myriad of integrated defense mechanisms, compensations, and adaptations that the organism organizes to protect itself from the effects of pathophysiology during the disease episode. For example, at a very basic level this response can be seen in the property of autoregulation in the vascular beds. When cells become hypoxic, various metabolites, such as lactic acid and adenine, accumulate, as well as hydrogen ions and carbon dioxide. These substances exert a vasodilatory effect on the arterioles and precapillary sphincters that supply the tissue beds, thus increasing the blood delivered to the hypoxic cells. This adaptation allows the cells to survive during any pathophysiologic process that produces hypoxia. Thus, a characteristic of health is the ability through complicated regulatory and compensatory mechanisms to respond to threats against homeostasis or the steady state, and disease can be thought of as a threat to the steady state.

Pathophysiology is the study of mechanisms by which disease occurs in living organisms, the responses of the body to the disease process, and the effects of these pathophysiologic mechanisms on normal function. It is a science that seeks to coordinate the signs and symptoms of disease with an understanding of the biology of the disease process at all levels of organization: molecular, cellular, tissue, and so on. Pathophysiology brings together the science of laboratory research with the clinical signs and symptoms that are observed at the bedside. The two sets of observations are intimately entwined. While much basic research has led to broad clinical applications in the understanding, diagnosis, and treatment of disease, the converse process has also been extremely important. Much basic research has been the direct result of clinical observations of the characteristics of a disease state. The unraveling of the immune system resulted from astute observation of the relationship between increased plasma cells and immunoglobulin proliferation in patients with multiple myeloma. From this observation came the impetus to study at the primary level the properties of plasma cells and immunoglobulins, which are now known to be a major foundation of immunity.

Since pathophysiology is such a complex science, involving not only the pathogenesis of disease and the response of the organism to the disease but also the effects of the disease process on normal physiology as a whole, one can say that pathophysiology is a relatively new science. The further development of this science requires not only basic research into the biology of disease but also continuing observations by trained and prepared minds. Those who care for the sick and injured are in the best position to make major contributions to the knowledge of pathophysiology.

It is the purpose of this chapter to introduce the student to the concept that knowledge of diseases is more than memorization of signs and symptoms. When mechanisms by which disease occurs are understood and the nature of the compensatory and adaptive response are clear, then the signs and symptoms are predictable. It should be obvious that pathophysiology cannot be comprehended unless the student has an excellent knowledge of normal physiology. It is not the purpose of this book to present normal physiology except for an occasional review of pertinent material. It is, however, a fortunate circumstance that many times an in-depth understanding of pathophysiology will clarify the normal physiology. Several excellent textbooks on normal human physiology are listed at the end of this chapter for the student to use as review material and in conjunction with this book.

This textbook is organized around the concept of the human organism as an open system, constantly seeking the steady state. Systems theory, which describes this approach, has many applications to physiology and pathophysiology. First used in engineering and computer science, it has since been applied to chemistry, biology, psychology, sociology, and other disciplines with great success. The elements of systems theory will be discussed below. Next various disease states will be described in terms of systems theory. This chapter concludes with a detailed model of pathophysiology not only to illustrate the application of systems theory to pathophysiology but

also to introduce the reader to the possibilities of interacting factors that may be involved in the pathogenesis and propagation of a disease.

SYSTEMS THEORY AND MAN AS AN OPEN SYSTEM

General systems theory was first proposed in 1928 for living organisms by Ludwig von Bertalanffy. The theory deals with the peculiarities of living organisms that interact greatly with the environment and that at first glance then seem to be thermodynamically unique. The systems theory explains the nature of the incredible organization found in life with regard to thermodynamics and the dynamic equilibrium that is maintained in living things and that is required for the organism to ·remain whole, functional, and alive. Thermodynamics had been used to explain physicochemical reactions prior to von Bertalanffy's work.

The second law of thermodynamics states that in a closed or isolated system the *entropy* (Fig. 1-1), which is basically the randomness or disorder of a system, tends to reach a maximum. This is not difficult to understand if one imagines a chemical reaction such as the ionization of sodium chloride in water. A crystal of salt has more structure and therefore a higher degree of energy and lower level of entropy before it is placed in water, but after it dissolves in water the Na^+ and Cl^- ions disperse freely and evenly throughout the water, and the disorder of the sodium chloride is obviously much greater than before dissolution. It also takes much less energy to maintain the dissolved and dispersed state of the sodium chloride as compared to that required to maintain the organization of the sodium chloride crystal. It is a tendency then of this system, which consists of sodium chloride and water, to reach a level of maximum entropy according to the second law. Such a system does not exchange freely with the environment and is isolated or *closed*. In contrast, biologic systems are open in that a constant exchange with the environment is absolutely required in order for the living organism to maintain its special equilibrium. The open system does not tend toward the true equilibriums of closed systems, which implies the tendency toward maximum entropy,

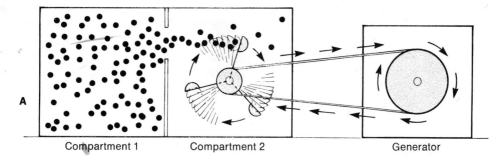

Compartment 1   Compartment 2   Generator

Molecules move in same general direction from compartment 1
to compartment 2, causing wheel to turn and run generator.

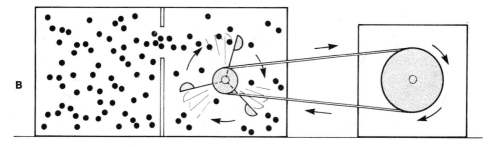

As distribution becomes more random, motion slows.

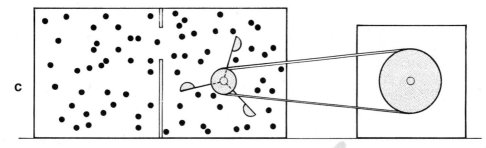

System becomes equalized and motion stops.

Fig. 1-1. Entropy and energy model. When there is order and organization in system, **A,** in which molecules are localized to compartment *1,* movement of molecules generates energy. As entropy of system increases, **B,** there is less and less energy generated. **C,** No energy is generated due to a totally random state of maximum entropy for this system. In living systems there is structure and tremendous organization, such that entropy is balanced by large inputs of free energy, and a steady state is maintained. As system ages or becomes diseased, the overall entropy tends to increase.

but rather toward dynamic equilibriums, which Hill defined as the *steady state*. This does not imply, however, that the second law is violated by living organisms but only that the open system must be analyzed in the context *of its environment*. Since living organisms take up and release energy and matter, which are necessary for the metabolism of the organism, the taking up of molecules that have much free energy available for work by the organism will eventually result in the metabolism of these molecules and release of heat or work by the organism that is thermodynamically equivalent to that originally used. If the open system is in a steady state, the entropy level is maintained in constant balance since the positive entropy that results from irreversible catabolism is equally balanced by the input of food molecules, which are high in free energy. In the open system of humans, the entropy of the living organism may be low, while the overall entropy of the environment with which humans interact may be increasing. In a sense humans deplete the environment of order and organization in order to maintain the steady state. However, all organisms die eventually, thus in a sense returning to the environment in highly entropic states.

Disease, when it interferes with the steady state of the open system, can be interpreted as increasing the entropy levels of the organism. Entropy and free energy are quantifiable terms, and a knowledge of the derivation of these terms is useful when discussing such diverse phenomena as biologic transport, osmotic work, action potentials, and pathophysiologic breakdowns of the steady state. A simple formula for calculating any change in free energy or entropy in a reaction is:

$$\Delta F = \Delta H - T\Delta S$$

where ΔF is change in free energy, ΔH is change in heat content or *enthalpy*, ΔS is change in entropy, and T is temperature.

The ΔH is always constant at a given temperature, so it can be seen that the ΔF becomes more negative as entropy increases. It is also apparent in this formula that entropy is temperature dependent. A reaction that increases free energy requires the input of energy and is termed *endergonic*, whereas reactions that decrease free energy release energy (in forms such as heat) and are termed *exergonic*. Another formula that relates the ΔF to the equilibriim constant of a reaction is

$$\Delta F = -RT \ln K$$

or

$$\Delta F = -2.303 \, RT \log K$$

where R is gas constant, K is equilibrium constant, and T is temperature.

The relationship of these formulas to pathophysiology is quite simple. If disease is thought of as increasing the entropy of the organism,

then it can be seen that the change in free energy becomes more and more negative. To maintain a balance the organism must increase its free energy through mechanisms that increase the order of the system. Compensatory mechanisms and adaptations do precisely this, but if they are inadequate in the face of progressive pathophysiology, the entropy levels will continue to increase, the order and organization of the organism will be progressively compromised, and death will eventually occur.

What has traditionally been known in physiology as homeostasis is in reality the steady state. Living organisms are made up of component parts, which all act to maintain dynamic equilibriums. This steady state is governed by the tendency of the biologic system to maintain itself, to regulate processes that are constantly fluctuating, and to generally preserve the organism in the changing environment. An important characteristic of the steady state is the property of *equifinality*, which means that the end result of biologic pathways can be reached through a variety of ways. Systems are able to adapt through various physiologic processes to alterations in the environment and thus maintain the steady state such that particular characteristics of the organism are always the same. For example, the blood glucose concentration must be maintained within certain limits. There is not just one route or mechanism by which the body regulates this. It is only when disease is present that these regulatory processes may be greatly interfered with, and the blood glucose level may not be regulated carefully. A disease such as *diabetes mellitus* interferes with the steady state of the organism by disrupting blood glucose regulation; the ramifications of this disease process are manifold and could eventually result in death (maximal entropy) if treatment is not instituted.

CYBERNETIC REGULATION OF THE STEADY STATE

There are a variety of mechanisms by which organisms act to maintain the steady state, and terms have been borrowed from cybernetics to explain these various phenomena. Regulation of metabolic functions is an obvious requirement of the steady state if an open system requires a balance in the flow of energy and matter between the organism and the environment. Two types of *feedback loops,* positive and negative, operate in the regulation of metabolism. These feedbacks are mechanisms whereby metabolic reactions, hormonal action, and concentrations of critical substances are controlled. Feedback loops may be open or closed; in biologic regulation most feedback loops are closed loops. These are illustrated in box at right; it can be seen that in the open loop, the system operates in a one-way direction and thus acts quickly. The level of the last component is controlled only by the level of the first component in the chain. The closed loop offers the advantage of "fine tuning" of the concentrations of the various components in the chain. It is called a feedback system in that information is fed back to other components in the chain such that the system "knows" at what rate the reactions of which it consists must proceed. The example of negative feedback that is often easiest to understand is that involving the production of an endocrine hormone by a trophic hormone (Fig. 1-2).

Open loop feedback

$$\boxed{1} \rightarrow \boxed{2} \rightarrow \boxed{3} \rightarrow \boxed{4}$$

In this model the concentration of $\boxed{1}$ and the reaction rate of $\boxed{1} \rightarrow \boxed{2}$ will determine the concentration of $\boxed{4}$.

Closed loop feedback

$$\boxed{1} \rightarrow \boxed{2} \rightarrow \boxed{3} \rightarrow \boxed{4}$$

In this simple model the concentration of $\boxed{2}$, $\boxed{3}$, and $\boxed{4}$ is determined by the concentration of $\boxed{2}$, in that the production of $\boxed{2}$ and the reaction of $\boxed{1} \rightarrow \boxed{2}$ is regulated. "Information" about the concentration of $\boxed{2}$ is fed back to $\boxed{1}$. This is also an example of negative feedback, since the concentration of $\boxed{2}$, when it reaches a certain level, will act to inhibit $\boxed{1} \rightarrow \boxed{2}$ as indicated by the $\ominus$.

The blood levels of substance X (Fig. 1-2) must be carefully regulated to maintain the steady state. Therefore, it is the blood level of X that controls the release of the trophic hormone. Without the stimulation of the trophic

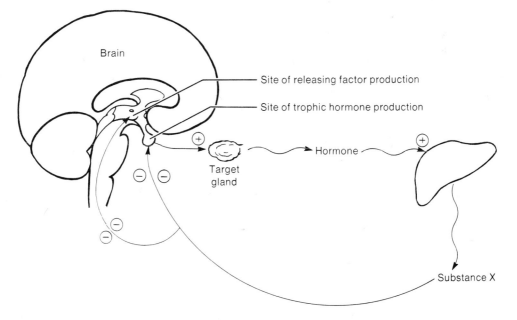

Fig. 1-2. Negative-feedback regulation. Negative-feedback regulation of substance X, product of target organ, is achieved by inhibitory effect of substance X (output of free target organ) on production and release of both releasing factor (which stimulates release of trophic hormone) and trophic hormone (which stimulates target gland to secrete its hormone); $\ominus$ indicates inhibition.

hormone, the hormone from its target gland cannot stimulate the production and release of substance X from the organ. The trophic hormone production is stimulated by a releasing factor from the brain. Imagine then what would happen if disease prevented the negative feedback of substance X on both the glandular source of the trophic hormone and the releasing factor source. The system would continue to produce trophic hormone, which would act on the endocrine gland, which would continue to produce the hormone. The ultimate result would be higher and higher levels of X. If X is osmotically active, great problems could arise with regard to cellular dehydration and electrolyte balance. It is apparent that this interruption would result in a tendency of this open system to increase its entropy and to disrupt the steady state. Thus, the operation of negative feedback is essential to the maintenance of the steady state. It can be said that negative feedback loops have inherent in them some sort of set-point sensor, so that the system "recognizes" the optimal levels of the substances it is regulating. This kind of information is genetically determined, and the processes by which it is sensed by the system are not well understood at this time.

Positive feedback loops also occur in biologic organisms. They are reactions in which the later components in the chain (see box below) perpetuate the production of the first components. Such loops could occur in processes such as autocatalysis or in metabolic pathways that are used as energy sources such that catabolism exceeds anabolism. These loops would result in a temporary increase in entropy of the system.

Positive feedback loops are common in pathophysiologic perpetuation of disease. It can be seen that the example of atherosclerotic hypertension discussed later in this chapter results finally in positive feedback mechanisms that enhance and propagate the initial step in the chain of events, which is hypertension.

INTERRUPTIONS OF THE STEADY STATE

This textbook will examine pathophysiologic mechanisms as disorders of steady state regulation. Therefore, it is important for the student to understand these mechanisms and to be able to relate them to disease. A number of common disease entities will be examined as disorders of normal regulation that result in disruption of the steady state. These are meant as illustrative models rather than as detailed discourses on pathogenesis and pathophysiology. The reader is referred to the appropriate chapters for further information.

Interruptions of mucosal integrity

The box below illustrates the normal negative feedback control on the secretion of hydrochloric acid by the parietal cells of the stomach lining. Hydrochloric acid is a highly ionized strong acid, and the lining of the stomach is protected by autodigestion through the secretion of an alkaline layer of mucus, through dilution of the acid by food and other secretions, and by regulation of hydrochloric acid production. Hydrochloric acid secretion is regulated through negative feedback control of the antral cells, which release gastrin when food is present in the stomach. When the pH reaches a

---

Positive feedback

$$\boxed{1} \rightarrow \boxed{2} \cdots \boxed{3} \rightarrow \boxed{4}$$

In this model the concentration of $\boxed{4}$ is also regulated, not by inhibition of the various reactions in the sequences, but by stimulation. Thus, as $\boxed{4}$ accumulates, it acts to stimulate $\boxed{3} \rightarrow \boxed{4}$, and so on, such that as $\boxed{4}$ builds up, it continually acts to increase its own production on and on.

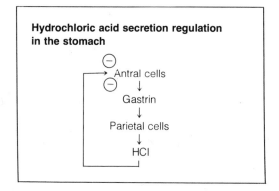

Hydrochloric acid secretion regulation in the stomach

certain set point, the antral cells become inhibited and no longer release the hormone. A decrease in gastrin leads to a decrease in parietal cell secretion, and thus the pH is regulated.

It is thought that ulceration of the stomach or duodenum can result either from hypersecretion of hydrochloric acid or from a breakdown in the normal protective barriers to autodigestion. Hydrochloric acid production is regulated by the release of a hormone, gastrin, from certain cells in the antrum of the stomach. This hormone is released into the bloodstream and ultimately reaches the parietal cells, causing them to secrete hydrochloric acid into the lumen of the stomach. The antral cells are sensitive to the stomach pH and respond in a negative feedback manner when the pH set point of 2.0 is reached. Further regulation of these cells is through parasympathetic stimulation, and vagal

activity is known to be increased in patients with peptic ulcer. The regulation of vagal parasympathetic outflow is at the level of the cerebral cortex and hypothalamus. Stress is thought to be associated with the development of peptic ulcer partly through this mechanism, although cortisone may also be pathogenic and is released by the adrenal cortex in stress situations. Distension of the stomach and certain food substances known as *secretagogues* also stimulate these antral cells to produce gastrin. A potent stimulant found in high concentration in the stomach lining is histamine, which is believed to act directly on the parietal cells to stimulate hydrochloric acid release. When the regulation of hydrochloric acid is disturbed, resulting in hypersecretion, peptic ulceration in the stomach or more commonly in the duodenum may result. It has also been shown that

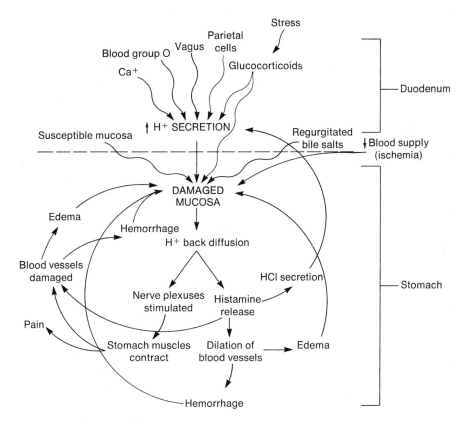

Fig. 1-3. Pathophysiology of peptic ulcer. Either an increase in H^+ secretion or a decrease in integrity of stomach mucosa can lead to ulcer formation. Once an actual ulcer forms, damaged mucosa is perpetuated by back diffusion of H^+, edema, and hemorrhage.

peptic ulcer patients have higher than normal nocturnal secretion of hydrochloric acid, when the stomach is empty.

When ulceration of the stomach or duodenal mucosa does occur, there are a number of pathophysiologic consequences (Fig. 1-3). Edema and interstitial hemorrhage may result, leading possibly to histamine release as part of the overall inflammatory reaction that occurs as back diffusion of hydrochloric acid through the broken tissue barrier occurs. Plasma and blood proteins leak into the interstitium and may be lost to the gastric or duodenal lumen. Excavation of the normal tissue may be so severe that perforation of the stomach or duodenal wall, massive hemorrhage, and shock result. It can be seen then that the slightest breakdown in the wall of the stomach or duodenum may lead to further pathophysiologic phenomena, which aggravate the ulceration even further.

Interruption in mitotic division

A characteristic of malignant cancer cells appears to be the loss of regulation of cell division, which is normally regulated by both tissue and humoral factors such as *chalones, antichalones,* and a phenomenon known as contact or density-dependent inhibition. Cell division within tissue appears to be controlled in part by the actual physical *crowding* of the tissue by the cells and ground substance that compose it. In cancer, both in vivo and in vitro, this regulation is lost, and cell division continues in an uncoordinated and uncontrolled manner. Can-

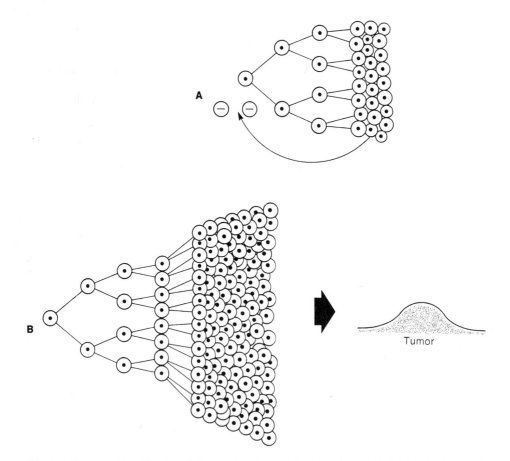

Fig. 1-4. Cancer cell proliferation. **A,** Increasing density of cells as they divide inhibits further cellular division. **B,** Negative feedback is lost in malignant cells as they divide, producing an accumulation of anaplastic cells known as a *tumor.*

cer cell proliferation therefore is at least in part perpetuated by the lack of negative feedback (Fig. 1-4) on mitosis.

Sodium ion concentration

Na⁺ concentration is carefully regulated around the average value of 140 mEq per liter in the blood serum. A major mechanism for this control lies in the juxtaglomerular apparatus (JGA) of some of the renal tubules. These cells are somehow able to sense the Na⁺ concentration in the tubular filtrate, which is usually a reflection of the serum value. This complex of cells releases renin, which ultimately causes aldosterone to be released from certain cells of the adrenal cortex. Aldosterone then acts on the Na⁺ permeability of cells in the distal tubule, stimulating the uptake or *reabsorption* of Na⁺ from the filtrate into the blood and thus conserving Na⁺. When serum Na⁺ concentration falls below a certain set-point value, the JGA will release renin, and serum Na⁺ will be reabsorbed. Thus, the system maintains the

blood Na⁺. Many diseases can interrupt this sequence of events (Fig. 1-5). Glomerulonephritis is a kidney disease that could interrupt the feedback at the level of the tubule, and essential hypertension is thought to result from JGA abnormal function. Addison's disease will cause aldosterone release to be depressed, while Cushing's disease may do the opposite. Thus, pathophysiology resulting in abnormal Na⁺ concentration is seen in this case to arise through many possible different mechanisms, which all ultimately interrupt the normal *regulation* of Na⁺ concentration.

A MODEL OF PATHOPHYSIOLOGY: HYPERTENSION

It is only when homeostasis cannot be maintained that disease ultimately results in death of the organism. A model that illustrates this pathophysiology is hypertension. Hypertension is generally defined as an elevation in the systolic blood pressure of over 140 mm Hg and in the diastolic blood pressure of over 90 mm Hg.

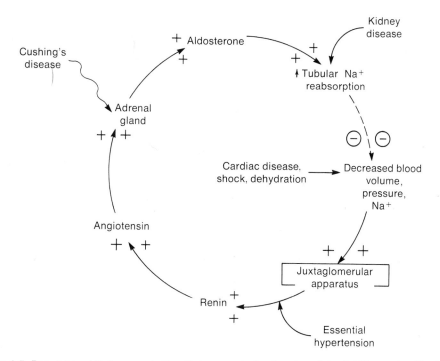

Fig. 1-5. Regulation of Na⁺ concentration. Na⁺ concentration in extracellular fluid is regulated by kidney through renin-angiotensin-aldosterone mechanism. Various disease states can interrupt this regulation, leading to abnormally low or high Na⁺ concentration.

Essential hypertension is the most common variety (over 90%), and its etiology is unknown, although recent research has led to speculation that the disease process may originate in the kidney. However, other authorities believe that defective catecholamine metabolism or deposition of sodium in the arteriolar wall may be the initiating lesion. Goldblatt showed that renal ischemia, which he caused by clamping the renal artery, resulted in the release of *renin* from the juxtaglomerular apparatus. Renin causes the eventual formation of *angiotensin II,* which is a pressor substance that elevates the blood pressure by constricting arterioles. Other evidence that the kidney is the initial site of essential hypertension is the constant finding of *renal arteriolosclerosis* in patients with essential hypertension. Debate exists, however, on whether this is the cause or the result of the disease process. Sclerosis of many other vessels is found in essential hypertension, and it is believed that prolonged exposure to elevated blood pressure *itself* can damage blood vessels, causing them to become thickened and sclerotic and even hemorrhagic and necrotic. There is a strong genetic tendency toward essential hypertension, and in all probability the etiology may be multifactorial. The development of arteriolosclerosis is a significant factor in the pathophysiology of hypertension. While the initiating lesion is not known, the most common pathologic finding in hypertension is increased peripheral resistance to blood flow, a phenomenon with a variety of effects which acting together set up and reinforce mechanisms that perpetuate and aggravate the disease process. Such mechanisms are often called vicious cycles or positive feedback loops.

A number of factors can cause peripheral resistance to increase. The most important one physiologically is the action of the sympathetic nervous system, which releases norepinephrine, causing constriction of arterioles. These small precapillary vessels are responsible for most of the peripheral resistance to blood flow. Thickening of these vessels through sclerosis effectively decreases the size of the arteriolar lumen and impairs the elasticity of the vessels. These vessels are then more resistant to the flow of blood through them. It is more difficult for the heart to push enough blood through the arterial tree to adequately perfuse and oxygenate the tissues. Therefore, the pressure of the blood and the work of the heart must increase. This is apparent in the following formula:

$$P = CO \times R$$

To maintain flow or cardiac output (CO) the pressure (P) of the blood pumped from the heart must increase as resistance (R) increases. However, the consequence of the increased blood pressure is often pathophysiologic, even though the increased blood pressure is a normal compensation that allows for survival and maintenance of homeostasis. The additional pressure can lead to cerebrovascular hemorrhage and exudation and hemorrhage of the retina of the eye; the heart becomes susceptible to myocardial infarction; and vascular damage to the kidneys may lead to eventual renal failure.

Debate exists as to whether the initiating lesion in essential hypertension is increased total peripheral resistance (TPR) or a normal TPR in the face of increased cardiac output, for which some evidence does exist. Perhaps the susceptibility of stressed executives to hypertension might be partly explained by an initial catecholamine hyperactivity or hypersensitivity.

The heart must work harder to pump the blood with adequate pressure through the narrowed arterioles. The mechanism by which this is accomplished is through hypertrophy of the myocardium. According to Starling's law of the heart, cardiac muscle increases its work production as it is stretched (the length-tension relationship of skeletal muscle is analogous). However, there are limitations placed on how far the muscle fibers can be stretched. When the blood supply of the myocardium becomes insufficient to oxygenate the hypertrophied heart, Starling's law of the heart no longer holds true, and in fact the heart becomes more and more ineffective with further stretching or dilation. This occurs in individuals with prolonged hypertension. When the critical limit of the myocardial stretch is reached, pathophysiologic mechanisms are set up: the heart is not able to pump effectively, and *forward congestive heart failure* occurs. The heart has a larger volume of blood left in it after each systole, and the pressure inside the chambers of the heart increases. This pressure will be reflected into the vessels that lead to the left side of the heart. Therefore a buildup of pressure occurs in the pulmonary veins and capillaries of the lung. Eventually the pressure is reflected into the pulmonary artery, the right ventricle, and the atrium, and the right side of the heart becomes dilated and ineffective, causing *backward failure,* which means that the pressure of the blood remaining in the heart is reflected back into the venae cavae and veins of the body.

These pressure changes are accompanied by *signs* and *symptoms* in the patient (a sign of a disease is a characteristic that can be observed by the onlooker, such as edema; a symptom can only be felt and observed by the patient, such as pain). For example, when the pressure increases to a level in the pulmonary capillaries where filtration pressure exceeds osmotic pressure, fluid will transude into the pleural spaces. This effusion will result in *pulmonary edema.*

The signs and symptoms of this condition are quite predictable if the normal physiology of the lung is kept in mind. Gas exchange is impaired, and the patient has air hunger and struggles for breath. There will be a cough, and fluid can be heard moving in the lungs with each breath. The patient may have *orthopnea* (the need to breathe in an upright position). The dyspnea may even be accompanied by *cyanosis,* a bluish coloration of the mucous membranes, nail beds, and skin due to poor oxygenation of the arterial blood. When right-sided backward heart failure occurs, the increased pressure in the veins is reflected into the venules and capillaries and a net outward filtration of fluid may then occur from these vessels, causing tissue edema, which is an accumulation of fluid in the interstitial space. These effects act together to further aggravate the hypertension (Fig. 1-6). Arteriosclerosis, which is a long-term complication of hypertension, may result in decreased cerebrovascular flow and

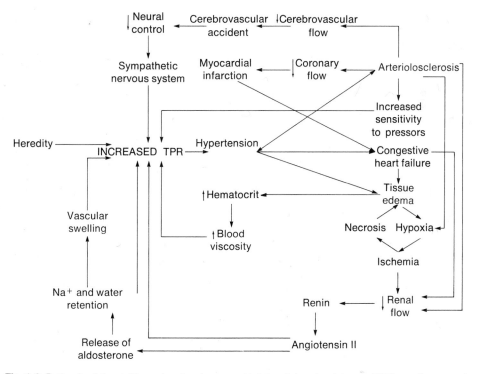

Fig. 1-6. Pathophysiology of hypertension. Increased total peripheral resistance (TPR) may be caused by many factors (vascular disease, hereditary factors, sympathetic nervous system activity, excessive pressor substances or increased sensitivity, and increased blood viscosity). Hypertension itself, acting through a variety of pathophysiologic mechanisms, can further perpetuate increased TPR.

cerebrovascular hemorrhage, which could interrupt central nervous system control of systemic blood pressure. The sclerotic arterioles and arteries appear to be more sensitive to the action of pressors, thus contributing to TPR, and, of course, tissue hypoxia may result from narrowing and hardening of vessels, aggravating the hypoxia that develops in consequence to congestive heart failure. The transudation of fluid from the blood into the tissues increases red blood cell concentration, elevating the hematocrit and causing the blood to become more viscous, a factor that also increases the total peripheral resistance. Renal ischemia may develop, releasing angiotensin II and aldosterone, with both substances acting via different mechanisms to increase the TPR. Angiotensin II is a direct pressor substance, while aldosterone release causes distal-tubule and collecting-duct retention of Na^+ and water. It can be seen in Fig. 1-6 that these mechanisms set in motion by hypertension are pathophysiologic, disturbing homeostasis so profoundly that without medical intervention, death seems inevitable.

It is obvious that a number of factors must be considered in the example given. The first factor is that a living organism is subject to the same laws of physics that govern matter anywhere in the universe. If pressure of a fluid is increased inside one part of an open system of tubes, that pressure will be distributed equally throughout the open system. The major difference between a system of connected rubber tubes and the cardiovascular system of a living organism is the ability of the organism to *regulate* the size of the tubes, the force of contraction of the heart, the osmotic pressure of the fluid, and other phenomena. An important point is that this regulation is achieved within certain physiologic parameters, and when the regulation becomes ineffective, the eventual result must be disease and death of the organism. The aim then of medical intervention is often not only to treat the initial cause of the disease but also to allow the normal compensatory mechanisms of the body to function in an optimal manner. Thus, the individual with hypertension may be advised to stop smoking, lose weight, eat less saturated fat, and avoid stress.

He may also be given drugs that act to increase the size of the arterioles, thus decreasing TPR. If heart disease develops, then a salt-and fluid-restricted diet may be indicated, so that the fluid load on the heart is reduced and pressure decreased. The individual may be given *diuretics,* which are drugs that act on the kidney to increase urinary output.

MOLECULAR BIOLOGY OF DISEASE

The conceptualization of pathophysiology through the use of feedback models based on steady state thermodynamics is useful on a broad scale. Most students of pathophysiology are eager to learn the details of disease processes, however, and this is an essential part of the study of pathophysiology. More and more work on the molecular bases of many diseases has been done in recent years, and new vistas of research and understanding are opening. Deviations on the molecular level have been described for hereditary diseases such as sickle cell anemia, in which the exact amino acid substitution on the hemoglobin molecule that results in this disease is known. Eventual identification of the location of the mutated gene is not an impossibility. Molecular membrane defects have been identified for a variety of blood diseases such as vitamin E–deficient hemolytic anemia of the premature infant, hereditary spherocytosis, and spur cell anemia. The molecular bases of metabolic disorders ranging from hyperthyroidism to phenylketonuria have been studied. These are only a few examples of diseases that involve known molecular alterations. It is certainly conceivable that all pathophysiology in biologic organisms is ultimately related to molecular events.

The following chapters will focus on the molecular biology of disease as well as the physiologic disruptions that occur as part of the disease process. When appropriate, disease mechanisms will be discussed in light of systems theory and models of representative diseases presented. The physiology of treatment for a number of disorders will also be part of the text.

SUGGESTED READINGS

Anthony, C., and Kolthoff, N. J.: Textbook of anatomy and physiology, ed. 10, St. Louis, 1979, The C. V. Mosby Co.

Blasius, W.: Problems of life research, Berlin, 1976, Springer Verlag.

Guyton, A.: Textbook of medical physiology, ed. 6, Philadelphia, 1979, W. B. Saunders Co.

Keale, C., and Neil, E.: Samson Wright's applied physiology, ed. 12, New York, 1971, Oxford University Press.

Laszlo, E.: The relevance of general systems theory, New York, 1972, George Braziller.

Mountcastle, V. B., editor: Medical physiology, ed. 13, St. Louis, 1974, The C. V. Mosby Co.

Pask, G.: An approach to cybernetics, New York, 1961, Harper & Row, Publishers.

Vander, A., Sherman, H., and Luciano, D.: Human physiology—the mechanisms of body function, ed. 3, New York, 1979, McGraw-Hill Book Co.

von Bertalanffy, L.: Perspectives on general systems theory, New York, 1975, George Braziller.

PART TWO

Pathophysiology caused by cellular deviation

CHAPTER 2

Genetic and teratogenic disease mechanisms

AT THE COMPLETION OF THIS CHAPTER THE STUDENT WILL BE ABLE TO:

- Describe normal meiosis and mitosis and predict the effects of alterations in these mechanisms.
- Explain the interaction of natural selection with the human gene pool and discuss why certain abnormal disease-producing genes have been retained in the human gene pool.
- Differentiate between hereditary and teratogenic mechanisms.
- Describe ways in which hemoglobinopathies characterize the general pattern of genetic disease.
- Describe how the major autosomal and sex chromosome trisomies arise and discuss possible effects of these abnormalities on the structure and function of the affected individual.
- List the major theoretic ways that teratogens might act on developing tissue and discuss congenital diseases with known etiology in relation to these possibilities.
- Predict the possibilities of prevention of common congenital diseases and discuss the relationship of present genetic research to future modes of treatment.

HUMAN GENE POOL

Each individual's appearance, body structure, intellectual capacity, and biochemistry is controlled in large part by the up to 40,000 possible gene pairs on the 23 pairs of human chromosomes. Every living species can be considered to have a pool of possible genes, and the combination of these genes through reproduction allows for the incredible variety that is observed in all the individuals of the species. Nevertheless, there is a constancy in the gene pool so that the characteristics of the species itself are preserved from one generation to the next. The expression of the *genotype,* which is the individual's unique set of genes, through the transcription of deoxyribonucleic acid (DNA) into ribonucleic acid (RNA) and finally into proteins, results in a specific *phenotype* for each member of the species. Each individual, while possessing traits that are spe-

cies specific (e.g., fur, limbs, erythrocytes), has the possibility for great variety in the nature of these traits through mutations that have occurred during the course of evolution and that have been retained by the species and form part of the gene pool.

Mixing of the parents' genes allows for individual variation as well and occurs during the processes of oogenesis and spermatogenesis through meiosis. Meiosis is a type of cellular division in which the normal or *diploid* chromosomal number (46 in the human) is reduced to half or to the *haploid* number. The basic difference between mitosis and meiosis is that in meiosis the centromeres do not divide as in mitosis, so that whole chromosomes move to the poles of the cell and thence into the daughter cells. This process is illustrated in Fig. 2-1. The final result of spermatogenesis and oogenesis is the production of four haploid gametes, which

19

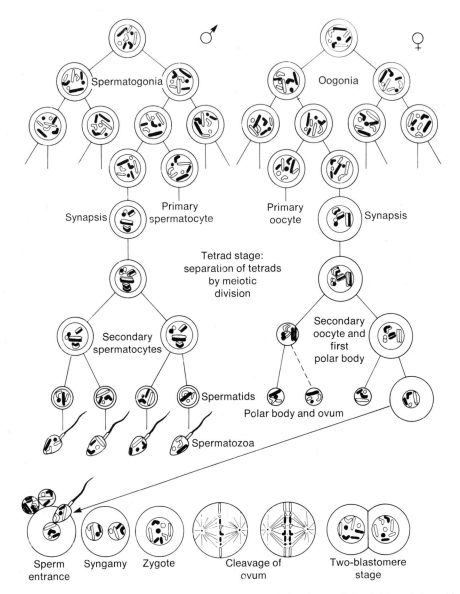

Fig. 2-1. Meiosis. Process of spermatogenesis and oogenesis involves meiotic division, during which whole chromosomes move to daughter cells. Primary spermatocyte and oocyte undergo synapsis, in which pairs of chromosomes line up and bits of genetic material may be exchanged between chromosomes. Chromosomes line up on spindle (tetrad stage), and then each member of a pair of chromosomes moves to a daughter cell of division. In this way, diploid number of chromosomes is reduced to half (haploid) in spermatozoa and ovum. Result of sperm entrance (fertilization) is indicated, with fertilized egg containing diploid number of chromosomes.

have the potential to unite with gametes from the opposite sex and form diploid embryos. In the case of oogenesis only one haploid gamete, the ovum, is produced, the three other products of meiosis forming *polar bodies,* which cannot be fertilized. The process of meiosis, when con-

sidered in light of the tremendous number of possible gene combinations from the species gene pool, ensures that no two individuals can ever be exactly the same except, of course, in the case of *monozygotic* (from one ovum) twins.

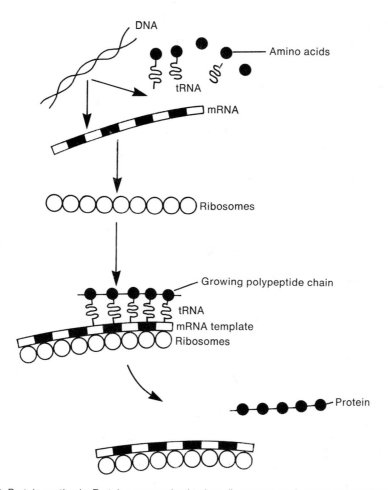

Fig. 2-2. Protein synthesis. Proteins are synthesized on ribosomes, and component amino acids are assembled according to sequence dictated by the code on mRNA. Sequence of mRNA is determined by transcription of nuclear DNA code. Amino acids are brought to ribosomes by the tRNA, which attaches via complementary bases, to mRNA, ordering amino acids in proper sequence.

Mutations

Mutations are alterations in the sequence of bases in the DNA molecule, which forms the genetic code. They may be caused by such agents as viruses, radiation, chemicals, and the aging process. Some mutations are lethal, some sublethal, some beneficial, and probably most are inconsequential. The cell has an elaborate and efficient system of enzymes that repair DNA damage in most cases. Mutations that occur in somatic (body) cells, if not repaired, may cause damage or change in that organism's functional integrity, but the mutation will not become part of the human gene pool, as it is lost when the individual dies. Mutations in germ (sex) cells that are retained can be passed on to viable progeny and could eventually become part of the gene pool.

During the course of the millions of years of evolution, mutations constantly occurred within the genetic material of all species and were, in fact, necessary for speciation and survival. The possibility of mutation is required for Darwin's theory of natural selection to have any validity. Mutations will cause a change in either the nature or the amount of the protein coded for by the DNA segment that has mutated. Fig. 2-2 illustrates the normal coding of DNA for RNA and protein. A change in a protein may not affect the protein's function to any measurable degree, and many minor differences in amino acid composition of particular proteins have been discovered in individuals. The amino acid variations represent mutations that have occurred in the distant past and have been retained as part of the gene pool. Generally speaking, a mutation that results in a deformity or a disease confers a selective disadvantage upon the individual, which in the competitive struggle for survival will make it more difficult for that individual to find food, shelter, and a mate. Thus, through the process of natural selection, undesirable traits are weeded out, and the strongest and healthiest of the species will continue to survive, bearing the most offspring for the further propagation of the species and parent-specific traits. Mutations that confer a selective advantage upon the individual will also be retained through the same process.

Natural selection is extremely slow, however, and many deleterious mutations within DNA presently exist and form part of the human gene pool. The reasons for this are obscure and complex. Theoretically any disease-causing mutation should be eliminated by natural selection, unless it somehow confers a selective advantage. Diabetes mellitus is a disease that has not only been part of the human gene pool for as long as recorded history but has actually appeared to increase in incidence over this time. It has been speculated therefore that diabetes, along with accompanying obesity, conferred a survival advantage in past times of uncertain food supplies and shortages, in the face of continuing hard physical labor, and has only caused severe disease in the majority of those so afflicted during the last 100 years, when the food and labor factors were drastically changed in many parts of the world.

It has been pointed out that certain areas of the world, the endemic malaria belts, coincide with the distribution of the sickle cell anemia trait. It has become apparent that the presence of the sickle cell trait, which is the asymptomatic heterozygous state of the mutated gene that codes for the abnormal hemoglobin of sickle cell disease, confers a resistance to malarial infection that results in a selective advantage in the carrier. Thus, the sickle cell trait has persisted in 10% of the black people in the United States in spite of the fact that the homozygous condition, which is the disease sickle cell anemia, is a serious and often fatal disease.

Most perfectly healthy people probably have three to five mutated genes for which they are heterozygous and which cause no symptoms of disease. If found in the homozygous state these genes would result in an inborn error of metabolism that could seriously affect the individual's potential for a healthy and productive life. A problem facing modern medicine lies in the treatment of people with hereditary conditions who live a long and healthy life, bearing offspring who may inherit the trait if not the disease. The mechanisms by which natural selection operate in nature can no longer ensure that the members of a species who survive are the strongest and most well adapted to the environment. This alone has implications for the future of mankind, and the growing ability of man to manipulate genetic material itself presages an entirely new direction for evolution in the future.

NORMAL DIFFERENTIATION

The human being develops from a single fertilized ovum into an incredibly complex, multicellular organism. The fertilized ovum or zygote is diploid and begins to divide by mitotic division shortly after fertilization. Mitosis (Fig. 2-3) produces two identical daughter cells with the same amount and type of DNA. Very early in the division or *cleavages* of the embryonic cells, certain cells begin to differentiate into different tissues, and three primitive germ layers are formed: the ectoderm, mesoderm, and endoderm. The ectoderm will further differentiate into major structures such as the skin and nervous system. The mesoderm differentiates into structures such as bone and muscle, while the endoderm will form the gastrointestinal tract and major abdominal organs. This process is known as *organogenesis* and takes place primarily in the first 3 months or first trimester of the human gestational period. The sequence and extent of organogenesis is precisely "programmed" in all animals. The first trimester as a whole is considered to be a critical period in terms of organ structure and function in that the developing human embryo is most sus-

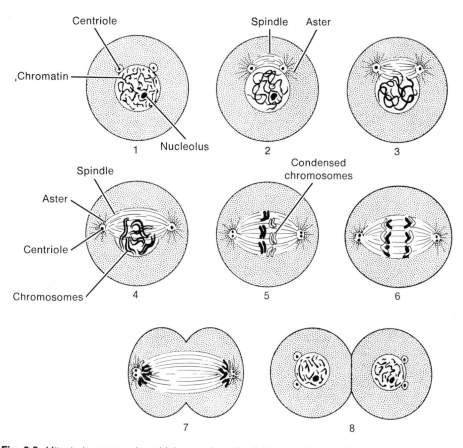

Fig. 2-3. Mitosis is process by which somatic cells divide. In mitosis individual chromosomes are pulled apart at centromere when cell divides, with chromatids moving to opposite poles and ultimately to daughter cells. Chromatids eventually duplicate, thus preserving diploid number of chromosomes.

ceptible to the damaging effects of agents known as *teratogens*. Teratogens cause developmental or *congenital* anomalies when put in contact with differentiating and growing embryonic tissues. Major teratogens include physical agents (trauma, irradiation), chemicals (drugs such as thalidomide), and microorganisms (rubella virus: German measles). The basic processes of teratogenesis will be discussed later, but there are several principles that it would benefit the reader to know at this point.

1. There are critical periods during organogenesis when teratogens will cause the most damage. The preimplantation period (days 1 to 10 following conception) is the time during which damage to the conceptus will interfere with implantation of the embryo into the uterine wall. The embryonic period (until the end of the first trimester) is the period of major organogenesis. Teratogens will cause a great variety of structural defects during this period. The fetal period, which spans the time between the end of the first trimester and birth, is a time of major growth, and teratogens may interfere with this process as well. Physiologic abnormalities may also result.

2. Many teratogens appear to have a proclivity for certain tissues. The rubella syndrome, which will be discussed later, illustrates this phenomenon.

3. Teratogenesis is a process involving not only the teratogen and fetus but also the mother. The mother's health, nutrition, and prenatal care are of great importance in determining the final outcome of teratogenesis on the fetus.

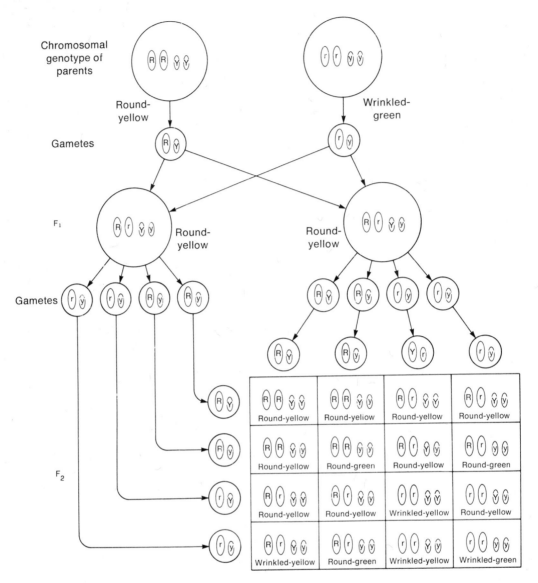

Fig. 2-4. Mendelian genetics. Crosses between pea plants illustrate segregation of genes in gametes and resultant phenotypes expected in F₁ and F₂ generations. If genes for color and texture are thought of as existing on separate chromosomes, then pattern of meiotic division can be understood.

4. It is often impossible to identify the teratogen that caused a deformity in a newborn. Furthermore, many conditions are hereditary rather than acquired in utero.

HEREDITARY MECHANISMS

Basic laws of mendelian inheritance require that any trait be governed by pairs of genes, which are located on pairs of chromosomes. This is illustrated schematically in Fig. 2-4,

which shows a mendelian experiment on pea plants. The 46 human chromosomes consist of 22 pairs of autosomes and 1 pair of sex chromosomes. One member of each of the 23 chromosomal pairs was initially contributed by the father's haploid sperm and one by the mother's haploid ovum. The individual chromosomes can be identified by the preparation of slides of certain cells such as stimulated leukocytes in metaphase, and a karyotype (a photograph of

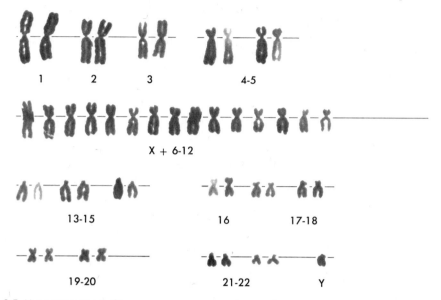

Fig. 2-5. Normal karyotype. Chromosomes are grouped according to size and centromere position. (From Reisman, L. E., and Matheny, A. P.: Genetics and counseling in medical practice, St. Louis, 1969, The C. V. Mosby Co.)

the matched chromosome pairs, Fig. 2-5) allows the geneticist to categorize the 46 chromosomes into seven groups, which are based on size, shape, and certain special characteristics.

Human karyotyping has become more accurate. Techniques for *banding* the individual member of each chromosome pair with Giemsa stain or fluorescent dyes have been developed. This banding is characteristic. Large numbers of syndromes and abnormalities have now been linked to chromosomal defects, some of them identifiable only by banding, so that geneticists believe that every human chromosome can be structurally altered, producing various defects, without necessarily affecting the viability of offspring.

GENETIC LOCI

The technology for ascertaining the location of certain genes on particular chromosomes is becoming available but is extremely complex. It, along with the technology involved in the construction of DNA in the laboratory, has opened a scientific frontier that is both awe inspiring and frightening in its possibilities. Basic research into cell *hybridization* has led to the identification of the loci for 50 genes

on 18 chromosomes controlling various enzymes; for example, enolase, adenylate kinase, phosphoglucomutase, and peptidase genes have all been localized to chromosome 1 in the human. The gene for malate dehydrogenase has been identified on chromosome 2, and the gene coding for glucose 6-phosphate dehydrogenase is on the X chromosome. Elegant experiments involving human cells and other species cells in hybridization result in fusion of cells in tissue culture with the resultant production of hybrid cells, which contain the genetic material of both cells (Fig. 2-6). Experiments in which human fibroblasts and mouse hepatoma cells were fused resulted in cells containing between 41 and 55 chromosomes. All 40 mouse chromosomes were invariably present; the human chromosomes that were present in different hybrid cells were variable and appeared to be present on a random basis. Identification of the mouse and human chromosomes can be carried out by Giemsa or fluorescent staining and by electrophoresis of the protein gene products. The amino acid composition of proteins of mice and humans is sufficiently different to allow separate identification. When genes coding for different proteins are either lost together or ex-

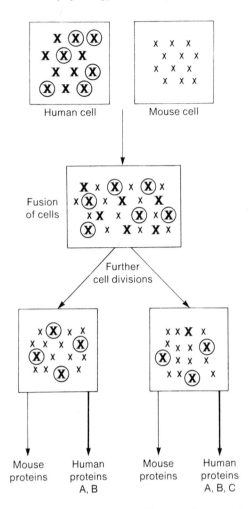

Fig. 2-6. When mouse cells and human cells are made to fuse under experimental conditions, cells that are formed contain both human and mouse chromosomes. These cells therefore produce both human and mouse proteins. All mouse chromosomes are retained, but a *variable* number of human chromosomes can be found in hybrid cells. Study of karyotype and protein products of fused cells has led to localization of genes on chromosomes.

pressed together in hybridization experiments, it can be assumed that these genes are *syntenic* or on the same chromosome. Thus, through careful study of the karyotype and the proteins coded for by the hybrid cells the location of various genes has been elucidated. Refinement of these basic techniques is leading to exciting discoveries in both the basic biology of genetics and in the understanding and treatment of diseases. It is now known, for example, that the polio virus receptor protein is coded by chromosome 5 and that the antiviral substance *interferon* requires two genetic loci for its production. Malignant transformation may be studied using these hybridization techniques. It has been demonstrated that genes can be repressed by repressor proteins and derepressed if present in the proper environment. Normally human leukocytes do not produce albumin. If hybrids of these cells and mouse hepatoma cells are made, some of the hybrids produce human albumin (as well as the normally produced mouse albumin). This would indicate that factors from the mouse hepatoma cells can possibly unmask the repressed gene for albumin in the human leukocyte chromosome. This experimental result has great implications for medical research. Gene expression and modulation in human cancer cells and in fetal cells derived from amniotic fluid may be studied, yielding knowledge that can be applied to the prevention and treatment of acquired and congenital diseases.

Recombinant DNA experiments are similar to the hybridization experiments, but biologic combination takes place at the molecular level, with the production of strands of DNA made up of pieces of DNA from different species. Thus, it has been possible in the laboratory to produce bacterial cells that contain *plasmids* made up of the bacteria's own DNA and foreign DNA from another species (Fig. 2-7). Plasmids are extrachromosomal pieces of DNA found in bacterial cells; plasmids sometimes participate in the exchange of genetic material between bacterial cells. The recombinant DNA produced by the enzymatic fusion of the different segments of DNA is able to code for the proteins of both types of DNA. Furthermore, when the bacterial cell divides, the plasmids containing the recombinant DNA are retained in the daughter cells, producing a new *clone* of cells. Such genetic engineering opens many possibilities for the treatment of disease. Manipulation of bacterial DNA so that certain synthetic capabilities are guaranteed and the insertion of this genetic material into the cells of individuals with various deficiency diseases (diabetes mellitus being only one of many examples) is one future possibility.

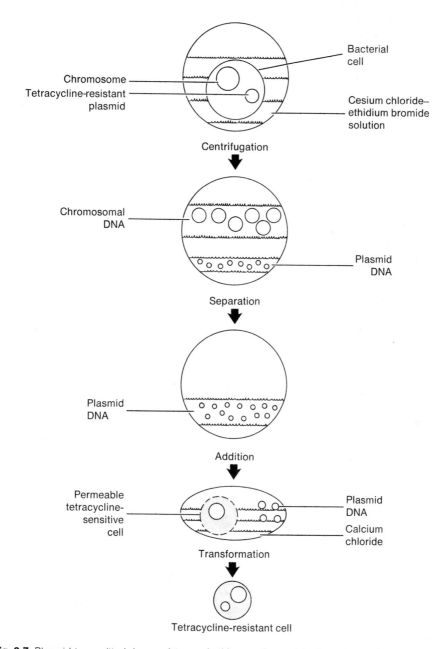

Fig. 2-7. Plasmid-transmitted drug resistance. In this experimental design, plasmid DNA is separated by differential ultracentrifugation from a bacterial cell. Plasmid DNA confers resistance to tetracycline on cell. When this plasmid DNA is added to permeable, tetracycline-sensitive cells it is incorporated into cell, becomes part of genome, and confers tetracycline resistance.

Genetic engineering also carries potential danger. The possibility of creating organisms that could play microbiologic and ecologic havoc on the planet has not been overlooked by scientists and concerned citizens. Careful control and regulation of recombinant DNA research is now legislated.

GENETIC EXPRESSION

Traits inherited as *dominant* are the expression of either the homozygous or heterozygous state. Homozygous genes are present in two copies, one each member of the chromosomal pair, while heterozygous genes are only present on one chromosome. *Recessive* inheritance requires that the homozygous condition of the gene be present. Therefore, the possibility of a homozygous individual's being born to heterozygous parents is one in four, and of a heterozygous child, one in two. Certain traits are carried on the sex chromosomes and are either X-linked recessive or dominant traits. Since males have only one X chromosome and females have two, the presence of an X-linked gene is always expressed in the female if she is homozygous for the particular gene.

The *penetrance* of a gene refers to the degree with which that particular trait occurs in the general population. Penetrance of hereditary disorders may be greatly influenced by environmental factors.

Furthermore, potential genetic diseases may not be apparent in affected individuals if the diseases require that other genes be inactive or altered, and it certainly is true that many traits are controlled by multiple genetic loci. The actual genetic cause of a disease may also be obscured by compensatory mechanisms that take place. For example, a genetic deficiency in a particular protein might be so well compensated for by the overproduction of an alternate protein that no actual disease appears. Another factor, particularly in diseases that result in the accumulation of a potentially toxic substance in the body, is the concept of a threshold. A threshold is a critical value above which a substance will cause disease but below which disease is inapparent. Thus, for a number of genetic diseases, for example, galactosemia and phenylketonuria, the threshold value is reached

over a period of time, and symptoms are absent until it is reached.

Diagnosis of a hereditary disease is based primarily on study of the individual's family tree. The appearance of the disease in ancestors and relatives with a mendelian pattern is convincing evidence of a genetic basis. Thus, a fetus with an inherited disorder has not been directly affected by a teratogen during embryogenesis but from the moment of conception has had an altered genetic code. Furthermore, the individual may pass traits on to offspring. Many such disease conditions require that the individual carry the altered genes in the recessive *homozygous* state. For this to occur the affected individual must be the progeny of the mating of heterozygous parents. In many cases the heterozygous parent will have no symptoms of the disease or will have symptoms only during very unusual circumstances. Thus, heterozygote carriers of the disease *thalassemia* are asymptomatic unless they become subject to severe hypoxia, such as might occur at high altitudes. The homozygote, on the other hand, suffers anemia, growth retardation, jaundice, and a great variety of other debilitating effects of the disease without any added environmental stress. Many laboratory tests have been developed recently for the detection of heterozygous states of hereditary diseases, which is of great importance for the genetic counseling of people contemplating childbirth.

Hemoglobinopathies

The hemoglobinopathies or abnormal hemoglobin conditions, provide an excellent illustration of the pathophysiologic mechanisms whereby altered DNA eventually produces the signs and symptoms of disease. To understand these conditions the normal genetic control of hemoglobin synthesis will be discussed.

Hemoglobin, a protein molecule containing iron, is produced by immature red blood cells. Mature erythrocytes cannot produce any protein molecules, as these corpuscles lack the necessary nuclear and cytoplasmic protein-synthesizing machinery, having lost it during maturation from the reticulocyte stage. Hemoglobin is a buffer molecule; it plays its major physiologic role in the carriage and transport of oxygen in arterial blood. The hemoglobin molecule actually consists of four polypeptide strands, two alpha (α) chains and two beta (β) chains. This form of hemoglobin is the predominant form in most people and is called hemoglobin A_1 (Hb A_1). A minor fraction of hemoglobin, hemoglobin A_2 (Hb A_2), is also normally present. Hb A_1 is commonly notated as $\alpha_2^A \beta_2^A$, which indicates that it is Hb A_1 and consists of two alpha chains and two beta chains. Fetal hemoglobin, which is normally present only in fetal life and early infancy, is notated as $\alpha_2^A \gamma_2^F$, indicating that two alpha chains and two gamma chains (rather than beta chains) make up its composition. The differences between the types of polypeptide chains lie in the sequencing and kinds of amino acids that make up the protein strand. Great differences in physiologic functioning of hemoglobin occur when even a single amino acid is altered on a strand. For example, sickle cell anemia is caused by the substitution of valine for glutamine at position 6 on the beta chain. It is thought that this is the result of a single mu-

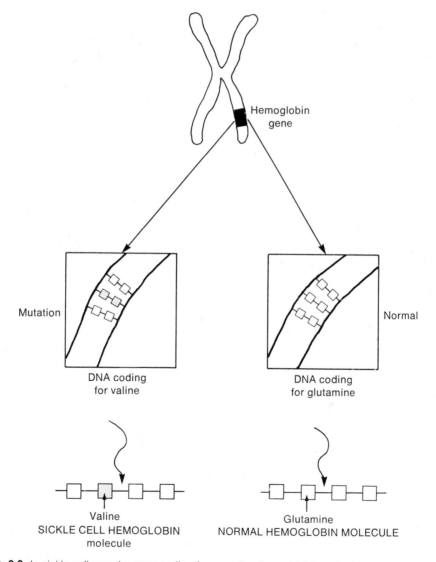

Fig. 2-8. In sickle cell anemia, gene coding for normal amino acid (glutamine) at position 6 of beta chain is substituted for by valine, leading to altered and abnormal hemoglobin (Hb S).

tated gene, which is responsible for the coding of the amino acid at this particular position on hemoglobin. Fig. 2-8 shows the production of the abnormal hemoglobin in a cell containing such a mutated gene. The valine substitution greatly alters the ability of this hemoglobin, called hemoglobin S (Hb S), to transport oxygen. Erythrocytes that contain Hb S have a shorter life span, are more fragile than normal erythrocytes, and tend to form a sickle shape, particularly under hypoxic conditions. The sickling process can be observed in vitro when red blood cells containing Hb S are observed under a coverslip with a microscope.

The signs and symptoms of sickle cell anemia can be explained by the physiologic disturbances caused by the abnormal hemoglobin. Chronic anemia, arthralgia, and episodes of acute pain are the most striking symptoms of this disease. Hb S has a low solubility at low oxygen tension and thus tends to form a gelatin-like mass *(tactoid)* inside the erythrocyte when the oxygen concentration is reduced, and the red blood cell thus becomes deformed into the sickle shape. The sickling of the erythrocytes increases the blood viscosity, and eventually stasis of the blood occurs within capillaries, decreasing oxygen and nutrition supplied to the involved tissue and thus producing anoxic pain.

The course of the disease is marked by episodes of acute crisis that may follow infection but that often are without an identifiable precipitating cause. The crisis is usually due to vascular occlusion and is identified by severe, often excruciating pain in the limbs or abdomen. If the circulating blood volume is significantly reduced by the removal of sickled red blood cells by the reticuloendothelial system, shock may ensue and cause death. Children with sickle cell anemia often die during the first 10 years of life because of infection, heart or kidney failure, or complications of crisis.

Carriers of the sickle cell trait usually show no signs of the disease in normal circumstances other than perhaps a mild anemia but can be identified from the general population by a mixture of Hb A_1 and Hb S in their circulating red blood cells. Carriers of the trait and those affected by the disease are almost always

of the black race, although there is evidence that the trait originated outside of Africa, perhaps in India.

Sickle cell anemia is but one hereditary hemoglobinopathy. Cooley's anemia (thalassemia) is another. A multitude of other conditions are caused by the great variety of possible abnormal hemoglobins. It is also quite common for an individual to have a mixture of several abnormal hemoglobins. Conditions such as these have allowed geneticists to speculate on the location and types of genes that control the ultimate configuration of the hemoglobin molecule. The genetic control of alpha and beta chains appears to be entirely separate, and genes that regulate the production of hemoglobin chains (operons) also have been suggested. Thalassemia may be due to a mutation of an operon gene that normally controls the rate of chain synthesis. Either alpha or beta chains may be involved, leading to α- or β-thalassemia. In one type of β-thalassemia, Hb A_1 concentration is very low or absent, and fetal hemoglobin (Hb F) and Hb A_2 are the chief hemoglobins found. These hemoglobins are physiologically inferior to Hb A_1 in the adult individual, and anemia and other signs and symptoms of the disease are present. Many different types of thalassemia are constantly being described, but the classic Cooley's anemia is β-thalassemia major and is a homozygous condition that causes impaired beta chain synthesis and a blood level of as much as 90% Hb F, which is distributed unevenly in the erythrocytes. β-Thalassemia minor is the heterozygous condition, and these individuals have few symptoms but can be identified by examination of the blood. The thalassemias appear to affect persons of Mediterranean origin primarily and may also confer a selective advantage with regard to malarial resistance when present in the heterozygous state. The homozygous α-thalassemia appears to be incompatible with life, while homozygous β-thalassemia may cause death during early childhood. A typical clinical picture of the child with thalassemia major is one in which profound anemia, splenomegaly and hepatomegaly, pallor, growth retardation, skeletal abnormalities, and a very characteristic mongoloidlike facies due to cranial and facial bone abnormalities is found.

Other known genetic diseases

The hemoglobinopathies are perhaps the best characterized genetic diseases in that the expression of the altered gene is a protein molecule that can be easily discerned by laboratory techniques such as electrophoresis. Furthermore, this group of diseases is fairly common, and therefore many patients are available for study. Phenylketonuria (PKU), another genetic disease, is notable in another regard. Through modern methods of mass screening of newborn infants the serious side effects of this disease can now be nearly totally prevented. PKU is an inborn error of metabolism in which the affected individual is unable to metabolize phenylalanine. It is inherited as an autosomal recessive trait, so that both parents are heterozygous for the defective gene. The gene that is defective normally controls the formation of an enzyme, *phenylalanine hydroxy-*

lase, which is responsible for the hydroxylation of phenylalanine to tyrosine. Without the treatment, which is simply restriction of phenylalanine in the diet, the infant accumulates phenylalanine in the blood and excretes phenylketones. Eventually neurologic damage occurs, resulting in severe mental retardation.

The pathophysiology of PKU is extremely interesting in that the infant is normal at birth, and the signs and symptoms develop as phenylalanine accumulates and causes damage over the first year of life. The mother may be the first to observe abnormalities in the child, such as a peculiar odor and slow development. The major damaging effect of excessive phenylalanine is deficient myelination of the nervous tissue during the first year of life. The brain is still developing during that time and must construct proteins from the amino acids that are available in the blood and tissue fluids. Because of the liver enzyme deficiency phenylalanine concentration increases tremendously, and the general amino acid pattern of the blood

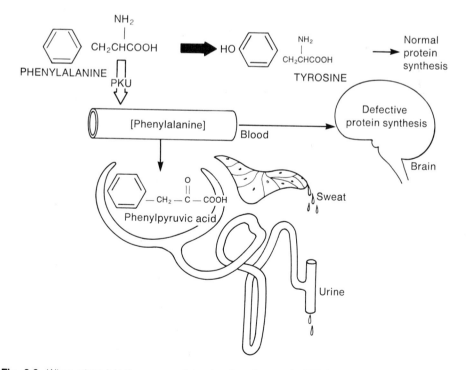

Fig. 2-9. When phenylalanine accumulates in phenylketonuria (PKU), increased concentration of this amino acid results in defective protein synthesis in developing brain. Large amounts of phenylpyruvic acid are excreted in sweat and urine.

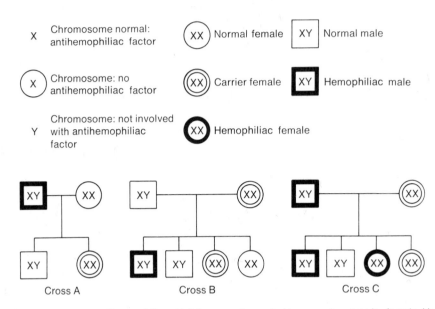

Fig. 2-10. Transmission of hemophilia, which is generally carried in recessive state by female. Hemophiliacs are generally male (cross B) since the Y chromosome does not code for antihemophiliac factor. If a hemophiliac male marries a hemophiliac carrier female, both male and female offspring may have hemophilia (cross C).

GENETIC DISEASES

Disorders of carbohydrate metabolism
Diabetes mellitus
Pentosuria
Glycogen storage diseases
Galactosemia

Disorders of lipid metabolism
Familial lipoprotein deficiency
Familial lecithin-cholesterol acyl-transferase (L-CAT) deficiency
Tay-Sachs disease
Gaucher's disease

Disorders of protein metabolism
Familial goiter
Phenylketonuria
Albinism
Alkaptonuria
Tyrosinosis

Disorders of purine and pyrimidine metabolism
Gout
Lesch-Nyhan syndrome

Disorders of metal metabolism
Wilson's disease
Hemochromatosis

Disorders of connective tissue, bone, and muscle
Familial periodic paralysis
Muscular dystrophies
Mucopolysaccharidoses

Disorders of the hematopoietic system and blood
Sickle cell anemia
Glucose 6-phosphate dehydrogenase deficiency
Thalassemias
Hereditary spherocytosis

and cellular and cerebrospinal fluid is distorted, and the maturation of the brain may be irreversibly impaired as a consequence. Fig. 2-9 describes the pathogenesis of phenylketonuria in the untreated individual.

Other possible genetic diseases that can result in abnormalities at birth or later in life include disorders of carbohydrate, protein, lipid, purine or pyrimidine, and mineral metabolism. Diabetes mellitus is an example of a condition with a striking hereditary background, which often requires the presence of environmental factors in order for penetrance of the genetic disorder into a phenotypic abnormality. Hemophilia is also hereditary in nature and is an X chromosome–linked recessive trait. The pattern of inheritance is diagramed in Fig. 2-10. It is usual for the hemophiliac to be male, having inherited the gene on the X chromosome from his mother. The other X chromosome in the carrier mother is able to code for sufficient antihemophiliac factor for her, but in the male the Y sex chromosome does not contain genes coding for this factor. Thus, the coagulation cascade is interrupted in the hemophiliac, and excessive bleeding following injury is likely to occur.

The box (p. 32) gives a partial listing of diseases known to be due to hereditary factors. These diseases are classified as to the metabolic pathways that they most profoundly affect.

TERATOGENIC MECHANISMS

While the importance of heredity in determining conditions at birth and susceptibility to diseases throughout life cannot be underestimated, most of the obvious structural organ and tissue defects and many syndromes of the newborn are caused mainly by environmental teratogens acting on the dividing cells of the developing embryonic tissues in utero. These congenital anomalies may range in severity and occasionally result in death of the infant before or shortly after birth. It is likely that many embryos with gross genetic errors and developmental defects do not survive and are aborted early in the pregnancy. It has been reported that at least 30% of all embryos spontaneously aborted during the first trimester have chromosomal abnormalities.

Many defects that are present in newborns may be repaired surgically with total recovery and a normal life span possible. It is quite common, however, for one congenital anomaly to occur along with another, indicating that the teratogen affected different developing structures during embryogenesis. Thus, the care of such an infant may be extremely complicated and challenging.

It is possible to categorize congenital defects into those associated with gross chromosomal abnormalities of either autosomes or sex chromosomes, those associated with structural defects of tissues and organs, and those associated with syndromes (a group of specific signs and symptoms observed in relationship to a particular pathogenesis).

CHROMOSOMAL DEFECTS
Trisomies of the autosomes

Autosomal defects of the chromosomes are identified on the basis of both karyotype and phenotype. Such anomalies appear to occur as the result of improper separation of chromosomes during meiosis. The most common example of a gross autosomal anomaly is a *trisomy,* which is the presence of three rather than two chromosomes at one of the 23 possible pair positions in the human karyotype. The most common trisomy is at the G group of chromosomes at 21 and results in mongolism or Down's syndrome. The phenotypic expression of a chromosome 21 trisomy is very characteristic, as is the facies (Fig. 2-11) and karyotype of such an individual (Fig. 2-12). The condition is always characterized by mental retardation and accounts for 10% of the institutionalized retardates. Mongoloid individuals suffer not only mental retardation but also disordered bone growth, altered dermatoglyphics (as exemplified by the presence of the simian crease), and anomalies of other organs and tissues; they are usually susceptible to upper respiratory infection and have a significantly decreased life span. Furthermore, the incidence of leukemia in these children is 15 times the normal.

Other congenital abnormalities are also found in Down's syndrome, as illustrated in Fig. 2-13.

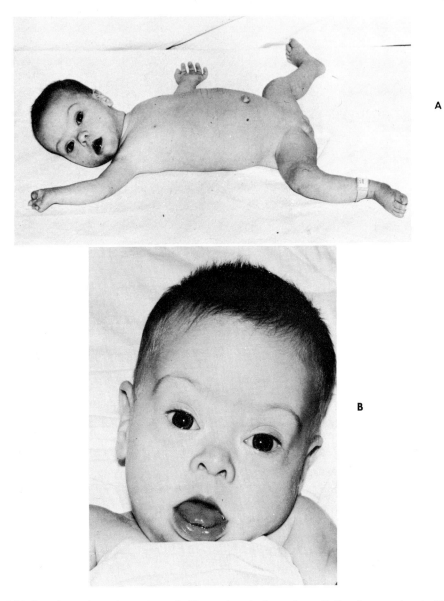

Fig. 2-11. Down's syndrome in newborn. **A,** Floppy, hypotonic newborn. **B,** Small square head with mongoloid slant to eyes, flat nasal bridge, and protruding tongue. (From Reisman, L. E., and Matheny, A. P.: Genetics and counseling in medical practice, St. Louis, 1969, The C. V. Mosby Co.)

The pathogenesis of Down's syndrome is probably the result of a *nondisjunction* during meiosis, so that a whole chromosome rather than a chromatid moves into a gamete (Fig. 2-14). The resulting gamete, if fertilized, will have 47 rather than 46 chromosomes, three chromosomes being at the chromosome 21 position. The incidence of mongolism increases strikingly with maternal age, indicating that ova from older women are subject to a chromosomal aging effect. This appears to be the cause of the meiotic abnormality, as other factors such as frequency of coitus and paternal age have been ruled out by epidemiologic research.

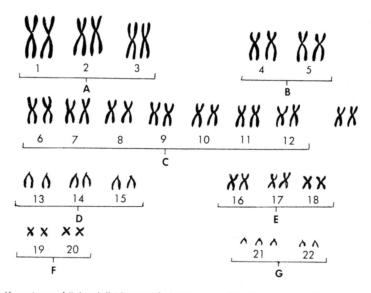

Fig. 2-12. Karyotype of "classic" trisomy of chromosome 21. There is an extra chromosome 21 in Down's syndrome probably due to nondisjunction during meiosis. (From Whaley, L. F.: Understanding inherited disorders, St. Louis, 1974, The C. V. Mosby Co.)

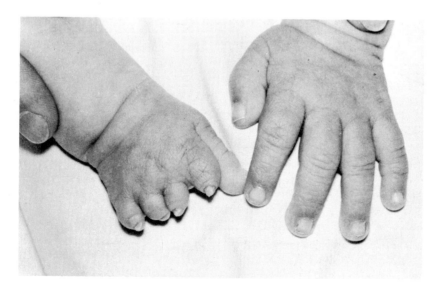

Fig. 2-13. Micromelia in child with Down's syndrome. Various types of such birth defects are commonly found in Down's syndrome. (From Reisman, L. E., and Matheny, A. P.: Genetics and counseling in medical practice, 1969, The C. V. Mosby Co.)

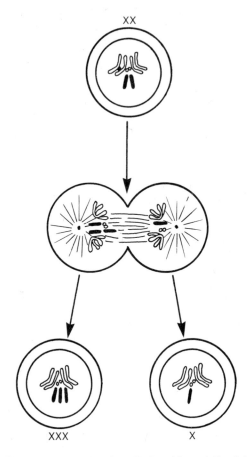

XX

XXX   X

Fig. 2-14. Nondisjunction. During this meiotic division, chromosome pairs do not move equally to daughter cells. In this case, one cell contains three chromosomes, while other contains only one.

Young women who give birth to a child with Down's syndrome often show a *translocation* of an extra chromosome 21 to a chromosome 15, so that the normal diploid number appears to be retained, but in essence an extra chromosome 21 is present.

Mongolism and many other genetic diseases can be detected by amniocentesis. Cells from samples of amniotic fluid that has been withdrawn from the pregnant uterus can be examined as early as the third month of gestation. The cells can be karyotyped, and the presence of abnormal numbers or structures of chromosomes can be determined with great accuracy.

Mongolism may be the result of a teratogen's acting on the ovum before fertilization or may be due to aging of the ovum such that the *meiotic efficiency* of the cell is impaired. The incidence rises with maternal age and is reported as occurring in 1 in 50 births in women over the age of 45, as compared to 1 in 2,300 for women between the ages of 15 and 19. The exact aging effect is not known but may be due to the general running down of the cellular enzyme systems that occurs with age of cells. There is also evidence that Down's syndrome is hereditary in certain cases, since there is a high incidence of the condition in the offspring of child-bearing mongoloids.

Trisomies of other autosomes, such as of groups D and E, have been well documented in the literature and produce characteristic phenotypes, but by far the most common viable autosomal trisomy is Down's syndrome. Trisomy E has been labeled as Edwards' syndrome, and chromosome 18 appears to be involved. The majority of these infants are postmature girls with low birth weights; they generally have round faces with small eyes, mouths, and jaws, low-set or poorly formed ears, altered dermatoglyphics, and extra skin folds on the neck and back. Congenital heart disease is also often present.

Many trisomies and other congenital anomalies are associated with altered dermatoglyphics; patterns of these abnormalities are illustrated in Fig. 2-15.

Other autosomal defects

Deletions of short or long arms of chromosomes have been described in association with various syndromes. However, deletions of the D group chromosomes can be found in 2% of the normal population. The cri du chat syndrome appears to be the result of a deletion of the short arms of the chromosome 5 pair of the B group. These infants are so named because of the characteristic mewing cry during infancy, which accompanies other phenotypic expressions such as microcephaly, failure to thrive, mental retardation, epicanthal folds, abnormal ears, and strabismus.

Duplication of chromosomal material results in a lengthening of the chromosomal arms. These defects also cause mental retardation and other anomalies.

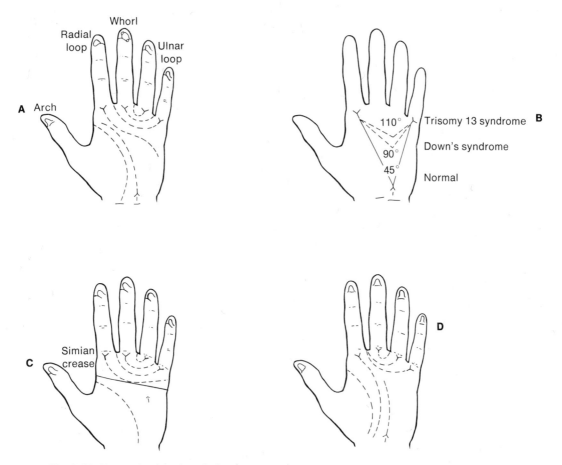

Fig. 2-15. Abnormal palm prints. **A,** Dermatoglyphic pattern of normal hand. **B,** Angles in normal person and in patients with Down's syndrome and trisomy 13 syndrome. **C,** Dermatoglyphic pattern in a patient with Down's syndrome. **D,** Dermatoglyphic pattern in a patient with trisomy 18 syndrome. (From Porter, I. H.: Heredity and disease. Copyright 1968 McGraw-Hill Book Co. Used with permission of McGraw-Hill Book Co.)

Translocation of one chromosomal segment to another chromosome has already been described for one type of Down's syndrome.

Ring chromosomes sometimes form and replace a normal chromosome. Again retardation and abnormal dermatoglyphics are often part of the clinical picture.

Additional small metacentric chromosomes have been found in human karyotypes and have not been clearly identified as members of any specific karyotypic group.

These abnormalities of the autosome usually are studied in an obviously malformed or atypical-appearing segment of the population,

and thus the true incidence of such defects is not known. Many malformed embryos are probably aborted even before implantation would take place, and many times a mother never realizes that a conception had occurred.

Abnormalities of the sex chromosomes

A number of fairly common disorders of both males and females can now be traced to abnormalities of the sex chromosomes. In the karyotype the human female sex chromosomes are designated as XX and the male as XY. The presence of at least one X chromosome is required for viability, and no sex chromosome disorders have been identified in living individuals in which the X chromosome was absent. However, a large number of disorders that involve either the *absence* or *multiplication* of the additional X or Y chromosome do occur. As in the abnormal autosomal defects, each of these disorders usually involves a specific karyotype.

The indifferent gonad. The normal embryogenesis of the gonad should be reviewed before disorders of sexual identity are discussed. Briefly, the gonad in the male or female embryo is *bipotential,* that is, it is capable of forming either male or female genitalia and internal organs, independent of the karyotype of the embryo. The major factor in sex determination is the hormonal environment of the embryo at the time of differentiation of the gonad. It has indeed been argued by women liberationists that all individuals are "basically" female, in that a karyotypically male embryo, if deprived of male hormones during gonadal differentiation, will develop as a female. The early human gonad consists of a cortex and medulla. Both contain primitive germ cells that have migrated into the structure during very early embryonic development. These cells will eventually give rise to either ova or sperm. If the gonad is destined to become a testes, producing male spermatogonia, the cortex regresses, and the medulla of the gonad differentiates into seminiferous and rete tubules, which are lined with epithelium containing the primordial sperm cells. If an ovary is to form, the cortex becomes germinal epithelium, which hypertrophies and produces follicles within which the primordial ova lie.

The usual sources of the hormones in the developing embryo are the organs and glands of the embryonic reproductive and endocrine systems. This production is under the control and regulation of both the sex chromosomes and autosomes. Without the proper hormonal balance as the gonads develop in the embryo, the indifferent gonad will differentiate in a direction that is not apparently dictated by the sex chromosome complement it has received at its conception. The importance of hormonal influence is shown by numerous animal studies.

The freemartin that is produced in cattle twinning has been shown to be due to the effects of male sex hormone on the developing female embryo. When cattle twins of different sexes share the same fetal circulation, so that the male sex hormone from the male twin can pass to the genotypically female twin, the female will develop into a basically male but sterile calf. Other evidence for the importance of the hormonal environment comes from hens. If the hen's ovary is removed at an early age or is destroyed by disease, the hen will develop a testes and become a rooster.

The influence of the genotype is, of course, profound. The presence of a Y sex chromosome will stimulate the indifferent gonad to form testes, even in the presence of multiple X chromosomes. Without a Y chromosome present to exert its masculinizing control on the immature gonad, the normal course of development will be to produce female structures. There is evidence that elements on other chromosomes, possibly the X chromosome, may be additionally required to produce this male determination, but the controlling genetic element is itself regulated by the Y chromosome.

In the female, while only one X chromosome is necessary for the production of femaleness, including the development of an ovarian gonad, a second X chromosome appears to be required for later normal development of an ovary. Thus, in *Turner's syndrome,* which is characterized by the presence of only one X chromosome, germ cells and ovarian tissue are present in fetal life and after birth, but by puberty all signs of ova and normal ovarian tissue have disappeared.

Turner's syndrome. Turner's syndrome, found in its pure form only in females, is caused by the absence of the second X sex chromosome and is therefore expressed karyotypically as 45, XO. It occurs in 0.45 of 1,000 live births. This disorder is characterized by *ovarian dysgenesis,* which is the absence of germ cells and mature ovaries, resulting in primary amenorrhea or absence of menstruation. A variety of somatic aberrations often accompany the sexual sterility and absence of secondary sexual characteristics. These include short stature, webbed neck, broadly spaced nipples, occasionally mild mental retardation, abnormal dermatoglyphics, an increased incidence of kidney anomalies, and coarctation of the aorta. Variants of ovarian dysgenesis syndromes have been described, and occasionally *mixoploidy* is observed. This is sexual mosaicism in which some cells of the body follow an XO cell line, while other cells may have an XY karyotype, an XX, or even XYY or XXX. In the case of mixoploidy the proportion of cells containing XY sex chromosomes to those with only X is crucial in determining whether the individual will be of male or female phenotype. Females with ovarian dysgenesis also may have an abnormally shaped second X chromosome rather than a complete absence of it as in the classic Turner's syndrome. The pathogenesis of Turner's syndrome appears to be the loss of the paternal sex chromosome in the zygote. The vast majority of such fetuses die in utero, and those that do survive may develop cardiac or renal disease of a life-threatening nature.

Klinefelter's syndrome. Klinefelter's syndrome is a eunuchlike condition found in males with one or more extra X chromosomes; it has an incidence of 2.13 per 1,000 live births. Phenotypically these individuals have small testes, enlarged breasts, a feminine distribution of pubic hair, and frequently mild mental retardation. Moreover, these boys grow rapidly after puberty and have proportionately longer legs. This disorder is associated with advanced maternal and paternal age. Klinefelter's syndrome is characterized by a 47, XXY sex chromosomal complement in 82% of the cases. Mixoploidy occurs in 11%, and 7% have either 48, XXYY, 48, XXXY, or 46, XX chromosomal complements. As in a normal female only one X chromosome remains genetically active within all cells, so that multiples of X chromosomes do not result in multiple copies of the genes that are present on the X chromosome. Multiple Y chromosome disorders also do not confer a great redundancy of genetic information, since the Y chromosome's only apparent function is to regulate embryonic sexual differentiation. The origin of the XXY sex chromosomes in Klinefelter's syndrome appears to be, in about two thirds of the cases, the result of *maternal meiotic nondisjunction*

(Fig. 2-14). The occasional Klinefelter's syndrome patient with an XX or female karyotype but with external and internal male genitalia represents an interesting case. The origin of such individuals remains only a matter for speculation. It is possible that these men began from a mixoploid cell line that contained a Y chromosome, which was able to exert its masculinizing effect on the embryo before being entirely lost in the individual. It is possible too that the missing Y chromosome had become translocated onto the X chromosome and is thus not identifiable. One intriguing possibility is that the XX Klinefelter's male is the result of a sex-linked autosomal recessive gene that could lead to complete sex reversal by stimulating the medulla of the indifferent gonad to differentiate into a testis. Animal studies bear out this possibility.

Sex chromosome polysomies. A number of situations have been described in which the X or the Y chromosome becomes duplicated. For example, 47, XXX females have been found in chromosomal surveys, and the incidence of this condition is about 0.65 in 1,000 live births. Such females have no particular phenotypic anomalies or congenital defects and are often fertile. An even rarer polysomy is 48, XXXX, of which five cases have been reported. All of these females are severely retarded but show no common phenotypic abnormality or aberrations of sexual developments. The origin of X chromosome polysomies may be correlated with the advanced maternal age of the mothers of these children. The most common origin is the fertilization of an XX ovum by an X-bearing sperm, or in the case of 48, XXXX, successive meiotic nondisjunction during oogenesis.

Among males, duplication of the Y chromosome has been reported and implicated in behavioral and phenotypic abnormalities. The origin of these males is probably *paternal nondisjunction,* which results in fertilization of an X-bearing ovum with a YY sperm. The frequency of XYY males among tall, violent, and criminal or psychopathic individuals may be as high as 24%. The general portrait of the XYY male is a person who is mentally deficient, tall, tending toward antisocial or criminal behavior, often suffering from acne, and often alcoholic. General sexual development and maturity seem unimpaired.

Intersexuality. XX males with Klinefelter's syndrome and XY females are examples of individuals with complete reversal of their sexual genotype. *Hermaphroditism* represents conditions in which sex reversal is only partially present. These conditions are described as intersexual. True hermaphrodites are classified on the basis of sexual mosaicism (gynandromorphism), in which both male and female cell lines can be found. Male and female cell clones may also be present in the gonadal tissue. Ovarian and testicular structures are both found in true hermaphroditism, while in *pseudohermaphroditism* the gonads are of one type only. The male pseudohermaphrodite has testes, but the internal genitalia are ambiguous; the external genitalia are male but poorly developed or feminized. The female pseudohermaphrodite usually has ovaries but rudimentary and masculinelike external genitalia and often a male phenotype. The common intersexual urogenital systems are diagramed in Fig. 2-16.

It should be mentioned that virilization of a female fetus could be effected by external sources. Tumors of the adrenal gland in the fetus or ovary in the mother might result in overproduction of male androgens, which in turn could act on the indifferent gonad. Administration of male androgens to the pregnant mother may also result in the same phenomenon.

GROSS STRUCTURAL ORGAN DEFECTS

It is beyond the scope of this book to describe in detail the many types of organ malformations and the pathophysiologic mechanism operating in these conditions. Other chapters in this book deal with various mechanisms of disease in the different organ systems, and these principles can be applied to the pathophysiology of defective organ structure. Birth defects have been catalogued in atlases, and detailed descriptions can be found in medical textbooks of pediatrics. This chapter's task is to define the pathogenic mechanisms through which such defects occur during embryogenesis.

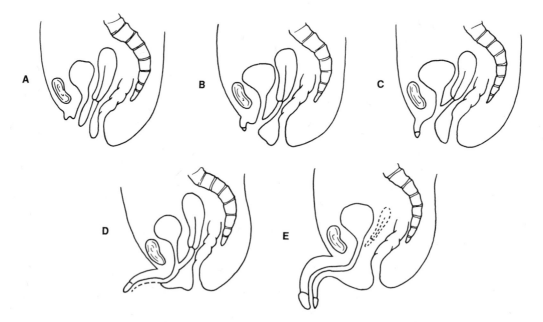

Fig. 2-16. Abnormal sexual development. **A,** Normal female. **B** to **E,** Deviations in structure of external genitalia. **B** and **C,** Rudimentary penis is present along with female structures. **D,** Penis is large, and bladder and vagina merge to form male-type urethra. **E,** Uterus is rudimentary.

Congenital anomalies

Fig. 2-17 lists various structural organ defects and the times during embryogenesis at which these structures were most susceptible to the action of teratogens. While it is theoretically possible for any organ to be malformed those that are most commonly seen are defects in the fusion of the lips and palate, abnormalities in the formation and rotation of the heart, central nervous system defects in brain, spinal cord integrity, and cerebrospinal fluid circulation, abnormalities in kidney structure, and defects in the formation of the gut.

Modes of action of teratogens

The end result of teratogens acting on developing embryonic tissue is either death, mal-

formation, retardation of growth, or functional disturbance. The vast majority (over 80%) of anomalies that an infant may be born with are caused by unknown factors acting during pregnancy. For a great variety of animal and human disorders it would appear that multiple factors may be required before the abnormality occurs. A teratogen known to cause cleft lip and palate may only do so in certain strains of mice and then only when the maternal diet is altered. Thus, genetic, teratogenic, maternal, and nutritional factors must operate together at a very specific time in the gestation of the embryo in order for the congenital anomaly to appear in the progeny. Other human development disorders that appear to follow this multifactorial threshold model include congenital

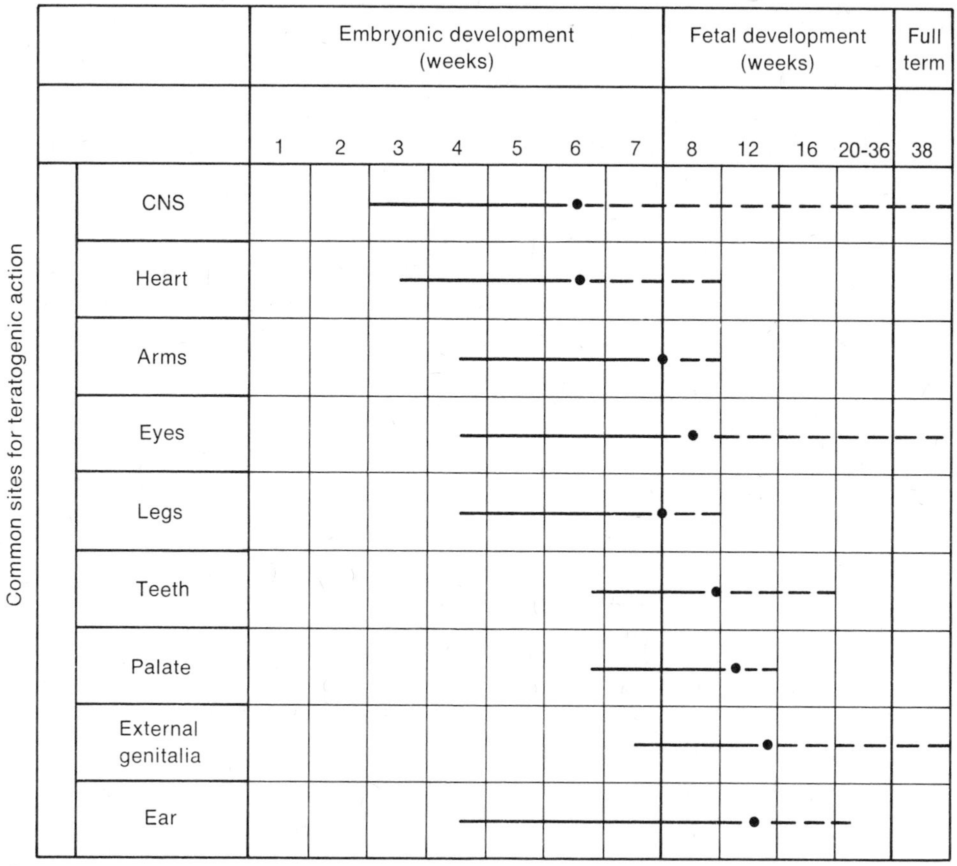

Fig. 2-17. Critical periods in human embryogenesis. Teratogens may act on a developing embryo at any time, but for any given teratogen, different tissues exhibit different sensitivity. For example, CNS anomalies in general are more likely to occur between the third and fifth weeks than at other times in embryogenesis.

hypertrophic pyloric stenosis, various congenital heart diseases, anencephaly and spina bifida, and Hirschsprung's disease. It can be said that for disorders with a known genetic background, such as cleft palate, the penetrance of the disease may be greatly affected by modifiers in the environment.

Most of our knowledge of the mechanisms of action of teratogens is derived from animal studies in which the processes of normal and abnormal embryogenesis can be followed very carefully. Extrapolation to humans is often made but has been shown many times to be invalid. Powerful teratogens in mice may have no effect on the human embryo and vice versa. The well-known thalidomide tragedy, in which a tranquilizer given to pregnant women resulted in lack of limb development and other anomalies in the offspring, is a case in point. Human teratogenesis presents an enormous problem for scientific investigation, and the application of the multifactorial threshold model to human anomalies has been made on the basis of study of the frequency of the disorder generally, in the families of those affected, and mathematical fitness to the model, based on these studies.

Table 2-1 lists some of the known human teratogenic substances. No common underlying similarity can be found among these agents at first glance. It would appear that the mode of action can be different with the end result in the fetus being the same. A number of theoretic mechanisms have been summarized by Wilson in the recently published *Handbook of Teratology*. There is some experimental evidence to support each of these mechanisms in malformation induction.

1. *Mutation* has been discussed as the original cause of all defects known to be hereditary; it can be caused by a number of known teratogens, such as irradiation, viruses, and a number of chemicals. Mutations in germ cells are usually implied when speaking of teratogenesis, although mutations in somatic cell lines are possible.

2. *Chromosomal nondisjunction and breaks* also have been discussed and are related to maternal age and aging of spermatazoa in the genital tract as well.

Table 2-1. Common teratogenic agents

Teratogens	Effects
Chemicals	
Alcohol	Fetal alcohol syndrome
Androgens	Masculinization of female fetus if administered to mother
Antibiotics (e.g., tetracycline)	Tooth defects
Cancer chemotherapy (e.g., aminopterin)	Central nervous system defects
Thyroid drugs (e.g., potassium iodide)	Congenital goiter
Tranquilizers (e.g., thalidomide)	Limb and other organ defects
Microbes	
Rubella	Rubella syndrome
Cytomegalovirus	Central nervous system and ophthalmic disorders
Toxoplasma gondii	Ophthalmic disorders
Radiation	
Therapeutic and possibly diagnostic radiation	Central nervous system and skeletal system abnormalities

3. *Mitotic interference* can be effected by a large number of teratogens, which can delay mitosis, prevent the spindle apparatus from functioning normally, or induce abnormalities in the formation or separation of the chromatids. Cells so interfered with usually cannot follow the developmental pattern of their particular cell line and thus delay or alter normal structure formation.

4. *Altered nucleic acid integrity or function* is the fourth possible mechanism by which developing embryonic cells can be affected. Drugs such as antibiotics and cancer chemotherapeutic agents are known to induce malformations in this manner and act basically by inhibiting purine or pyrimidine synthesis, crosslinking DNA, or binding with DNA to block RNA synthesis.

5. *Lack of precursors and substrates needed for biosynthesis* is another mechanism of teratogenesis, which has been well described for vitamin deficiency–induced malformations. Drugs that mimic required nutritional factors, thus taking

their place in metabolic processes, may result in developmental abnormalities. Furthermore, the role of the placenta is important in that the fetus must receive all nutrients from the mother's bloodstream through the extremely permeable placenta. Azo dyes and tissue antiserums in the placenta of experimental animals are able to interfere with the absorption of metabolites and nutrients into the fetus. However, this mechanism has not been documented for humans.

6. *Altered energy sources* may be an important mechanism of teratogenesis. Cells deprived of energy sources will not be able to generate ATP, which is required for all synthetic processes, and such phenomena common to the embryonic cell as division, differentiation, and motility.

7. *Enzyme inhibition* is the seventh possible mode of action by which teratogens affect growing embryos. Certain teratogenic drugs do inhibit the function of a number of critical enzymes, such as DNA polymerase or carbonic anhydrase.

8. *Osmolar imbalance* has been defined as a teratogenic mechanism based on the edema that results in chick embryos subjected to hypoxia. The accumulation of abnormal amounts of fluids and electrolytes in developing tissue could not only mechanically distort the tissue but also interfere with physiologic function. Osmotic changes could, of course, be secondary to a variety of teratogenic insults.

9. *Alteration in membrane characteristics* is the last conjectured mechanism and, while probably rare, is a theoretic mode of action. Ultrastructural membrane damage caused by vitamin A hypervitaminosis has been reported to be teratogenic in rodent embryos.

While the mechanisms described above may have different results in developing tissue, a search for a single, common, unifying process in teratogenesis would appear to implicate

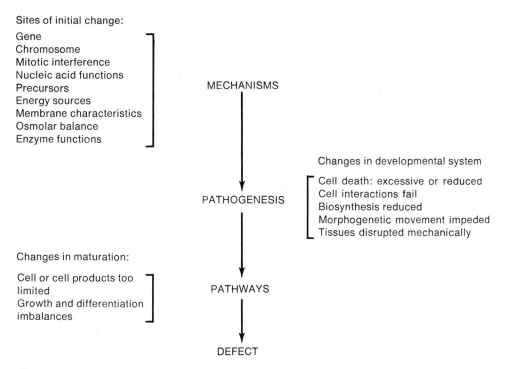

Fig. 2-18. Pathophysiology of developmental defects resulting from teratogenic insult. While teratogens may act at many possible sites, pathogenic pathways leading to defect are relatively few.

cellular necrosis in almost all teratogenic phenomena. Cellular necrosis at any stage of embryogenesis could interfere with normal formation, development, resorption, and growth. Cell death is one of the most common aspects of teratogenesis, no matter what mechanism has initiated the process. The pathophysiology of teratogenesis is shown in Fig. 2-18.

Maternal factors in teratogenesis

The interruption of pregnancy by childbirth must be considered as just another landmark in human development. Indeed, the first postnatal year is in many ways an extension of the fetal period as many organs and tissues are still developing and maturing during that time. Many congenital anomalies may not be evident at birth but certainly will be by the first birthday. A major difference between prenatal and postnatal life is the maternal influence on development while the fetus is in utero. There are two major ways that teratogens may affect the embryo. The first is directly, by crossing the placenta and interacting with embryonic cells at critical stages of development. The second mechanism is often given little attention but may ultimately prove to be just as important as the first. Teratogens may do their damage by altering the maternal physiology, so that the fetal development is impeded in a much more indirect way. For example, the degree and ease of the placental transfer of certain teratogens may be greatly affected by the maternal physiology, and it is one of the overriding principles of embryology that a teratogenic effect is almost always dose dependent.

Maternal malnutrition during pregnancy, while not directly related to major congenital anomalies, does result in low-birth-weight infants, and these infants have a higher incidence of perinatal mortality and developmental defects. Some authorities consider low birth weight to be a congenital anomaly in itself, and it has been associated with maternal viral infections. Maternal smoking is directly correlated with low birth weight and prematurity in offspring. Furthermore, a simian crease, a characteristic of mongolism and also often found in association with congenital heart defects and other anomalies, has been found in some children of heavy smokers.

The recent association of excessive alcohol ingestion during pregnancy and a characteristic syndrome in the offspring should also be noted.

The incidence of anencephaly and spina bifida has also been shown to be above average in countries such as Ireland and states such as Maine because of the mother's consumption of blighted potatoes. The antibiotic produced by the potato in response to blight has been particularly implicated as the teratogen responsible. Stored potatoes with any trace of blight should be scrupulously avoided by pregnant women during the first 4 weeks of pregnancy in particular.

Maternal vitamin deficiencies and excesses have been reported to be teratogenic in many animal species, but little information is available on these effects in humans. Vitamin A excess has been the best described vitamin teratogen in experimental animals. Other maternal nutritional factors that have been studied include the effects of undernutrition during the prenatal period on subsequent brain development and behavior. Whether humans are subject to *permanent* changes in brain function as the result of maternal undernutrition has not been clearly established.

Maternal age has been established in a causal relation with Down's syndrome, as previously discussed. The incidence of other congenital anomalies may be increased in younger women. An example is anencephaly and spina bifida, which occurs with an incidence of 1 in 1,000 total births in the United States. Its occurrence in miniepidemics is interesting, but no true relationship with environmental agents has as yet been established. The incidence of children with this defect is higher in short mothers than among the general population, and it is possible that malnutrition during the mother's childhood resulted in damage to germ cells or reproductive tract integrity, which was then later expressed as teratomas in the offspring. Anencephaly and spina bifida are also found with a higher frequency among mothers of lower socioeconomic status, among blacks, and in infants of low birth weights.

Maternal ingestion of potentially teratogenic drugs may result in defective offspring if the mother's own detoxification or metabolism of the drug is abnormal. The liver metabolism of thalidomide differs greatly among species, and this may account for the wide disparity of teratogenicity among species.

While not conclusively established, many case histories of mothers who have borne children with congenital abnormalities include maternal stress and psychologic imbalance, suggesting that maternal psychosocial well-being is somehow related to normal growth and development of the fetus.

Maternal rubella. The disease model for teratogenesis in this chapter is the rubella syndrome, which is the sequelae of maternal rubella during pregnancy. The relationship between congenital malformations and maternal rubella was first suggested by Gregg in Australia in 1941, following a rubella epidemic. Children born of mothers who had contracted rubella (which is itself a mild self-limiting illness) during pregnancy were observed to have an increased incidence of congenital cataracts, deafness, microcephaly, mental retardation, congenital heart defects, and evidence of chronic infection in many organs. The association of these signs with a history of maternal rubella came to be known as the rubella syndrome.

The risk of rubella syndrome in the offspring of an infected mother is greatly increased during the first trimester of the pregnancy, but it has recently become apparent that long-range sequelae from rubella infection in utero can occur even when the infection occurred later in the pregnancy. For fetal damage during organogenesis to occur, several events must proceed in an orderly fashion. An initial maternal viremia that may be so mild as to be undetected by the pregnant mother is followed by infection of the placenta with rubella virus. The fetus then becomes infected, and fetal viremia ensues. Many organs and tissues can become sites of local rubella infection with subsequent inflammation and necrosis. The virus often persists in these structures long after damage has occurred, and virus has been cultivated in the eye of a child with congenital rubella-induced cataracts after 3 years. Live virus may be shed through the nasopharynx and urine of infants born with congenital rubella syndrome for many months after birth and be a source of infection for others. The pathophysiologic mechanism whereby the fetal rubella infection subsequently causes the characteristic organ malformations may be due to an arteritis, which leads to hypoxia of developing parts. Of course, direct cell necrosis may play an important role. Often, too, the infection persists in the fetal cells and becomes chronic, and development can be interfered with on a long-term basis. Statistical likelihood of malformations in the offspring is highest among mothers infected during the first month of pregnancy, with an estimated risk of 50%. The probability decreases to 22% during the second month, and to 6% to 8% in the third through fifth months of gestation.

It should be mentioned that fetal rubella infection is not always associated with congenital anomalies and that a certain percentage of rubella-infected fetuses survive and appear to be

Table 2-2. Teratogenic effects of rubella virus by gestational age of fetus*

Gestational age	Congenital anomalies				No congenital anomalies		Deaths (false or fetal)
	No.	Severe	Moderate	Mild	? Normal	Normal	
Preconception	5	1					4
0-4 weeks	23	11	6				6
5-8 weeks	28	7	3	7	1	1	3
9-12 weeks	14	3	3	7	1		0
13-16 weeks	10	2	3	1	2		2
17-20 weeks	7	1		1	1	3	1
21-30 weeks	11	1	2	2	2	4	0
31-45 weeks	4			1	2	1	0

*From Hardy, J. B.: Immediate and long-range effects of maternal viral infection in pregnancy. In Bergsma, D., and Schimke, R. N., editors: Cytogenetics, environment and malformation syndromes. The 1975 Birth Defects Conference, New York, 1976, Alan R. Liss for the National Foundation—March of Dimes.

normal. Table 2-2 tabulates data from a major study (at Johns Hopkins) on maternal rubella and risk to offspring.

The long-range effects of maternal rubella infection on the affected offspring are becoming apparent continuously as these children are identified and followed over their lifetimes. IQ is definitely affected, and children with normal IQs frequently experience a variety of learning disorders. Many children have hearing difficulty, the organ of Corti being the auditory structure most often infected with the rubella virus. Little improvement has occurred with age in the children in the Johns Hopkins' study. Growth retardation, which is evident at birth in these children, is maintained during the early years of childhood. Recent reports also suggest that rubella syndrome children are subject to a variety of late onset diseases, particularly during the first year of life. These include chronic rashes, thrombocytopenia, failure to thrive, persistent diarrhea, and generalized interstitial pneumonia. Another condition that is appearing in the second decade of life in these children is a chronic panencephalitis, which is progressive and degenerative. Rubella virus has been isolated from the central nervous system in one of the four reported cases.

In 1969 a rubella vaccine was licensed for use, and massive immunization of children and women at risk for rubella was carried out. It is routine in many states to determine the rubella antibody titer before marriage and subsequently to carry out prophylactic vaccination. A decline in the incidence of rubella and rubella syndrome has been occurring since the widespread vaccination program was begun.

SUGGESTED READINGS

Anderson, W. A. D., and Kissane, J. M., editors: Pathology, ed. 7, St. Louis, 1977, The C. V. Mosby Co.

Bergsma, D.: Birth defects, atlas and compendium, Baltimore, 1973, The Williams & Wilkins Co.

Bergsma, D., and Schimke, R. N., editors: Cytogenetics, environment and malformation syndromes. The 1975 birth defects conference, New York, 1976, Alan R. Liss.

Boyce, A. J., editor: Chromosomal variations in human evolution, New York, 1975, Halsted Press.

Ciba Foundation Symposium: Intrauterine infections, Amsterdam, 1973, Associated Scientific Publishers.

Cohen, S. N.: The manipulation of genes, Sci. Am. **233**(1):25-33, 1975.

Hamerton, J. L.: Human cytogenetics, New York, 1971, Academic Press.

Huettner, A. F.: Fundamentals of comparative embryology of the vertebrates, New York, 1966, Macmillan Publishing Co.

Janerich, D. T., Skalko, R. G., and Porter, I. H., editors: Congenital defects, new directions in research, New York, 1974, Academic Press.

Moore, K. L.: Before we are born, Philadelphia, 1974, W. B. Saunders Co.

Nelson, W.: Textbook of pediatrics, ed. 10, Philadelphia, 1975, W. B. Saunders Co.

Ruddle, F. H., and Kucherlapati, R. S.: Hybrid cells and human genes, Sci. Am. **231**:36-44, 1974.

Stanbury, J., Wyngaarden, J., and Fredrickson, D.: The metabolic basis of inherited disease, New York, 1972, McGraw-Hill Book Co.

Wintrobe, M. M.: Clinical hematology, Philadelphia, 1967, Lea & Febiger.

Wilson, J., and Clarke Fraser, F., editors: Handbook of teratology, New York, 1977, Plenum Publishing Corp.

CHAPTER 3

Carcinogenesis

AT THE COMPLETION OF THIS CHAPTER THE STUDENT WILL BE ABLE TO:

- Differentiate between benign and malignant neoplasia and describe the structural and functional alterations that are observed in malignant anaplasia, as compared to the normal, embryonic, dysplastic, hyperplastic, and metaplastic states.
- Describe and compare the processes of invasion and metastasis and discuss these phenomena in relationship to the natural history of various cancers in man.
- Discuss common carcinogens, the possible mechanisms whereby they cause cancer, and models of carcinogenesis.
- Discuss research findings that support the carcinogenesis models presented.
- Describe the anorexia-cachexia syndrome, showing how various factors can reinforce and perpetuate this process.
- Analyze the immune response to cancer that is thought to occur and discuss how alterations in the immune response might be involved in carcinogenesis and how manipulation of the immune system may be used therapeutically.
- List the major characteristics of the various tumor types that were presented and be able to randomly choose any tumor type and relate its natural history in man to the general principles of carcinogenesis and the pathophysiology of malignancy.
- Relate how a knowledge of carcinogenesis and the pathophysiology of malignancy might be used in assessing a cancer patient.
- Contrast the physiologic bases of the four major modes of cancer treatment and describe the side effects that might be experienced in each case.
- Summarize the major areas of cancer research that have yielded information which has resulted in better care or lengthening of life span in cancer patients.

NATURE OF CANCER

No definition of cancer has been universally accepted, and no one common unifying theory of cancer causation scientifically validated. The nature of cancer appears to be one in which a genetic disease of somatic (body) cells occurs as the result of a mutation in a previously normal cell, producing an abnormal cell type, which is perpetuated in the body. The mutation produces a cell that has lost the normal regulatory constraints of the homeostatic steady state on mitotic division and that generally appears immature and poorly differentiated. The diagnosis of cancer can be made by examination of these cellular changes that occur. This is usually done by examination of the cells taken by biopsy from the tissue that is suspect. The morphologic cellular changes and the processes by which cancer causes disease and death are known and occur in a characteristic manner—regardless of the actual cause of the original change in the cells.

As more is learned about the process whereby a normal cell undergoes carcinogenic transformation and about the pathophysiology of the malignant cells, the less likely it appears that a single basic biologic phenomenon will be described for all cancers. The diseases classified as cancer probably result from many factors interacting in the host at the biochemical, cellular, tissue, organ, and organism level, and all factors interact again within the particular environment that the person finds himself.

The recognition of cancer as a group of chronic diseases of primarily environmental origin has been the single most important common result of cancer research and has provided various rationales for the prevention, detection, and treatment of certain kinds of cancer. Much further research needs to be carried out on the basic mechanism of carcinogenesis throughout the animal and plant kingdoms and on the natural history of the disease process in humans, in order to aid both the scientist and the health care provider in approaching cancer from phenomenologic and practical aspects.

The common pathophysiologic mechanisms that appear to operate in all cancer cells are (1) the loss of regulation of mitotic rate, (2) the loss of specialization and differentiation of the cell, (3) the ability of the cancer cell to move from the original or *primary* site and establish new malignant growths at other tissue sites *(metastasis),* and (4) the capacity to invade and destroy normal tissue in which the cancer grows.

Cancer can be found in either a diffuse disease state, such as in leukemia, in which the leukemic cells are widely dispersed, or in cellular associations called *tumors,* which form actual masses within tissues. Tumors or neoplasms (new growths) can be benign or malignant and can arise in any tissue or organ of the body. The tissue of origin of the primary tumor can be determined from tumor nomenclature, the Greek root for tumor being *oma.* For example, a sarcoma is derived from connective tissue, a carcinoma from epithelial tissue, an adenoma from glandular tissue, and a teratoma from embryonic tissue. Malignant tumors are distinguished from benign tumors by the morphology of the cells in the mass and the fact that benign tumors are generally noninvasive and encapsulated within a membrane and never metastasize. It is important to realize, however, that a benign tumor can be extremely pathologic to the host if it obstructs critical vessels, ducts, or tracts within the body, interfering with normal oxygenation, nutrition, or elimination, or if it has functional activity, such

as excess hormone production, which would disrupt the normal feedback regulation of the endocrine system. Conversely, occasional malignant tumors grow so slowly that there is little effect on the host for a considerable period. Many tumors do not have to reach a certain critical size before cells begin to break away and metastasize, however.

Although there are certain populations of individuals who are considered to be at high risk for the development of cancer, it is generally impossible to predict who will develop malignant disease within the general population. A typical example that characterizes the natural history of the malignant disease in humans is one in which the affected individual presents himself initially to the physician with malignant, metastatic, and invasive cancer, usually accompanied by vague generalized symptoms. The development of cachexia may be apparent. *Cachexia* is a syndrome characterized by muscle wasting, weakness, fatigue, anorexia (loss of appetite), and anemia. It is much less common for a malignancy to be discovered early in the disease process by a physician or screening clinic when the malignant mass is small and locally confined (in situ) and no metastatic dissemination has occurred. It is obvious that the detection of cancer in the early stages plays an important role in the efficacy of therapy and control of the advancement of the malignant disease process. Early detection of many tumor types results in a greater survival rate, and the possibility of cure is much more real when treatment is initiated early.

CANCER CELL
Predisposing factors

The cancer cell shows morphologic and physiologic deviations from normal. The anaplastic (without form) nature of the malignant cell is characterized by immaturity and lack of differentiation of the dividing cells. It may be difficult to distinguish structurally the cell type from which the malignancy was originally derived. Frequently hyperplasia and metaplasia precede the conversion of the normal tissue into neoplastic tissue. For example, the incidence of endometrial cancer is significantly increased in females who have a history of endometrial hyperplasia. *Hyperplasia* is a process in which cells respond to a stress by increasing in number through increased cellular division. The endometrium may respond to an increased concentration of estrogen, for example, by hyperplasia. The rising incidence of uterine cancer in postmenopausal women who have received replacement therapy with estrogen compounds has recently been established and may be related to this hyperplastic process. It is conceivable that hyperplasia predisposes to neoplasia by merely increasing the statistical likelihood of a cellular neoplastic transformation in that many more cells are dividing much more rapidly than in normal tissue and may therefore generally be more sensitive to carcinogens. *Metaplasia* is the process whereby one cell type changes to another cell type in response to stress and generally assists the host to adapt to the stress.

Dysplasia is another type of nonmalignant cellular growth, which again may precede neoplastic changes in the tissue. It is associated with chronic irritation of a tissue by a chemical agent, such as cigarette smoke, or by inflammatory irritation of a chronic nature, such as chronic cervicitis (inflammation of the cervix). The dysplastic tissue appears somewhat structureless and disorganized and may consist of atypical cells.

Dysplasia, hyperplasia, and metaplasia are intrinsically reversible in nature, and the tissue can revert to normal structure when the stress that initiated the changes is removed. Malignant neoplastic growth, on the other hand, is not usually reversible when the carcinogenic stress is removed but appears to be the result of a permanent alteration in the transformed cell, which is inherited by all the daughter cells from every division of the neoplastic cell.

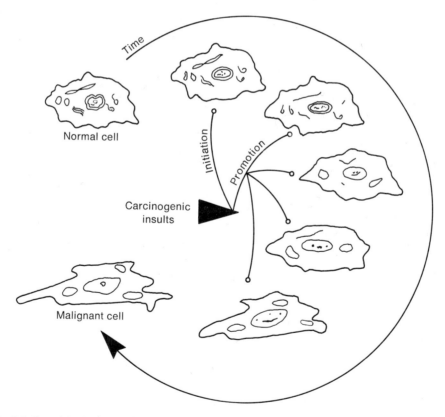

Fig. 3-1. Berenblum's theory of carcinogenesis: initiation and promotion. Several events are required for a normal cell to become transformed into a cancer cell. Initial event, initiation, will not cause cancer unless several promoting events occur over time.

Cellular pathophysiology of malignancy

Cancer appears to arise from an originally normal cell that is transformed. This transformation, according to the Berenblum theory, probably involves at least two steps: *initiation and promotion* (Fig. 3-1). Agents that initiate and later promote transformation are termed *carcinogens*. Carcinogens may be chemical agents, viruses, radiation, hormones, and perhaps physical irritation. Cocarcinogens may be required for the carcinogen to effect transformation or perhaps for promoting the growth of the cells once it is transformed. All carcinogens appear to act ultimately at the nuclear level of the cell and are able to damage or somehow alter the normal nucleic acids. It is not known whether carcinogenesis directly results from this type of damage, but it appears highly likely that the DNA of neoplastic malignant cells is mutated, as the malignant properties of the transformed cell are inherited by the daughter cells derived from every mitosis of the originally transformed cell and its daughter cells. Damage to the genetic material may result from a direct mutation caused by the carcinogen or may be a more indirect phenomenon in which the carcinogen acts to unmask hidden genetic information that is normally *repressed*. This repressed bit of genetic code, which has been added to human genetic complement sometime in the evolutionary past, has been termed the *oncogene;* when the oncogene is "turned on," the cells begin to produce proteins, which ultimately change the nature of the cell, causing it to become malignant. The oncogene may exist in all human cells or only in the cells of that 25% of the human population that will ultimately have cancer. The postulated existence of the oncogene forms the basis for one theory of cancer susceptibility from parents to children, which has been reported for certain cancer types. Viral DNA is also known to invade the host cell DNA and may remain latent for many years. Activation of a latent *virogene* may also result in malignant transformation.

It has been shown experimentally that the cancer process can originate in animals when a single malignant cell is injected. Nevertheless, cancer cells are not necessarily autonomous in nature but may require considerable immunologic, nutritional, chemical, and hormonal support from the host in order to flourish. This is demonstrated by the occasional reports of long intervals between the surgical excision of a primary tumor and the appearance of secondary metastases. This phenomenon may be due to the anoxic environment that results at the surgical site and that suppresses growth and metastasis of malignant cells left behind after surgery. Over a period of years the surgical site becomes revascularized and normoxic, and the cells are no longer suppressed by the host's hostile environment.

It is interesting to note that transmission of information through cellular mitosis in cancer cells is magnified not always by a rapid division rate but by the further division of every daughter cell of every mitosis, which is in contrast to the normal mitotic pattern. It has been shown that a single cell cycle, consisting of division, rest, and growth, is not shorter in many tumor cells and may, in fact, be longer than in the normal cell. Tumor formation may result when a normal pattern of division and growth within a tissue renewal system is altered. Many tissues renew themselves constantly when the normal physiology of that tissue consists of loss of cells from that tissue. This process occurs continuously in the skin, the gastrointestinal tract, the testes, and the blood. The originator of the new tissue replacement cells is an undifferentiated, unspecialized, immature cell known as the *stem cell*. This primitive cell is committed to divide and develop a new population of like cells through a progression of (1) mitosis and (2) differentiation of daughter cells. The stem cell divides a certain number of times, and then it appears that only one daughter cell continues to divide further, while the other daughter cell will differentiate into a specialized cell type. Malignant cells may not follow this pattern but will divide continuously without differentiation into very specialized or functionally integrated cells. The cells remain anaplastic and immature. Stem cells are themselves in general sensitive to the mutagenic effects of radiation. Malignancy may occur when a carcinogen, such as radiation, acts upon the sensitive stem

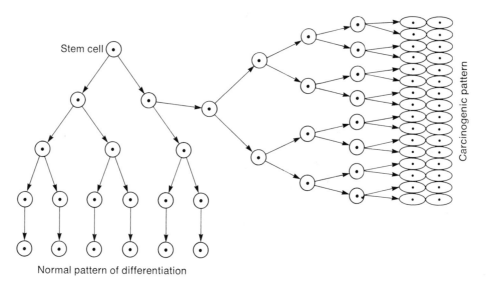

Stem cell

Carcinogenic pattern

Normal pattern of differentiation

Fig. 3-2. Carcinogenesis. Carcinogen acts on sensitive stem cell, which then produces malignant tumor through a loss of normal mitotic pattern and differentiation of daughter cells.

cell, which then divides and propagates the initial transformation of the cell into a malignant tumor mass (Fig. 3-2).

The growth of a tumor may also be influenced by the rate of cell loss from the growing cell mass whether or not the cell cycle is changed in duration. Some skin cancers grow extremely slowly over a period of years without a significant increase in size. This is probably due to rapid and constant *exfoliation* (loss of skin cells from the surface of the epithelium) from the malignant mass. Many solid tumors, as well, generally appear to grow to a defined size, which may, in fact, be maintained only by metastasis of cells away from the tumor rather than by a decrease in the actual growth.

The degree of malignancy produced by a given carcinogen may be dependent on the stage of differentiation of the target cell of the carcinogen. It is theorized that a benign tumor might be the result of a carcinogenic stimulus acting on the matured cells in a tissue renewal system (such as skin, gut, or blood), whereas the same carcinogen acting on a stem cell could give rise to a potently malignant cell. Tumors can generally be classified by biopsy into four grades of malignancy:

Grade 1   Tumors in which 75% or more of the cells appear well differentiated

Grade 2   Tumors in which 50% to 75% of the cells appear differentiated

Grade 3   Tumors in which 25% to 50% of the cells appear differentiated

Grade 4   Tumors in which 0% to 25% of the cells appear differentiated

Thus, tumors of higher grade would consist largely of anaplastic cells and would in general have the poorest prognosis for the patient.

Considerable evidence does exist that certain tumors are derived from transformed undifferentiated stemlike cells. Tumors originating from embryonic tissues (teratocarcinomas) in particular seem to have this characteristic. Indeed, carcinogenesis in the adult organism may be a pathophysiologic caricature of the normal histogenesis observed in the developing embryo as it differentiates toward a mature form. A carcinogen would then be seen to act by *derepressing* (i.e., unmasking) certain genes that are usually active only during embryonic life and repressing others. The activated genes would then code for a certain protein profile, which would characterize the cell as malignant. The search for particular embryonic proteins in cancer tissue is an important part of the research into carcinogenesis. Cancer of the colon and liver appears in many cases to produce embryonic proteins, which may be detected early in the disease process. Such cancer markers may aid in early cancer screening and detection.

If cancer can be regarded as a return of a differentiated cell to a state somewhat like the embryonic one, then the question arises, "Are embryonic cells similar in any way to malignant cells?" Certain characteristics of cancer are reminiscent of the embryo. The motility of cancer cells, the anaplasia, the production of fetal antigens, the release of angioblastic (blood vessel–forming) substances by tumors, and the invasiveness of cancer cells (which can be compared to the extraordinary invasive penetration of the endometrium by the trophoblast of the embryo) all point to certain similarities.

It has also been shown that prenatal exposure to radiation, stilbesterol therapy, and certain viral diseases, especially parainfluenza and chickenpox, increases the subsequent risk of cancer in the child. Furthermore, there is an observed association between congenital malformations and cancers in the fetus. These observations would lend credence to the theory that cancer develops more readily in undifferentiated tissue and may in fact represent a mimicking of embryogenesis, albeit uncontrolled and pathologic.

Morphology. The structural characteristics of most neoplastic cells resemble in certain ways the immature cells of the embryo. Indeed, the presence of anaplastic cells within a tissue specimen taken from a tumor is nearly pathognomonic of cancer. The degree of malignancy of a tumor is positively correlated with the degree of anaplasia. Anaplastic cells themselves are of abnormal size and shape, and the nuclei are usually large and contain grossly abnormal nucleoli. The nucleolus, a nuclear organelle that contains DNA and RNA, is not only pleomorphic (abnormally shaped) in malignant cells but is subsequently altered also by cancer chemotherapeutic agents such as actinomycin D, which causes the nucleolus in cancer cells to change both its shape and activity. The role of the nucleolus in both the transformation of a cell and the maintenance of the neoplastic processes has not been determined but remains an area of scientific speculation and research.

Malignant cells also contain *abnormal chromosomes* and unusual mitotic spindles, which produce bizarre cell divisions. It appears likely that the abnormalities of the nucleus and chromosomes are secondary to the intrinsic loss of regulation of cell mitosis and other physiologic processes rather than the direct result of carcinogenic injury or insult to the nucleus. The many cells of a given tumor do not usually exhibit absolutely identical karyotype and phenotype, although it is believed that a tumor does not develop in consequence to more than one initiating carcinogenic agent acting on a number of target cells. Thus, the changes seen in tumor cells do not always represent the direct effects of a carcinogen, even if a carcinogen can be identified. Indeed, the nature of the carcinogens for most tumors in humans is not known, and for those that are known the mechanism of action is still obscure.

Metabolism and protein synthesis. The cancer cell exhibits a general loss of the specialized protein synthetic capabilities that would identify it as a differentiated cell type. For example, a differentiated liver cell synthesizes only liver cell enzymes. Highly anaplastic cells from a hepatocarcinoma might synthesize few of these normal enzymes, and in fact a *fetal* liver protein may be produced. It seems that the enzymes and other proteins that cancer cells do produce allow only for the tumor cell mass to grow rapidly, and the "frills" of differentiated and specialized protein production are eliminated in this process.

The biochemical metabolism of neoplastic cells is usually more anaerobic than that of normal non–rapidly dividing cells. Thus, malignant cells may be able to withstand hypoxic conditions for prolonged periods. In terms of systems theory we can say that cancer cells have reached a uniquely more stable steady state than normal cells and are doing so at the expense of the host's steady state.

Nuclear changes. The chromosomes that constitute the *karyotype* (the chromosomal number, sizes, and shapes) of neoplastic cells generally are altered, and many of the known carcinogens are *mutagens* (i.e., able to cause mutations in the cellular DNA). Carcinogens therefore might act by causing direct mutations in the chromosomes of the cell, and this may constitute transformation. Carcinogens might also act in other ways, by membrane damage, for example, or by altering the general characteristics of the tissue in which the neoplasm is destined to arise. They may act by promoting complex intracellular relationships that result in genetic expression of repressed bits of DNA. The kinds of chromosomal aberrations that are commonly observed in the malignant cell are *nonspecific* in nature, except for a few cancer types. Chronic myelogenous leukemia is usually characterized by the appearance of an extra chromosome, known as the Philadelphia chromosome, in certain blood cells of the individual. There is also an increased incidence of leukemia in mongoloids, a condition that results from a trisomy of the chromosome 21 pair in humans. A genetic marker accompanying cancer seems to be the deletion of the long arm of chromosome 13, reported in 50 patients with retinoblastoma. Other tumors, such as osteogenic sarcoma, a tumor of bone, also appear in these individuals, thus indicating an association of a chromosomal defect with malignancies.

The presence of chromosomal aberrations by themselves does not indicate that cancer is the result of faulty DNA. Clearly factors other than the DNA code itself are involved in the expression of genetic traits in both normal and malignant cells. This is exemplified by an experiment in which two populations of malignant cells were fused, with a resultant mixing of the cellular DNA. The cells produced by the fusion were not malignant. Certain genes may be repressed in normal cells and expressed in cancer cells by cytoplasmic and non–nucleic acid nuclear factors.

Membrane changes. There are conflicting reports regarding the nature of the cancer cell membrane (the membranes of cancer cells have been reported to have increased passive and active permeability and drastically decreased permeability). Cancer cells in tissue culture usually have increased glucose and amino acid uptake. There may be an altered calcium ion concentration in the malignant cell membrane, which may in part be responsible for the lack of *contact* (or density-dependent) *inhibition* and cohesiveness in neoplastic cells.

In tissue cultures of cancer cells, the transformed cells clump together and pile up on one another instead of forming the typical cellular monolayer usually seen in tissue cultures. This can be viewed as an in vitro microtumor. Normally cell division in a population of cells is impeded by cell surface-to-surface contact.

Cellular membrane communication appears lost in cancer cells, so that movement of materials and cell membrane–mediated transmission of biologic information is impaired, and cellular cohesion is interrupted as well. The malignant transformation process may be accompanied by the revelation of normally masked membrane components, such as antigens, channels, or binding sites. The membranes of neoplastic cells also do not turn over the lipoprotein components with the same rapidity as normal cells. This may indicate that the membrane is the site of initial carcinogenic insult and injury. Disruption at the membrane could be magnified by a cascade of events throughout the cell, eventually resulting in modifications of DNA synthesis, protein synthesis, and cell mitosis.

Electron microscopy of cancer cells has shown that the cell membrane, surface coat, and cytoplasmic projections may be abnormal, and cancer cells are known to be intensely phagocytic and mobile. Cancer cell surfaces may have electric charge alterations as well.

Invasion. Cancer cells have increased motility, and this appears to be a factor in the property of invasion and infiltration of normal tissue by malignant tissue. Invasion may be aided by the production of lytic enzymes, which are increased in neoplastic cells. Invasion is not well understood, but experiments indicate that there is a preferential destruction of the normal tissue by the malignant cells, as has been demonstrated in vitro. Invasion is defined as the penetration of adjacent tissue by a neoplasm. Normal invasion of a tissue by another tissue can occur and is characteristic of implantation of the zygote in the uterine wall. Neoplastic invasion appears random and unchecked, however. It has been shown that normal tissue interactions that maintain histologic structure are disturbed in malignant invasion. Invasion of epithelial malignant tumors into the underlying connective tissue is accompanied by structural and functional changes in the cell surfaces, which allow the malignant cells to more easily penetrate the dermal tissue. Tumor invasion may also be enhanced by the elaboration of angioblastic substances by malignant cells, which promote vascularization of the infiltrating tumor. The property of invasion of normal tissue can account for much morbidity in the cancer patient and in part can explain the development of cachexia (severe wasting) in terminally ill individuals with cancer.

Metastasis. Metastasis is the dissemination of malignant cells from the primary cancer site to other tissues in the body and the establishment of secondary malignancies that have many of the same characteristics as the primary tumor. Cells or tissue fragments from a malignant growth can break away at any time from the primary tumor and travel through lymphatic vessels, veins, or interstitially through the tissue spaces. Lymphatics appear to be the most common method of metastatic spread. The presence of cancer cells or cancerous tissue fragments in the circulating blood does not constitute metastasis. There is no correlation between the presence of these cells in the bloodstream and the ultimate prognosis of the cancer patient. The malignant cells that leave the primary tumor must find a favorable tissue environment in which invasion and growth is facilitated. It is well known that certain primary tumors metastasize preferentially to specific organs. Such spread does not seem related to such known tissue characteristics as location or vascularity. Establishment of secondary cancer in a tissue is also aided by the elaboration of an angioblastic substance that promotes a microcirculation in the growing tumor mass. The *selective affinity theory* of metastasis describes the spread of the neoplastic cells to certain organs as a function of the organ to which the cells travel and flourish in. Some unknown character of the tissue is therefore involved in establishing a favorable environment for the primary tumor cells. The *mechanical theory* of metastasis relates metastasis only to factors such as metastatic cell size, pressure, vessel size, and other purely physical factors. *The transformation theory* of metastasis corre-

lates cancer cell spread with the transformation of secondary tissue cells by cancer cell DNA. Generally most metastatic invasion can be described by the selective affinity theory, but mechanical factors do seem important in some cases.

Metastasis occurs most commonly to the lymph nodes, lungs, liver, bones, kidneys, and adrenal glands. Individual cells can travel through the lymph or blood, or actual cancer cell thrombi can seed an organ. These tissue fragments become coated with fibrin, and anticoagulant therapy has been used recently for the prevention of metastasis. Often cancer cells metastasize to areas that have been physically injured. Growth of cells along the puncture wound of a needle biopsy site has been described. Secondary carcinoma has also been observed along the suture line of a surgical incision resulting from cancer surgery. The trauma of surgical manipulation has been shown to release a shower of malignant cells into the tissue spaces and bloodstream. The release of cancer cells from a primary tumor has even resulted from manual diagnostic examination of a tumor.

Certain tumors are more likely to metastasize than others. For example, the basal cell carcinoma of skin rarely metastasizes. Metastasis generally occurs away from the primary tumor via the lymphatic vessels. These vessels end in blind, thin walled, and highly permeable capillaries. Lymph is filtered by the lymph nodes, which are dispersed along the lymphatic channels. The lymph nodes are thought by many authorities to be an important barrier to cancer spread, and the routine removal of lymph nodes during cancer surgery is now being questioned by some. Degenerating and necrotic cells can sometimes be found in these nodes, as well as *histiocytes* (macrophages that act to phagocytose debris and foreign material), indicating that a defense reaction of the body occurs in response to the neoplastic cells. Cancer cells can grow in the lymph nodes, however, resulting in localized hard and painful tumor masses that must be removed. The presence of malignant cells in the lymph nodes surrounding and draining a malignant cancer indicates that metastasis has begun, and the extent of lymph node involvement can be correlated with the patient's ultimate prognosis.

Malignant cells can also infiltrate into veins, while arterial invasion is rare. The tumorous tissue erodes into the veins and propagates by growing along the endothelium. Vessels can actually become obstructed with plugs of neoplastic cells. The tumors of higher grade are more anaplastic and show the greatest incidence of venous spread.

Metastasis is the most lethal property of cancer cells and ultimately causes death in patients with incurable cancer. Much cancer therapy is aimed toward preventing or retarding this process.

THEORIES OF CARCINOGENESIS AND COMMON CARCINOGENS

Basic research and epidemiologic investigations have resulted in a number of prominent theories of carcinogenesis. Most theories recognize that as much as 85% of all human cancers are of environmental origin. Known environmental carcinogens include radiation, chemicals, viruses, hormones, and irritation.

Chemical carcinogenesis

Tar-induced production of skin cancer in the rabbit was first described at the beginning of this century. Since then many other naturally occurring and synthetic compounds have been shown to have carcinogenic potential, and the list grows constantly. The identification of chemicals that are carcinogenic in humans is complicated by long latent periods between exposure and the first appearance of cancer. Thus, man may now be exposed to carcinogens that may ultimately result in cancer 20 years hence. The ubiquity of latency in neoplastic development is a poorly understood phenomenon. The length of the latent period appears to be a function of the carcinogen as well as the host; it may be the time required for a transformed committed cell to grow or for a sequence of cellular changes that ultimately result in cancer. The latter possibility has the most experimental support.

Chemical carcinogenesis seems to follow a concentration pattern. Many substances that are components of the atmosphere, soil, and food and drink have been shown to induce tumors in experimental animals when used in high concentrations. Some of these agents are listed in the box on p. 56. Little is known about the effects of these carcinogens when the host is exposed to minute amounts in the environment over a period of many years. The same is true for the effects of very low doses of ionizing radiation. Controversy reigns over whether there exists a threshold for biologic damage by chemical carcinogens or radiation below which the organism is able to repair damage and above which irreparable injury of a dose-dependent nature occurs.

The mechanism by which chemical carcinogens cause neoplastic transformation is not known. It is clear that the host cells themselves must interact with most carcinogens for cancer to occur, by enzymatic activation of these compounds. For example, the derivatives of human metabolism of the polycyclic hydrocarbons (chemicals found in oxidizing smogs of the Los Angeles type) yield cancer-inducing entities, as do the aromatic amines. Individuals vary in their abilities to activate chemical carcinogens, and this genetically determined difference may be correlated with cancer susceptibility. Carcinogens or the metabolites of carcinogens are often mutagenic, but it is not known if all carcinogenesis proceeds from an initial mutational change in the host cell DNA. However, alkylating agents are mutagens as well as carcinogens, and the degree of carcinogenesis is directly correlated with the degree of binding of the agent to DNA. A number of known carcinogens bind covalently to DNA and RNA. All chemical carcinogens have an *electrophilic* (electron-loving) nature in common or will produce electrophilic compounds in vivo. These structures contain electron-deficient atoms, are highly reactive, and can interact with DNA, RNA, and certain cellular proteins. The postulated mechanisms by which chemical carcinogens transform normal cells include (1) *mutations* in the host cell DNA or modifications of RNA, (2) heritable changes in the *expression* of the host cell DNA, (3) *activation* or release of part or all of a latent integrated viral genome, and (4) *selection* of a latent tumor cell.

Common chemical carcinogens for human

CHEMICAL CARCINOGENS AND REPRESENTATIVE MOLECULES

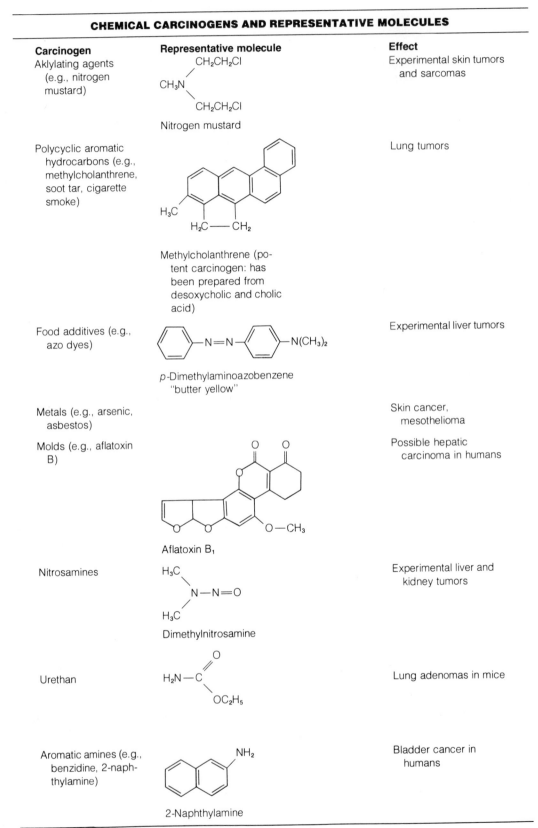

Carcinogen	Representative molecule	Effect
Aklylating agents (e.g., nitrogen mustard)	Nitrogen mustard	Experimental skin tumors and sarcomas
Polycyclic aromatic hydrocarbons (e.g., methylcholanthrene, soot tar, cigarette smoke)	Methylcholanthrene (potent carcinogen: has been prepared from desoxycholic and cholic acid)	Lung tumors
Food additives (e.g., azo dyes)	p-Dimethylaminoazobenzene "butter yellow"	Experimental liver tumors
Metals (e.g., arsenic, asbestos)		Skin cancer, mesothelioma
Molds (e.g., aflatoxin B)	Aflatoxin B_1	Possible hepatic carcinoma in humans
Nitrosamines	Dimethylnitrosamine	Experimental liver and kidney tumors
Urethan		Lung adenomas in mice
Aromatic amines (e.g., benzidine, 2-naphthylamine)	2-Naphthylamine	Bladder cancer in humans

CHEMICAL CARCINOGENS AND REPRESENTATIVE MOLECULES—cont'd

Carcinogen	Representative molecule	Effect
Hormones (e.g., diethylstilbestrol)		Genital cancers

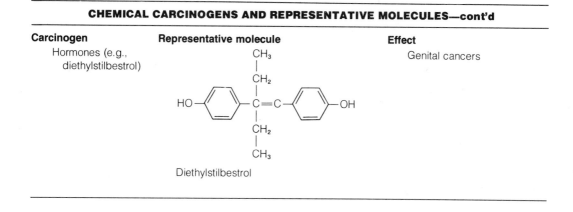

Diethylstilbestrol

cancer include aniline dyes (bladder cancer), polycyclic hydrocarbons (skin cancer), asbestos (mesothelioma), amphetamine sulfate (leukemia), and cigarette smoke (lung cancer). Other carcinogens commonly found in the environment include nitrites, coal tar, aromatic amines, and aflatoxin B (a product of a common food mold). An important carcinogen appears to be cigarette smoke, which contains a number of chemicals experimentally demonstrated to be carcinogenic. Cigarette smoking not only increases the probability of lung cancer but also acts in a synergistic manner with asbestos in the production of mesothelioma (a rare tumor, except among asbestos workers) and with radon in the production of lung cancer among uranium miners. It is interesting to note that while the crocidolite form of asbestos appears to be the form most clearly implicated in the etiology of mesothelioma (its use has been restricted in Great Britain since 1970), its importation to the United States has been steadily increasing. This form of asbestos is used in the production of artificial fireplace coals.

Other occupational groups that are at high risk for the development of certain forms of cancer include furniture workers, electroplaters, cannery workers, book binders, jewelers, zinc mixers, and tanners. The list is lengthy, indicating the prevalence of chemical carcinogens within the industrial environment. The general population's exposure to carcinogens is more difficult to quantitate, but some generalizations can be made. Food preserva-

tives and food additives that are in common usage have been shown to be carcinogenic in laboratory animals when used at high concentration. Furthermore, certain chemicals found naturally in food, such as caffeine, have been identified as carcinogens. Pollution of the air with potential carcinogens represents a possible threat to humans, which is as yet difficult to determine. Certainly a person's defenses and barriers must be called into play in order to protect the steady state.

Since the process of carcinogenesis is commonly characterized by a period of latency between the initial carcinogenic exposure and the appearance of actual malignant disease, one can only speculate on the incidence and types of future cancers caused by carcinogens presently acting on human cells.

Many substances have been shown to be carcinogenic in the laboratory. Transformed cells injected into an animal host cause malignant disease in the animal, but such an experiment, of course, cannot be done in humans. While transformation of human cells in tissue cultures has been shown for many chemical carcinogens, much of the evidence for chemical carcinogenesis in humans has been gathered from epidemiologic investigations, which can only infer a cause-and-effect relationship from statistical evaluation. It must also be mentioned that transformation in vitro by a chemical agent does not always imply carcinogenesis, as many cell lines, human and otherwise, that are grown as tissue cultures in laboratories all over the world commonly undergo spontaneous transformation into neoplastic cells. It is not known why this process occurs, but it could theoretically be because of cell age, reactivation of a latent virus within the tissue culture cell's own DNA, or exposure of the cells to the essentially abnormal in vitro environment, which is, of course, devoid of the normal hormonal, physiologic, and chemical regulation by the total organism.

Radiation carcinogenesis

Ionizing radiation is a known mutagen in all living organisms, and almost from its earliest use radiation was correlated with an increased incidence of cancer among those who were exposed to it. The carcinogenic effects of radiation in all its high-energy forms (ultraviolet, x-ray, alpha, beta, and gamma) have been demonstrated both in tissue culture and in whole animals. Human radiation carcinogenesis has been studied in groups of people accidentally or purposefully exposed to high levels of radiation. These include the survivors of the atomic bombings of Hiroshima and Nagasaki, groups of patients who received radiation therapy for a variety of conditions, and groups of individuals who ingested radioactive materials, such as the radium–watch dial painters who ingested radon when they tipped their paint brushes with their lips.

The incidence of leukemia, particularly myeloid leukemia, was greater in the Hiroshima and Nagasaki populations than in the nonexposed Japanese and correlated with the distance of the exposed individual from the hypocenter of the bomb and therefore with radiation dosage. Thyroid tumors also appeared in this population and were characterized by a latency period of 15 to 20 years after exposure. The increased thyroid cancer may have been due to radioactive iodine fallout after the bombing, which was taken up by the thyroid gland, as is normal iodine, when it was absorbed into the body. Another observation in the exposed Japanese population is the presence of one or more abnormal chromosomes in the circulating blood cells in certain groups. It is not possible to correlate this directly with carcinogenic transformation, however.

Individuals treated with therapeutic irradiation for conditions such as ankylosing spondylitis in general appear to develop leukemia with greater than average frequency. The incidence peaks 4 to 8 years following the irradiation and then falls in incidence to a relatively low level after 15 or more years. Another group of radiation-exposed individuals received thymus gland irradiation as children. They have been recently identified as having a high risk for thyroid tumors, both benign and malignant.

Ingestion or therapeutic injection of bone-seeking radioactive isotopes such as ^{224}Ra also leads to a high incidence of cancer, most commonly osteogenic (bone-forming) tumors.

In summary, radiation is a potent carcinogen in humans. Its mechanism of action in carcinogenesis is basically unknown, but certainly its

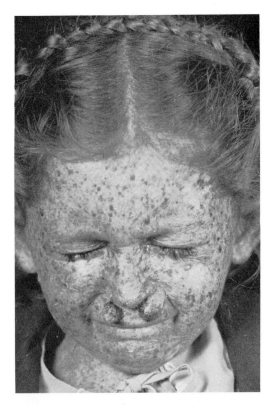

Fig. 3-3. Child suffering from xeroderma pigmentosum. Such a patient inevitably dies of multiple skin carcinomas. (From del Regato, J. A., and Spjut, H. J.: Ackerman and del Regato's cancer: diagnosis, treatment, and prognosis, ed. 5, St. Louis, 1977, The C. V. Mosby Co.)

mutagenic property may be inherent to the transformation process. In support of this theory is the frequent occurrence of multiple skin tumors in individuals with xeroderma pigmentosum (Fig. 3-3), a rare hereditary defect in which the cellular enzymes that repair ultraviolet light–induced mutations within cellular DNA are missing. Reduced repair of DNA from xeroderma pigmentosum cells has also been observed following exposure to a chemical carcinogen. The etiology of this disease supports the concept that cancer is the result of mutations in the host cell DNA. In xeroderma pigmentosum cells it may be that the initial irreparable mutation allows further transforming events to occur, leading to neoplasia.

Further support also comes from the high incidence of cancer in individuals affected with *Fanconi's anemia,* a hereditary disease characterized by a defect in DNA repair and in which many spontaneous and chemically induced chromosomal breaks have been identified in the cells.

Viral carcinogenesis

Viruses identified as causative agents in the production of tumors are known as *oncogenic viruses.* Many have been implicated in animal cancers, but the identification of tumor viruses in humans has been extremely difficult. Oncogenic viruses can transform cells in tissue culture, including human cells, but this is not adequate evidence for viral oncogenicity in the total organism. When viruses have been observed by electron microscopy inside cancer cells, it has not been possible to show whether the viruses caused the malignancy or were merely nonintrusive passengers in the cell. Other means of identification of oncogenic viruses include biochemical determination of viral antigens (proteins specifically coded for by viral DNA), which can be considered as ''footprints'' of viral presence, or viral nucleic acids, isolation of the virus from the cancer cell, and experimental demonstration of oncogenicity in cell cultures or whole animals.

The viruses that have been identified in association with human cancers include the C type RNA viruses (oncornaviruses), B type RNA viruses, and certain DNA viruses, including

herpesvirus II and the Epstein-Barr virus. The oncornaviruses contain *reverse transcriptase,* an enzyme that allows RNA to transcribe for DNA, thus permitting exogenously introduced viral RNA to act as a template for the formation of DNA. The viral DNA can then code for specific viral proteins, using the host cell protein-synthesizing machinery. The oncornaviruses have been implicated in the etiology of feline leukemias and appear to be infectious, that is, horizontally transmitted rather than vertically transmitted from parents to offspring through the genes. Oncornaviruses are also associated with leukemias, sarcomas, and carcinomas of chickens, mice, and cats. While C type RNA viruses have been identified in human cancer cells, no clear-cut relationship between their presence and the carcinogenic process has yet been established. All RNA viral transformed cells produce changes in the antigenic makeup of the cell surface. Furthermore, human cancer cells produce virus-specific antigens. Recent identification of C type viruses in human leukemic cells grown in tissue culture and the observation that leukemic cells contain DNA and RNA with base sequences identical to known primate and murine leukemic viruses has further implicated oncornaviruses in human leukemia. Additional evidence is garnered from the occurrence of a nonspecific illness characterized by fever, malaise, leukocytosis, and upper respiratory symptoms that sometimes precedes the onset of acute leukemia. This infectious insult may initiate the leukemic process directly or may simply decrease the immunologic competency of the individual, allowing cancer to occur. Hodgkin's disease (a lymphoma, or malignancy of the lymphatic glands) also appears to have an infectious, possibly viral, background. Clustering of cases of Hodgkin's disease within families, schools, and communities has also been reported, further substantiating the viral theory.

Human breast cancer is another malignancy for which much evidence has accumulated to implicate a virus, specifically known as a B type RNA virus or the *Bittner factor.* This virus has been identified in mouse mammary gland carcinoma and can be transmitted through the mother's milk to the suckling mice or vertically from parents to offspring through the gametes. If virus-free mice of a certain strain are injected with the Bittner factor, the virus concentrates in the mammary gland, which then proceeds to produce virus particles in large quantities. When these mice eventually lactate at 8 to 10 months of age, many will have developed mammary tumors. Identification of a similar virus in association with human breast cancer has been attempted, and a small amount of Bittner factor can be found, but human milk also contains factors that destroy it. A virus like the Bittner factor has been found replicating in a line of tissue-cultured cells derived from a human breast cancer. Human milk also contains an RNA-directed DNA polymerase, which is perhaps of viral origin. Additional evidence for a viral origin in human breast cancer is provided by the discovery that there are nucleic acid base sequences in human breast cancer that are nearly identical to those of the murine mammary tumor virus. It has also been shown that the leukocytes from many human breast cancer patients are immunologically sensitized to their own tumors and to *other* breast cancer patients' tumors. As a further note, immunization of many strains of laboratory mice by formalin-inactivated mouse mammary tumor virus has been carried out successfully with a resultant dramatic drop in the incidence of mammary tumors among the mice.

DNA viruses have been even more definitively linked with human cancers. The best documented relationship is between *Burkitt's lymphoma,* a malignancy of the jaw region found with striking predominance in malarial belts of Central Africa, and the Epstein-Barr virus (EBV), the causative agent of infectious mononucleosis. EBV is a herpeslike virus that infects only B lymphocytes and may remain in a latent state in the cells after the initial infection. Some environmental factors may then interact with the latent virus, causing it to become oncogenic. The EBV can transform lymphocytes in vitro, and continuous lymphoblastoid cell lines can be easily established in vitro from Burkitt's tumor tissue. Nucleic acid like that of EBV has been detected in 98% of African Burkitt's lymphoma biopsies. The antibody titer against the viral antigen falls and

rises with tumor regression and recurrence.

Other herpesviruses have also been strongly implicated. The herpes simplex virus is well known as the causative agent of cold sores and fever blisters in humans and is highly prevalent among the human population, existing in a latent state that is subject to reactivation by a variety of agents, such as exposure to high temperature or radiation. Another member of the herpesvirus family, herpesvirus II, also infects man and can lie dormant, subject to reactivation. The virus can cause genital infection, which has been shown in females to be associated with the later development of cervical cancer. Patients who develop malignancy have a high titer of antibodies to the virus, and the malignant cells contain viral DNA, RNA, and proteins. Preinvasive cervical cancer cells have also been reported to contain herpesvirus antigens.

Hormones, nutrition, and physical injury

Hormones, nutritional habits, and physical injury have all been implicated in neoplastic transformation. Estrogen may play a role in the development of both male and female breast cancer. Progesterone acts as a cocarcinogen with viruses or chemicals in the production of murine mammary tumors. Recent evidence suggests that uterine cancer can be associated with postmenopausal hormone replacement therapy, suggesting a role for female sex hormones in carcinogenesis. Another hormone, *diethylstilbestrol,* administered to women threatening to abort a pregnancy, has been linked to a high incidence of vaginal cancer in the female offspring and testicular cancer in the male offspring of the pregnancies as these individuals reach puberty.

It is difficult to imagine that physiologic levels of hormones can be carcinogenic. It seems more likely that hormones act indirectly when elevated, by enhancing normal cellular proliferation until neoplastic transformation occurs, and when depleted, by failing to inhibit target cells such that uninhibited cells proliferate and become neoplastic. Hormones may also potentiate the conversion of normal cells to malignant cells when carcinogenesis has been initiated by another agent, and lastly, hormones may support the growth and spread of an established tumor.

Irritation and physical injury may also play a role in carcinogenesis. The early experiments on tar-induced skin cancer in the rabbit demonstrated that cancers developed frequently around injured areas of the skin. Some investigators have suggested that the neoplastic process itself is a response to injury and represents a wild and uncontrolled "overhealing" reaction. Continuous irritation of a premalignant lesion may result in transformation. The development of malignant melanoma from a previously benign pigmented mole that has been subject to irritation of a prolonged nature supports this concept of carcinogenesis. Ulcerative colitis, polyposis coli (a familial disease characterized by polyps of the colon that frequently become malignant), and a high meat diet all predispose to cancer of the colon, and all may act by continual irritation. When *20-methylcholanthrene* is applied to animal skin, followed by weekly treatment of the site with an irritant, neoplasia may result in malignancy. However, 20-methylcholanthrene alone does not cause cancer. The irritant may act by promoting the malignant change initiated by the chemical. Lung cancer, according to this concept, could theoretically be initiated by chemical carcinogens in the environment and promoted by the highly irritating as well as carcinogenic components of cigarette smoke.

Nutritional factors have been implicated in carcinogenesis. One observation is that nutritionally restricted young mice develop significantly fewer cancers than do their well-fed counterparts. A leukemia virus genome that is vertically transmitted in both wild and inbred strains of mice can be prevented from expression and causing leukemia in the wild mice by dietary restrictions. Some dietary factor appears to precipitate the cancerous process in this particular case. A further observation is that food, food preservatives, and food mold all can contain carcinogenic agents.

Models of carcinogenesis

The known carcinogens, the population they affect, and the pathophysiologic processes that occur in carcinogenesis all lead to several theories of cancer.

Berenblum's two-stage initiation and promotion theory is one of the most widely accepted and unifying theories, but little is known about the actual molecular mechanisms by which a cell is transformed. The prevalent notion is that genetic changes must take place in order for a cancer to appear in previously normal tissue, and controversy reigns over the actual number of sequential mutational events that must occur before a cell can be considered malignant. Mathematic models of chemical carcinogenesis suggest that three steps are involved in malignant transformation. Radium-induced human tumors also may occur when three nuclear "hits" by radioactive emission from the bone-incorporated radium transform a bone cell.

Burch's model of carcinogenesis suggests that every cell has several restraining genes that act independently to prevent the development of cancer in the cell. When all these genes are inactivated by carcinogenic insults, the cell is released from the effects of these genes and becomes malignant. Thus, all carcinogens would act by a common mechanism, that of inactivation of the restraining genes. The probability that all the restraining genes in a given cell will become inactivated would naturally be a function of how long the cell has been subject to carcinogenic threats. For many cancers this would be dependent on the individual's age. When a mathematic plot of cancer incidence and age is done, the slope of the plotted line suggests that five mutations must occur during the individual's life span before a malignancy will develop. Thus, cancer can be considered to have an "incubation period" that begins with the first mutation, which is the initiating step, and ends with the fifth, which preludes the onset of a malignant growth. This theory not only explains the increased incidence of cancer with age but also elucidates the long latency period that characterizes many cancers. Furthermore, it suggests that by middle age, many individuals will have small nests of potentially neoplastic cells in many tissues and organs. Rampant malignancy may never occur in these sites, due to the long latency of the tumor and the limitations imposed by the life span in the host. The theory also implicates environmental factors in the causation of cancer, which are potentially avoidable threats to the human organism.

The oncogene and virogene theories of cancer have been alluded to previously. According to these theories cancer is caused by a segment of repressed endogenous DNA or a latent viral genome inserted into the host cell DNA. Theoretically this genetic information could be passed from generation to generation, causing cancer only when the DNA is released from inhibition, or derepressed. Carcinogens would then act by altering in some manner the expression of the oncogene or virogene. Certainly these theories dovetail very well with the initiation and promotion theory.

Research indicates that a single model cannot adequately explain the great diversity of the many diseases that are classified as malignant.

PATHOPHYSIOLOGY OF MALIGNANT DISEASE IN HOST
Immunologic responses to cancer cells

The provocation of an immunologic response by the host to cancer cells growing within his body has been well documented. Cancer cells produce proteins, known as antigens, which are specifically associated with the tumor cells and which elicit a cellular and humoral response by the immune system, with antibodies produced in response to the tumor-specific antigens. Two antigens that have been well characterized are the carcinoembryonic antigen (CEA) and alpha fetoprotein. Malignancies produced by oncogenic viruses appear to produce the same antigens in a variety of hosts, while tumors that result from chemical- or radiation-induced carcinogens produce nonspecific antigens that are different in every host. The normal immunologic surveillance system would recognize the tumor-specific antigens as abnormal proteins and react against them. Up to 10 million cancer cells could be totally destroyed by the normal host defense response. However, a clinically detectable neoplasm, 1 cm in diameter, contains approximately 1 billion cells. Thus, even in individuals with apparently in situ palpable lesions of a barely detectable size, the immune system has likely been overwhelmed by the malignant mass.

Tumors constantly shed antigens that circulate in the bloodstream as antigens or antigen-antibody complexes. The soluble antigens may block the destruction of the malignant cells by T-lymphocytes. Tumor growth may be further enhanced by a generalized suppression of the immune system, which is commonly observed in the cancer patient. This phenomenon may itself be part of the natural malignant process in humans. The self-enhancement of tumor growth may also be perpetuated by a host response in which the B-lymphocytes produce blocking antibodies that act to protect the tumor cells from attack by T-lymphocytes (Fig. 3-4).

Suppression of the immune system can result in increased tumor incidence or enhancement of

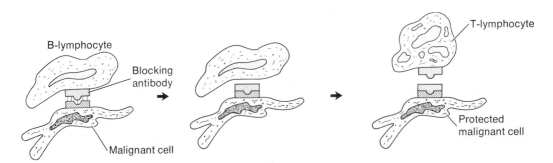

Fig. 3-4. Blocking antibodies and malignancy. Tumor cells may be protected from immune recognition by and interaction with T-lymphocytes by an initial B-lymphocyte reaction with malignant cell. B-lymphocyte may transfer blocking antibody to malignant cell as illustrated. T-lymphocyte receptor thus is blocked and cell protected.

an existing tumor's growth, as has been reported for a number of oncogenic virus-induced cancers. Furthermore, individuals with immunodepressive diseases or those treated with immunosuppressive drug therapy have an extraordinarily high rate of cancer. Depression of the immune system by such entities as a simple viral infection in a normal individual may allow a transient loss of immunocompetence that is sufficient to permit cancer cells previously held in check to grow and spread. When immunologic suppression occurs, the T-lymphocyte "killer cells'" surveillance becomes inadequate, and malignant cell antigens will drain into the bloodstream. Cancer therapy initiated at this time may reduce the number of tumor cells to a number manageable for the immune system, and the malignant disease may be eradicated. However, a second immunodepressive event occurring before the dissemination of the malignant cells has been controlled might result in an overwhelming release of the cells from immunologic surveillance and control, and widespread metastasis would then occur.

It is also possible that carcinogens themselves, by being *intrinsically* immunodepressive, enhance their cancer-producing effects. There have been reports of depressed cellular immunity in patients with cancer. It may also be that the individual who develops cancer may not be able to launch a sufficiently great enough immune response to tumor antigens, a phenomenon that would perhaps be genetically determined.

Immunotherapy, combined as an adjuvant with other forms of cancer therapy, has been used successfully with many patients in the last 10 years. The incidence of spontaneous regressions of neuroblastomas, Burkitt's lymphomas, and choriocarcinomas and the relationship of such regressions to reported immunologic reactions in the host certainly justify further exploration and expanded use of immunotherapy in cancer. Three major types of immunotherapy are currently in use. A general stimulation of the immune system, a response that is nonspecific and poorly understood, by BCG (Bacille Calmette Guerin) a bacterial material used for the prevention of tuberculosis for many years, has resulted in clini-

cal improvements in patients with malignant melanoma and leukemia. *Passive immunization,* or immunization of an individual with material from another host previously immunized with cancer-specific antigens, has not been successful in human recipients, but animal studies have shown that passive immunization with antiserums or lymphoid cells is possible. *Active immunization* in humans with certain tumor vaccines that have been inactivated by such techniques as irradiation, heat, or treatment with mitomycin C so that the tumor cells contained in the vaccines cannot proliferate in the recipient also holds considerable promise in cancer therapy. A drawback to immunotherapy is the possible transfer of antibodies to the individual with cancer, which can inhibit the host's own immune response to tumor antigens, resulting in a stimulus to tumor growth.

Anorexia-cachexia syndrome

Cancer provokes many responses in the host apart from an immunologic one. Most systemic and organ-specific responses are poorly understood. The most damaging and debilitating systemic response to cancer is the development of cachexia, which is observed in at least two thirds of all cancer patients. Cachectic wasting is the most common cause of death in patients with cancer of the breast, stomach, and colon or rectum. It is, nevertheless, not exclusively a terminal symptom but may actually be the reason that an individual with undiagnosed cancer presents himself to the doctor. Weight loss of unexplained origin is often the first sign of cancer. Cachexia is manifested by weight loss, wasting, weakness with resultant loss of mobility, anemia, fluid and electrolyte disturbances, malnutrition, increased basal metabolic rate, and anorexia. It appears that anorexia is so intimately related to the development of cachectic wasting that together they comprise the *anorexia-cachexia syndrome* (Fig. 3-5). It has long been thought that cachexia results from special nutritional demands of the tumor that compete with the host for those specific nutrients. The resultant lack of these nutrients within the host's normal system could directly affect the hypothalamic satiety and feeding center regulation of food intake and feeding ac-

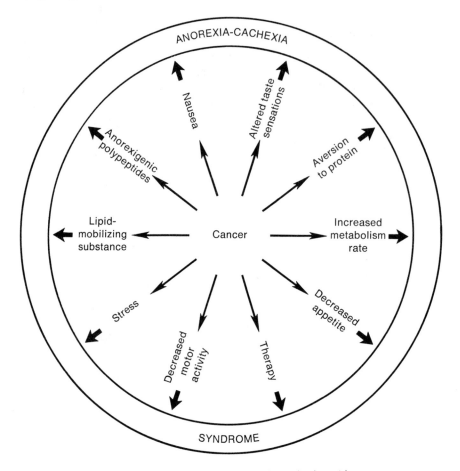

Fig. 3-5. Factors contributing to anorexia-cachexia syndrome.

tivity, resulting in anorexia. The evidence for a specific competitive uptake of substances by malignant tissue or specific lack of nutrients in the host is sketchy. The evidence for a direct hypothalamic effect is also controversial.

Voluntary food intake does decline in the cancer patient, and this anorexia appears to be the major cause of the cachexia. Many cancer patients are temporarily aided by a technique known as hyperalimentation, in which cancer patients are tube fed a rich nutrient mixture during periods when they are experiencing profound anorexia.

The anorexia is probably caused by a multifactorial profound disturbance in the host's metabolism. The anorexia not only contributes significantly to the development of cachexia, but the cachexia appears to act in a positive feedback manner to reinforce the anorexia. For example, it is thought that the tumor may release an anorexigenic substance, which stimulates the hypothalamic satiety center, causing loss of appetite.

The development of cachexia is enhanced by other pathologic processes disturbing the normal physiology of the cancer patient, such as obstruction of the gastrointestinal tract by a malignant mass, hemorrhage, necrosis, ulceration, infection, nausea, and impaired tissue or organ function from tumor invasion and destruction. It is also further reinforced by the physiologic and psychologic stress that is so common in the patient with cancer and that may initiate a nonspecific stress alarm syndrome, which may result in anorexia. The tumor may also produce amino acids and polypeptides that inhibit food intake, such as those seen in patients with uremia. Furthermore, the chemotherapy and radiation given for the malignant disease may itself cause an aversion to protein foods in the cancer patient, enhancing and perpetuating the anorexia-cachexia syndrome.

The major effect of the host on the tumor appears to be the attempt by the immune system to destroy the tumor, which for most individuals with cancer is an inadequate response. The major effect of the tumor on the host is the development of cachexia, immunologic suppression, and specific symptoms related to the type of tumor and its location in the body.

It is common to consider cancer as a group of often chronic diseases. The specific signs and symptoms of each cancer are related not only to the basic pathophysiology of the cancer cell and the host's response but also to the tumor type. Great variability exists between individuals and between tumor types. The following discussion will present some common forms of cancer as disease models. An understanding of these disease processes must be underscored by a knowledge of the pathophysiology of malignancy as previously presented.

TUMOR TYPES

While an exhaustive description of the common malignant diseases of humans is not possible in a book of this type, some tumor types will be described as illustrative models of cancer. The reader is referred to textbooks of clinical oncology for further reading.

Skin cancer

Skin carcinomas arise from the epithelium and are of two basic types: basal cell carcinoma and epidermoid or squamous cell carcinoma. These represent the most common form of all cancers, increasing in incidence with age. These malignancies rarely metastasize, and cause damage mainly through invasion of underlying structures. They respond extremely well to treatment, with a 90% or higher cure rate. Skin cancers usually occur more frequently on exposed surfaces such as the hands, head, and face. A number of factors predispose to the development of skin cancer. These include a history of chronic sun, radiation, or

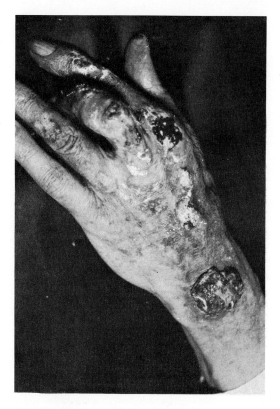

Fig. 3-6. Skin cancer and radiation. X-ray dermatitis and multiple carcinomas of 5 years' duration in 83-year-old male physician after 15 years of repeated small exposure to x-ray irradiation. (From Anderson, W. A. D., and Kissane, J. M., editors: Pathology, ed. 7, St. Louis, 1977, The C. V. Mosby Co.)

arsenic exposure, particularly in fair-skinned people. A long latency period before the cancer appears is characteristic. Fig. 3-6 shows the effects of radiation carcinogenesis on the skin. *Senile keratosis* (a thickening and pigmentation of the skin that occurs with age) also predisposes to skin malignancy.

Basal cell carcinoma usually begins as a painless, pearly gray nodule, often on the face. It almost never metastasizes but can grow and ulcerate and eventually invade underlying tissue, bone, and cartilage.

Squamous cell carcinoma appears initially as a slow growing, scaly, raised lesion resembling a wart. The tumor usually arises from a previously hyperkeratotic patch on the hands, cheeks, or ears. The lesion will eventually ulcerate and become painful and invasive. Metastasis can occur through the lymphatics but does so only rarely.

The treatment is excision of the lesion and occasionally radiation. There is always a possibility of recurring skin cancer after treatment as well as the appearance of new primary tumors in susceptible individuals. Follow-up of patients treated for skin cancer should therefore be done on a regular basis.

Another form of skin cancer is *malignant melanoma,* which arises from melanocytes (pigment cells) in a previously benign pigmented nevus. This mole is usually present for many years before malignant transformation takes place, and it has been suggested that exposure to sunlight and chronic irritation may play precipitating roles in the transformation. Malignant melanoma is the rarest form of skin cancer and by far the most pathologic. It is most common in whites between 40 and 70 years of age. The usual history is of a sudden increase in the growth of a mole on the head, neck, or lower limbs, which becomes elevated and more pigmented and often bleeds. The gross appearance of the melanoma is of a heavily pigmented, firm, ulcerated lesion, which may be surrounded by elevated satellite nodules or dark fingerlike projections. The malignant cells have often infiltrated the lymphatics before the diagnosis is made and treatment instituted. The 5-year survival rate ranges from 70% to 0% depending on the size, depth, and location of the lesion and the extent of local and distant metastasis. The treatment for malignant melanoma is wide, local, surgical excision of the tumor and surrounding lymphatics, and this is often followed by chemotherapy and immunotherapy.

Other forms of skin cancer do occur, but over 90% of all skin malignancies are of the three types that have been discussed. Aside from malignant melanoma, skin cancer represents the most curable form of cancer and one in which the disease process is best understood.

Cancers of the gastrointestinal tract

Malignancy can occur in all parts of the gastrointestinal tract, but the most common types are cancer of the stomach and cancer of the colon. It can be stated generally that the prognosis for gastrointestinal tract cancer improves for cancers of the lower part of the tract as compared with the upper alimentary canal. For example, cancer of the esophagus carries with it a 5-year survival rate of only 4%, whereas cancer of the colon has a 50% 5-year survival rate, and this could be vastly improved with earlier diagnosis.

Stomach cancer. Cancer of the stomach has been decreasing markedly in incidence over the last 30 years. No explanation for this phenomenon has been forthcoming, but some unknown dietary factor may be responsible. The decrease in incidence has been most noticeable in the United States. A diet that is high in starch and low in fresh fruits and vegetables may cause stomach cancer. Japan has a much higher death rate from stomach cancer, and the incidence is high among the American Japanese ethnic group. In general among all races and countries, there is a 2:1 male prevalence of occurrence.

There are a number of predisposing conditions, which include chronic gastric ulcers, pernicious anemia, and polyposis (multiple stomach polyps). Almost all cancers of the stomach arise from glandular cells and are adenocarcinomas. The signs and symptoms of this type of cancer are often vague and include epigastric pain, weight loss, anorexia, iron-deficiency anemia, and melena (blood in the stool). It is common for the symptoms to be so mild as to warrant no concern on the part of the patient until liver and peritoneal metastasis has occurred.

Ulcers that do not respond to the conventional forms of treatment should be suspected of malignancy. Diagnosis is made by barium studies of the upper gastrointestinal tract, gastroscopy and biopsy, and laparotomy. The usual treatment is surgical excision of the tumor and a large part of or the entire stomach, procedures known as subtotal and total gastrectomies. The prognosis for patients with cancer of the stomach is not good, as approximately 42% will be inoperable at the time of surgery. Of the remaining, the 5-year survival rate ranges from 8% to 25%. Distant metastases to the liver (Fig. 3-7), peritoneum, lung, and bone are the most common sites. When the

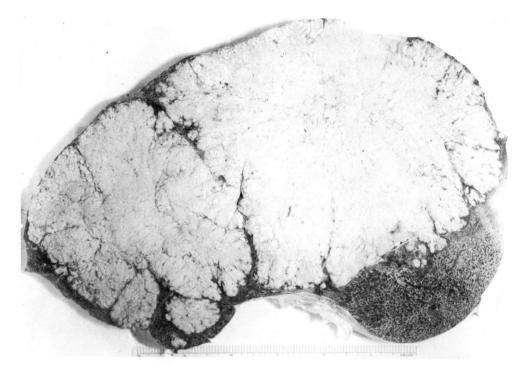

Fig. 3-7. Section of liver showing almost complete replacement of parenchyma by metastatic carcinoma. Primary tumor was in colon. (From Anderson, W. A. D., and Kissane, J. M., editors: Pathology, ed. 7, St. Louis, 1977, The C. V. Mosby Co.)

regional stomach lymph nodes show no evidence of malignant cells, the 5-year survival rate may reach 67%, but with positive lymph nodes the chances for survival are small.

Cancer of the colon, rectum, and anus. Colon and rectal cancers carry with them the second highest death rate of any cancers in the United States and are the most prevalent internal cancers in this country. Both men and women are equally affected. Remarkably low incidence among the general population is reported in Japan and Finland.

This type of cancer generally appears after the age of 50, except in individuals who have been predisposed to this malignancy by ulcerative colitis and familial polyposis coli. *Chronic colitis* (inflammation of the colon, often associated with ulceration and bleeding) places individuals at a definite risk for colon cancer. This is particularly true if the chronic colitis began in adolescence. *Familial polyposis coli* is an hereditary condition that is inherited by mendelian dominant transmission. Polyps develop in the colon of affected individuals, and over a period of years the colon becomes a virtual bed of polyps, which have a marked tendency to undergo malignant transformation, the incidence of occurrence being virtually 100% as the affected individuals grow older.

Diet has been implicated as a major factor in cancer of the colon. The incidence of this cancer is high in countries that have diets high in meat and low in undigestible cellulose. It is thought that the length of time of contact of fecal material with the colonic wall may be an important etiologic factor. Breakdown products of bile may be carcinogenic, and long exposure to these products may initiate carcinogenic transformation.

The signs and symptoms of lower gastrointestinal tract tumors depend upon the location and size of the tumor. Generally, rectal bleeding may be the first sign and is often attributed to hemorrhoids, which are often present concurrently. A change in the normal bowel habits is another significant sign, and many pa-

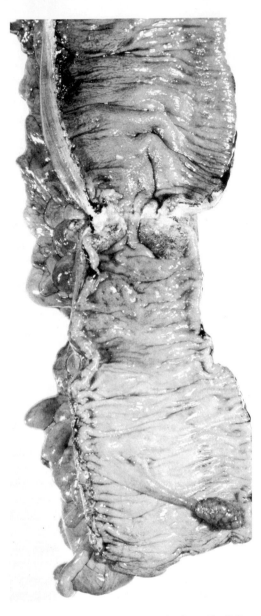

Fig. 3-8. Constricting carcinoma of colon with dilation of bowel proximal to tumor. Pedunculated polyp is incidental finding. (From Anderson, W. A. D., and Kissane, J. M., editors: Pathology, ed. 7, St. Louis, 1977, The C. V. Mosby Co.)

tients also report abdominal cramping or pain. A small percentage of patients have no symptoms at all. Bowel obstruction can occur (Fig. 3-8) but may be so well compensated for by hypertrophy of the muscular lining of the large intestine that tumors may reach a fairly large size before producing significant symptoms, particularly if the tumor is located in the right colon. Many patients with colonic cancer develop a profound anemia, which may be the first sign of the disease.

It is important to note that 50% of all cancers of the colon and rectum can be detected by digital examination through the anus, and two thirds can be diagnosed through the use of the sigmoidoscope. This procedure should be part of the routine physical examination for all patients in high-risk groups. Diagnosis of cancer is made by sigmoidoscopy, barium enema, and biopsy. It is believed that this tumor grows quite slowly in situ, and early detection before metastasis and invasion have occurred would result in an excellent prognosis. The usual treatment for colonic cancer is removal of the colon segment containing the cancer and subsequent anastomosis of the adjacent ends of the intestine. A permanent colostomy may be necessary if the tumor is low and involves the rectum. The 5-year survival rate ranges from 25% to 50%. Fig. 3-9 shows the contrast of malignant cells with normal cells in the colonic mucosa.

Cancer of the pancreas. Cancer of the pancreas should be mentioned, as its general incidence is increasing rapidly, and it now can be considered among the five major sites of cancer for men, and the most common gastrointestinal gland cancer. No known etiologic factors have been found for this carcinoma. The presenting symptoms are often pain, anorexia, weight loss, indigestion, and nausea. The tumor may invade other abdominal structures such as the duodenum and cause obstructive disease with enlargement of the gallbladder and jaundice. Metastasis to the liver is common, and the disease process is extremely morbid and rapid, so that only 10% of these patients are still alive 1 year from the time of first diagnosis. The treatment is surgical with palliative chemotherapy.

Reproductive tract cancers

Cancer of the prostate. Cancer of the prostate gland is the most common form of cancer in men over the age of 50 aside from skin cancer. It is most common in the United States,

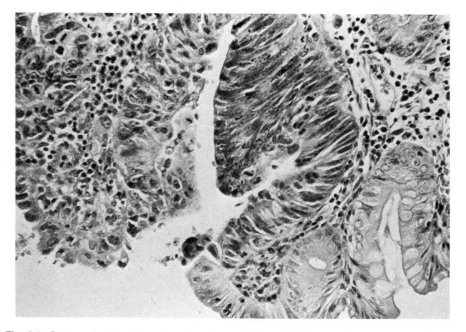

Fig. 3-9. Cancer of colon. Area of malignant anaplastic cells is found adjacent to normal mucosa. (Courtesy Department of Pathology, University of Tennessee, Memphis.)

and the etiology is unknown but may be hormonal in nature. Most prostatic tumors are adenocarcinomas and almost always involve the posterior lobe of the gland. The early symptoms of this malignancy are easily confused with benign prostatic hypertrophy, which is common in older men. These symptoms include dysuria, hematuria, dribbling, and retention of urine in the bladder, which may cause cystitis. Pain may also be present and is referred to the bladder, urethra, rectum, perineum, and occasionally to the sacrum and legs, where it may be confused with sciatica. This cancer can be diagnosed by rectal examination followed by biopsy. Treatment is radical prostatectomy, which may be followed by radiation therapy. Patients may be treated nonsurgically if the stage of the malignancy or the general age and condition of the patient warrant it. This involves the administration of estrogens as a palliative measure. The metastasizing cells apparently require male hormonal support, which is masked by the administration of estrogen. Estrogen therapy often significantly relieves pain and anorexia-cachexia in incurable patients with advanced disease.

The 5-year survival rate ranges from 25% to 70%, depending on the stage of advancement of the disease at the initial time of diagnosis. The most common sites of metastases for prostatic cancer are the bone and lungs.

Cancers of the cervix and uterus. Cancer of the cervix represents that rare carcinoma that can be easily detected while in situ, before invasion or metastasis can take place and by a relatively simple and inexpensive screening procedure known as the *Papanicolaou smear*. Cytologic examination of the cells obtained by this smear of the cervix can detect not only carcinoma but also premalignant dysplasia, a condition that may be present 5 to 10 years before frank invasive carcinoma develops. It is thought that the natural progression of this cancer is from cervical epithelial dysplasia, to carcinoma in situ (of the squamous cell variety), to invasive carcinoma. Treatment of cervical carcinoma in situ yields a nearly 95% cure rate, and therefore the importance of yearly Papanicolau smears in all women over 21 years of age cannot be stressed enough. The general incidence of this cancer is high, making up 20% of all female cancers. Known predisposing factors include frequent and early coital experiences, low socioeconomic class, and a history of venereal disease. The low incidence of this type of cancer among Jewish women has been attributed to genetic factors rather than circumcision among the males. The role of previous herpes infection has not as yet been clearly elucidated, but much evidence indicates that this virus is etiologic.

The early signs and symptoms of cervical carcinoma are often considered inconsequential by women and may be ignored until frank invasion occurs. These signs and symptoms include heavy menstruation, watery discharge, postcoital bleeding, and occasionally menstrual-type pain. Later symptoms include hemorrhage, pain, foul discharge, leakage of urine and feces from the vagina, anorexia-cachexia, nausea and vomiting, and signs of uremia when compression of the ureters occurs. The growth of the cervical tumor is into the vagina, toward the pelvic wall, and into the bladder and rectum. Metastasis occurs through the lymphatic channels and frequently involves the bone, lungs, or liver. Treatment is surgical removal of the cervix and uterus and frequently other pelvic organs that have become involved. In stage 0 (early carcinoma in situ), surgical intervention is generally the only form of treatment. With stages I, II, III, and IV (the stages indicating increasing levels of invasion and lymph node metastasis) the preferred method of treatment is radiation therapy, which may be delivered externally or by insertion of a radioactive source such as radium into the cervical cavity.

Cancer of the uterus is much less common than cervical carcinoma. It is more frequent in postmenopausal women and among Jewish women. Etiologic factors may involve hormonal imbalance. Estrogen therapy in postmenopausal women may be associated with an increased incidence of endometrial uterine cancer. Ninety percent of these cancers are adenocarcinomas. The major presenting symptom of uterine cancer is postmenopausal bleeding, and the major form of treatment is hysterectomy and intracavitary radiotherapy for inoperable patients. Chemotherapy may be used in women with advanced carcinoma and debilitated women and includes the use of specific hormone regimens.

Cancer of the breast

Carcinoma of the breast is the most common form of cancer among women over the age of 40 and the leading cause of death from all causes in women between the ages of 40 and 44 years. The incidence appears to be increasing, and the prevalence (number with breast cancer in a given year) is approximately 100 per 100,000 women. It is more common in single, divorced, or widowed women than in married women and also in women who have given birth for the first time at the age of 35 or over. The incidence is low among Japanese women, and this disparity is retained among Japanese ethnic groups who have emigrated to other countries with higher breast cancer incidences. Breast cancer does occur in males but is 100 times less frequent. It is more common among women whose mothers and maternal aunts have had breast cancer. Chronic cystic mastitis is believed by some to predispose the affected individual to breast cancer. Cystic mastitis is seen with higher frequency in the breasts of women with diagnosed carcinoma, but this is, of course, not definitive proof that benign cystic mastitis tissue undergoes malignant transformation more readily than does normal breast tissue. The presence of multiple cysts in the breasts makes the early detection of a malignant tumor extremely difficult. Ninety-five percent of all breast cancers are discovered by the woman herself, either accidentally or by routine breast self-examination. Early masses are poorly movable, hard, painless lumps, half of which occur in the upper outer quadrant of the breast. Possible etiologic factors in breast cancer include viruses, hormonal factors, particularly estrogen levels, genetics, and immunologic abnormalities.

Breast cancer is diagnosed by a number of techniques that utilize x-ray films (mammography, xerography) and by thermography (which can detect "hot spots" of tissue, the increased temperature due to increased metabolic activity and mitotic index). Recent attention to the risk of carcinogenic transformation by these soft diagnostic radiation exposures may limit the use of these procedures to women in high-risk groups. Biopsy confirms carcinoma and may be done by excision or aspiration of the mass.

Most breast carcinomas arise in the epithelium of the glandular ducts of the breast and give rise to lesions with infiltrating edges, which invade the normal breast tissue. They can become large enough to cause nipple retraction such that the skin overlying the breast resembles the skin of an orange. Ulceration and hemorrhage of the breast is common if the tumor is not treated. The major pathophysiologic mechanism whereby breast cancer causes morbidity and death is through metastatic dissemination of the malignant cells, usually through the axillary lymphatics. Prognosis is vastly better when regional lymph nodes show no evidence of metastasis, but 50% of those tumors that have been detectable for a period of 1 month will have spread to the lymph nodes. Some undetectable or barely detectable lesions may, on the other hand, remain small and nonmetastatic for up to 2 years. The 5-year survival rate is 84% when no lymph node involvement is found at surgery and on the average 56% when lymph node involvement does occur. The more lymph nodes positive for malignant cells at the time of operation, the less favorable the prognosis.

Treatment of breast cancer is by removal of the lesion (lumpectomy), the breast (simple mastectomy), and most commonly the breast, lymphatic drainage, and underlying pectoral muscles (radical mastectomy). A complication of radical mastectomy is *lymphedema* of the shoulder and arm on the affected side, which results from the removal of the normal channels for lymphatic drainage. Radiotherapy is also frequently used postoperatively in an attempt to kill any tumor cells left at the site, thus preventing metastasis. Radiotherapy is also used in the treatment of metastasis to the bone, which is common with breast cancer. Dramatic relief of pain, prevention of fractures, and prolongation of life can be achieved with radiotherapy.

Hormone therapy is also a major mode of treatment in metastatic breast cancer. These malignant cells appear to have cytoplasmic hormone receptors that allow an initial binding to hormone molecules to take place, which then causes cellular division and growth to ensue. The type of endocrine therapy carried out is dependent on the nature of the tumor cell receptors, as some are androgen dependent and some are estrogen dependent. Estrogens may be administered if the cells are androgen dependent so as to compete with and mask the effects of androgen and inhibit tumor cell growth and vice versa. Irradiation and surgical removal of the ovaries (oophorectomy) may also be done, and occasionally even the pituitary gland may be extirpated (hypophysectomy) so that estrogen production may be blocked entirely.

Chemotherapy has been used in metastatic breast cancer (cyclophosphamide [Cytoxan], 5-fluorouracil, adriamycin) with patients who are not helped by hormonal treatment. Drugs are administered as part of a treatment regimen but have not been as successful in the treatment of breast cancer as they have been in some other forms of cancer.

Breast cancer mortality has not been changed dramatically with the advent of the treatments presently at hand, but the duration of life has increased for those individuals with metastatic disease.

Lung cancer

Lung cancer is a highly malignant, morbid disease that has been increasing dramatically in incidence over the past 60 years, with men being affected four to five times as frequently as women. There are 80,000 deaths per year from lung cancer, and bronchial cancer is the leading cause of cancer death among American men.

Most lung cancers arise from the main bronchus and are therefore termed *bronchogenic carcinomas* (Fig. 3-10). They may be of the squamous cell, oat cell, anaplastic, or adenocarcinoma type. The relationship of cigarette smoking to the development of both squamous cell and oat cell carcinomas has been demonstrated repeatedly in epidemiologic studies, the most notable being Doll and Hill's study of 40,000 British physicians. The 1964 US Surgeon General's report on smoking and

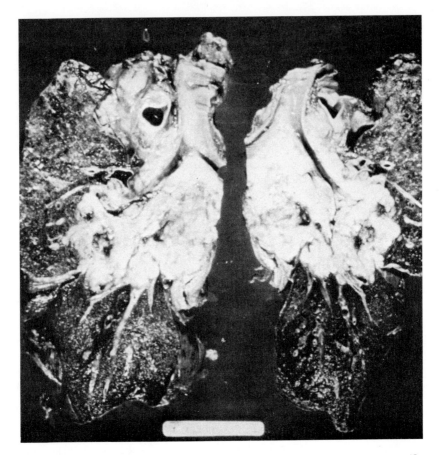

Fig. 3-10. Bronchogenic carcinoma. Extensive malignancy of bronchial tree is observed. (Courtesy Department of Pathology, University of Tennessee, Memphis.)

health supported the belief that cigarette smoking is the most important etiologic agent in the causation of lung cancer among men and probably also among women. The risk of lung cancer is 60 times greater for a man who smokes two packages of cigarettes per day as compared to a man who has never smoked.

Identification of the actual carcinogenic agent in cigarette smoke has not been possible thus far. A number of carcinogenic components of smoke have been isolated and shown to cause cancer in laboratory animals. These include various hydrocarbons, including benzopyrenes. Other factors in the environment appear to increase the incidence of lung cancer among smokers by acting synergistically with cigarette smoke. Thus, environmental pollution and exposure to radon, asbestos, and coal tar have been linked to lung cancer.

The lower incidence of lung cancer among women has been attributed to their past smoking habits, which included not only a smaller number of smokers but also fewer women who actually inhaled the cigarette smoke into the lungs.

The mortality for lung cancer is around 90%. Half are inoperable by the time the patient is first seen by a physician. The early symptoms are often ignored and interpreted by the patient as the symptoms of a prolonged cold. These symptoms include a heavy cough, particularly at night, hemoptysis (coughing up of blood), loss of weight, and sometimes chest pain. The symptoms progress to dyspnea, dysphagia, clubbing of fingers, pleural effusion, and sometimes signs of superior vena cava obstruction. Often the first signs of lung cancer are related to metastatic spread, particularly to the brain.

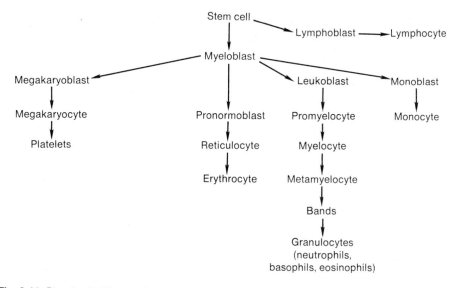

Fig. 3-11. Blood cell differentiation. All blood cells are produced from bone marrow stem cell, which differentiates into lymphoblasts and myeloblasts, primitive cells that are precursors for lymphocytes, granulocytes, monocytes, erythrocytes, and platelets.

Other common sites of metastases include endocrine glands, skin, and bones. The route of metastasis is through the lymphatic channels, and scalene node biopsy is often performed to determine if metastasis has occurred once lung cancer has been diagnosed. The usual diagnostic tools for lung cancer include x-ray films, bronchoscopy, sputum cytology, and bronchial brush or needle biopsy. Surgical exploration of the thorax (thoracotomy) is done when no evidence of metastatic spread is evident. Removal of a lobe of the lung (lobectomy) or an entire lung (pneumonectomy) is carried out.

If the tumor is inoperable, various chemotherapeutic regimens and radiation therapy may be carried out as palliative measures. The drugs most commonly used are alkylating agents, but generally the response of metastatic lung cancer to chemotherapy has been disappointing. Radiation therapy is successful in the alleviation of symptoms in the inoperable lung cancer patient, and some cures of bronchogenic carcinomas that have been treated by supervoltage radiation have been reported.

Leukemias and lymphomas

Leukemias and lymphomas are classified as malignant proliferative diseases of the hemato-poietic system, particularly the bone marrow and lymph nodes. This is based on the fact that abnormal proliferation of one cell type occurs, often at the expense of the normal production of other hematopoietic cells. In leukemias incredibly high numbers of immature cells are found in the bloodstream and bone marrow, while in lymphomas the abnormal cells tend to remain more confined to the lymphoid organs rather than being disseminated into the circulation.

Fig. 3-11 indicates the pattern of hematopoiesis in humans and shows that all blood cells (erythrocytes, white blood cells, and platelets) are ultimately derived from a single cell, the stem cell, which then differentiates into different cell lines entirely distinct from each other. Erythroid, platelet, and leukocytic diseases could theoretically arise through a number of possible mechanisms operating at any stage in hematopoietic differentiation. The leukemias are disorders mainly of leukocytes and can be either acute or chronic in nature and lymphocytic or myelogenous in origin. The abnormal cell type that appears in the bone marrow and bloodstream identifies the cell of origin of the leukemia.

The pathophysiologies of all forms of leukemia are very similar, with duration of survival and severity of symptoms being the most common variables between the acute and chronic forms. All leukemias cause an extensive infiltration of leukemic cells into the hematopoietic organs. This is a major cause of the various decreases or *cytopenias* that invariably accompany leukemia. Normal hematopoiesis is interfered with, resulting in an often profound anemia and thrombocytopenia. These account for the pallor and easy bruisability of the leukemic patient. Often the cause of death in leukemia is hemorrhage into a vital organ such as the brain. The mechanism whereby the leukemic cells prevent normal hematopoiesis is not clear at the present time. It may be due to an actual mechanical overcrowding of the marrow spaces or perhaps may be caused by unknown inhibitory factors released by the leukemic cells.

The leukemic cells infiltrate the liver and spleen as well as other organs, giving rise to tremendous hypertrophy of these structures, signs that are often the first evidence of leukemia in the patient. Leukemic infiltration, no matter at which site it occurs, may interfere with the normal function of the tissue or organ, giving rise to particular signs and symptoms. Furthermore, the leukemic cells themselves may be either too immature to assist the organism in fighting infection or may be immunologically incompetent, as is the case in the lymphocytic leukemias.

Acute leukemia. *Acute lymphocytic leukemia* is the form of leukemia common in children, accounting for the most frequent cancer of childhood. The cell type that is abnormal is a leukemic lymphoblast (the suffix blast indicates that it is an immature form of lymphocyte). The carcinogenic transformation probably takes place in a bone marrow stem cell, which then gives rise to the malignant proliferation. The lymphoblasts cannot be identified as T cells or B cells in the majority of the cases. The leukemic cells crowd the bone marrow, bloodstream, and lymph nodes; anemia, granulocytopenia, and thrombocytopenia all are side effects of the disease process. The onset of this disease is usually abrupt, with a rapid course lasting about 4 months until death, unless treated. The early symptoms are fever, lymphadenopathy, pallor, fatigue, purpura, and general malaise. It is common for the leukemia to have run one third of its typical course before the child is diagnosed.

Acute myelogenous leukemia is more common in adults than in children and involves the proliferation of immature blast cells derived from the bone marrow. Commonly the disease process involves the granulocytes (neutrophils, basophils, and eosinophils). Occasionally erythroid or monocytic blood elements become leukemic, thus confirming the concept of a stem cell transformation by the carcinogenic process. As with acute lymphocytic leukemia, the onset is abrupt, and the symptoms are similar. It is more common for splenomegaly to occur with this form of acute leukemia, while hepatomegaly and lymphadenopathy are generally more pronounced in the acute lymphocytic variety. Although the total white blood cell count is enormously elevated, the immature blast cells are inadequate defense against infection, and a major complication of acute leukemia is infection. Thrombocytopenia and anemia are also often pronounced, thus contributing to susceptibility to infection. Leukemic cells infiltrate normal tissue and may cause severe disorders related to the site of infiltration.

Both acute forms of leukemia are considered fatal, although treatment of the childhood form has recently yielded some long-term remissions and possible cures. Treatment consists of intensive chemotherapy.

Chronic leukemias. Chronic leukemias are also of two major categories: lymphocytic and myelogenous. Both forms have slower onsets than acute leukemia and are initially characterized by general malaise and loss of weight. Anemia is often the first presenting symptom, and the leukocytosis is discovered at that time. The course of the disease is much more prolonged than in the acute forms, with the median age of survival around 3 to 4 years.

Chronic lymphocytic leukemia occurs in individuals usually over the age of 35. The cell type involved in most patients is the immunoglobulin M–secreting B-lymphocyte, which appears to be immunologically incompetent and which does not seem able to give rise to other immunologically competent cells. The carcinogenic transformation that occurs in chronic lymphocytic leukemia apparently occurs after the stem cell has differentiated into an identifiable B-lymphocyte. The leukemic process is similar if perhaps not identical in etiology to lymphosarcoma, except that in the latter disease the malignant cells are predominantly confined to lymphoid tissue, while in leukemia the white blood cell count in the peripheral blood is often greatly increased. The cells do invade the lymphoid tissue in the leukemic process, however, and thus may present a pathology similar to that of lymphosarcoma, which is classified as a lymphoma. The lymph node enlargement and splenomegaly that can accompany the leukemia are often great, and patients with these signs and symptoms may be treated with chemotherapy and radiotherapy. Patients who are apparently well (even though the circulating lymphocytes may be increased to levels close to 1 million WBC/mm³) are generally not submitted to any form of cancer therapy until the symptoms become indicative of more acute disease.

Chronic myelogenous leukemia is nearly always associated with the presence of a small acrocentric chromosome (derived from the long arm of chromosome 22) in the malignant leukocytes of the bone marrow and peripheral blood. Known as the *Philadelphia chromosome,* it has been detected in blood smears of individuals who subsequently developed chronic myelogenous leukemia many years later. The origin of the chromosome is entirely unknown, but there is no question that it is somehow associated with the carcinogenic process. The cells usually affected in this form of leukemia are the granulocytes and sometimes the megakaryocytes, and the cell of origin for this cancer is thought to be a stem cell. These cells present a more mature morphology than do those cells in the acute form of this leukemia. Patients with chronic myelogenous leukemia have early symptoms that have been present for many months before the diagnosis is made. Very often the spleen is greatly enlarged, and the patient complains about a dragging, full abdomen. The typical course of the disease runs about 3½ years and is controlled by chemotherapy. As the disease progresses, the leukemic process becomes more typical of acute myelogenous leukemia, and a blast crisis invariably occurs. The immature blast cells also contain the Philadelphia chromosome, and these cells may actually be lymphoblasts rather than myeloblasts. Once the blast crisis occurs, the response to chemotherapy may be poor, and survival is usually only a matter of weeks or months. The steady state can no longer be maintained as the body defenses and barriers are overwhelmed in the crisis.

Malignant lymphomas and Hodgkin's disease. Malignancy of the lymphoreticular system can take many forms. Hodgkin's disease was formerly classified as a malignant lymphoma but is now considered to be a different neoplastic process and will be discussed separately.

Malignant lymphomas arise initially in the lymph nodes and may then involve other organs of the reticuloendothelial system. The pattern of the disease may be either nodular or diffuse, and the involved cell type is used to categorize these lymphomas into lymphocytic, histiocytic, or reticular stem cell. It has been speculated that the origin of these malignancies involves some type of interference with the normal feedback regulation of lymphocyte proliferation, such that immature and poorly functioning lymphocytes are produced. Many patients with lymphomas have impaired B-lymphocyte (humoral) immunity and general hypogammaglobulinemia. Occasionally the disease will change into a typical lymphocytic leukemia, and there is some thought that the two disease processes involve the same mechanisms, with chronic lymphocytic leukemia being a disseminated form of lymphocytic lymphoma. The role of the Epstein-Barr virus in Burkitt's lymphoma has been discussed previously. All lymphomas may have a viral or infectious etiology either with the virus producing an immune system depression that then allows a secondary carcinogenic transformation to ensue or with the virus itself acting as the carcinogen. The usual treatment of lymphomas involves radiotherapy and chemotherapy.

Hodgkin's disease also may have an infectious origin. The epidemiologic evidence for this has been previously presented. It is further supported by the pattern of morphologic and pathophysiologic disruption of the lymph nodes and other tissue that appears to present both an inflammatory and malignant picture. The diagnostic criterion for Hodgkin's disease is the presence of Reed-Sternberg cells in the lymphoid tissue. These cells may be found in other disease conditions, but they are always found in Hodgkin's disease. There are several histologic patterns to Hodgkin's disease. These are characterized by (1) lymphocyte predominance, (2) nodular sclerosis, (3) mixed cellularity, and (4) lymphocyte depletion. All forms of Hodgkin's disease, while probably arising at a single origin, may eventually result in invasion of any organ in the body. The disease is thought to arise in the thymus gland or thymus-dependent areas of the lymph nodes and may be a T cell disease. $HL-A_5$, a component of a system of leukocyte antigens, is increased in Hodgkin's disease, perhaps linking the presence of an altered histocompatibility gene to the oncogenic process. Cellular immunity is definitely impaired. The course of the disease varies, depending often on the histologic type. The form characterized by lymphocyte predominance has the best survival rate, with the 5-year survival greater than 50% and the 15-year survival over 45% when adequate high-voltage radiation has been used as the principal form of treatment. The disease often begins as a painless swelling in one node, which may be accompanied by night sweats, fever, and weight loss. The progression of the disease may result in invasion of other lymphoid tissue and organs such as the bones and lungs, with the symptoms then being related to the extent of involvement of these organs. Hodgkin's disease may have long periods of disease-free remissions, and cures are possible with adequate treatment at every clinical stage of the disease. Occasionally the disease manifests itself as an acute or chronic process, but most cases are of an intermediate variety.

Conclusion

The tumor types that have been discussed in this section represent those forms of primary cancer that are most commonly seen in clinics and hospitals. Metastatic cancer has not been discussed in great detail, but it should be noted that cancers of the brain, bone, and liver are often the sites of metastases from primary tumors at other origins. The signs and symptoms of cancer in these or any organ or tissue affected are often easily predictable if the normal physiology of that organ or tissue is understood. The pathophysiologic manifestations of disease in an organ or tissue can also be predicted once the student has gained a knowledge of the principles of pathophysiology both generally and for each organ system. Thus, uremia may be a complication of obstruction, no matter what the actual cause of the obstruction in the urinary tract (malignant growth, heavy metal deposition, glomerulonephritis, hemorrhage, etc.).

The following discussion will present some principles that underlie the usual treatment of malignancy.

PHYSIOLOGY OF CANCER TREATMENT

The major treatment modalities used for malignant disease are surgery, radiation therapy, chemotherapy, and immunotherapy. The physiologic bases of these treatments will be discussed in this section, but it should be recognized from the outset that for most cancers no one mode of treatment is used exclusively. Rather, a combined interdisciplinary approach, using methods and techniques from each area of treatment, is used. The aim of all treatment is to reduce the tumor load and to assist the patient in restoring and maintaining the steady state. The oncology team usually consists of specialists from a number of professional disciplines: oncologist, surgeon, pathologist, radiologist, biochemist, nurse, social worker, and so on.

Surgery

The rationale for the use of surgery may seem quite obvious at first. However, surgery may not always be the best treatment for the patient. The effects of a pneumonectomy on a patient with metastatic lung cancer do not warrant this surgery in this particular situation, and other forms of treatment are used. While surgery was for many years the only treatment widely used for cancer, basic research into cell biology, the pathophysiology of cancer, chemotherapy, radiation therapy, and immunology has led to other forms of treatment that can be used instead of or along with surgical excision.

Some principles that govern the use of surgery in cancer are related to the extent of surgical excision when surgery is done. Normally a tumor and surrounding tissues are removed, along with the primary lymphatic drainage of the tissue involved (block dissection). The extent of this type of surgery is governed by whether the tumor is localized or has invaded the tissue, fixing tissue to the tumor; by whether widespread inflammation is present; and by whether palpable tumor can be felt in the lymph nodes. Local excision of the tumor alone may be done if the tumor is not highly malignant or metastatic, such as for skin carcinomas. Special surgical techniques are also used in cancer therapy. These include cryosurgery, lasers, and surgical isolation of vessels for perfusion or infusion.

Radiation therapy

One of the basic laws of radiation biology is that the more undifferentiated or immature a cell is, the more susceptible it is to the damaging effects of ionizing radiation. Thus, compartments of cells constantly undergoing renewal and therefore containing populations of stem cells and cells in various stages of differentiation and maturity are affected by radiation at much lower doses than are mature and fully differentiated cells. Radiation acts basically on cellular targets, causing death of the cell when a critical number of targets have been hit by radioactive particles or waves. "Hits" of the targets are theoretic requirements of this target theory of radiation damage, and it is not known exactly what cellular components correspond to the targets, but DNA is suspect. There is no question that the genetic material of the cell is vulnerable to radiation damage and can be altered by a number of well-described mechanisms. Furthermore, the stage of the cell cycle during which the radiation impinges is also critical. These properties of radiation are considered when radiation is used in the treatment of cancer.

When a malignant tumor is irradiated, the radiologist hopes to kill as selectively as possible, relying on the fact that the malignant cells are more radiosensitive than are the normal tissue cells around the tumor. The aim of radiation therapy is to kill cancer cells selectively, with as little damage as possible to underlying tissue and blood vessels, although in practice this may be difficult to achieve; tumor cells are generally more radiosensitive than is the tissue around them, and also malignant cells are not as well able to repair radiation-induced damage as are normal cells. This is also true at the tissue level, in that fibrous repair of normal tissue is very effective, whereas it is not in tumorous tissue. The determination of the radiosensitivity of a tumor and thus of the dose of radiation required is related to three major factors. The various tissues of the body have different degrees of radiosensitivity, which is reflected also in tumors that may arise in these tissues. Thus, one of the most radiosensitive tumors is testicular cancer, and one of the most radiosensitive compartments of cells is the spermatozoan series. Another factor is the cellular radiosensitivity itself, which is related to such things as cell type, cell cycle, mitotic rate, age, differentiation, and DNA synthesis rates. The third factor is the tissue environment. The *oxygenation* of tissue is an important factor, in that radiation causes the formation of oxygen and peroxide free radicals, which are highly reactive and can peroxidate lipids and other molecules in the cell, thus causing radiation damage indirectly. It should be recalled that tumors are often quite hypoxic in comparison to other tissues, and modification of radiosensitivity may be attempted by methods that increase tumor oxygen tension. The vascularity of the tissue also is important in regard to oxygenation and radiosensitivity itself, in that blood vessels can become very permeable at fairly low doses of radiation.

Radiation can be curative for a number of malignant tumors provided the selection of the dose, the way the radiation is administered and focused on the tumor, the fractionation of the dose over time, and the type of radiation used are all optimum.

It is a striking observation that radiation not

only cures cancer but also causes cancer. The radiation dose that is usually administered to malignant tissue is extremely high and is administered at very high voltages. The radiation is directed to a small area of tissue, so that maximum cell death occurs in that focus. It is nevertheless possible that normal cells around an irradiated tumor may receive carcinogenic doses of radiation, and although the original tumor may be completely eradicated, a second and entirely different tumor may appear at the site many years later. The source of this tumor is likely to have been a carcinogenically transformed cell that originated at the time of the therapeutic radiation. Both the cell-killing and the cell-transforming effects of radiation probably reflect the ability of radiation to damage nucleic acids. The concept of a threshold of radiation dose below which no irreparable damage occurs to cells and above which damage accumulates and causes effects such as cancer or teratogenesis is a much debated matter in radiation biology. There is evidence that even very low doses of radiation can be carcinogenic, and some would extrapolate down to the background and zero levels of radiation dose. The incidence of leukemia in the offspring of mothers pregnant at the time of diagnostic radiation to the abdominopelvic area has been shown to be significantly higher than the normal incidence. Leukemia in the offspring of pregnant women irradiated by the bombing of Hiroshima has been linearly related down to very low doses with distance from the hypocenter. Very low doses of diagnostic radiation received by women at the time of mammography have recently been correlated with later appearance of breast cancer in these women.

While radiation is an extremely potent and effective tool in the arsenal of weapons against cancer, it is one that should be handled with extreme care. Knowledge of both the immediate and long-term effects of radiation is necessary to health care workers who are assessing patients undergoing radiation therapy. The most obvious effect may be the erythema of the overlying skin at the site of the radiation therapy. The skin becomes red and warm due to vasodilation, simulating a severe sunburn. It even-

tually becomes very hard and brown. Many patients undergoing radiation therapy also have severe gastrointestinal symptoms. The epithelium of the gut is a tissue renewal system that turns over rapidly and is therefore highly sensitive to radiation damage. Depending on the extent and area of radiation therapy, some gastrointestinal tract damage and symptoms may occur if the gastrointestinal tract is irradiated. The hematopoietic system is another tissue renewal system and is the most radiosensitive system. Exposure of the bone marrow and lymph nodes to very low doses will result in a depression of hematopoiesis. The lymphocytes particularly are radiosensitive, but erythrocyte, granulocyte, and platelet precursor cells are all affected by radiation. Therefore, anemia, leukopenia, and thrombocytopenia may all develop as the result of radiation to the bone marrow. This greatly increases susceptibility to infection, a process that may be life threatening in the cancer patient. The reproductive tract of men is another tissue renewal system that is profoundly sensitive to radiation; the cells most easily damaged by radiation are the spermatogonia, particularly type A spermatogonia, which are the most primitive. Sterilization can occur as the result of radiation exposure to the testes. Ova are radiosensitive as well, and sterility can occur with radiation of the ovaries. All the preceding effects of radiation on the patient are potentially reversible, however, with time. Some permanent changes in the organ systems mentioned may occur, such as might be caused by ischemia and necrosis resulting from any cause. The effects of radiation on different organ systems are more fully discussed in Chapter 6. It is important to realize that radiation damage to an organism is dependent on a number of factors. These include the dose of radiation, the volume of tissue irradiated, and the time over which the radiation is administered. A much larger dose of radiation can be administered to a patient if it is distributed over time (fractionated) so that the patient can recover between doses. The volume of tissue can be extremely small if the radiation is focused on a tiny area, and therefore very high dosages can be given. For example, 10,000 rads over a period of 1 month might be given to an organ. A dose of 450 rads given at one time as whole body irradiation (from a bomb or accidental exposure) would cause death within 30 days to 50% of those humans receiving it.

The long-term effects of radiation might not be manifested for many years after the exposure. Carcinogenesis has been discussed before. Radiation is also known to affect life span by either accelerating the aging process or producing deleterious degenerative changes in the previously irradiated tissues, which increase the possibility of a variety of disease processes taking place. Other long-term effects of radiation include infertility, inhibition of bone growth, and cataractogenesis.

Chemotherapy

Only rarely can drugs be considered curative measures for cancer. For most patients the drugs are given to relieve discomfort and prolong life. Chemotherapeutic agents can be generally classified into four main groups: alkylating agents, antimetabolites, hormones, and antibiotics and plant alkaloids. Use of these drugs is in large part experimental, and recent research has indicated that combining drugs

rather than giving them singly as part of a drug regimen may be more effective for many cancers. A major problem with chemotherapy is the fact that a drug can usually only be given in one course of therapy. Tumor cells apparently are subject to the same laws of natural selection and survival of the species that all living organisms are. Selection of tumor cells resistant to the action of the chemotherapeutic agent occurs, and the drug being used then becomes ineffective against the growth and metastasis of the malignancy. A new drug must then be initiated, until the same process occurs all over again (Fig. 3-12). The alkylating agents, plant alkaloids, antimetabolites, and antibiotics used to combat cancer all have profound side effects, which are primarily related to the mechanism of action of these drugs at the cellular level. These drugs interact in some way with the DNA, RNA, and protein-synthesizing machinery of the cell (Fig. 3-13). Such interruptions will inhibit either division or protein synthesis of the cell, eventually resulting in cell death. These drugs act not only on cancer cells but on all rapid turnover cell compartments (much as radiation does), and the side effects in some ways mimic the effects of radia-

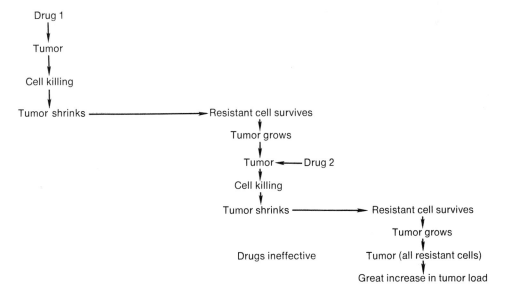

Fig. 3-12. Development of resistance to cancer chemotherapeutic agents occurs through a process of natural selection in which resistant cells are selected in presence of drug, grow, and produce clones of resistant cells.

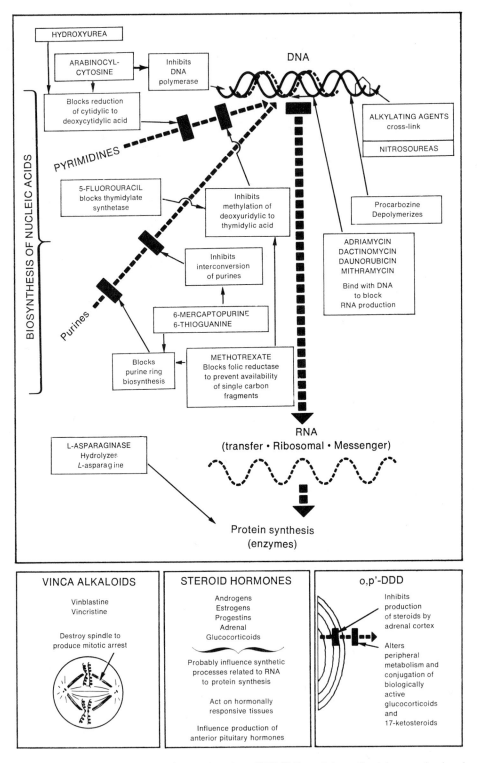

Fig. 3-13. Cancer chemotherapeutic agents act on DNA-RNA protein-synthesizing mechanism in various ways. Other agents act at different levels on cellular division or metabolism as indicated. (From A Cancer Journal for Clinicians **23:**208-219, 1973.)

tion sickness. These include bone marrow depression, nausea, vomiting, diarrhea, lesions and hemorrhage of the mucous membranes, and alopecia. The reproductive tract may be affected, and liver toxicity may occur. The active chemotherapeutic agents have a further specificity of action, in that some are cell-cycle specific, perhaps acting only during mitosis (vincristine) or only at the S (synthesis) phase of the cell cycle (arabinosylcytosine, hydroxyurea). Table 3-1 lists the major cancer drugs, their uses, dosages, and toxicities.

Table 3-1. Cancer chemotherapy*

Drug	Common dosages	Examples of use	Signs of toxicity
Antimetabolites			
Methotrexate	PO 2.5-5.0 mg/day; IV 25-50 mg once or twice a week	Acute lymphocytic leukemia; cancers of testes, cervix; lymphosarcoma; choriosarcoma	Mouth and gastrointestinal tract ulcerations; hematopoietic depression; more toxic in patients with decreased kidney function
6-Mercaptopurine	PO 2.5 mg/kg/day	Leukemia	Nausea; vomiting; hematopoietic depression
5-Fluorouracil	IV 12 mg/kg/day for 3 days	Colon, pancreatic, ovarian, and breast cancers	Nausea; vomiting; hematopoietic depression
Alkylating agents			
Chlorambucil	PO 0.1-0.2 mg/kg/day	Chronic lymphocytic leukemia; Hodgkin's disease; lymphomas	Hematopoietic depression with decreased leukocyte, erythrocyte, and platelet counts; alopecia; cystitis dermatitis; hepatotoxicity; nausea and vomiting
Cyclophosphamide	IV 40-60 mg/kg/day for 10 days; PO 50-200 mg/day	Acute leukemia, chronic lymphocytic leukemia; lung cancer; multiple myeloma	
Antibiotics			
Adriamycin	IV 50-75 mg/m² every 3 weeks	Bone, breast, lung, ovarian, bladder, and thyroid cancers; acute leukemia; Hodgkin's disease	Stomatitis; alopecia; hematopoietic depression; cardiac toxicity
Dactinomycin	IV 0.01 mg/kg/day for 5 days	Osteogenic sarcoma; Wilms' tumor; testicular cancer	Stomatitis; gastrointestinal disturbances; acne; alopecia; hematopoietic depression
Vinca alkaloids			
Vincristine	IV 0.02-0.05 mg/kg weekly	Acute lymphocytic leukemia; Hodgkin's disease; neuroblastoma	Peripheral neuritis; areflexia; weakness; paralytic ulcers; hematopoietic depression
Vinblastine	IV 0.1-0.2 mg/kg weekly	Hodgkin's disease; lymphomas	Nausea; vomiting; areflexia; hematopoietic depression
Steroids			
Androgens		Breast cancer	Masculinization
Estrogens		Breast cancer	Sexual impotence in males
Progestins		Endometrial, prostate, kidneys, and breast cancer	Edema; altered menstruation
Adrenocorticoids		Hodgkin's lymphomas; multiple myeloma; leukemia; breast cancer	Salt and water retention; edema; ulcers; diabetes; infection
Other drugs			
L-Asparaginase	IV 200 to 1,000 IU/kg 3 to 7 times weekly for 28 days	Acute lymphoblastic leukemia	Nausea; vomiting; anorexia; weight loss; abnormal liver metabolism; hyperglycemia; hyperlipidemia
Hydroxyurea	PO 20-40 mg/kg/day	Malignant melanoma; chronic granulocytic leukemia	Hematopoietic depression

*Modified from Krakoff, I. H.: Cancer **23:**209-219, 1973.

POLYFUNCTIONAL ALKYLATING AGENTS

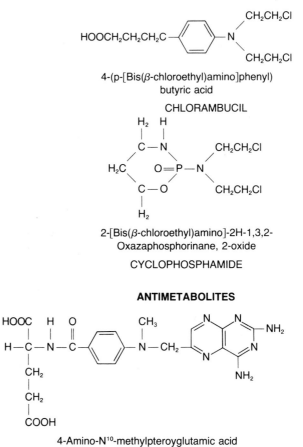

4-(p-[Bis(β-chloroethyl)amino]phenyl)
butyric acid

CHLORAMBUCIL

2-[Bis(β-chloroethyl)amino]-2H-1,3,2-
Oxazaphosphorinane, 2-oxide

CYCLOPHOSPHAMIDE

ANTIMETABOLITES

4-Amino-N^{10}-methylpteroyglutamic acid

METHOTREXATE

5-Fluorouracil

5-FU

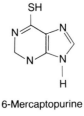

6-Mercaptopurine

6-MP

Fig. 3-14. Selected common chemotherapeutic agents used in treatment of cancer.

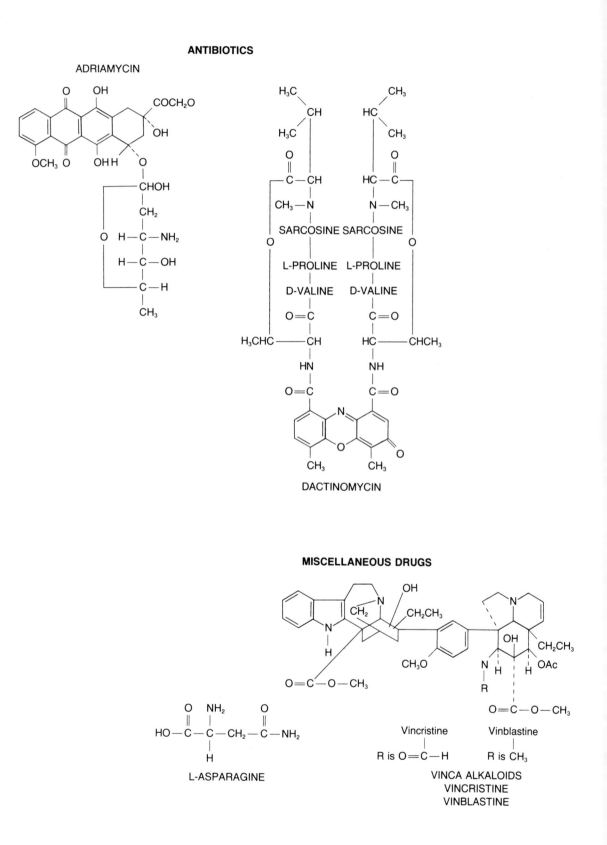

ANTIBIOTICS

ADRIAMYCIN

DACTINOMYCIN

MISCELLANEOUS DRUGS

L-ASPARAGINE

Vincristine — R is O=C—H

Vinblastine — R is CH_3

VINCA ALKALOIDS
VINCRISTINE
VINBLASTINE

Fig. 3-14 shows the molecular structure of some chemical agents used to treat cancer.

Cancer immunotherapy

The field of cancer immunotherapy has been undergoing rapid growth in recent years. The reader is referred to the discussion in the early part of this chapter on the host's immune response to malignancy. Manipulation of the immune response underlies immunotherapy, and there are three major modes of action of immunotherapy intervention. The first method is by active immunization of the host by tumor cells that have been first irradiated. The irradiated tumor cells may invoke a stronger immune response, thus destroying both injected and native tumor cells. Often this therapy is done in conjunction with chemotherapy, radiotherapy, and the administration of BCG, which appears to be a nonspecific immune system stimulant. It is possible also to separate leukocytes from peripheral blood samples, activate them with phytohemagglutinin, and then reinject the cells. A second method of immunotherapy is through passive immunization, with antilymphocyte serum in chronic lymphocytic leukemia, with lymphoid cells from donors who have previously submitted to grafting of the host's tumor, and with transfer factor, a substance produced by leukocytes, which can transfer delayed hypersensitivity reactivity from one person to another. The third mechanism of immunotherapy is through the use of agents known as immunologic adjuvants (BCG, corynebacterium parvum), which appear to act nonspecifically but have been very successful in the treatment of malignant melanoma.

CONCLUSION

It should be apparent to the reader that the major areas discussed in this chapter (basic pathophysiology of cancer, tumor types, and modes of treatment) are prominent areas of research, and new discoveries are being made constantly. Cancer will develop in one of every four individuals, and a true cure for this disease may never be discovered until the basic biology of the cancer cell is unraveled. Inroads into this kind of knowledge and understanding have been made with remarkable speed in only the past 10 or 20 years, and most cancer researchers feel great optimism that all cancers will eventually be curable.

SUGGESTED READINGS

American Cancer Society: A cancer source book for nurses, 1975, The Society.

Anderson, W., and Kissane, J., editors: Pathology, ed. 7, St. Louis, 1977, The C. V. Mosby Co.

Bechar, F., editor: Cancer 2, New York, 1975, Plenum Press.

Bucalossi, P., Veronessi, V., and Cascinelli, N., editors: Proceedings of the XI International Cancer Congress, New York, 1975, American Elsevier Publishing Co.

Busch, H., editor: The molecular biology of cancer, New York, 1974, Academic Press.

Cairns, J.: The cancer problem, Sci. Am. **233**(5):64-72, 77-78, 1975.

Carter, S. K.: Immunotherapy of cancer in man, Am. Sci. **64**:418-423, 1976.

Casarett, A.: Radiation biology, Englewood Cliffs, N.J., 1968, Prentice-Hall.

Clark, R., Cumley, R., McCay, J., and Copeland, M., editors: Oncology 1970, Chicago, 1971, Year Book Medical Publishers.

del Regato, J., A., and Spjut, H. J.: Ackerman and del Regato's cancer: diagnosis, treatment, and prognosis, ed. 5, St. Louis, 1977, The C. V. Mosby Co.

Emmelot, P., and Muhlbock, O., editors: Cellular control mechanisms and cancer, New York, 1974, American Elsevier Publishing Co.

Everson, T., and Cole, W.: Spontaneous regression of cancer, Philadelphia, 1966, W. B. Saunders Co.

Foulds, L.: Neoplastic development, New York, 1969, Academic Press.

Fry, R., editor: Recent results in cancer research, New York, 1969, Springer-Verlag New York.

Grundmann, E., and Tulinius, H., editors: Recent results in cancer research, New York, 1972, Springer-Verlag New York.

Harris, R., Allen, P., and Viza, D., editors: Cell differentiation, Copenhagen, 1972, Munksgaard, International Booksellers Publishers Ltd.

Klein, G., and Weinhouse, S., editors: Advances in cancer research, vols. 17 to 22, New York, 1973, 1974, 1975, Academic Press.

Krakoff, I. H.: Cancer chemotherapeutic agents, Cancer **23**:209-219, 1973.

Marshall, J., and Groer, P.: A theory of the induction of bone cancer by alpha radiation, Radiat. Res. **71**(1):149-192, 1977.

Mehlman, M., and Hanson, R., editors: Control processes in neoplasia, New York, 1974, Academic Press.

Moore, D., and Charney, J.: Breast cancer: etiology and possible prevention, Am. Sc. **63**(2):160-168, 1975.

Morrison, S. D.: Generation and compensation of the cancer cachectic process by spontaneous modification of feeding behavior, Cancer Res. **36**:228-233, 1976.

National Cancer Institute: Carcinogenic abstracts, vols. 12-15, 1974-1977.

National Cancer Institute: The national cancer program and international cancer research, Monograph, DHEW Publication no. (NIH) 74-351, 1974.

Pierce, G., Nakane, P., and Mazurkiewicz: Natural history of malignant stem cells. In Differentiation and control of malignancy of tumor cells, Baltimore, 1974, University Park Press.

Robbins, S., and Angell, M.: Basic pathology, Philadelphia, 1976, W. B. Saunders Co.

Rubin, P., editor: Clinical oncology, ed. 5, 1979, American Cancer Society, Inc.

Smith, P. G., and Pike, M. C.: Case clustering in Hodgkin's disease: a brief review of the present position and report of current work in Oxford, Cancer Res. **34:** 1156-1160, 1974.

Southam, C. M.: Evidence for cancer specific antigens in man, Prog. Exp. Tumor Res. **9:**1-34, 1967.

Stevens, L. C.: Testicular teratomas in fetal mice, J. Natl. Cancer Inst. **28:**247-267, 1962.

Tarin, D., editor: Tissue interactions in carcinogenesis, New York, 1972, Academic Press.

Theologides, A.: The anorexia-cachexia syndrome: a new hypothesis, Ann. N.Y. Acad. Sci. **230:**14-22, 1974.

Tomati, L.: The role of prenatal events in determining cancer risks in progeny, Biochem. Soc. Trans. **4:**703-705, 1974.

Weinhouse, S.: Differentiation and control of the malignancy of tumor cells, Fed. Proc. **32:**2162, 1973.

Zervas, J., Delamore, I., and Israels, M.: Leucocyte phenotypes in Hodgkin's disease, Lancet **2:**634-635, 1970.

PART THREE

Pathophysiology of body defenses and barriers

CHAPTER 4

Inflammation

AT THE COMPLETION OF THIS CHAPTER THE STUDENT WILL BE ABLE TO:

- Describe the ways in which man defends himself against invasion and injury from biologic, chemical, and physical agents.
- Discuss the concept of inflammation as a nonspecific response and list a number of specific responses that occur in various types of injury.
- Discuss the three major stages in acute inflammation and compare simple acute inflammation with delayed hypersensitivity inflammation.
- Describe some of the current theories regarding the role of local and systemic chemical mediators in the inflammatory process.
- Discuss normal and abnormal types of healing and the basic nature of regeneration and replacement.
- Contrast acute and chronic inflammation, particularly with regard to cellular events occurring at the site.
- Describe the differences between banal and granulomatous inflammation and cite examples of each.
- Contrast gouty arthritis and rheumatoid arthritis with regard to pathophysiologic mechanisms that initiate and perpetuate the two conditions.
- Choose any disease at random and discuss the role of inflammation in the disease process.

NORMAL PROTECTIVE MECHANISMS

The major vertebrate defenses are structural and functional components that serve to protect the organism from the potentially deadly effects of mutagens, carcinogens, microorganisms, teratogens, foreign bodies, and physical and chemical trauma. These agents are part of the normal environment, and through the process of natural selection humans have evolved elaborate mechanisms by which they are able to survive and function optimally in a hostile world.

Environmental threats may be handled in a human being by such a discrete mechanism as an enzymatically mediated detoxification of a drug by the liver or by the more obvious barrier that the integument physically presents to noxious agents. The integument and its accessories (e.g., hair, glands, nails, and pigment) and the mucous membrane linings of the respiratory and digestive tracts are the first line of defense that the body poses against the attack of potentially dangerous agents. Although it is apparent that these structures are physical barriers across which a chemical or a microorganism would have to pass, there are also other phenomena, which function in a coordinated manner with the other defenses of the body, operating in these tissues. There is, for example, the integrated and directional movement of the cilia of the columnar epithelium of the bronchial tree, which sweeps particles and mucus toward the external orifices of the nasopharynx. Another example is the cellular enzyme system in the skin, which acts to repair DNA damage caused by the mutagenic effect of ultraviolet radiation.

A further defense system, more diffusely

scattered than the tissue of the integument, is the reticuloendothelial system (RES). This widespread network of phagocytic cells, many of which are found in contact with the circulating blood, is responsible for the recognition, removal, and disposal of microscopic particulate matter such as cellular debris, damaged, old, or foreign cells, immune complexes, and microorganisms. The immune system intimately participates with the RES in this vigilant guard against outside invasion and damage. Unwanted material may be "tagged" by the immune system so that the cells of the RES will recognize it as foreign or unwanted and remove it, usually by phagocytosis.

A further protective mechanism is the inflammatory response that results whenever vascular tissue is damaged, such as when infection or trauma occurs. This reaction is both local and systemic in nature. The inflammatory response involves the "walling off" of the site, attack of invading substances by leukocytes, disposal of the invader and the necrotic debris left by the acute inflammatory response, and finally repair of defects left at the inflammatory site. The inflammatory response is extremely complex in nature and involves finely tuned cellularly and humorally mediated feedback controls on the release of a great variety of substances throughout the body. It can be viewed as a protective mechanism, but the inflammatory response itself may result in pathophysiologic processes, and its aftermath may actually cause deformity and further disease.

The nonspecific response of the body to stressors is activation of the pituitary-adrenocorticotropic axis with release of glucocorticoids such as cortisone. This is the mechanism

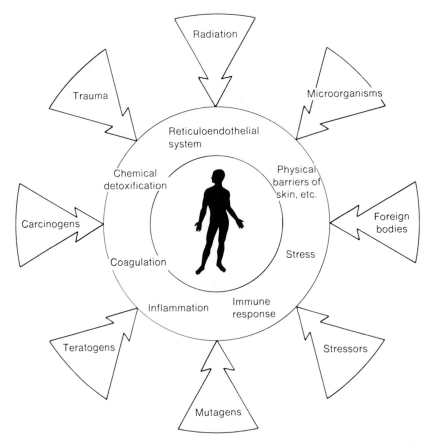

Fig. 4-1. Human lines of defense. Humans are constantly assaulted by environmental factors. In healthy state, organism is able to respond through the many defense mechanisms.

by which the body adapts to stress, but it has been speculated to eventually result in diseases of maladaptation. Nevertheless, the stress-adaptation response can be viewed as a nonspecific defense response.

The immediate reaction to stress, which involves instantaneous activation of the sympathetic nervous system, allows the individual to respond to threats by the well-described fight or flight reaction and thus is another defense mechanism of the body to outside dangers. The body defenses and barriers are illustrated in Fig. 4-1.

When pathophysiologic patterns emerge in these many mechanisms by which the body protects itself, it is evident that the individual becomes extremely vulnerable to attack not only from without but also from within.

In this chapter the inflammatory response will be described, and the interaction of the immune system with inflammation will be discussed.

NATURE OF INFLAMMATION

Found only in vertebrates, inflammation is a complex, integrated host response to a great variety of threats from the internal and external environment. It is basically a nonspecific response to any cell and tissue injury or death. In other words it is not a response to an irritant per se, and the nature of the response does not depend directly on the causative agent. Chemicals, heat, microorganisms, foreign bodies, irradiation, trauma, immune complexes, and many other agents and threats to the body's steady state may stimulate an inflammatory response. An acute reaction is an immediate response to these stressors. This inflammatory process usually resolves itself entirely if no complicating circumstances interfere with healing. Normal simple acute inflammation has a usual time course of 8 to 10 days between the onset of the acute response and the ultimate healing of the inflamed site. Inflammation that does not follow this pattern but instead pursues a course of weeks, months, or even years is considered chronic inflammation.

While the inflammatory response itself is nonspecific in nature, any agent that causes it may also cause a specific response in the host.

For example, radiation causes inflammatory changes, which are essentially the same as those that arise from chemical trauma, heat, or infection. Radiation also causes very specific effects in the host, such as alopecia, bone marrow depression, and nausea and vomiting. Thus, there is superimposed on any injury that causes an inflammatory response a wide variety of other possible interacting factors that may contribute to the development of pathophysiologic mechanisms.

Essentially there are three broad categories of inflammation: (1) simple acute, (2) immunologically mediated delayed hypersensitivity, and (3) chronic. The simple acute type involves the typical signs of inflammation: pain, redness, and swelling. The second type differs from simple acute inflammation in that it is directly caused by an antigen-sensitized lymphocyte reaction, so that the inflammation is a direct response to this interaction and thus takes longer to develop. The delayed hypersensitivity reaction is a typical inflammatory response; that is, it also is characterized by pain, redness, and swelling. Thus, the major difference between simple acute and delayed hypersensitivity inflammation lies in the initiating factors. Although simple acute inflammation occurs the most quickly, both processes are acute reactions, as compared to the third type of inflammation, chronic inflammation. Chronic inflammation is also characterized by pain, redness, and swelling; however, it differs from the first two forms in that it does not subside in a period of days but may instead have a relentless, damaging course of weeks, months, or years. Certain acute inflammatory responses appear to be able to develop into chronic inflammation, while other forms of chronic inflammation appear in a sense to have been destined to be chronic from the beginning of the process. Chronic inflammation seems to be a process in which healing becomes impaired.

Acute inflammation

Simple acute inflammation is characterized by three major phenomena, which occur in the following order: (1) increased vascular permeability, (2) leukocytic cellular infiltration, and (3) repair.

An inflammatory exudate is formed because of the increased permeability of the blood vessels at the inflammatory site and the leukocytic infiltration that occurs secondary, to a degree, to the increased permeability. This exudate is rich in protein and has a high specific gravity. As the inflammatory process proceeds, the exudate changes from a clear serous fluid to a thick, creamy fluid, which contains necrotic debris. The exudate formed by the common cold illustrates this change and is well known to all of us. The exudate in the tissue increases the tissue pressure, and sensitive pain nerve endings are stimulated. Furthermore, chemicals found in the inflammatory exudate can directly stimulate these nerve endings, so that pain usually accompanies acute inflammation. Another sign of inflammation is increased temperature and a reddish coloration of the inflamed site. These properties are due to vasodilation and stasis of the blood at the site.

The signs of inflammation then are *rubor* (redness), *calor* (heat), *dolor* (pain), *tumor* (edema), and *loss of function*. Loss of function occurs as the aftermath of acute inflammation and could actually result in more debility and deformity than that which would have been produced by the original irritant had the inflammatory process not occurred! There are certain clinical conditions for which pharmacologic agents are administered to suppress the inflammatory response. These drugs include the corti-costeroids, penicillamine, and aspirin. The inflammation associated with rheumatoid arthritis can cause so much joint destruction, pain, and disability that a normal life is impossible without the aid of these drugs.

Vascular permeability increase. In 1927 Lewis described the triple response to a firm stroking of the skin. This can best be seen in very light-skinned individuals but occurs in everybody. The initial response is a very transient vasoconstriction, which is immediately followed by dilation of small blood vessels along the line. The second response is thought to result from the local axon reflex; it occurs because of a dilation of neighboring arterioles. The third response is a whealing of the skin. Lewis identified *histamine* as the cause of the triple response that results from vasodilation and increased vascular permeability. The result of these blood vessel alterations is stasis of blood at the inflammatory site, hemoconcentration, and increased viscosity and decreased colloid osmotic pressure of the capillary blood. Inflammatory exudate is formed entirely because fluids and proteins leak through the capillary walls into the inflamed tissue site. The mechanism by which permeability increase occurs is through a widening of the junction between adjacent endothelial cells (Fig. 4-2). Thus, more fluids, as well as proteins and blood cells, can filter into the tissue, resulting in tissue edema that contains a highly cellular exu-

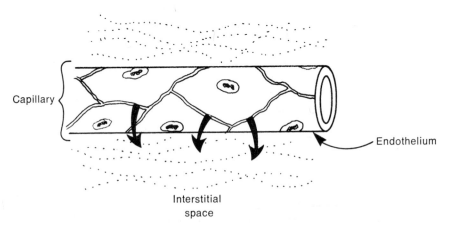

Capillary

Endothelium

Interstitial
space

Fig. 4-2. Fluid movement in inflammation. Capillary permeability is vastly increased during acute inflammation mainly because of a widening in gaps between adjacent endothelial cells.

in notes

date. Furthermore, *hyperemia* may be obvious. Hyperemia is the engorgement of tissue with blood; it may be active or passive. Active hyperemia occurs when the blood flow to a tissue increases dramatically as, for example, in exercising muscle. Passive hyperemia, on the other hand, could be the result of venous stasis in a tissue, which then, of course, leads to hypoxia of the tissue and a reflex vasodilation of arterioles. The increased volume of blood at the inflammatory site, coupled with vasodilation, hemostasis, capillary engorgement, increased vascular permeability, and the resultant decreasing colloid osmotic pressure of the blood as protein leaks into the tissue all act to promote formation of the exudate.

Recent research has indicated that histamine alone is not responsible for the increased permeability that accompanies early inflammation. Many other substances have been identified, but the most important agents appear to be kinins and prostaglandins. Two distinct phases of increased permeability, which appear to be different in nature and cause, have been well characterized.

Early phase. The increased permeability of blood vessels at an inflamed site has two phases; the first appears almost immediately after the application of an irritant, such as a toxin or heat, and disappears 30 minutes later. The second phase of permeability increase occurs about 2 to 4 hours later and lasts for approximately 10 hours. The first phase appears to involve mainly venules. The increased leakiness of these minute postcapillary vessels is probably greatly affected by histamine. Histamine is formed by the enzymatic decarboxylation of histidine, an amino acid, and is stored primarily in mast cells. These are basophilic tissue cells that release histamine into the inflammatory site soon after inflammation begins. Antihistamine drugs, if given at this time, reduce the first phase of the increased permeability response. Antihistaminic drugs act by preventing histamine from combining with its receptors. These drugs are *substituted ethylamines,* which mimic the molecular configuration of histamine and may be able to combine with histamine receptors and thus block histamine attachment.

The phenomenon of increased permeability is also a tissue response rather than solely a vascular reaction. Events occur in an apparently coordinated manner in the blood vessels, interstitium, and lymphatics.

Delayed phase. The delayed or second phase of the permeability increase, which involves small venules and capillaries, occurs by the same mechanism as that illustrated in Fig. 4-2 but is of much longer duration. The nature of this response is different than the first phase, and it is not clear what chemical mediators are involved and in what sequence. There is evidence that bradykinin and prostaglandin E may play roles, but both of these mediators do not seem to have a long enough duration of action. The changing nature of the tissue at the inflamed site may itself play a major role in the development of the second permeability increase. For example, the pH of the tissue changes from neutral to acidic during the acute inflammatory response as venous stasis leads to anoxia, and this may then affect the local blood vessel permeability.

When injury is extremely severe, such as might occur with deep burns of the skin or extensive traumatic injury that results in tissue death and blood vessel destruction, the biphasic nature of the increased permeability is lost, and the excessive permeability results from total destruction or great damage to blood vessels. Loss of blood from the damaged vessels into the tissue spaces will continue until a clot forms and closes off the vessel.

Bradykinin is considered by many authorities to be a major vasodilator in the inflammatory process. The extent of its involvement in the later increased permeability phase remains unclear. It is known to transiently increase the permeability of microcirculation. In addition, bradykinin is now known to stimulate pain nerve endings at the inflamed site and is responsible for the "dolor" of inflammation. It is a nine–amino acid peptide produced in the plasma by the action of *kallikrein* on a precursor substance, *bradykininogen.* The origin of kallikrein is through the action of activated Hageman factor, the same factor responsible for the coagulation cascade. Blood clotting at the inflamed site, which helps to wall off the

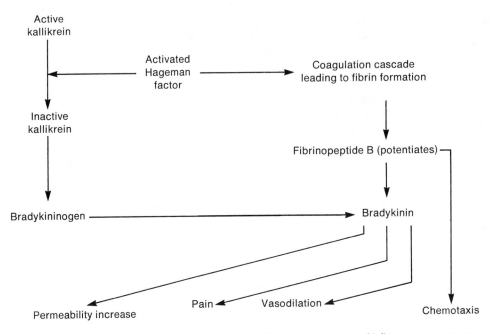

Fig. 4-3. Formation and role of bradykinin. Bradykinin is a major mediator of inflammatory response and is formed through action of activated kallikrein. Its action is further potentiated by fibrinopeptide B, formed in coagulation process.

area with a mesh of fibrin strands, creating a minienvironment, also aids in the bradykinin action, as a peptide formed in coagulation (fibrinopeptide B) potentiates bradykinin's permeability effect. Fibrinopeptide B is also a chemotactic substance that attracts leukocytes into the site. This complex interaction of precursors and activated agents is depicted schematically in Fig. 4-3.

Prostaglandins E_1 and E_2 are also suspected to be important in causing the increased permeability of inflammation, although their action may be short lived. Prostaglandins are lipid-like substances that were first isolated from gonadal tissue. They have been implicated in a number of processes, including smooth muscle contractility and cell membrane interactions. The source of prostaglandins in inflammation may be mononuclear white blood cells, and these chemicals appear to perpetuate the permeability changes of inflammation. Prostaglandins have been shown to disrupt rat cells, so it is possible that their mechanism of action on permeability may be through the release of histamine. It has recently become clear that aspirin

and other nonsteroidal antiinflammatory agents, which have been in wide usage for years, block the synthesis of prostaglandin E. The mechanism of action of aspirin in inflammatory diseases such as rheumatoid arthritis has long remained a mystery, but this line of research may find answers to this important question.

Other chemical mediators have been shown to increase permeability, but their separate roles and the possible interaction with the damaged tissue as it changes in nature during inflammation is not clear.

Leukocytic cellular infiltration. The second major hallmark of inflammation is the migration and proliferation of leukocytes. The cells of the exudate, which are derived from the blood and ultimately the bone marrow, race to an injured area almost as soon as the tissue damage occurs. The increase in permeability that occurs almost simultaneously probably plays a major part in facilitating the escape of these cells from the bloodstream, but cellular infiltration is not merely a passive phenomenon. The leukocytes initially appear to stick to the endothelial lining of the capillaries and marginate (or line up around the circumference of the vessels) before moving through the wall. This process occurs independently of the permeability changes of the vessels.

Generally the first cell type that is found in great abundance at the inflamed site is the neutrophil, a polymorphonuclear granulocytic cell with great phagocytic capabilities. These cells appear to be especially attracted to the injured tissue through *chemotaxis,* a chemical attraction of tissue substances for the leukocytes. Chemotaxis is an important aspect of inflammation in that certain substances are produced by inflamed tissues, which are chemotactic for particular cell types. Numerous substances have been identified as chemotactic for neutrophils and macrophages and possibly for lymphocytes, which are leukocytes that form the basis of the immune response and are present at inflamed sites whenever antigenic material stimulates these cells to produce antibodies. Lymphocytes, rather than neutrophils, may be the first inflammatory cell type to enter virally infected tissue, and occasionally eosinophils may predominate in allergic or parasitic inflammation. The neutrophils that typically enter the inflamed site are accompanied by mononuclear phagocytes, but neutrophils are the major cell type present during the first 12 hours of the inflammatory response. They are actively phagocytic at that time and may eventually leave the site; more commonly they rupture (lyse) and die, releasing their cytoplasmic lysosomal enzymes into the interstitium. These lytic enzymes digest the connective tissue matrix and help to excavate the inflamed site in preparation for healing. Furthermore, these enzymes act as an additional chemotactic stimulus for macrophage infiltration. The major chemotactic agents for neutrophils appear to be the breakdown products of complement, particularly C5a, which becomes chemotactic through the action of a serum peptide, *cocytotoxin.* Other known chemotactic favors may actually require that complement be present for maximal activity. The term *complement* really describes a series of 11 enzymes, which are basically antibacterial in nature and which move quickly to injured tissue when vascular permeability is increased. Complement activation is somewhat

similar to the coagulation cascade in that sequential activation of the complement proteins occurs in response to an initiating step, such as the reaction of antigen with complement-fixing antibody (such as immunoglobulin M), which precipitates along the walls of blood vessels. The Arthus reaction is typical of this kind of inflammatory reaction. When activated, certain portions of the complement chain can attack and lyse foreign cells. The C3 and C5 segments of the chain are extremely chemotactic for polymorphonuclear leukocytes. Furthermore, lysolecithin, which is released by complement, is thought to participate in the permeability increase associated with inflammation. The presence of complement usually indicates that the body's immune system is participating in the inflammatory response. Figs. 4-4 and 4-5 illustrate the complement system.

The major role of the neutrophil at the inflamed site is to dispose of invaders, foreign bodies, and cellular debris through phagocytosis (Fig. 4-6) and enzymatic dissolution. Phagocytosis is a mechanism that requires energy input from the cellular metabolism.

Before a neutrophil can phagocytose a microorganism a process known as *opsonization* must occur. Opsonins are proteins formed in the body that coat microbes in such a way that the neutrophils recognize them as foreign. Opsonization prepares the microorganism for phagocytosis by neutrophils. During the process of phagocytosis of the microbe the neutrophil activates a specialized, oxygen-consuming metabolic pathway, which makes large amounts of hydrogen peroxide, and this substance then plays a role in peroxidative killing of the microorganism. The importance of this process is demonstrated by chronic granulomatous disease, in which the affected patients are subject to recurrent pyogenic infections. It has been shown that there is defective phagocytosis in these patients so that phagocytosed microbes persist and proliferate inside neutrophils and other phagocytic reticuloendothelial cells. It appears that this results from a defect in the cellular metabolic pathway that generates hydrogen peroxide.

In the normal cell, once the material is encapsulated by a phagosome inside the cyto-

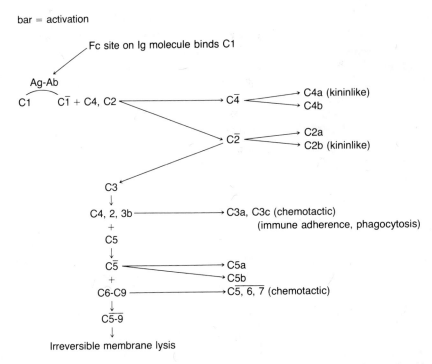

Fig. 4-4. Classic complement cascade. Once activated, complement sequence proceeds with successive activation of complement components, which may produce indicated effects. End result of complement activation on a cell membrane is cell lysis.

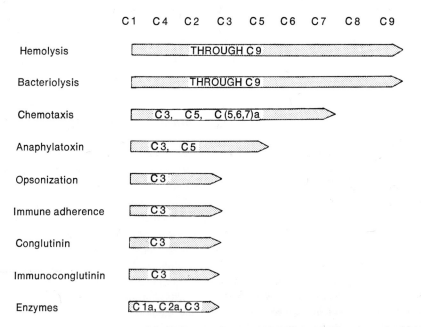

Fig. 4-5. Functions of components of complement. Arrows end at last component required for that particular reaction. (From Barrett, J. T.: Textbook of immunology: an introduction to immunochemistry and immunobiology, ed. 2, St. Louis, 1974, The C. V. Mosby Co.)

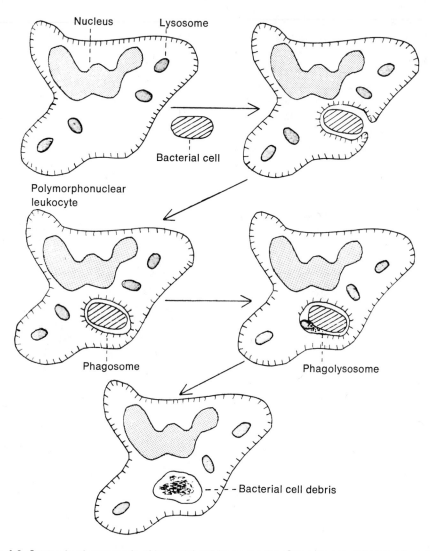

Fig. 4-6. Stages in phagocytosis of bacterial cell by neutrophil. Chemotoxins elaborated by cell attract neutrophil, which then begins to surround bacterium. After engulfment, bacterium is retained in a phagosome. On contact of phagosome with lysosomes, enzymes from lysosomes are released into structure, which is now termed a *phagolysosome,* or *phagolysome.* Undigested debris from bacterium is eventually egested. (From Barrett, J. T.: Textbook of immunology: an introduction to immunochemistry and immunobiology, ed. 3, St. Louis, 1978, The C. V. Mosby Co.)

plasm, the membrane fuses with the lysosomal membrane, and the hydrolytic enzymes of this organelle spill into the phagosome. These enzymes can break down bacterial cell walls and dissolve other materials. Certain organisms and foreign bodies are not destroyed very well by the neutrophils and macrophages and may persist intracellularly in giant cells that form at the site. The causative organisms of tuberculosis and leprosy typify this reaction, which will perpetuate a chronic inflammation. Occasionally bits of wool or steel remain inside giant cells as part of a foreign body reaction.

Phagocytosis may be inhibited in certain disease conditions, as described above, or by immunosuppressant drugs.

The monocytic series of cells begins to predominate within inflamed tissue after 12 hours as the neutrophils die off. The major cell type is the macrophage, which appears to rise from the monocyte. If the inflammatory lesion becomes subacute or chronic, then the cellular infiltrate remains high in macrophages throughout the life of the inflammation. Activation of the macrophage appears to occur at the site and probably is the result of immune mechanisms. Once activated the macrophage is an extremely phagocytic, mobile cell. It secretes enzymes such as collagenase and elastase, which may allow it to pave its way through connective tissue to reach the inflamed site.

While the character of the cell type is thought to be dependent on the nature of the tissue at a specific time and on the release of appropriate chemotactic substances, the circulating blood leukocyte composition and concentration may also play a major role. Fluctuations in the blood neutrophil concentration occur during the inflammatory response, with an increase occurring at 6 hours and a decrease at 12 hours. This coincides with the concentration of these cells at the site. This may be a secondary effect of certain leukopoietins released by the inflamed tissue that stimulate the bone marrow to produce the appropriate white blood cells.

Repair is the third phase of inflammation and will be discussed later in this chapter.

Systemic responses. While the acute inflammatory process appears to result in a localized phenomenon, there are many systemic changes observed during the acute phase. There are changes in the blood levels of certain proteins, which may in turn be due to altered synthetic rates of these proteins by the liver. For example, albumin may decrease in the plasma during the acute response, while α_1-acid glycoprotein may increase to 20 times its normal concentration. Anti-inflammatory plasma protein, which appears to be produced by the liver, rises in concentration after an injury; these proteins, many of whose functions are known, are called _acute phase reactants_. Fibrinogen functions in clotting and repair, and α_2-acid acute phase glycoprotein is antiinflammatory. Kininogen and kininogenase allow the release of bradykinin, and complement fragments C3 and C5 play major roles in immune processes and chemotaxis. Other proteins' functions are not

so well characterized. The role of C-reactive protein is not clear, nor is the role of many glycoproteins that increase in concentration during the acute phase of inflammation. The changes in plasma proteins may affect the outcome of drug therapy in an individual with an acute inflammation. Aspirin, for example, binds to albumin, and only the unbound fraction is responsible for the drug action. A decrease in albumin may allow for more aspirin's becoming available to the inflamed site, but it also increases the possibility of toxicity.

Certain disorders have been traced to abnormal acute phase reactant concentrations. Patients deficient in an antitrypsin are subject to pulmonary emphysema. Hereditary angioneurotic edema may be associated with a decrease in a C1 esterase inhibitor.

Other systemic effects of inflammation include fever (pyrexia), malaise, increase in the white blood cell count (leukocytosis), fibrinolysis, shock, and endocrine and metabolic dysfunctions. The development of fever during acute inflammation is not well understood. It is speculated that leukocyte pyrogen produced by dying cells is liberated into the bloodstream and eventually reaches the temperature-regulating center of the hypothalamus. The pyrogens then "reset" the internal thermostat so that the set point for the body's core temperature increases above the normal 37 C (98.6 F). The increase in the body temperature speeds up metabolic operations throughout the body and may aid in the resolution of the inflammation. Once this occurs the leukocyte pyrogen is no longer released, and the temperature returns to normal.

The elevation in the circulating white blood cell count that is usually observed during an episode of acute inflammation (although certain inflammations may be associated with leukopenia) may be due to stimulation of the bone marrow by substances such as leukocytosis-promoting factor (LPF), neutropoietin, or leukopoietin G, which are released by dying leukocytes at the inflamed site. These substances then become blood borne, eventually reaching the bone marrow. In an acute inflammatory response as much as 90% of the circulating leukocytes will be neutrophils, and the total white blood cell count may increase to three or four times the normal value. Certain viral diseases are not accompanied by a neutrophilic leukocytosis but rather a lymphocytosis, and in parasitic and allergic inflammation, an eosinophilia. A differential white blood cell count is therefore important in diagnosing the cause of the inflammation.

Delayed hypersensitivity inflammation

Inflammation caused by a delayed hypersensitivity response differs from acute inflammation in that the inflammatory response is dependent upon an *antigen-sensitized lymphocyte reaction,* and the initial cellular infiltrate is predominantly lymphocytic. Acute inflammation may have an immune component but is not directly caused by a reaction of antigenic material with the lymphocytes of the blood and tissue. A brief review of the nature of the immune system may help the reader identify more clearly the complex reactions that take place in the delayed hypersensitivity response.

Immune mechanisms. Any foreign protein or substance that becomes protein bound in the body, as well as certain purified polysaccharides, can stimulate the immune system. The basis of the immune response is the antigen-antibody reaction, in which foreign material (antigen) binds to antibody. This effectively ''removes'' this material from the host, generally marking it for disposal by the phagocytic cells of the reticuloendothelial system. Antibodies (immunoglobulins) are produced by lymphocytes, which are mononuclear white blood cells that are originally produced in the bone marrow but travel to the lymphoid tissues early in life. The problem of how lymphocytes are able to produce appropriate antibodies for all the millions of antigens that exist has not been solved.

It is even more difficult to explain the self-recognition of the body's own proteins, a phenomenon called self-immunity. Somehow individuals learn to tolerate their own proteins through processes that occur early in fetal life, which may produce blockage or destruction of those lymphocytes that produce antibodies to those antigens.

It has been shown that certain proteins which have been sequestered from the blood and body fluids by anatomic or physiologic properties of the host are not recognized by the immune system as self-antigens. In sympathetic ophthalmia the proteins of the lens of the eye escape into the humoral fluids after injury or surgery to the eye. This stimulates the immune system to produce antibodies that may cause lens protein to be destroyed, wherever it is found. Thus, injury to one eye may eventually result in injury and perhaps blindness in the other eye.

A number of diseases appear to have an autoimmune component. Autoantibodies to particular tissue proteins have been identified in many of the collagen diseases, such as systemic lupus erythematosus (SLE), rheumatoid arthritis, scleroderma, dermatomyositis, and polyarteritis nodosa.

The problem of how recognition of the antigen by the appropriate antibody molecule occurs has not been resolved. Formerly it was thought that an antigen could induce the formation of a specific antibody with which it could unite. Most authorities now believe that the body produces the trillions of antibody molecules more or less randomly by amino acid substitution at regions on the antibody molecule called the *combining sites.* This region can then combine with the *epitope* (or antigenic-determining site) of one particular antigen. Thus, the antigen selects the proper antibody with which it can then combine when it enters the body. The immune system then amplifies the response by producing a clone of lymphocytes, which ''remember'' the antigen and can immediately produce the right antibody if confronted by the antigen again. In the case of some antigens this is a lifelong memory that confers immunity to the antigen.

The immune system reacts in one of two ways when confronted by antigenic material. The *cell-mediated response* involves the T-lymphocytes derived from leukocytic cells that have passed through the thymus gland on their way from the bone marrow to seed the lymph nodes. Some unknown interaction occurs in the thymus gland, which may involve a thymus-derived hormone (thymosin) and which makes the T-lymphocyte capable of reacting directly with antigenic material on its cellular surface. The second way in which antigenic materials are handled by the immune system is by *humorally mediated* immunity. This response involves B-lymphocytes (bone marrow dependent), which have the capability of producing immunoglobulins and antibody molecules that react with dispersed antigens in the bloodstream. These B-lymphocytes become plasma cells upon stimulation by a recognizable antigen. Plasma cells then begin to synthesize and release specific antibodies, which can react with the antigen in the bloodstream or other tissue spaces. The T-lymphocyte is responsible for the phenomenon of delayed hypersensitivity (sometimes referred to as cellular hypersensitivity), the basis of an inflammatory response. A good example of delayed hypersensitivity is the positive skin reaction of a previously exposed individual to a tuberculin test.

A model of delayed hypersensitivity: the positive tuberculin test. When tuberculin is injected into the skin, specific lymphocytes in the skin and in adjacent lymph nodes that bear receptors for this particular antigen are attracted to the tuberculin, react with it, begin to divide, and produce *lymphokines.* These are chemical substances manufactured by T-lymphocytes that play a major role in the perpetuation of this inflammatory process. Known lymphokines include (1) *chemotactic factors,* which act to attract lymphocytes, neutrophils, and macrophages to the inflamed site, (2) *mitogenic factors,* which stimulate leukocyte division, and (3) *macrophage inhibiting factor,* which acts to inhibit the movement of macrophages away from the inflammatory site, thus prolonging their action.

Cellular infiltration is a hallmark of all inflammation, including the delayed hypersensitivity reaction. The positive tuberculin test is a swollen, red, itchy, and sometimes painful induration. The classic signs of acute inflammation (redness, heat, swelling, and pain) are all evidenced by the tuberculin reaction. This reaction reaches a peak between 48 and 72 hours and then slowly subsides. Tuberculin is a readily digestible irritant, and young macrophages and granulocytes can ingest and destroy this material quickly. When the tuberculin is removed from the skin by the macrophages, the irritation is also removed, the inflammation subsides, and repair begins. The delayed hypersensitivity reaction, typified by the positive tuberculin test, is thus a localization of antigenic tuberculin material through (1) recognition by T-lymphocytes and (2) the resultant recruitment by lymphokines of more sensitized lymphocytes and macrophages, which migrate into the skin and react with the tuberculin at the site. Thus, the tuberculin can be destroyed in situ before it can enter the systemic circulation.

Many other factors are involved in this reaction. The macrophages that are chemotactically attracted to the site by lymphokines become activated by interacting with T-lymphocytes that have been previously sensitized by tuberculin. These T cells appear to be able to transfer antigen receptors from their surface to the surface of macrophages and other lymphocytes.

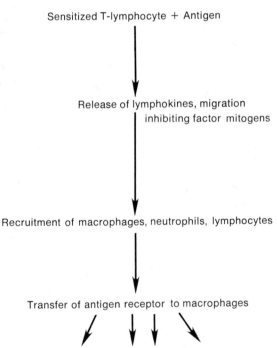

Fig. 4-7. Production of delayed hypersensitivity inflammation. Activation of killer macrophages in delayed hypersensitivity inflammation is believed to be caused by a transfer of antigen receptors from T-lymphocytes to macrophages.

This activated macrophage then becomes an extremely potent killer cell that can phagocytose a variety of antigenic materials (Fig. 4-7). The process of phagocytosis by macrophages involves the encapsulation of the antigenic material by a membrane contiguous with the cell membrane. This forms a vacuole, which enters the cell and fuses with a lysosome, which then pours its hydrolytic enzymes into the vacuole and breaks down the foreign material into its components. The macrophage can then either cytolyze (break apart or lyse) at the inflammatory site or travel away from the site via the lymphatics. Eventually the macrophage may be destroyed by the RES. The macrophage has recently been identified as a major cell in the initiation of the immune response of the body. Before antigen reacts with T- or B-lymphocytes, it appears to be "processed" by an initial reaction with macrophages. The nature of this processing is not clear at this time. Thus, the role of the macrophages in delayed hypersensitivity inflammation is complex, involving both presentation of antigen to the lymphocytes and interaction with these sensitized lymphocytes, so that ultimately the macrophages can phagocytose the antigen.

The delayed hypersensitivity inflammatory reaction is responsible for the rejection of foreign tissue transplants, which is a serious problem accompanying heart, kidney, and other organ transplants. The T-lymphocytes recognize the transplanted organ cells as foreign and react with them, becoming activated and capable of killing all cells that carry the foreign antigens. The cell-killing effect may be due to direct killing or may be due to, or augmented by the release of lymphokines, which would attract other cells to the inflammatory site. Rejection of cancer cells is also a T-cell response.

Tumor patients generally show cellular immunity to their tumor antigens, but this is blocked by factors in their serums. These factors are thought to be antigen-antibody complexes.

Chronic inflammation

Occasionally acute inflammation does not become fully resolved, and healing is not evidenced, even after a period of weeks. It is not known whether an inflammatory process, by its nature, is destined in certain cases to become chronic, or whether any acute inflammation has the potential to become chronic. The nature of a chronic inflammation is certainly different than the acute type, and the systemic effects on the host are not the same. An acute inflammatory response is protective and immediate, and when the source of the injury is removed by the inflammatory process, healing restores structure and function in many cases, or repair with scar formation will at the very least result in structural integrity. A chronic inflammatory process, whether local or systemic, is debilitating and damaging and has long-term, far-reaching effects on the host's well-being.

Chronic inflammation can be caused by a great variety of agents, such as infection by bacteria and viruses, physical factors such as trauma, irritation, or the actual size or solubility of a foreign body, and biochemical factors, such as an unresolved immune reaction. Rheumatoid arthritis is characterized by a chronic inflammatory course and is thought to be of an autoimmune nature. Many investigators believe that prolongation and chronicity of any inflammation are ultimately due to aberrant immunologic mechanisms.

Cellular infiltrate. The nature of the inflammatory site changes as the inflammation becomes chronic. The macrophage becomes the major cell type, although plasma cells and lymphocytes are also found. It functions as an activated phagocyte that contains microbicidal substances and hydrolytic enzymes. Activated macrophages also release a number of enzymes, such as plasmin activator and collagenase, as well as pyrogens, which will cause a febrile response. Occasionally the inflammation is best characterized as subacute rather than chronic, and this usually occurs when an irritant remains at the inflammatory site after the acute response has passed. Continuous migration of macrophages occurs into the area, and these cells may divide at the site. They are eventually killed by the irritant and spill cytoplasmic enzymes into the site. The vaccines, namely, BCG (bacille Calmette Guerin), pertussin, and typhoid will all produce a subacute lesion, which will be resolved only when the vaccine material is either destroyed, removed, or effectively sequestered by cells.

A chronic inflammation, on the other hand, has a *slow* macrophage turnover. The cause is often a fairly nontoxic but not readily digestible irritant. The macrophages may react to the substance by forming multinucleated giant cells. The irritant may cause the macrophages to release biologically active substances, which act to further perpetuate the inflammatory process.

Chronic inflammation is more *proliferative* than exudative, as compared to acute inflammation, and necrosis commonly occurs and recurs. Granulation tissue will form in response to this, and then connective tissue will follow. Thus, increasing amounts of fibrous scar tissue will characterize a persistent, long-term chronic process.

Types of chronic inflammation. Two types of chronic inflammation have been characterized, *granulomatous* and *banal*. A granulomatous inflammation is highly cellular and destructive and is typified by tuberculosis, leprosy, syphilis, sarcoidosis, or rheumatoid arthritis. The first three diseases are all characterized by infection of the host by large, facultative, intracellular bacteria, while sarcoidosis and rheumatoid arthritis are of unknown origin. Many fungi, minerals, and foreign bodies will stimulate a granulomatous reaction, and antigen-antibody hypersensitivity reactions themselves may also be important causes.

The granulomas may be of a high or low turnover type with regard to the recruitment, division, and death of macrophages, which are found in great numbers at the site. Fibroblasts can form part of the cell population in both types, particularly at the periphery of the granuloma where organization and attempts at repair are occurring. This may be observed, for example, at the border of a tubercle or in silicosis, which stimulates a fibrogenic response by itself. The tubercle is the characteristic pulmonary lesion of tuberculosis (Fig. 4-8). The granuloma consists of macrophages and epithelioid giant cells at the center of the lesion, the core of which is often necrotic. Lymphocytic infiltration can be seen at the periphery of the lesion, which is further edged by fibroblasts and connective tissue. The tubercle reaches a size of

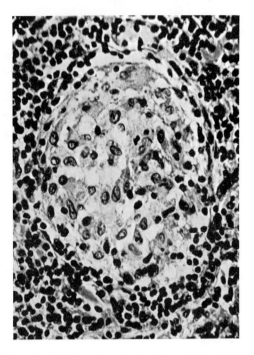

Fig. 4-8. Chronic tuberculosis. Macrophages in tubercle, which is circumscribed ovoid focus in center. Peripheral cells mostly lymphocytes. Caseous necrosis subsequently developing at center of tubercle. (×510.) (From Anderson, W. A. D., and Kissane, J. M., editors: Pathology, ed. 7, St. Louis, 1977, The C. V. Mosby Co.)

approximately 1 mm, and as the disease advances the tubercles begin to merge, and extensive fibrotic changes in the tissue further complicate the disease process.

Granulomatous infection may or may not be marked by the typical focal lesions that have been described. The systemic effects of the disease may be the more obvious clinical manifestation of the inflammation. Furthermore, the granulomatous histology for any given disease varies.

Banal chronic inflammations are generally not highly cellular and produce relatively smaller lesions. They may produce severe illness in the affected individual, however. Examples of banal chronic inflammation include chronic glomerulonephritis, cholecystitis, and many skin inflammations.

In general a chronic inflammation is caused by the persistence of an irritant after the acute response. That irritant may be of a biologic, physical, or chemical nature. The irritant remains at the site due to an inability of the macrophages to digest it. The cycle of cellular infiltration, necrosis, and fibrosis will continue as long as the irritant remains. Very often there is a delayed hypersensitivity response associated with the chronic irritation and inflammation, and there is also a great variety of systemic responses (fever, lymphoplásia, leukocytosis), which may contribute to the debility and further susceptibility of the host to other diseases.

HEALING AND REPAIR

The processes of healing and repair at the inflamed site begin with the removal of the agent that caused the original perturbation, usually through the already described mechanisms of phagocytosis and enzymatic dissolution. Healing will be uneventful if the inflammatory process does not become complicated by excess necrosis, hemorrhage, ulceration, abscess formation, or cellulitis.

Necrosis is always part of the inflammatory picture in that individual cells die and remain at the site. Certain infections are particularly characterized by necrosis caused by bacterial toxins. Gas gangrene, a clostridial infection, is an anaerobic process characterized by overwhelming local sepsis and tissue destruction. The affected part, often a limb, becomes extremely edematous, discolored, and noxious smelling and may have to be amputated.

When the necrotic debris in the exudate at the inflamed site is purulent and very localized so that the pus is confined to a space in which hydrostatic pressure can increase, an *abscess* forms. The pressure eventually will result in a track forming in the area of least resistance, and the pus will drain out in this direction. Rupturing of the abscess in this manner results in the formation of a fairly large defect, and scarring may be marked. Many times this can be partially eliminated if the abscess is drained surgically.

Ulceration at an inflamed site can occur, particularly when the inflammation is complicated by vascular obstruction or infection. The inflammation than may become chronic. An example of this process is a peptic ulcer. An ulcer is an excavation in the lining of the stomach or duodenal mucosa, surrounded by inflamed, infiltrated tissue. Continuous irritation of the site perpetuates the inflammation. Healing can be accompanied by *regeneration,* which is repair of the defect left by an injury or by the aftermath of the inflammatory process; this repair is accomplished through replacement of the tissues with cells of the same type as those that were destroyed. However, more commonly healing is accompanied by *replacement* of the lost cells with connective tissue cells, a process that results in scar formation.

Regeneration

The ability of cells to regenerate is dependent on whether they are labile, stable, or permanent, cell types. Labile cells, which divide constantly during their life span, such as the cells lining the gastrointestinal tract, epithelial cells of the skin, or cells of the bone marrow, are in a sense less specialized than the permanent cell types, such as nerve cells. They are more capable of regeneration than nerve cells, and injury to the skin epithelium can be followed by regeneration and healing without scar formation. The liver and kidney parenchymal cells do not divide constantly as part of their normal physiology, but nevertheless they do retain the capacity to regenerate when the organ becomes damaged or lost through injury or disease. Lower animals have the capacity in certain instances to replace an entire limb, and theoretically every cell in the human body has the memory within its nuclear DNA to replace an amputated limb, but this code is suppressed or somehow lost in the cells of higher animals.

Replacement

Most injuries heal by connective tissue repair and second intention. *First intention* healing occurs when wound margins are nicely apposed, such as in surgical repair of a surface wound. Little scar formation occurs if there is no secondary infection, trauma, or vascular obstruction. *Second intention* connective tissue repair occurs when the wound is large and exudative, with a large amount of necrotic tissue formed as part of the inflammatory process. The site first fills in with a highly vascular, pinkish tis-

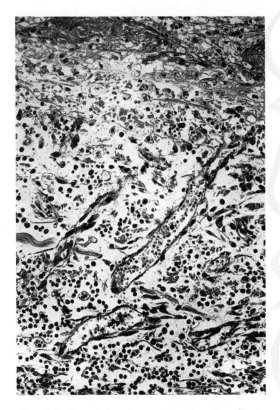

Fig. 4-9. Granulation tissue in pericarditis. Newly formed blood vessels are supported by loosely arranged connective tissue, in interstices of which lie inflammatory cells. Fibrinous exudate *(top)* obscures outline of serosal pericardium. (×170.) (From Anderson, W. A. D., and Kissane, J. M., editors. Pathology, ed. 7, St. Louis, 1977, The C. V. Mosby Co.)

sue known as granulation tissue (Fig. 4-9). Fibrin, which was formed in the initial inflammatory exudate, serves as a scaffolding for migrating fibroblasts from the neighboring connective tissue and a matrix upon which the granulation tissue is laid down. Fibrin eventually undergoes fibrinolysis (or liquefaction) through the action of fibrinolytic agents released by the lysosomes of leukocytes, or more usually through the action of *plasmin,* which is a blood protease. The fibroblasts move into the granulation tissue and lay down an initially disordered array of collagen fibrils, which later become remodeled into an organized structure that will form a scar. Granulation tissue receives an excellent blood supply from capillary buds that form new vessels, which bend and loop into the defect. This vascular supply later regresses, so

that the final scar *(cicatrix)* is less vascular than normal tissue (accounting for its whitish coloration). Collagen formation by the fibroblasts is dependent on adequate amounts of vitamin C (ascorbic acid), which is required in the hydroxylation of lysine and proline, subunits of the collagen molecule. Granulation tissue not only is a compact sealer of the wound but is also resistant to infection and contains macrophages that assist in the removal of debris and necrotic cells. It later contracts greatly in the healing process, and this allows the wound edges to move together, facilitating the repair.

DISORDERS OF INFLAMMATION

It is difficult if not impossible to isolate direct disorders of inflammation from those classified as immune system abnormalities. There are disturbances of leukocyte chemotaxis that impede the inflammatory response and that account for some human diseases, but it is likely that such diseases in turn cause a suboptimal immune response during inflammation. Conversely an abnormal immune response is associated with a great variety of systemic inflammatory disorders, neoplastic diseases, and a generally increased likelihood of infection. For example, patients born with congenital thymic dysplasia have an absent T cell response and are extremely susceptible to fungal and viral infections. T cell immunity appears to regulate susceptibility to this type of microorganism, while B cell or humoral immunity regulates bacterial response.

It is obvious too that inflammation is a sign of a great many disorders that would not ordinarily be classified primarily as inflammatory disorders. Inflammation accompanies any injury or insult to vascular tissue and thus is seen in conditions ranging from acute appendicitis to cirrhosis of the liver to a herpetic coldsore. Indeed, in all these conditions the inflammation secondary to the cellular damage wrought by the pathogen or toxin causes the greatest discomfort to the patient.

Gouty arthritis is classified as an inflammatory disorder, a metabolic error, a genetic disease, and an arthritis. This typifies the manner in which many diseases can be classified, and an understanding of pathophysiology must be underscored by a knowledge of these interrelationships.

Two disease models, gout and rheumatoid arthritis, will be presented here as disorders of inflammation, the first being nonimmune in nature and the second having a strong immune component. Both disease models are of an arthritic (joint inflammation) process.

Gout

Gouty arthritis is a complication of prolonged uric acid elevation in the blood, which ultimately results in the deposition of uric acid deposits in the joints, kidneys, and subcutaneous tissue. The basic cause of the hyperuricemia may vary from patient to patient, but the primary form is an inborn metabolic defect in purine metabolism or in uric acid excretion. The disease is typified by acute attacks, which are precipitated by such factors as trauma, drugs, and possibly overeating. The first attack of gout involves only the great toe in most patients, 90% of whom are male. Later attacks may involve other joints.

The inflammation that characterizes gouty arthritis is immediate and results in great pain, swelling, and redness. It is treated medically, usually by the administration of salicylates, allopurinol, or colchicine, or it may resolve itself. The mechanism of action of colchicine is obscure, in that it relieves the pain of only this condition. It does not act by increasing the urinary excretion of blood concentration of uric acid, as do the salicylates. It does not alter the function of xanthine oxidase as does allopurinol, nor does it reduce the amount of uric acid that is formed through purine metabolism. The most plausible mechanism for colchicine action is through interruption of the leukocytic response to the uric acid crystals, so that the characteristic inflammation is halted.

The inflammation of gouty arthritis is initiated by the precipitation of uric acid crystals, which occurs at lowered pH levels in the acidic joint capsules. This results when the serum uric acid increases above 6.5 mg/100 ml. The uric acid crystals can activate Hageman factor and the kinin system, which have previously been described, and an acute effusive inflammation in the joint ensues. Repeated attacks of gout lead to the collection of large crystals, which initiate a chronic granulomatous response. These granulomas, known as *tophi,* can seriously impair joint function and if formed in the kidney may result in obstruction and renal damage. Tophi can often be demonstrated in the earlobe of the gouty individual and may ulcerate in any location. Thinning of the cartilage and pitting of the bony surfaces may result when chronic inflammation characterized by tophi formation occurs.

Rheumatoid arthritis

Rheumatoid arthritis is a systemic, chronic, inflammatory disease, involving tissues throughout the body. While there is little question that the inflammation itself appears to perpetuate both the disease process and the resultant deformity, much research on the basic mechanisms of inflammation is needed before the nature of the abnormality in rheumatoid arthritis is known. Rheumatoid arthritis may strike people of all ages, as compared to osteoarthritis, which is the inevitable stiffening of the joints accompanying old age. The cause of rheumatoid arthritis is unknown, but much evidence has accumulated to indicate an autoimmune etiology, which may be precipitated by a severe infection, a drug reaction, or stress. The presence of *rheumatoid factors* (RFs) in almost all patients is the most striking evidence in this regard. RFs are antibodies (of the IgG and IgM classes of immunoglobulins) to gamma globulin. It is speculated that antibodies to one's own proteins may occur if the structure is altered so as to "fool" the immune system. Such a configurational change might be due to a viral infection, an abnormal metabolic reaction, or a previous antigen-antibody reaction. Rheumatoid arthritis is classified as a collagen disease, implying that connective tissue, which produces fibrils of collagen protein, is involved. Other collagen diseases include scleroderma, polyarteritis nodosa, dermatomyositis, and systemic lupus erythematosus (SLE). The autoimmune nature of SLE has been the most definitively described of all the collagen diseases. In this particular disease a somatic mutation in the antibody-forming lymphocytes is thought to occur, resulting in a clone of cells that produce antibodies able to react with the host's own cells. The presence of the characteristic *LE cell,* which is a neutrophil containing immune complexes of DNA–anti-DNA antibodies, in the bone marrow and blood of patients with this disease indicates that an autoimmune attack on cellular DNA has occurred. Antinuclear antibodies and antibodies to cytoplasm, erythrocytes, platelets, and clotting factors have all been described in SLE. Furthermore, lesions that occur throughout the connective tissues may be equivalent to the LE cells. The disease is strikingly exacerbated by sunlight, presumably because photo-denatured DNA is potently immunogenic in this disorder.

Rheumatoid arthritis may be caused by a similar mechanism or may, like chronic glomerulonephritis and rheumatic fever, be the possible result of a cross-reactivity of human antigens with bacterial antigens. Bacterial antigens like those of the *Streptococcus,* would be so similar in structure to the human antigens that the immune system's bacterial antibodies would also attack and destroy certain human antigen-bearing cells. Collagen fibrils or connective tissue ground substance may become altered in rheumatoid arthritis, so as to be immunogenic. It is possible that these immune phenomena are only the result of the disease process of rheumatoid arthritis, rather than initiating causes of the disease, however.

It is thought that complement is activated as part of the initial inflammation in rheumatoid arthritis, and consequently leukocyte infiltration ensues. These cells, as well as the synovial membrane cells of the joint capsule, then release lysosomal enzymes, which themselves act to perpetuate a chronic synovitis, leading to eventual destruction of the articular cartilage, and the typical pain, stiffness, and loss of function. Serum complement often is not decreased in rheumatoid arthritis, but the synovial complement concentration often is decreased, possibly indicating that it has been used up in the activation of the complement cascade that has previously been described.

In this condition it would seem that the inflammation itself, which normally serves a protective and self-limiting function, leads to the disease process and is in a sense a protective

mechanism gone awry. In fact, the major pharmacologic treatment for this disease is suppression of the inflammatory process with both nonsteroidal antiinflammatory agents and glucocorticoid steroids. The physiology of corticosteroid treatment in inflammatory disease is based on the fact that corticosteroids increase the vasomotor activity of the vascular bed such that capillary dilatation is decreased, and the reactivity to epinephrine-induced vasoconstriction is increased. These effects would thus oppose the normal increases in vascular supply and permeability during inflammation. Corticosteroids also alter the permeability characteristics of blood vessels directly. Thus, inflammatory edema and tissue swelling are decreased by the administration of these drugs.

Corticosteroids also inhibit polymorphonuclear chemotaxis, decrease granulocyte adherence, and decrease fibroblast proliferation and collagen production and blood vessel growth at the inflamed site.

The onset of symptoms of rheumatoid arthritis is often preceded by an infectious illness. The precipitating cause leading to persistent inflammation may be a transient infection of the joint lining by an organism such as a latent virus or mycoplasma. This results in the conversion of gamma globulin to a form that then stimulates autoimmunization. RFs certainly appear to play an important role in the pathophysiologic propagation of the rheumatoid disease process. The RFs themselves may provoke tissue damage, causing vasculitis, histamine release, and kinin activation. Phagocytosis may be enhanced or depressed in the presence of RFs, and complement fixation to RFs also has been reported.

Rheumatoid arthritis may be characterized by an initial attack, which is then followed by a complete disappearance of symptoms or by a course characterized by remissions and exacerbations and occasionally by a relentless, progressively destructive, and irreversible destruction of the joints. Synovial membranes are the most commonly affected tissues, but blood vessels, pericardium and pleura, and subcutaneous tissue can all show inflammatory changes. Connective tissue nodules occur in at least 15% of the cases and may themselves cause pain and disability, depending on location. These nodules are granulomatous inflammatory reactions of the connective tissue of the derma. Gradual deformation and contracture of the joints can occur, particularly without early and continued treatment. The principal symptoms begin usually as morning stiffness, often of the fingers (although one or many joints can be initially involved), which gradually clears with movement. The involved joints become red, hot, and swollen, and the individual is usually fatigued and debilitated during the acute stages of the disease. The swelling of the fingers is described as fusiform, or spindle shaped, and is quite characteristic. In addition, muscular atrophy may develop and become quite marked. Further diagnostic criteria include an elevated erythrocyte sedimentation rate, a positive test for rheumatoid factor, and a variety of systemic symptoms such as fever, anemia, and lymphadenopathy. On x-ray examination a thinning of the cartilage may be seen, as well as the presence of small punched out areas of bone.

The tendency to avoid movement of a painful joint may lead to contracture and ankylosis of the joint, and this, coupled with progressive synovitis and joint damage, may lead to severe deformity. In the most severe forms of the disease, vasculitis can lead to tissue anoxia, necrosis, and gangrene. In the acute form of rheumatoid arthritis pulmonary and cardiac inflammation may also produce overt signs of distress.

Often rheumatoid arthritis follows a relatively benign course with periods of long remission. Treatment with rest and moderate exercise, physiotherapy, and administration of drugs such as the salicylates, penicillamine, and corticosteroids often allows the arthritic to function optimally in spite of his disease. Joint surgery may be required when severe deformity leads to pain and loss of function.

SUMMARY

This chapter has presented the topic of inflammation in the light of cellular, humoral, systemic, and immune events, which the host is able to coordinate in a remarkable way to present a combined front against possible injurious agents. Thus, the interaction of these body defenses and barriers helps to preserve the steady state when the organism is threatened. Various classes of inflammation (simple acute, delayed hypersensitivity, and chronic) have been described, and the processes involved in healing, regeneration, and repair have also been discussed. Two disease models of inflammation have also been presented in order to acquaint the reader with different mechanisms of pathophysiology; nevertheless, both disease models cause inflammation and pain in the joints. The concept of inflammation then as a nonspecific response, which is normally protective but occasionally destructive in itself, underscores these disease models. Thus, we can view inflammation as a steady state mechanism that ultimately may turn against itself and become pathophysiologic.

SUGGESTED READINGS

Anderson, W. A. D., and Scott, T. M.: Synopsis of pathology, ed. 9, St. Louis, 1976, The C. V. Mosby Co.

Barrett, J.: Textbook of immunology: an introduction to immunochemistry and immunobiology, ed. 3, St. Louis, 1978, The C. V. Mosby Co.

Cheson, B. D., Curnette, J. T., and Balor, B. M.: The oxidative killing mechanisms of the neutrophil. In Progressive clinical immunology, vol. 3, New York, 1977, Grune & Stratton.

Dannenberg, A. M., Jr.: Macrophages in inflammation and infection, N. Engl. J. Med. **293:**489-493, 1975.

Ferriera, S. H., and Vane, J. R.: New aspects of the mode of action of non steroid anti-inflammatory drugs, Ann. Rev. Pharmacol. **14:**57-73, 1974.

Forscher, B. K., editor: Chemical biology of inflammation, Oxford, Eng., 1967, Pergamon Press Ltd.

Future trends in inflammation II, Agents actions **6**(1-3), 1976.

Henson, P. M., and Cochrane, C. C.: The effect of complement depletion on experimental tissue injury, Ann. N.Y. Acad. Sci. **256:**426-440, 1975.

Hollander, J. L., and McCarty, D. S.: Arthritis, Philadelphia, 1974, Lea & Febiger.

Houck, J. C.: Inflammation: a quarter century of progress, J. Invest. Dermatol. **67:**124-128, 1976.

Kaj Jerne, N.: The immune system, Sci. Am. **229:**52-60, 1975.

Kaplan, A. P., and Austen, K. F.: Activation and control mechanisms of Hageman factor-dependent pathways of coagulation, fibrinolysis and kinin generation and their contribution to the inflammatory response, J. Allergy Clin. Immunol. **56:**491-506, 1975.

Mayer, M. M.: The complement system, Sci. Am. **224:** 52-66, 1973.

Perper, R. J., editor: Mechanism of tissue injury with reference to rheumatoid arthritis, Ann. N.Y. Acad. Sci. **256,** 1975.

Robbins, S., and Angell, M.: Basic pathology, ed. 2, Philadelphia, 1976, W. B. Saunders Co.

Silverstrinj, B., and Tura, S.: Inflammation: proceedings of an international symposium, Amsterdam, 1968, Excerpta Medica Foundation.

Snader, T. C.: Inflammatory disorders, Am. J. Pharm. **146**(4):113-125, 1974.

Snyderman, R., Pike, M. C., and Altman, L. C.: Abnormalities of leukocyte chemotaxis in human disease, Ann. N.Y. Acad. Sci. **256**:386-401, 1975.

Williams, D. M., and Johnson, N. W.: Alterations in peripheral blood leukocyte distribution in response to local inflammatory stimuli in the rat, J. Pathol. **118**:129-141, 1976.

Zweifach, B. W., Grant, L., and McCluskey, R. T., editors: The inflammatory process, ed. 2, New York, 1974, Academic Press.

CHAPTER 5

Disorders of body defenses and barriers

AT THE COMPLETION OF THIS CHAPTER THE STUDENT WILL BE ABLE TO:

- Relate the disorders of the immune system, the infectious process, and coagulation disorders to systems theory and state how each disturbs the steady state.
- Describe how the normal immune response functions as a body defense.
- Cite the possible mechanisms of immunodeficiencies with reference to normal T cell and B cell function and predict the symptoms of these conditions.
- Discuss the possible modes of therapy for various immunodeficient diseases.
- Relate how atopy is an alteration of normal immunity, describe the forms it takes, and discuss possible treatment modalities based on the pathophysiology.
- Describe the process of complement activation and relate it to immune complex disease and the pathophysiology of inflammation and coagulation.
- Describe the normal development of self-immunity and discuss factors that influence its development.
- Cite the possible interruptions in normal physiology that might result from autoimmune disease.
- Discuss the identification of histocompatibility antigens and the implications of research in the association of tissue antigens with disease.
- Relate the interactions of the body's defenses and barriers to infectious diseases.
- Discuss the differential leukocyte response to various infectious agents and the normal pattern of leukocyte response in an acute infection.
- Describe the general properties of common antibiotics with regard to their bactericidal activity.
- Cite the interacting factors that are responsible for normal coagulation and the ways that this normal pattern can be altered.
- Discuss common abnormalities of coagulation and state how abnormal coagulation can interfere with maintenance of the steady state.
- Describe the normal role of platelets and ways in which their function may be disturbed.

This chapter considers disruptions in important body defenses and barriers that lead to pathophysiologic processes and overt disease states. Within this category are classified specific disorders of the immune system, infection, and coagulation. The immune system is discussed first as disease states often originate within it and it provides a basis for understanding the infectious process in humans. Its nature is discussed in Chapter 4; also in Chapter 4 one particular type of immune system phenomenon, delayed or cell-mediated hypersensitivity

inflammation, is described in detail. This process can become pathophysiologic when the normal protective functions of the response become disruptive to the host. For example, the destruction of an organ transplant is the result of this normal T-lymphocyte response, and the catastrophic effects of a focus of immunologically mediated necrosis in the host are obvious. Therefore, transplant patients must be treated aggressively with immunosuppressive drugs, so as to halt this normal response. This, of course, leads to tremendous problems in the ability of these patients to withstand infection, as immunologic defense is so depressed. There are other immune phenomenon that lead to pathophysiology, including (1) atopy and anaphylaxis, (2) autoimmunity, and (3) immune complex disease.

Human beings are constantly assaulted by environmental and internal microorganisms, which are usually adequately disposed of by the immune system, the reticuloendothelial system, and the acute inflammatory response. Occasionally these systems fail, often for reasons that are not clear, and infection occurs. It is important to distinguish infection from the acute inflammatory response, which is always part of infection; acute inflammation is a nonspecific protective response to any cell injury or necrosis. Infection always involves cell injury or death caused by microorganism invasion and is a process that is specific to the organism causing the infection. Infection is such an important pathophysiologic phenomenon that it is discussed separately from inflammation and immunity. The essential destruction of the host by microorganisms is an important cause of disease-related death, but much of the former morbidity and mortality has been eradicated by antibiotics.

Coagulation is a normal protective response of the body to injury that might otherwise result in the loss of large amounts of blood and body fluids. Normal coagulation may become disrupted in a number of ways, and when this occurs, pathophysiologic mechanisms may be set up, causing signs and symptoms of disease.

PATHOPHYSIOLOGY OF THE IMMUNE SYSTEM

The basic physiology of the immune system has been described, but the details of immunopathology require a more elaborate description of the immune system. Basic to all immune reactions, whether cellular or humoral in nature, is the antigen-antibody reaction.

ANTIGEN-ANTIBODY REACTIONS
Antigens

The initiation of any immune response is carried out by the introduction of an antigen,

which is usually a protein, a protein-bound molecule, or a polysaccharide that the body recognizes as foreign. This antigen is recognized by the immune system, which produces antibodies to combine with it and react with it in specific ways, depending on the nature of the antigens, the antibodies, and the general functioning of the immune system. It is obvious that the immune system does not function in isolation from the rest of the body but is an open system that is constantly affected by occurrences elsewhere. For example, the integrity of the reticuloendothelial system and the phagocytes of the blood is required if immune capability is to be complete.

Antigens are generally macromolecules, exceeding molecular weights of 10,000. These molecules are usually complex, and their stereochemistry confers upon them a specific identity. This molecular configuration is important, as it elicits the release of specific antibodies. Foreign antigens are soluble in body fluids and are different in structure than self-antigens and tissues. The immune system tolerates self-antigens except in diseases of autoimmunity (see Chapter 4). *p 125*

Antibodies (immunoglobulins)

Antigens react with antibodies, which are proteinaceous molecules known as immunoglobulins. These are produced by B-lymphocytes. There are five classes of immunoglobulins in humans: IgG, IgM, IgE, IgA, and IgD. Only the functions of the first four classes are known. Immunoglobulins are composed of heavy and light chains of protein (Fig. 5-1). The active binding site of the antibody molecule is part of a region of variable amino acid composition, which gives the antibody its specificity. Amino acid composition of the heavy and light chains has been delineated for some immunoglobulins and has been shown to differ from one immunoglobulin to another. *Multiple myeloma* is a malignancy of the plasma cells (Fig. 5-2) that results in tremendous overproduction of immunoglobulins, sometimes of one particular type and sometimes of a number of different types. These immunoglobulins are usually of the IgG class. Individuals with multiple myeloma often excrete

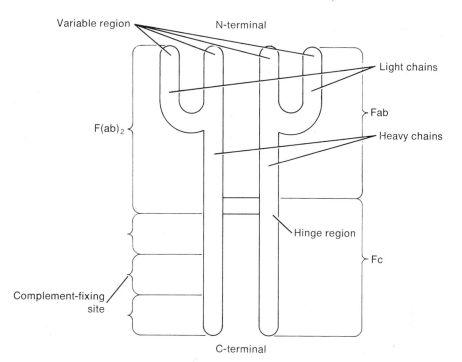

Fig. 5-1. Immunoglobulin molecule. Immunoglobulins are proteins made up of heavy and light chains of amino acids. Regions of variable amino acid composition are indicated. This determines which antigens immunoglobulin will bind to. Complement-attaching (-fixing) site also exists.

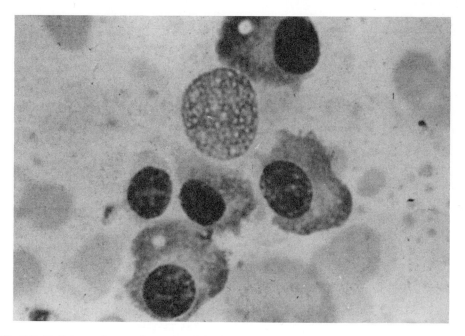

Fig. 5-2. Multiple myeloma cells are found in abundance in blood and lymphoid tissue of patients. They produce Bence Jones proteins and are malignant plasma cells. (Courtesy Department of Pathology, University of Tennessee, Memphis.)

Bence Jones proteins, which are in reality light chains of immunoglobulin molecules. Thus, a source of light chains for study is provided by the blood and urine of these individuals. Heavy chains are also produced in a specific disease state known as *heavy chain disease,* which is also a neoplasm of the plasma cells.

IgA (immunoglobulin A). IgA makes up only 5% to 10% of the serum immunoglobulins and has a half-life of 7 days. It is composed of two light and two heavy chains. IgA is concentrated in the respiratory and gastrointestinal tracts, namely, in saliva, tears, and gastrointestinal secretions. It has a specific configuration, which differs from its structure in the interstitial tissues, when it is found in the exposed surfaces of the respiratory and gastrointestinal tracts. This specific configuration results from the attachment of a *secretory component,* thought to be synthesized in epithelial cells, to IgA. This allows IgA to attach to exposed surfaces and to withstand the harsh environments where it is usually found.

IgG (immunoglobulin G). IgG is the major immunoglobulin of the blood. It is found in high concentrations within the lymphoid follicles, where it is secreted by B-lymphocytes. The structure of IgG is extremely similar to IgA, namely, two light and two heavy chains. It plays its major role in recognizing microorganisms and facilitating the removal of these invaders by phagocytes. IgG also has the ability to activate complement. It is able to pass from the blood into the interstitial space and also to pass quite easily through the placenta, thus providing the fetus and newborn with maternally acquired immunity until the infant is able to produce sufficient immunoglobulins to render it safe in a germ-filled world.

IgE (immunoglobulin E). IgE (formerly known as reagin) has been convincingly demonstrated to be the immunoglobulin involved in allergic, anaphylactic, and atopic reactions.

IgM (immunoglobulin M). IgM makes up about 10% of the serum immunoglobulins. Its structure has been postulated to be made up of ten heavy and ten light chains. Its size prevents it from traversing through capillary barriers, and it reacts therefore with foreign antigens in the bloodstream. It is also capable of activating complement. IgM is believed to be the major immunoglobulin produced during infancy, with colostrum and breast milk providing maternal immunoglobulins of the other classes.

IgD (immunoglobulin D). Although IgD has been definitively described in human serums, its function remains unknown at this time. It comprises about 1% of the total immunoglobulins in the serum, and it has an extremely rapid half-life.

Nature of the antigen-antibody reaction

The extraordinary ability of the immune system to react with at least 1 million different possible antigens during a human's lifetime is thought to be due to the production (by about 15% of the total DNA) of immunoglobulin molecules, which have the distinct capability of reacting with specific antigens. This specificity is the most striking characteristic of the immune system. It is not known how this specificity arises, but there are two schools of thought. One theory holds that antigens induce the formation of specific antibodies, and the second theory holds that all the immunoglobulins that could possibly be needed by a person are produced early in fetal life and are available whenever an antigen is presented to the system. Once the foreign antigen has been recognized, the response is amplified by the action of a B cell clone, which stimulates the production of the same immunoglobulin.

The reaction of antigen and antibody has been likened to a lock-and-key interaction. The lock-and-key reaction requires a tight molecular fit, which is specific to the two molecules that are reacting. Occasionally cross-reactivity occurs, when one antigen so closely resembles another that the same antibodies can attach to both antigens. This is believed to be the basis for certain streptococcal-induced diseases, such as glomerulonephritis and rheumatic fever. Generally, however, the antigen-antibody reaction is unique to its components.

Serologic responses

The serologic results of the antigen-antibody reaction are, however, not unique. A number

Table 5-1. Major serologic reactions involving the immune system

	Neutralization	Agglutination	Complement fixation	Precipitation
Reaction	Toxin-antitoxin reactions: bacterial exotoxin (powerful poisonous enzyme released from bacterial cells) reacts with specific antitoxin obtained from immune animal when both injected into host animal	Complexing of *insoluble* antigens to antibody	Complexing of antigen with antibody with result that complement is activated	Complexing of *soluble* antigen with immune antiserum At optimal ratios of antigen to antibody, a precipitate forms in the body
Example	Tetanus antitoxin administered to patients infected with *Clostridium tetani* neutralizes the exotoxin	Erythrocytes are hemagglutinated by antibodies against the erythrocyte's surface antigens	Arthus reaction and immune complex disease	Certain forms of glomerulonephritis

of possible phenomena may result from the combining of antigen with antibody in the blood. These include (1) neutralization, (2) agglutination, (3) complement fixation, and (4) precipitation (Table 5-1).

These serologic reactions in Table 5-1 are now explained at the molecular level in terms of immunoglobulin reactions, cell surface phenomena, and complement activation. They can occur in the test tube, in which case they are used as a diagnostic aid. For example, neutralization forms the basis of the antistreptolysin O (ASO) test; agglutination is observed in various antibody titration tests (e.g., Widal's test, Weil-Felix test); complement fixation is the basic phenomenon occurring in the Wasserman test; and precipitation occurs in the VDRL test, and in the *Streptococcus* grouping.

AGGLUTINATION
Blood transfusion reactions

An important blood transfusion reaction is agglutination in that it is the basis of blood group incompatibilities, which are experienced by newborns and by patients receiving incompatible blood transfusions. There are four major blood antigen types: A, B, AB, and O. Individuals with erythrocytes bearing A antigens have antibodies of the IgG type, which react with B antigens, and normally there would be no B antigen–containing erythrocytes present in this blood. However, if a transfusion of type B blood was received, the donor erythrocytes would react with the serum antibodies of the recipient, causing a massive agglutination or clumping of the donor cells. The reverse process is observed in patients with blood group B who receive a transfusion of type A blood. The type O designation is reserved for individuals whose erythrocytes bear neither A or B antigens. This blood, called the universal donor, is therefore acceptable blood for emergency transfusion since it does not often elicit a transfusion hemagglutination reaction. Individuals with type O blood have antibodies for both A and B antigens in their blood serum, but these antibodies are usually so diluted by the recipient's blood that no reaction occurs. The AB blood type contains no antibodies to A or B antigens, but the erythrocytes contain A and B antigens. Therefore, AB blood is considered the universal recipient. The antigens are produced as gene products, and the blood group is inherited from the parents as either the homozygous (OO, AA, BB) or heterozygous (AO, BO) state. It has recently been shown that type O blood does contain antigen which appears to be a precursor to the A and B antigens. This antigen is known as H substance, and thus the blood group genotypic system is referred to now as the ABO(H) system. Agglutination of incompatible blood results in a reaction that can be immediate and dramatic. The clumped red blood cells can obstruct vessels, and ischemia and necrosis may result. Patients experience pain and dyspnea; shock may occur. Renal failure may also result from obstruction of the glomerular vessels, leading to necrosis of the tubules and renal damage.

Erythroblastosis fetalis

An analogous situation to blood transfusion agglutination is the disease erythroblastosis fetalis, or hemolytic disease of the newborn. In this disease the presence of an Rh antigen on the erythrocytes of the fetus and the absence of this antigen on the erythrocytes of the mother lead to immunization of the mother such that she produces antibodies to the Rh antigen, which can traverse the placenta and which react with and result in lysis of the fetal erythrocytes. The fetus attempts to compensate for the excessive hemolysis by erythropoiesis, which results in an increased number of primitive erythroblasts in the blood. These cells are not as capable of oxygen transport, the blood is more viscous, and the hemolysis of the cells leads to jaundice and kernicterus (the deposition of bilirubin in the nervous tissue), which leads to irreversible damage. Many of these infants are spontaneously aborted or are stillborn. (If children with erythroblastosis fetalis do survive birth, they are usually high risk and may have to be exchange transfused a number of times.)

Since immunization of the mother with the infant's blood takes place during the first pregnancy and especially during the birth process itself, the first child is not at risk. It has been possible to prevent the development of this condition in susceptible families by the administration of RhoGAM to mothers after the birth of the first child. RhoGAM is anti-Rh_0 gamma globulin, which acts to destroy any fetal cells of an Rh-positive nature that enter the mother's circulation before they can produce an antibody response to the Rh antigen. Thus, infants of subsequent pregnancies usually are protected from erythroblastosis fetalis.

CELLS OF THE IMMUNE SYSTEM
B cells

T- and B-lymphocytes and their origins in humans have previously been discussed. While it is known that T-lymphocytes are thymus dependent, the B-lymphocytes are not presently known to require interaction with any glands or structures in order to assume their unique identity. Some possible sites through which the B cells may pass on their way from the bone marrow to the lymph nodes and peripheral blood include the fetal liver, Peyer's patches, and the appendix in the intestine. B cells are known to acquire identity in the bursa of Fabricius in the chicken, an animal that has provided us with a wealth of information about the immune system. Within the bursa the B cells develop during embryonic life and begin to produce immunoglobulins, and in fact if chicken embryos are "bursectomized," the chickens will develop a variety of immunodeficient states. The development of these immunoglobulin-producing cells is not dependent upon the introduction of any foreign antigenic material and thus must be considered genetically programmed. Once the immunoglobulin-producing B cell is formed in the bursa, further expansion of these compartments of cells requires stimulation by foreign antigens. Controversy exists over whether these B cells are multipotential before reacting with antigen or whether they become "committed" only upon exposure to the antigen. The induction of this antigen-requiring differentiation of B-lymphocytes requires T cells as "helpers," and the end product of this process is the differentiation of the B cell to an active immunoglobulin-producing plasma cell. It would appear that the antigen selects the B cells that are producing the specific immunoglobulin with which it can react, and once this system is activated by the reaction, the B cell differentiation proceeds rapidly, resulting in a clone of B cells, which differentiate to plasma cells. The plasma cells in turn pour out the specific immunoglobulin that binds to that antigen. Furthermore, the clone of cells often persists for many years, producing the antibody that therefore makes the individual immune to the antigen for as long as the plasma cells exist and produce sufficient antibody.

B cells cannot be morphologically distinguished from T cells except under close examination by electron microscopy (scanning electron microscopy of T and B cells shows that the B cells have longer microvilli). Within the peripheral blood smear there are no obvious differences, however. These cells have been identified in the 9-week-old human embryo, and thus the differentiation of this immune component occurs very early in intrauterine life. Both B cells and T cells are found in greatest abundance in the lymphoid tissue, which is found throughout the body in discrete accumulations known as lymph nodes or in other structures such as tonsillar tissue, spleen, bone marrow, and thymus. They also occur in the peripheral blood, constituting about 35% of the leukocytes, and they exist as well in the tissue spaces. B cells appear to be responsible for immunity to encapsulated pyogenic pathogens.

T cells

T cells or thymus-derived lymphocytes originate in the fetal hematopoietic tissue, as do all the blood cells, and then migrate during embryogenesis to the bone marrow. Those lymphocytes that will become committed as T cells leave the bone marrow and pass from the bone marrow through the thymus as "traffic" before passing on to seed the lymphoid tissues of the body, a process that takes several days. This system was originally described in chickens but is known to also occur in humans. The thymus gland is located in the mediastinum and is large in infancy and childhood, involuting greatly during adult life. Infants have occasionally been born without a thymus gland and are totally deficient in cellular immunity, entirely lacking T-lymphocytes. The thymus gland is known to have at least two functions, the first being differentiation of primitive lymphocytes into immunocompetent T cells, and the second being the further expansion of antigen-stimulated T cells, perhaps by the production of extracts or hormonal substances such as thymosin. The T cell is known to react with antigens on its cellular surface, but the nature of the cell membrane receptors of T cells is not clear at this time. While B cells certainly produce immunoglobulins and react initially with antigen by a surface immunoglobulin reaction, the same process has not been well described in T cells. The T cell may make immunoglobu-

lin, which then functions as its receptor molecule, or it may absorb antibodies onto its surface, possibly IgM produced by B cells, which then functions as the T cell antigen receptor. T cells can be identified by their ability to respond to certain chemicals known as *mitogens*. Mitogens such as phytohemagglutinin, a kidney bean extract, cause T cells to transform and divide. T cells also can be identified by their ability to form "rosettes" with sheep erythrocytes. Other more easily determined differentiating markers of T and B cells do not exist at the present time.

The nature of the T cell response to antigen was detailed in Chapter 4 in the discussion of delayed hypersensitivity. The complexity of the T cell reaction to antigen is becoming more apparent as further research is done. Macrophages appear to play an important role in identifying and processing antigen before presenting it to T- and perhaps B-lymphocytes. The macrophage's presence appears to be physically required for T cells to be stimulated by foreign antigens. Furthermore, macrophages are now known to secrete various substances such as enzymes, and molecules, which stimulate or modulate lymphocytes. Many of these substances have not as yet been characterized. Macrophages appear to interact initially with foreign antigen by phagocytosing the antigen and reacting it with a protein product of the immune responsiveness gene. This gene is linked to the major histocompatibility antigen genes, known as the HL-A system. The nature of the HL-A system will be discussed later in this chapter. The interaction of the immune responsiveness gene product with antigen alters the antigen, and then the macrophage presents the altered antigen, a process that appears to require physical contact, to the lymphocytes, which recognize it as "non-self," become sensitized, stimulated, and proliferative (Fig. 5-3). T cells are known to mediate cellular immunity, calling forth a typical inflammatory reaction, and are also required as helpers to B cells. This T cell requirement appears early in the life of the B cell, perhaps as early as its second stage of differentiation from an uncommitted to a committed immunoglobulin-producing plasma cell. The T cell–B cell inter-

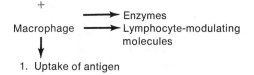

Foreign antigen

+

Macrophage → Enzymes → Lymphocyte-modulating molecules

↓

1. Uptake of antigen

↓

2. Interaction of immune responsiveness gene product with antigen

↓

Altered antigen formed

↓

Macrophage presentation of altered antigen to T cells and B cells

↓

T cell recognition of nonself; B cells produce Abs

↓

T cell proliferation

↓

Clone of sensitized T cells formed

Fig. 5-3. Macrophage processing of antigen. It is believed that macrophages "process" antigen, preparing it in some unknown manner, before presenting it to lymphocytes. After interaction with macrophages, antigen is then ready to be identified by immune lymphocytes. Abs = antibodies.

action may occur in an oblique rather than a direct cell-cell manner. For example, antigens may be processed by an interaction with macrophages, specific T cells, and then with B cells. DiGeorge's syndrome is a condition in which the patient is born without a thymus gland. These individuals do not possess T cells but are able to produce immunoglobulins quite adequately. Therefore, the significance of the T cell helper function is not clear at this time, at least in humans. T cell–suppressor function has also been described and appears to be involved in the development of self-immunity. Suppressor T cells may inhibit the production of certain immunoglobulins by B cells.

Transfer factor

T cell responsiveness is required (1) for maximal protection of the host from bacterial, viral, parasitic, and mycotic microorganisms, (2) for autoimmune phenomenon, and (3) for rejection of malignant cells and transplant tissue. One important characteristic of the T cell response is the ability of a cell-free leukocyte extract to transfer cellular immunologic reactivity to an antigen from one host to another. The nature

of the component in the cell-free extract remains obscure, but this elusive factor has been named transfer factor, and much recent research has been dedicated to identifying, characterizing, and therapeutically administering transfer factor. Transfer factor preparations have been used clinically in the treatment of many diseases; the first disease so treated was chronic mucocutaneous candidiasis. Since then immunodeficiency diseases such as thymic hypoplasia and Wiskott-Aldrich syndrome have been treated with transfer factor. The results of this treatment were transitory increases in delayed hypersensitivity, as measured by skin testing, and resistance to infection. Chronic viral, fungal, and certain facultative bacterial infections are extremely common in individuals with depressed T cell immunity, and treatment of these infections with transfer factor has been quite successful.

The use of transfer factor in the treatment of malignancies is becoming more and more common. Cancer cells have certain specific antigens against which the immune system attempts to react (see Chapter 3). The immune system is often depressed in the cancer patient as the result of both the disease process and the therapy. Immunodeficient individuals also have a greatly increased risk of cancer, and transfer factor for individuals with metastatic fatal cancers therefore seems justified. The source of transfer factor is often close contacts of the affected patient. Family members often show an immunologic reactivity to tumor antigens derived from the tumorous tissue of the patient. This has been described particularly in the families of patients with malignant melanomas. Some tumors that have been treated with transfer factor include malignant melanoma, breast carcinoma, Hodgkin's disease, nasopharyngeal carcinoma, and widely disseminated metastatic cancers of various types. The success of transfer factor in producing tumor regression is currently being evaluated, but for certain patients there is no question that transfer factor administration has been beneficial.

The action of transfer factor remains totally obscure, but one theory suggests that once injected, the transfer factor turns on a cascade of normally inactive events. This cascade causes unidentified immunologic phenomena to occur and results in an immune responsiveness that was formerly absent in the individual.

Null cells

A third class of immune lymphocytes, null cells, has been described. Little is known about the function of these cells, but they may be able to transform into B cells.

DISEASE STATES

While most categories of immune dysfunction will be presented here, a number of disease models will be elaborated upon as representative of immune disease. It should be obvious to the student at this point that essentially no disease state is isolated from some interaction with the immune system, but certain conditions share an actual intimate cause-and-effect relationship with the immune system. Best exemplifying this condition are the immunodeficiency diseases, some of which have been alluded to previously.

Immunodeficiency states

The first well-described immunodeficient state was X-linked infantile agammaglobuline-mia, in which patients lack B cells but have apparently normal T cell reactivity. Since that discovery, more than 20 immunologic disorders have been described. These disorders can be classified according to which cell type is affected and at what point in the development of the cellular system the disease process has intervened. Thus, stem cell, B cell, T cell, and combined B and T cell immunodeficiency diseases have been discovered in humans.

Stem cell immunodeficiency. Over 200 cases of a condition known as severe combined immunodeficiency (SCID) have been described. These children have a striking lymphopenia and overwhelming susceptibility to infections; this condition is now thought to be the most common immunodeficiency disease. It is believed that the disease process usually results from the early lack of a stem cell, which would normally give rise to lymphocytes in the bone marrow. Thus, the bone marrow contains very few lymphocytes, and the thymus is dysplastic, contains no or few lymphocytes, and is located in the neck rather than the mediastinum. There is an absence of cellular immunity, and antibody synthesis, and there is very little immunoglobulin in the blood. Lymphopenia may be profound, and the lymphocytes that are present are immature. This overwhelming disease invariably is associated with fatal infection. Half those affected with SCID have a marked deficiency in an enzyme, adenosine deaminase. It is possible that the lack of this enzyme results in the accumulation of adenosine, which may then act to inhibit T and B cell differentiation during early development.

Physiology of treatment. Treatment of these infants has been difficult. The hereditary nature of the condition is known, and certain infants have been isolated from birth in germ-free (gnotobiotic) chambers that protect them from the environment. Such measures are aimed at maintaining these children until appropriate treatment can be instituted. The most practical treatment is bone marrow transplantation, which is the intraperitoneal injection of bone marrow containing immunocompetent stem cells. The major difficulty in bone marrow transplantation is the use of completely histocompatible cells. Histocompatibility antigens of the HL-A system are a major basis for de-termining the tissue type of a donor and a re-cipient. These are cellular antigens, which are, of course, genetically determined, and there-fore the possibility of two individuals possess-ing the same or similar HL-A antigens is great-ly increased in relatives. It is interesting to note that the identification of HL-A antigens, which has been so useful for tissue typing, has also resulted in the discovery of certain associations of HL-A antigens with disease states.

Occasionally SCID patients have been treated with thymus transplants, and some have received fetal liver cells. Again the major prob-lem is graft versus host reactions, leading to severe disease and eventual death. Another form of therapy for patients with this disease who have not had transplants, due to lack of a suitable donor, is the use of thymosin, a hor-mone produced by the thymus gland, and trans-fer factor. The use of these agents requires that some lymphoid precursor cells be present.

B cell immunodeficiency. When the pro-duction of adequate numbers of B cells is dis-turbed, humoral immunity is impaired. The best example of this condition is infantile X-linked agammaglobulinemia. There is a delay between birth and the onset of signs and symptoms of this immunodeficient state due to the retention of maternal immunoglobulins by the child. By about 9 months of age, however, these children begin to develop severe infections caused by pyogenic organisms such as staphylococcus, pneumococcus, streptococcus, and *Hemophilus influenzae*. The children are not unusually sus-ceptible to viral or enterobacteria infections. The disease affects boys only, and in addition to recurrent infection a variety of collagenlike symptoms and signs are observed. There is also a high incidence of hemolytic anemia, eczema, and allergy.

The response of these patients to infection is often bizarre. Delayed hypersensitivity is either slightly reduced or normal, yet the blood lym-phocyte count is normal. The diagnostic cri-terion for this condition is the absence of plas-ma cells in antigen-stimulated lymph nodes. The lymphoid tissue is also often disorganized, and frequently tonsils are atrophic or absent. The physiology of treatment of these patients

is replacement of the missing immunoglobu-lins, particularly IgG. Gamma globulin is therefore given regularly, with antibiotics also occasionally being administered prophylac-tically. Commercially prepared IgA, IgE, and IgM are not presently available, and therefore a source of immunoglobulins of all classes is donor plasma infusion.

Several variants of infantile X-linked agam-maglobulinemia have been described. One such situation appears to be agammaglobulinemia caused by a block in the maturation of B-lymphocytes so that they never actually release immunoglobulins into the blood.

Other B cell disorders have been described in which there is a selective loss of some and retention of other immunoglobulin production capability. An example of this is IgA defi-ciency, in which there is a normal or increased number of lymphocytes, but the concentration of IgA in the blood and other secretions is minimal, and there is an absence of IgA-syn-thesizing plasma cells. There appears there-fore to be a maturation block in the develop-ment of IgA-synthesizing plasma cells. IgA de-ficiency is often found in normal individuals with no signs of disease (in fact, it was dis-covered by two healthy immunologists to be ab-sent in their own blood). Some cases are asso-ciated with steatorrhea and nontropical sprue (see Chapter 14). The lack of IgA in the gastro-intestinal tract may play an important role in the etiology of these conditions. There is also a lack of IgA in the disease ataxia-telangiectasia, which is a hereditary disease associated with a defect in cellular immunity. Ataxia begins dur-ing infancy, but the typical skin lesions do not appear until childhood.

T cell immunodeficiency. The best de-scribed disease that results from a defect in T cell–mediated immunity is DiGeorge's syn-drome. In this rare condition there is a con-genital anomaly that results in the partial or to-tal absence of the parathyroid and thymus glands. Both of these structures are derived from the embryonic pharyngeal pouches, and both glands arise simultaneously during em-bryogenesis. It is therefore believed that this syndrome results from the action of teratogenic influences on these developing structures. It is interesting to note in this regard that congenital heart disease, most commonly tetralogy of Fallot, is usually found as well. These infants usually are hypocalcemic and are extremely susceptible to infection. There is normal B cell humoral immunity, but cellular immunity is absent. In cases where some thymic and parathyroid tissue is present, the disease may follow a relatively less morbid course, and some T cell capability is acquired in both the severe and mild forms of the disease if the children survive to 4 or 5 years old.

Physiology of treatment. Fetal thymic transplants have been used to treat children with T cell immunodeficiency; even in children with 10% to 20% of the normal amount of thymic tissue, tiny amounts of fetal thymus can result in the production of a state of immunocompetence in the previously immunodeficient child. Therefore, it is apparent that the absolute amount of thymus gland tissue is not the sole criterion for the production of adequate T cell–mediated cellular immunity.

T and B cell immunodeficiency. The last category of immunodeficiency encompasses a large number of disease states that are associated with impairment of both B and T cell immunity. A disease model that illustrates this spectrum of complex disorders is the Wiskott-Aldrich syndrome. The immunologic defect that produces this disease appears to result from an inability of the immune system to initiate a response to antigen, rather than a primary defect in the immune cells' capability. There is usually a normal number of B and T cells, and in vitro tests indicate that the cells are able to launch an immune response to antigen. Therefore, the disease originates somewhere in the so-called afferent limb of the immune response, the efferent limb being that part of the immune response in which T and B cells are activated to react normally to antigen. The afferent limb then consists of the processing of antigen by lymphoid and accessory phagocytic cells before the antigen is presented to immunocompetent cells with which it then combines and initiates the typical immune response. The signs and symptoms of the Wiskott-Aldrich syndrome include thrombocytopenia, eczema, and repeated episodes of many different types

of infection. There is also an increased incidence of malignancy in these patients. The condition is genetically transmitted as an X-linked trait and is therefore found only in males. This disease has been successfully treated with transfer factor, the effects of which may last as long as a year.

Summary. Although many other immunodeficiency diseases do exist, all of these conditions are extremely rare. The most common types of immune disorder, in fact, cannot be easily classified. A discussion of the unusual disorders, such as has been pursued here, is justified for several reasons, however. Study of these conditions has led to a tremendous growth in the knowledge of the immune system function. From this understanding of the normal physiology have come better ways to treat a great variety of diseases, many of which are not primarily immune in nature. The common denominator in all disease may be the immune system, and the types of manipulation, including cellular engineering, that researchers are beginning to do is exciting and perhaps the most important of all applied medical research. Once an understanding of the graft versus host reaction is fully reached, and the nature of histocompatibility is clear, organ transplantations of all types are conceivable, thus extending the length and quality of human life. Furthermore, the aging process (see Chapter 18) may be the result of immunologic decay and as such may be significantly delayed by immunologic manipulation.

ALLERGY

An allergic condition is a pathophysiologic response of the immune system. Even within susceptible individuals, the pathophysiologic presentation of an allergic reaction differs remarkably, a phenomenon that in part may be due to inherent circadian (daily) rhythms in susceptibility. Many asthmatic patients, for example, suffer acute attacks at night. The manifestation of allergy in susceptible individuals varies, ranging from chronic rhinitis (inflammation of the nasal cavities) to sudden death from acute anaphylactic shock. The symptoms of all allergic disorders are, nevertheless, related to the release of substances such as histamine and slow-reactive substance of anaphylaxis (SRS-A). These mediators are released primarily as a result of mast cell and basophil stimulation by an IgE-antigen complex. The recent discovery of the importance of IgE in the allergic response has opened up new areas in research and treatment of allergies. IgE is present in only tiny amounts in the blood, but this concentration is increased in allergic diseases such as hay fever and asthma.

Mechanism of IgE-produced allergy

The role of IgE in normal, nonallergic individuals is not clear, but it would be surprising that nature has allowed this gene-determined antibody to persist unless there was some selective advantage to it. Evidence is accumulating to suggest that IgE and the immune allergic response it provokes in most susceptible people is pathophysiologic in civilized societies. In present-day primitive tribes and in humans' early ancestors, IgE plays and played a role in controlling parasitic, especially helminthic, infestations. This protective IgE-mediated reaction takes place mainly in the gut mucosa. An IgE reaction also results in the release of heparin from mast cells, and heparin is involved in protection of the host against certain infections, snake venoms, and microbial metabolites. Thus, atopic sensitivity is the bothersome expression of a potentially useful mechanism in certain environments. Humans as a species have not been freed from these types of parasitic and microbial threats long enough for natural selection mechanisms to operate in the elimination of the IgE reaction.

The term "atopy" implies a susceptibility to develop immediate hypersensitivity reactions, or allergies. Four factors are usually present in the atopic individual: (1) signs and symptoms, (2) a family history of atopy, (3) skin reactivity (usually a weal and flare) to injected allergens, and (4) eosinophilia. The atopic individual reacts to antigens in the environment by sensitization rather than immunization. Instead of producing an immune reaction that removes the antigen from the blood and tissues by an antigen-antibody complex, which can be phagocytosed or otherwise eliminated, the atopic individual continuously combines certain antigens, or allergens, with IgE. This antigen-antibody complex then attaches to the surface membranes of basophils, which are leukocytes, and mast cells, which are cells found along the walls of blood vessels and scattered throughout the tissues. There is then a concentration of the allergen on these cells, which respond by degranulation, or exocytosis of their large intracellular granules. The granules are believed to contain histamine, heparin, and other substances, and the degranulation process involves intracellular microtubules in a step that requires Ca^{++}. These mediators are then free to exert their effects. Histamine, for example, causes weal formation, itching, bronchoconstriction, and hypotension. SRS-A is also released during the degranulation process, although probably not from the granules per se. This mediator is believed to be the major substance in intrinsic asthma (see Chapter 8), and new evidence suggests that it may also be released from polymorphonuclear leukocytes. SRS-A is produced in great quantities by lung mast cells during an allergic respiratory reaction, and it is a potent bronchoconstrictor, which could account for wheezing, which is the major pathophysiologic manifestation of asthma. Various prostaglandins are also released with SRS-A. Their role was discussed in Chapter 4. It is believed that during allergic reactions these compounds may sensitize nerve endings to bradykinin, thus causing itching and pain.

The molecular events surrounding degranulation of the mast cells (Fig. 5-4) and basophils have not been completely described, but good evidence that cyclic AMP is involved has come from a number of sources. The target cells of the allergic reaction appear to have a number of different cell membrane receptors, one of which is a beta-adrenergic receptor for epinephrine. When epinephrine combines with the beta receptor, there is a rise in cyclic AMP concentration and a subsequent block in degranulation. Thus, a mode of action for epinephrine and other antiallergic agents in acute allergic reactions is suggested at the cellular level, in addition to their well-known bronchodilator and vasoconstrictor effects. Cyclic AMP is the "second messenger" for a number of

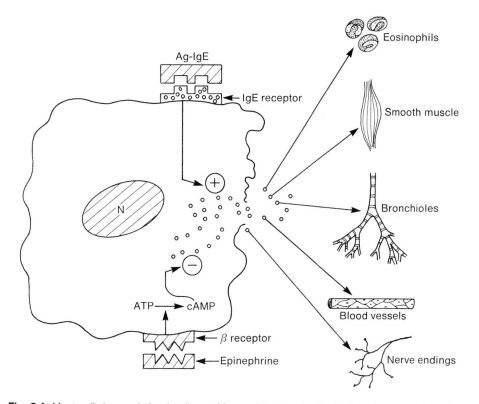

Fig. 5-4. Mast cell degranulation in allergy. Mast cell is target cell of IgE-antigen complex, shown schematically as attaching to membrane receptors and initiating events in mast cell that lead to degranulation. Granules contain histamine, slow-reactive substance of anaphylaxis, and perhaps other mediators, which act on nerve endings, blood vessels, bronchiolar and other smooth muscle, and eosinophils. Effects produced on these targets cause allergic responses such as eczema and asthma. Epinephrine acts in an inhibitory manner on degranulation by stimulating cAMP formation.

hormonal actions. It is converted from ATP by the action of membrane-bound adenyl cyclase, an enzyme that is activated by the "first messenger," which is the hormone. Thus, cyclic AMP signals the cell that hormonal stimulation is present, and a variety of phenomena, depending on the hormone and other factors in the cellular environment, takes place. In the case of mast cells and basophils, activation of adenyl cyclase by epinephrine blocks degranulation. Binding of the IgE-allergen complex to the cell membrane conversely causes a fall in adenyl cyclase, which appears to be associated in an unknown manner with initiation of degranulation.

Histamine itself, which is released in large amounts from the mast cells and basophils, may exert an autoregulatory influence on the degranulation process by acting in a negative feedback manner on these cells, inhibiting degranulation when present in sufficient quantities. Histamine cell membrane receptors have been suggested to exist on these cells.

Mast cells and basophils also release a substance that is chemotactic for eosinophils, and eosinophilia is a characteristic of atopy. This substance (ECF-A, eosinophil chemotactic factor in anaphylaxis) not only attracts eosinophils but also causes these cells to release the enzyme aryl sulfatase, which inactivates SRS-A. Other factors present in eosinophils may inhibit histamine release and function. Eosinophils then are thought to act as a "switch off" mechanism to the acute hypersensitivity response of allergen and IgE. Eosinophils are also mildly phagocytic, and their true function in allergy is just being discovered. They are increased in concentration in the blood of individuals with parasitic, particularly helminthic, infestations. This is an interesting corollary to the role of the IgE response to helminthic infections, which was previously described.

Theories of atopy. While the basic mechanism of atopy is the combining of particular antigens to IgE, it is not at all clear why certain individuals are more prone to atopy than others. About 20% of the United States population suffers from some form of allergy. Four major theories of atopy are presently being investigated. The first theory is that susceptible individuals are more prone to produce skin-sensitizing antibodies of the IgE type in response to repetitive low doses of antigens. In the second theory it is suggested that the atopic individual has an intrinsic enzyme deficiency or defect such that antigens that penetrate the body barriers are retained for longer periods than in normal people, and there is increased antibody formation in response. The third theory suggests that there is an enhanced reactivity to the mediators that are released from mast cells and basophils during an IgE-mediated reaction, and the fourth theory implicates the local defenses of the body, so that an increased concentration of antigen is absorbed into the body across mucous membranes.

It is possible that no single theory will be found to encompass all possible atopic reactions. The mechanisms involved in asthma, for example, appear to be somewhat different from those involved in allergic atopic dermatitis or eczema. There is some evidence to suggest that atopic individuals respond to antigens by secreting IgE, while the normal individual produces protective types of antibodies, such as IgA and IgG. Others believe that everyone has the possibility of developing atopy, but there is a genetically programmed threshold of antigen for each person, above which an allergic reaction will ensue. Another possibility is that the atopic response is due to a primary deficiency in the IgA system, which then causes an overstimulation of the IgE antibodies. Furthermore, it has been shown that IgG antibodies play some role in the regulation of the IgE response, as IgE falls when IgG rises, so that the primary defect may rest in the gamma globulins. The thymus may be involved as well in IgE regulation.

Whatever theory is finally accepted, medical management of atopy will always focus on prevention of damaging symptoms, such as wheezing, skin rashes, swelling, and hay fever.

Physiology of treatment. Common allergens exist for those who are atopic, including pollens, certain foods, drugs, dust, insect venoms, molds, and animal dandruff (dander). The most common allergic condition, hay fever, affects 20 million persons in the United States. It has an hereditary background in that at least the susceptibility to hay fever is apparent within families. Hay fever is seasonal, being most related to the environmental concentration of ragweed pollen. Treatment of hay fever involves the careful administration of antihistaminic drugs, which compete with histamine for specific cell membrane receptors, displacing the histamine molecule and preventing its action. Another approach to severe allergy, including hay fever, is immunotherapy. The individual is desensitized to the allergen by repeated injections of minute amounts of ragweed pollen extract. The antigen present in the extract causes the development of specific IgG over time, which can then function as a ''blocking'' antibody to the IgE-allergen combination, preventing target cell degranulation. Suppressor T cells may also be stimulated during long-term immunotherapy.

Although hay fever, with its accompanying swollen nasopharyngeal mucosa, rhinitis, sinusitis, headache, and general malaise is the purest model of immunologic allergy, three other conditions, which are in reality complex disorders, serve as good models of allergic processes: atopic dermatitis, asthma, and anaphylaxis.

Atopic dermatitis

Atopic dermatitis is allergic in nature and is caused by environmental allergens that are either ingested or inhaled. Most infantile eczema can be classified this way, but the condition can develop at any time in life. Lesions are often located in the skin creases and folds, on the face, genitalia, and antecubital and popliteal areas. They are scaly, dry, itchy lesions, which can be either nummular or diffuse. These lesions are susceptible to superinfection, particularly with vaccinia virus, herpes, and bacteria such as *Staphylococcus*. In infants, widespread, disseminated, infected skin lesions can develop after a smallpox vaccination, and the disease that results can be serious enough to cause death.

While allergic mechanisms are known to operate in the development of atopic dermatitis, it is certainly possible that contributory factors play just as important a role. For example, the atopic individual often perspires more than normal, and the sweat is less able to solubilize oil. The skin is often very dry as well. These factors may combine to produce a state in which the sebaceous glands become plugged with oil, resulting in local areas of skin breakdown at which eczematous lesions arise. Wool is extremely irritating to the skin of the atopic individual and provokes the typical lesions of atopic dermatitis. The increased incidence of exacerbations of the disease in the winter months is thought to be due to both dryness of heated indoor spaces and the heavy clothing required in the colder months. Eczema that develops in infancy often follows an irregular course characterized by periods of quiescence and then sudden flare-ups, which are thought to occasionally be due to emotional stress. In up to half of those children with persistent childhood eczema, respiratory manifestations of allergy develop later in childhood and adolescence. The penetrance of the genetic factors that control atopy are probably greatly influenced by environmental factors. For example, avoidance of certain notorious allergens in early infancy, such as chocolate, eggs, and even cow's milk, may prevent both skin and respiratory manifestations in the potentially atopic individual. An autosomal dominant gene or groups of genes with weak penetrance are postulated in most cases. There is evidence that the X chromosome carries these genes, which influence IgE synthesis. There is also further evidence of genetic factors as the atopic individual has increased levels of certain histocompatibility antigens, primarily HL-A3 and HL-A9. The general association of autoantigens and disease will be discussed later in this chapter. It should be mentioned that contact dermatitis caused by chemical irritants can be atopic.

Asthma

Atopic asthma is a respiratory distress disorder manifested within minutes after a second or subsequent exposure to a particular allergen. It is characterized by bronchial and bronchiolar constriction, which leads to acute dyspnea, in which expiratory stridor or wheezing is the major sign. SRS-A and histamine are thought to cause vasodilation, subsequent edema, and bronchoconstriction, producing symptoms of wheezing, itching, sneezing, and coughing. Bronchospasm, increased secretions and accumulation of secretions, aggravates the asthmatic attack.

The first exposure to the offending allergen usually is not noticeable, as it results only in sensitization of the individual. This process causes the immune system to be stimulated to secrete IgE antibodies, which will rise in titer over time, and when the second exposure occurs, the IgE is then available to combine with the allergen and cause the classic allergic response just discussed. Asthma in children is usually atopic in nature, but adults may have other forms of asthma, such as intrinsic or infectious asthma, which are not accompanied by an elevation of serum IgE. Children as well often develop asthmatic bronchitis during respiratory infections. The individual with asthma of an allergic nature exhibits the four major signs of atopy (see p. 120) in contrast to those with infectious or intrinsic asthma. The atopic reaction is localized to the respiratory tree and occurs in response to inhalants or ingested allergens. Allergens to which the atopic individual is hypersensitive may be determined by skin testing and thus avoided if possible. Generally, however, an atopic individual is allergic to many different substances, and the number of possible allergens tends to increase as the individual gets older.

Delineation of the underlying pathophysiology of intrinsic asthma, in which no allergen can be found, is more difficult. It has been suggested that under normal circumstances SRS-A and histamine may function to maintain normal respiratory tree muscle tone, and their effects may be held in check by epinephrine, as discussed previously in terms of cell membrane adenyl cyclase control in mast cell degranulation. If the beta-adrenergic-receptor response was inadequate, then the epinephrine regulation would be lost, and all the signs and symptoms of atopic asthma, in the nonatopic individual, would be present. This is the beta-blockade theory of intrinsic asthma, and there is good experimental support for this theory. Thus, the intrinsic asthmatic is characterized by hyperreactivity of the bronchial muscle tone.

Physiology of treatment. The presence of an acute asthmatic attack is serious and requires medical intervention. The physiology of treatment should be obvious, as the aim of therapy should be prevention of the effects of the mediators responsible for the symptoms. Thus, epinephrine or drugs that mimic epinephrine are usually given. Aminophylline, for example, is a bronchodilator that is thought to inhibit the enzyme that breaks down cyclic AMP, so that a rise in cyclic AMP then inhibits degranulation. Various inhalant sprays are now available so that the asthmatic may be able to control an impending attack through bronchodilation. Another aspect of therapy for the asthmatic is identification of the allergen(s) by skin testing and desensitization. The results of desensitization are often questionable, but research into the chemistry and ultimate purification of antigenic material may eventually result in effective prophylaxis against asthma and other atopic reactions. Another possible area of treatment may result from research into the role of the central nervous system in asthma, as it has been shown that there is interplay of nervous as well as hormonal and cellular aspects in the bronchospasm of acute asthmatic wheezing.

Anaphylaxis

The most dramatic and life threatening of all allergic diseases is anaphylactic shock. This results from the second or subsequent exposure to an allergen, usually in an individual known to be atopic. Common allergens that promote the attack are drugs, particularly penicillin, and insect venoms. Within minutes after exposure to the allergen, the individual becomes acutely ill, experiencing profound bronchoconstriction and vasodilation. The latter may be so severe as to result in shock characterized by decreasing cardiac output and falling blood pressure. There may or may not be skin urticaria, or "hives," which are skin manifestations of the IgE-allergen reaction. The mechanisms of anaphylaxis do not differ from those already described in asthma and atopic dermatitis. The manifestation of the allergic reaction is just much more pathophysiologic, and treatment is aimed at life-saving restoration of vasomotor tone and bronchial tree patency.

IMMUNE COMPLEX DISEASE

This category of immune system diseases includes serum sickness, SLE, and certain forms of glomerulonephritis; the diseases are associated with a precipitation reaction to a foreign protein and deposition of antigen-antibody complexes in the blood, kidney, and other organs to a sufficient degree that symptoms result. There is a typical allergic component to the disease, except that the reaction, which is typified by hives, or skin rashes, edema, fever, and joint pains, is not immediate in nature, typically not appearing for 7 to 10 days. The most common cause of serum sickness is the injection of bovine or horse antitoxins, or penicillin, particularly of the long-acting type. The systemic inflammatory nature of serum sickness is interesting. Aside from the deposition of immune complexes in joints, blood vessels, kidneys, and the heart, activation of complement also occurs in serum sickness. Complement activation is sufficient to produce the pathophysiologic alterations that result in tissue damage. A variety of possible processes could interact to cause the inflammation and necrosis associated with immune complex disease. Platelet aggregation is induced by the collection of immune complexes and complement along the blood vessel walls. Platelets are then stimulated to release vasoactive amines such as serotonin and histamine. Furthermore, coagulation may occur as the result of the platelet aggregation. Activation of platelet histamine and serotonin release can also be accomplished by the action of *anaphylatoxins,* which are released during the activation of the complement system. It has recently been realized that anaphylatoxins play an important role in the tissue destruction so often associated with inflammation. They are thought to be released as fragments of C3 and C5 and are therefore known as C3a and C5a. These mediators are ten times more potent than bradykinin, and thus their role in inflammation should be appreciated. Their biologic activity includes histamine release from basophils and mast cells, although the mechanism is not known, smooth muscle contraction, leukotaxis, particularly for neutrophils, eosinophils, and monocytes, and stimulation of the release of lysosomal enzymes from human neutrophils. Thus, the action of complement and the production of anaphylatoxins, along with the mechanical effects of immune complex formation and deposition, are probably sufficient to cause the pathophysiologic alterations associated with immune complex disease.

Autoimmunity

The development of tolerance to self-antigens is believed to occur very early in embryonic life, although the basic mechanisms by which this occurs have not been completely described.

It is obvious that individuals tolerate their own cells and tissues and do not form antibodies to them. When autoantibodies arise, a pathophysiologic process ensues that impairs function and ultimately destroys the individual's own cells. Diseases in which this occurs are known as autoimmune diseases. They appear generally to be acquired rather than congenital. The incidence rises with age and is greatest in immunodeficient individuals. Some diseases considered to be primarily autoimmune in nature include systemic lupus erythematosus (SLE), Hashimoto's thyroiditis, autoimmune hemolytic anemia, juvenile diabetes, rheumatoid arthritis, and multiple sclerosis.

The basic pathophysiology involves the production of autoantibodies, which can be found in the blood and tissues, to DNA, RNA, red blood cell membrane, platelets, muscle cells, gamma globulin, thyroglobulin, and brain tissue. Complexing of these autoantibodies to self-antigens results in several manifestations, depending on which type of antigen-antibody reaction occurs and which tissues are involved. Hemolysis of red blood cells occurs when the autoantibody-antigen reaction occurs on the surface of the erythrocyte. Thrombocytopenia may result if this occurs on the surface of the platelet. Chronic thyroiditis develops when the autoantibody reacts against thyroglobulin.

To understand the development of autoimmune disease, the normal production of self-tolerance should be reviewed. This is a complex and theoretic area of research. Several possible mechanisms for the development of self-tolerance have been suggested. One theory, originally put forth by Burnet, is the *forbidden clone theory*, which explains tolerance on the basis of events in early embryonic life that destroy or inactivate any lymphocytes that produce immunoglobulins against or are capable of reacting with self-antigens. Thus, self-antigens are permitted to exist within the adult. This is the classic theory of self-tolerance, and while there is much experimental evidence to support it, there are also conflicting findings in the literature. It is clear, however, that self-tolerance develops during embryonic and early neonatal life, and foreign antigens that are presented to the fetus can "fool" the primitive immune system such that they are subsequently treated as self-antigens by the adult immune system. When the animal is exposed to the same antigen later in life it does not produce antibodies against it.

It has recently been shown that the T cell system is extremely important in the development of self-tolerance. Long-lived T suppressor cells, which are capable of inhibiting B cell production of immunoglobulins, particularly IgG, are thought to be produced during early life.

Other mechanisms of immune inhibition include the production of blocking factors, which are known to exist in the serum and are probably complexes of antigen and antibody. They may compete for membrane receptors on immune cells and thus suppress certain immune responses. Their presence and the presence of unblocking factors are suggested to be important in carcinogenesis as well. These suppressive and inhibitory phenomena are thought to involve mainly cell-bound antigen reactions.

Soluble antigens in the blood and other body fluids are also recognized as self-antigens in the normal individual. Two types of tolerance may develop in response to soluble antigens injected into experimental animals, and these same types may also occur in the development of self-tolerance during the ontogeny of the immune system. These are low-dose and high-dose tolerances, both of which are mediated by the cells of the immune system.

Low-dose tolerance appears to involve only the T cells, but both T and B cells are implicated in the development of high-dose tolerance. It has been observed that when antigens are injected they are sometimes immunogenic only within a narrow dose range. Repeated injections of low doses of soluble antigenic material or administration of very high doses induces a tolerant state, such that no specific antibodies are produced in response to subsequent injection of the antigen. The low-dose effect is thought to be due to the elimination of T helper cells so that specific immunoglobulin production by B cells is inhibited. Low doses of certain antigens also result in small amounts of IgG being produced, which is thought then to act in a negative feedback manner on the production of further specific IgG. It is possible too that low doses of certain antigens may not be sufficient to produce a significant immunoglobulin production stimulation.

High doses, on the other hand, may result in paralysis of both T and B cells and may form aggregates in the body fluids, which then are not able to bind with receptors and initiate an antibody response. High-dose tolerance is often characterized by the presence of antigen in the serum, which is continually being removed by antibody. In some cases the tolerance is reversible once the antigen is eliminated by the body. It is believed that the affinity of lymphocyte receptors for different antigens may be important in low- and high-dose tolerance. Lymphocytes with high-affinity receptors are more easily stimulated by low concentrations of antigen than are lymphocytes with low-affinity receptors, but they can be inactivated by extremely high doses of antigen. In self-tolerance the lymphocytes with high-affinity recep-

tors to self-antigens may be eliminated or inactivated, while the low-affinity lymphocytes may actually persist. Certainly high-dose tolerance to a protein such as serum albumin (normal value 40 mg/ml) can be understood in this framework as a high-dose switch off. Low-dose tolerance to a protein such as thyroglobulin, which is present in the minute concentration of 100 ng/ml, can also be explained in terms of elimination of T helper cells.

B cells with the capability of reacting against self-antigens have been shown to exist in normally immune individuals. These cells react against low concentrations of certain antigens, such as thyroglobulin and human growth hormone. Cells able to react against high concentrations of human self-antigens are not found, however. The persistence of these B cells argues against the forbidden clone theory and is more in line with the low- and high-dose tolerance induced by soluble antigens on low- and high-affinity lymphocyte receptors.

Although the theoretic background for the development of self-tolerance is complex and confusing, certain unifying concepts are apparent. Immunity is a protective and at times a pathophysiologic process. A finely balanced steady state defines immunocompetence, and deviation of one component of this giant system can have far-reaching effects. One example of this is the development of autoimmune diseases, which may arise through a variety of possible perturbations of the normal immune system. Normally sequestered self-antigens may be exposed to the surveillance of the immune system, causing autoaggressive destruction. Normal self-antigens may be so changed by processes such as viral infection that anti-self B cells begin producing immunoglobulins to the altered antigens. A third possibility is cross-reaction, in which foreign antigens structurally akin to certain self-antigens provoke an immune response, which in turn reacts not only with the exogenous antigens but also with certain self-antigens. Fourth, the immune cells themselves may mutate and begin to produce antibodies to self-antigens.

A model of autoimmune disease: systemic lupus erythematosus. Systemic lupus erythematosus (SLE) illustrates autoim-

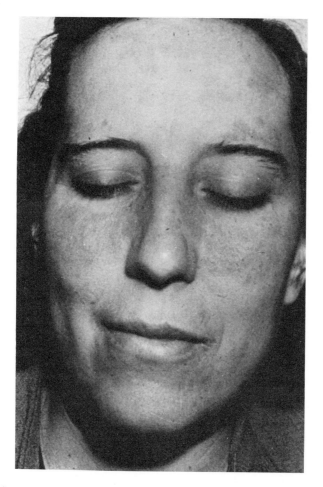

Fig. 5-5. "Butterfly" rash of SLE. Skin manifestations, including butterfly-shaped rash over cheeks and nose, are extremely common in SLE. (Courtesy Department of Pathology, University of Tennessee, Memphis.)

munity. This is primarily a disorder of young women, and in many cases it is associated with a butterfly rash on the nose and cheeks, the sign of the "red wolf" (lupus erythematosus) (Fig. 5-5). This rash is but one of many possible manifestations of the basic pathophysiology. The disease is not only autoimmune in nature but can be considered an immune complex disorder as well. Deposition of complexes of autoantibodies and self-antigens in tissues such as the kidneys, joints, blood vessels, and central nervous system occurs.

Central to the diagnosis of SLE is the presence of LE cells (Fig. 5-6), which were described in Chapter 4. LE cells are neutrophils containing one or more LE bodies, structures

that may occasionally be found free in the blood as well. The LE body is formed from anti-DNA antibody of the IgG class of immunoglobulins. Thus, the immune system is reacting an autoantibody against its own nucleoprotein, forming a structure that the phagocytes of the blood attempt to remove, as evidenced by LE cells. These immune complexes cannot be totally removed from the blood by phagocytosis, and they cause an immune complex disease pattern. SLE is associated with the presence of autoantibodies of all types. The antigenic stimulus for the development of these autoantibodies is not known, but many investigators have suggested that a viral infection may precede and cause SLE. A disease that is

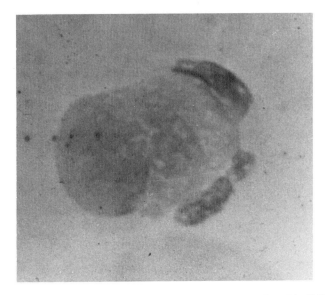

Fig. 5-6. LE cells, which contain inclusions and abnormal nuclei, are found in SLE. They are considered evidence of an autoimmune pathogenesis. (Courtesy Department of Pathology, University of Tennessee, Memphis.)

likely viral in a specific strain of mice appears to be identical to SLE in humans. Furthermore, viral-antiviral complexes have been identified in the cytoplasm of glomerular endothelial cells from SLE patients. Certain drugs are also known to induce an SLE-like syndrome, which is usually reversible when the drug is withdrawn. Procainamide in particular has been implicated in the development of serologic abnormalities usually found only in SLE. The virus or the drug that might cause SLE could act by altering self-antigens and thus provoking the production of autoantibodies. The virus could also presumably act by antigenically combining to antibodies, attaching to cells, at which site the immune reaction then causes cell lysis and release of intracellular constituents, which react with autoantibodies. The production of self-antigen-autoantibody complexes would then ensue, causing immune complex deposition, complement activation, and cell destruction and lesion formation. Thus, SLE results in inflammation and necrosis throughout the body. Another theory of pathogenesis of SLE suggests that T suppressor cells, which normally suppress clones of B-lymphocytes capable of reacting with self-antigens, are inactivated. It has been reported that patients with SLE have a decreased number of T cells and an increased number of null cells. Also present in SLE serum is a substance toxic to lymphocytes. These factors may then contribute to a depletion in available T suppressor cells and allow B-lymphocytes to recognize and react with self-antigens, causing an autoimmune disorder.

The autoantibodies found in SLE include antibodies to nucleoprotein, cell cytoplasmic protein, red blood cell and platelet membranes, and plasma proteins, including some of the factors involved in the coagulation cascade. The deposition of the immune complexes formed by the reaction of these various autoantibodies with self-antigens, and the diverse number and nature of the autoantibodies lead to the major characteristic of SLE—its protean nature and course. This has led to the name "the great imitator," for many tissues of the body may be involved, and the course is generally characterized by remissions and exacerbations. Often SLE is not diagnosed for years, because the signs and symptoms are often vague in the early stages of the disease. Often it is only when renal and cardiovascular involvement becomes severe that the disease

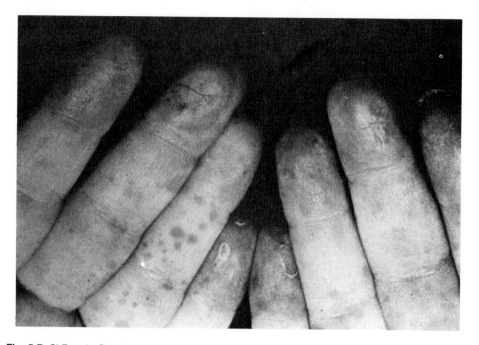

Fig. 5-7. SLE rash. Skin lesions on fingers of patient with SLE. (Courtesy Department of Pathology, University of Tennessee, Memphis.)

is recognized. The presence of rheumatoid factors and LE cells is then determined, and treatment is instituted. Much of the serious pathophysiology that develops in these patients can be related to the deposition of immune complexes in the renal glomeruli and blood vessels. In this regard SLE greatly resembles serum sickness. Serum complement levels are greatly decreased during the acute stages of the disease, suggesting that complement has been used up in the development of the lesions in susceptible tissues.

SLE affects many different organs and tissues but causes serious pathophysiologic interruptions in mobility, oxygenation, and elimination through involvement of the joints, the kidneys, the heart, and serous membranes throughout the body. Skin involvement occurs in 80% of the patients but in most cases is not disfiguring (Fig. 5-7). One remarkable aspect of the skin involvement is the photoreactive nature of the skin rash. Exposure to sunlight often precipitates the development of the typical SLE rash. The SLE rash may develop into discoid rashes, which are elevated erythematous patches that can occur anywhere on the body.

Involvement of the heart and blood vessels is extremely common. Blood vessels of involved organs are usually inflamed (acute vasculitis), which appears to be caused by immune complex deposition and activation of complement. Occasionally this will proceed to necrosis and scarring, with great damage to the hypoxic organ over time. Renal failure is the major cause of death in SLE and is due to glomeruloneneritis, which ultimately results from capillary necrosis caused by immune complex deposition. The heart is involved in about 50% of SLE cases and shows signs of lesion formation, resulting in small growths on the valves and endocardium. The inflammation may subsequently produce scar formation. The vessels of the heart may be involved as well, and cardiac signs and symptoms may become severe as the disease progresses. Serous membranes such as the pleura and pericardium can be involved, with exudation and effusion causing symptoms. Joint involvement is common but unlike rheumatoid arthritis is not associated with great pain and deformity. The synovial membranes of the joint capsule are most particularly affected.

The general course of SLE is variable, and

treatment is based on the stage of the disease and the severity of organ involvement. Generally the corticosteroids form the major arsenal against SLE, and immunosuppressive drugs are also used. Thymosin may be used in the future as it appears able to transform null cells into T cells and may then restore T suppressor function.

ASSOCIATION OF HL-A ANTIGENS AND DISEASE

It has long been suspected and recently confirmed that immune responsiveness and general resistance to certain diseases is genetically determined. With the advent of techniques to identify certain human tissue antigens in order to match donor and recipient in transplant procedures, a great number of tissue or histocompatibility antigens have been described. The vast majority of these make up part of the HL-A system of tissue antigen genes. These are genetic determinants located on chromosome 6 at four different loci. The HL-A complex is made up of many different alleles and is genetically polymorphic. The nomenclature of the four linked loci of the HL-A system is described in order on the chromosome as HLA-A, HLA-C, HLA-B, and HLA-D. Making up these four loci are many genes, which code for tissue antigens.

Fifty tissue antigens of the HL-A system are now known. These tissue antigens can be identified in vitro and used to match donor organs and recipient tissues, thus preventing major graft versus host reactions in many cases. The actual function of these tissue antigens in the living person is not known. Beside coding for the histocompatibility antigens, the HL-A complex also appears to be involved in immune responsiveness to a variety of antigens and also may play some role in the complement system.

The HL-A pattern is extremely variable in any given individual, but patterns of similarities exist within ethnic groups and in geographic areas. Within groups of individuals with certain patterns of HL-A antigens it has recently been noted that some disease states are much more prevalent than in the normal population. This phenomenon had been observed in laboratory animals and has now been confirmed in humans.

The disease that has the best correlation to a given HL-A antigen is ankylosing spondylitis. It has been shown that 90% of these patients have the histocompatibility antigen HLA-B27, while the frequency of this antigen among the general population is only 9%.

Other diseases that have now been correlated to specific HL-A antigens include multiple sclerosis, SLE, myasthenia gravis, juvenile diabetes mellitus, Addison's disease, chronic hepatitis, celiac disease, and herpes labialis. Other associations are continually being made, particularly with regard to various malignant diseases, and there is great optimism among researchers in this field that early and better differential diagnoses as well as possible prevention of diseases may result from this research.

The actual mechanism whereby the association exerts its effect on resistance or susceptibility to various diseases is unknown. It is speculated that immune responsiveness genes are linked to various HL-A determinants, and these genes in turn exert a regulatory effect on the T cell immune system. Another possibility is that certain disease agents are antigenically similar to the HL-A antigens and thus are not aggressively attacked by the immune system if they infect an individual. Another suggestion is that the HL-A antigens may themselves be involved in the mechanisms of various diseases. HL-A antigens may function as complement receptors on certain cell membranes. Furthermore, the Epstein-Barr virus, which causes infectious mononucleosis and Burkitt's lymphoma, binds to the C3 receptor of lymphocytes, thus suggesting that HL-A antigens may actually be important in the propagation of certain diseases, including certain viral diseases, autoimmune diseases, and cancer. Another possible explanation for the association of HL-A antigens with various diseases is that infecting viruses that cause a given disease act to alter the HL-A complex and modulate its genetic expression in terms of antigenic types.

Whatever mechanism or mechanisms are finally shown to be important in the pathophysiologic functioning of this association, there is no doubt that they will shed much light on a great variety of human diseases.

SUMMARY OF IMMUNE SYSTEM PATHOPHYSIOLOGY

A review of the normal development and function of the immune system has been presented. With this background, the student is then introduced to a survey of the major categories of immune system pathophysiology. The immune system is seen as an open system attempting to maintain the steady state in the face of a great number of external and internal variables, which constantly threaten the organism. Aberration and alteration in immunocompetence lead to pathophysiology when the open system cannot maintain the equilibrium. As a new equilibrium is reached when the organism copes with the disease process, survival is assured at least for a time. Perpetuation of the pathophysiologic mechanisms often continues, however, and eventually the organism can no longer cope with the abnormalities in normal function. Treatment can often halt or retard the disease process and therefore is discussed in terms of the physiologic processes that are involved.

INFECTION

The next major category to be discussed in this chapter is the infectious process. Again, the same systems principles apply to the pathophysiology of infection. It is assumed that students using this book have had a college level course in introductory microbiology. Therefore, little emphasis will be placed on agents of infectious disease but rather on the response of the body to infection, both pathophysiologic and restorative.

It has been implicit in the discussions concerning immunity and inflammation that the infectious process may trigger the responses that have previously been detailed. Any infection will elicit both an inflammatory and an immune reaction. However, in order for the infection to be clinically apparent these defense mechanisms must be overcome by the agent causing the infection. The susceptibility to infection and the manifestation of infection within the host depend on a great number of possible interacting factors. These factors include the virulence, invasiveness, and organ preference of the infecting organism, the health and age of the host,

the presence of other infection, which would increase the host's susceptibility to additional infection, the general integrity of the natural defense and barriers that have been discussed, the nutritional status of the host, and other factors such as sex, occupation, race, drugs, radiation exposure, temperature, and fatigue.

Infection then can be defined as the successful attack and growth of microorganisms in a particularly suitable host. Survival of microbes demands that these living organisms find an appropriate environment in which to implant, divide, and multiply. Thus, a parasitic relationship has developed between the microorganisms and the human body. In the vast majority of instances this parasitic relationship can be thwarted in its early development by human defenses, such that the microorganisms do not overwhelm and destroy cell and tissues. In fact, many infections are inapparent in that no overt signs and symptoms ever develop. As the severity of the parasitic attack increases, so also do the signs and symptoms in the host. The human body serves as a limited reservoir in which microorganisms grow, producing progeny, which can leave one host and attack another. The evolution of both human beings and microbes has proceeded in such a way that most invasions of human tissue do not cause significant damage to the host and allow the continued propagation of the various species of microorganisms that attack humans.

Major infecting organisms of humans

Briefly those organisms that are responsible for infection in humans are the bacteria, mycoplasmas, rickettsiae, viruses, chlamydiae (bedsonia), fungi, protozoas, and larger parasites such as roundworms and flatworms. The process of infection differs for each of these classes. Some can infect directly; others require animal vectors or reservoirs. A great many environmental factors must operate together in order for an actual infection to occur, and thus infection must be considered multicausal.

Pathophysiology of infection

When infection is clinically apparent there are several fairly common findings indicative of a unified pathophysiology. Each organism will, of course, cause specific symptoms, such as the rash of measles, the tubercle of tuberculosis, or the parotitis of mumps. Nevertheless, the acute inflammatory response and the immune system will predictably react and cause certain phenomena, such as fever, leukocytosis, general malaise, and lymphadenopathy. Of course, not all infections will result in all these signs, but these four responses are the most common signs and symptoms of the general pathophysiology of infection. Most of the damage wrought by infectious organisms is related to the production of endotoxins and exotoxins. Other effects may be produced by obstruction of vital structures, bacterial enzymes, invasion, virulence, and organ preference.

Fever. This sign of infection is variable and may appear at any stage of an infectious process, depending on the agent and the host. Generally, however, infection causes fever, and fever does not appear until the infecting organisms have caused an acute inflammatory reaction and cellular necrosis has occurred.

The hypothalamus is the temperature-regulating center of the central nervous system. It is believed that neurons sensitive to the core temperature of the body supply information to the hypothalamus. Changes in the core temperature produce regulatory responses to return the core temperature to the normal value—in humans, approximately 37 C. It is believed that temperature regulation is achieved by negative feedback mechanisms determined by the set point of the sensor in the hypothalamus. This set point is genetically determined and is different for each species. There is a range of normal values for any given species, and the temperature itself is subject to internal circadian rhythms, such that in humans the temperature is low in the morning and high in the evening. It is also believed that during infection the hypothalamic set point is "reset" so that the central and peripheral nervous systems respond as if the higher core temperature is normal and acceptable. In other words, certain factors released during an infection reset the normal core temperature to a higher value, for example, 40 C (104 F), and the body operates not by decreasing this value through mechanisms for heat loss but rather by allowing this temperature to be maintained. While this response is beneficial to the host in that the higher temperature increases the basal metabolism, thus aiding in the response to and elimination of the pathogens, fever is usually considered to be pathophysiologic. Fever may produce convulsions in the young child, which may cause irreversible damage to the brain. Fever can damage other tissues directly by interfering with certain enzyme activity, transport processes, division, and general metabolism. Hemorrhage, especially of the brain, may also occur. There is a limit to the amount of fever that a person can tolerate for any length of time, and often the fever will "break" by itself before this limit is reached.

Mechanism of fever production. It has been suggested that fever is caused by bacterial pyrogens, which may be endotoxins, as well as by pyrogens released from the host's own infected and necrotic cells. The endogenous pyrogen may be a lipoprotein derived from the cellular membranes of neutrophils and monocytes. Prostaglandins may also be fever producing.

Leukocyte changes in infection

Neutrophilia. An increase in the percentage of circulating white blood cells is found in many infections. All leukocytes are produced in the bone marrow and probably originate from a single progenitor cell or stem cell. The continuing process of leukopoiesis provides for renewal of the various cellular populations when cells are depleted, usually through cell death, from the circulating blood and tissue spaces. It is believed that the neutrophils, which make up approximately 55% of the total leukocytes of the blood, are the major phagocytic cells of the blood, and they are known to increase early in the infectious process. The stimulus to the production of neutrophils is thought to be mediators such as neutropoietin, which are released from infected and necrotic tissue. Neutrophils are granulocytic, polymorphonuclear cells, which can freely move from the blood to the tissue and back. They are mobilized early in an acute inflammatory reaction, (see Chapter 4). Neutrophils mature into their adult multilobulated nuclear structure from cells with only slightly indented nuclei. Thus, the presence of these immature or *band* cells in the bloodstream indicates that neutrophil production has been stimulated and that juvenile neutrophils are being released from the bone marrow in response to the infection. The term *shift to the left* has arisen to describe an increase in the immature neutrophils in comparison to the normal percentage, which is about 7.9%. This term is used because the table of cells used for differential counting of blood smears indicates the immature neutrophils toward the left of the table and the mature forms toward the right. The term *neutrophilia* indicates an increase in the percentage of neutrophils and is usually accompanied by some degree of shift to the left in acute infections, particularly of the pyogenic type. Pyogenic, or pus-producing, infections are the result of infections by microbes, which kill the neutrophils that phagocytose them. This cytolytic property results in the accumulation of cellular debris, which thus accumulates as pus. Infections caused by organisms that persist within macrophages and do not form pus differ from infection by pyogenic organisms. The former do not cause the death of the macrophage, but result in chronic, low-grade infections. Examples of pyogenic microbes are the cocci bacteria such as *Streptococcus, Staphylococcus,* and *Pneumococcus;* nonpyogenic organisms include the *Mycobacterium, Salmonella,* and *Brucella.*

Other causes of neutrophilia include certain fungal *(Actinomyces),* viral (rabies, poliomyelitis, herpes zoster), and parasitic (liver fluke) infections. Neutrophilia is particularly common in localized infection, such as in an abscess, furuncle, osteomyelitis, tonsillitis, and otitis media, and in certain generalized infections, including rheumatic fever, scarlet fever, chickenpox, diphtheria, septicemia, appendicitis, peritonitis, meningitis, and gonorrhea. Other noninfectious processes can cause neutrophilia as well, including intoxications, hemorrhage, surgery, thrombosis, neoplasms, hemolysis, leukemias, and exercise; also neutrophilia is present physiologically in the normal newborn.

Generally speaking the degree of neutrophilia in an infection indicates the degree of resistance of the host. It is critical to determine the absolute number of neutrophils, the percentage increase, and the percentage of immature forms that are found. Neutrophilia is the normal physiologic response to certain infecting organisms and certain types of infections. It is only when the demands of the infection are so great that the bone marrow is unable to effectively respond that pathophysiologic mechanisms are perpetuated. A severe infection that is well handled by the host is indicated by a neutrophilia, leukocytosis (increase in the total number of leukocytes), and a moderate shift to the left, which could be as much as 25% immature forms. The presence of toxic granules in the immature neutrophils is another important indicator of the adequacy of the bone marrow response to the infection. These large or small granules indicate that the cell is an inadequate phagocyte and may in fact be a damaged cell. Some toxic granulation is still compatible with an effective response, but if an increase in toxic granulation is accompanied by a fall in the total leukocyte count and a great increase in the number of immature neutrophils, it indicates that the neutrophils' response is probably inadequate to handle a severe infection. Some extremely severe infections such as septicemia are in fact accompanied by a leukopenia, indicating that the bone marrow has been overwhelmed. The actual mechanism for the production of this phenomenon is not known, however.

Leukopenia. Leukopenia may be the normal response to certain infecting agents, especially the viruses and rickettsiae, in which leukocytosis may not occur unless bacterial infection occurs along with the viral process. Again, the cause of the leukopenia is obscure but is an important aid in the differential diagnosis of an infection.

Lymphocytosis. An increase in the normal percentage (35%) of lymphocytes occurs in response to certain acute infections, such as pertussis and infectious mononucleosis, in some exanthem-causing diseases, such as rubella, in a large number of chronic infections, in leukemias, in infancy, and during the recovery stage of an acute infection. The role of the lymphocyte in inflammation has previously been discussed.

Monocytosis. Mononuclear cells may increase

above normal values (6.5%) in infections such as tuberculosis. They are also commonly elevated in rickettsial infections such as Rocky Mountain spotted fever and typhus. The monocyte is the chief cell in the formation of the tubercle of tuberculosis; its interaction with the bacilli in the pathogenesis of a chronic tubercular condition was discussed in Chapter 4.

Eosinophilia. The role of the eosinophil in atopy has been described, and it is therefore not surprising that these granular polymorphonuclear cells increase in percentage value above normal (3%) in allergy, such as asthma, hay fever, and eczema. They are also increased in skin diseases such as pemphigus and dermatitis herpetiformis and in parasitic infestations such as trichinosis and ascaris. Certain infections such as scarlet fever are also characterized by eosinophilia, and eosinophilia may be present in chorea.

Basophils. The function of the basophils, which make up about 0.5% of the total leukocyte count, is not known, and variations of basophils with disease states and infections are not noteworthy.

Summary. In general, infection can be characterized by three phases. The first phase is progressive and acute and is accompanied by neutrophilia, a shift to the left, and some toxic granulation. During the stage of recovery from an acute infection the monocytes begin to reappear and increase in number while the neutrophilia decreases. Eosinophils also reappear at this time. During the convalescent stage of acute infection the lymphocytes begin to increase in number, the neutrophils drop to their normal percentage, and the shift to the left disappears. Different organisms may produce different patterns as have been described; this is therefore only a general picture of the stages of the leukocyte response to all infection.

General malaise. General malaise is a nonspecific but extremely common symptom of many infections. It is difficult to trace pathophysiologically. The feeling of ''sickness'' may be the result of the stress response (see Chapter 6). It may also be produced through the release of various substances by necrotic cells that can act on many organ systems of the body. In a sense malaise serves a useful purpose, since the individual is forced to confine himself to bed, not having the inclination nor the stamina to engage in daily activities. Thus, the organism's myriad defenses can be recruited in one major direction, that of combating the infection. However, there is little research in the area of general malaise, albeit the most common symptom of any sickness, and there is little that can be done to alleviate it.

Lymphadenopathy. Most moderate to severe infections are accompanied by some degree of palpable enlargement of the lymph nodes. Often the involved nodes drain the infected areas of the body, but they may also be enlarged generally, as in a systemic infection. Nodular enlargement may be so severe that pain and impairment of mobility are serious side effects. Lymphadenopathy indicates immune responsiveness to the infecting agents and is therefore a reassuring sign of an adequate response. It can also be a pathophysiologic sign in certain malignant diseases, such as Hodgkin's disease. During an inflammatory response there is an increase in the flow of lymph, which is carried in the lymphatic channels from the inflammatory site. The lymph nodes then mount a response to the agents that may be carried in the lymph. However, if there is not an effective response, the lymph itself may be the major mechanism by which an infection is carried from one site to another. Reticuloendothelial phagocytes line the lymphatic channels and are found as well in the nodes, liver, spleen, bone marrow, lung, and tissues throughout the body. Thus, the liver and spleen may also be significantly enlarged in an acute infection. The hypertrophy of lymph nodes, liver, and spleen is the result of increased numbers of lymphocytes, histiocytes, and other cells.

Disease model of acute infection: otitis media

Suppurative infection of the middle ear is common in the young child because of the high incidence of nasopharyngeal infections in this age group and because of the structure of the eustachian tube and ear in the young child. The eustachian tube is much shorter and straighter in the child, and thus infecting organisms have an easier transit to the middle ear than in the adult. The development of otitis media is often preceded by a respiratory tract infection. The child complains of pain or if too small to so indicate, often pulls on the affected ear. He is irritable, anorexic, febrile, and may appear to have pain on swallowing. Often the fever will be as high as 40 or 41 C (104 or 105 F), and the infant must be carefully watched for the development of febrile convulsions. There is usually a leukocytosis with neutrophilia. Upon physical examination, there is often lymphadenopathy, and otoscopic examination of the tympanic membrane indicates the presence of inflammation and exudate behind the membrane. There can be perforation of the tympanic membrane due to a buildup of exudate and therefore pressure. The membrane, which is normally pearly gray, may be reddish or yellow when infected. The light reflex may be lost in otitis media.

Pathogenesis of otitis media is thought to require blockage of the eustachian tube. This may occur in any respiratory tract infection. When the tube is obstructed any microorganisms present can multiply and thus become a potent localized source of infection. It is interesting to note that the most common agents of otitis media are components of the normal bacteria of the respiratory tract and under normal circumstances are nonpathogenic. These include *Streptococcus, pneumoniae, S. pyogenes,* and *Hemophilus influenzae.*

Treatment of otitis media is with decongestants and antibiotics, usually broad-spectrum types such as ampicillin. Culturing the fluid of the middle ear is not usually done, but if otitis media is found in the newborn, it usually is advisable, as the microorganisms responsible are usually of a different nature than in the older infant or child. It may also be necessary to perform a therapeutic myringotomy, or puncturing of the ear drum, when the tympanic membrane is bulging and close to perforation in both the infant and older child. If the infection is not treated, the organisms may multiply and spread to the mastoid process and then to the meninges, causing meningitis.

Physiology of treatment. As in the disease model described above, treatment of infec-

Table 5-2. Mode of action of antibiotics*

Mode of action	Representative antibiotics
Inhibition of bacterial cell wall synthesis	Penicillins Cephalosporins Bacitracins
Alteration of membrane permeability	Polymyxin B Amphotericin B Nystatin
Inhibition of microbial DNA translation and transcription	Erythromycin Tetracyclines Streptomycin Lincomycin Kanamycin Chloramphenicol
Inhibition of essential metabolite synthesis	Para-aminosalicylic acid Sulfonamides Isoniazid

*Adapted from Top, F. H., and Wehrle, P. F.: Communicable and infectious diseases, ed. 8, St. Louis, 1976, The C. V. Mosby Co., p. 38.

tion is aimed at alleviating specific signs and symptoms, for example, by the use of myringotomy, but whenever the microorganism is susceptible, antibiotics are also used. Most bacterial but few viral infections can be treated with antibiotics; drugs also exist to treat rickettsial, fungal, and other types of infection as well. Briefly the mechanism of action of the various types of antibiotics includes inhibition of the synthesis of the bacterial cell wall, alteration in the bacterial cell membrane permeability, inhibition of the genetic coding of bacterial proteins, and inhibition of the synthesis of essential metabolites. Table 5-2 lists various antibiotics according to these modes of action, and Table 5-3 categorizes organisms in relation to antibiotics that are effective in eradicating them.

The efficacy of antibiotic therapy in a given host with a specific infection depends on a great many variables, including the host's defenses and barriers. Simply stated, the more severe the infection, the more difficult to cure with appropriate antibiotics. Furthermore, many microorganisms have become resistant to certain antibiotics. A strain of gonorrhea has recently been described, supergonorrhea, which is resistant to most known antibiotics. There are many other

Table 5-3. Usefulness of sensitivity tests with various microorganisms to different agents*†

	Sulfonamides	Sulfamethoxazole-trimethoprim	Penicillin	Methicillin, oxacillin, nafcillin, and the cloxacillins	Cephalothin and other cephalosporins	Clindamycin	Erythromycin	Ampicillin
Streptococcus pyogenes, group A	—	—	S	O	O	E, O	E, O	S
Groups B, C, and G streptococci	—	—	S	O	O	O	O	S
Enterococci	—	—	E	R	R	R	O	E
Pneumococci	—	—	S	O	O	E, O	E, O	S
Staphylococcus aureus	—	—	O	S	S	O	O	O
Gonococci	—	?	E	O	O	R	E, O	S
Meningococci	R	?	S	O	O	R	O	S
Microaerophilic and anaerobic cocci	R	—	S	O	O	S	O	S
Clostridium species	—	—	S	O	O	S	O	S
Bacteroides species	R	—	O	—	R	S	O	O
Corynebacterium diphtheriae	—	—	O	—	—	O	S	O
Escherichia coli	O	O, ?	—	—	O, R	—	—	O
Klebsiella pneumoniae	O	O, ?	—	—	O, R	—	—	O
Enterobacter species	R	O, ?	—	—	R	—	—	R
Serratia species	R	O, ?	—	—	R	—	—	R
Proteus mirabilis	R	O, ?	R	—	R	—	—	E
Other *Proteus*	R	O, ?	—	—	R	—	—	R
Pseudomonas aeruginosa	R	R	—	—	—	—	—	—
Acinetobacter species	R	O, ?	—	—	—	—	—	R
Salmonella species	R	E, O	—	—	—	—	—	E, O
Shigella species	O	E, O	—	—	—	—	—	E, O
Listeria monocytogenes	—	—	E	—	O	—	O	E
Francisella tularensis and *Yersinia pestis*	—	—	—	—	—	—	—	—
Pasteurella multocida	—	—	E	—	—	—	—	O
Bordetella pertussis	—	—	—	—	—	—	—	O
Haemophilus influenzae	—	O, ?	—	—	—	—	—	E
Brucella species	—	O, ?	—	—	—	—	—	O
Vibrio cholerae	—	O, ?	—	—	—	—	—	—
Treponema pallidum	—	—	S	—	—	—	S	S

*From Top, T. H., and Wehrle, P. F.: Communicable and infectious diseases, ed. 8, St. Louis, 1976, The C. V. Mosby Co., p. 45.
†S = Uniformly susceptible; sensitivity testing not required. E = Drug of choice for empirical use, but sensitivity should be checked. O = Occasionally sensitive; results cannot be predicted without sensitivity tests. ? = Clinical data not available. R = Organism usually resistant; drug should not be used without sensitivity tests. — = Sensitivity tests not indicated; uniform resistance or other agents proved more effective in severe infections.

resistant strains of common microorganisms, and the mechanism of resistance development within microbes is dependent on natural selection of the hardiest, most enduring strains of microorganisms in the environment. Thus, those strains least affected by antibiotics will be the most likely to survive and propagate, creating a large population of resistant organisms capable of infecting humans. New antibiotics to destroy the new strains of microbes must continually be developed.

There is also some evidence that certain antibiotics themselves can alter the cell wall of certain bacteria, making them resistant. Some instances in which antibiotics actually stimulated the growth of colonies of bacteria have also been described.

Superinfection is a problem that can affect the efficacy of antibiotic treatment. In this process the normal flora of the respiratory tract, gastrointestinal tract, vagina, and perhaps other systems is disrupted by the bactericidal activity of the antibiotic, and normally small populations of potential pathogens are then allowed to grow

Streptomycin	Tetracyclines	Chloramphenicol	Polymyxin and colistimethate	Kanamycin and amikacin (A)	Gentamicin and tobramycin	Nitrofurantoin	Nalidixic acid	Vancomycin	Carbenicillin
—	O	—	—	—	—	—	—	O	—
—	—	—	—	—	—	—	—	O	—
R	O	R	—	—	—	—	—	O	O
—	O	—	—	—	—	—	—	—	—
—	R	O	—	O	O	—	—	O	—
—	E, O	O	—	O	O	—	—	—	—
—	O	O	—	—	—	—	—	—	—
—	O	O	—	—	—	—	—	O	O
—	O	O	—	—	—	—	—	—	O
—	O	S	—	—	—	—	—	O	O
—	O	—	—	—	—	—	—	—	—
—	O	O	E	E	E	O	O	—	O
—	O	O	E	E	E	O	O	—	O
—	O	O	R	E	E	R	O	—	R
—	R	R	E	E	E	O	O	—	O
—	R	R	R	E	E	R	O	—	O
—	—	—	E	E (A)	E	R	R	—	O
—	O	O	E	E	E	O	O	—	O
—	—	E, O	—	—	—	—	—	—	—
—	O	O	—	—	—	—	—	—	—
E	E	O	—	O	—	—	—	—	—
—	O	—	—	—	—	—	—	—	—
O	E	—	—	O	—	—	—	—	—
O	E, O	E	—	—	—	—	—	—	—
S	S	O	—	—	—	—	—	—	—
—	S	S	—	O	—	—	—	—	—
—	S	—	—	—	—	—	—	—	—

rapidly, since the competition for nutrients has been decreased. Thus, removal of the normal flora may allow resistant strains that are present to flourish, making the treatment of infection extremely problematic.

Summary

The discussion of the infectious process and the physiologic and pathophysiologic responses has been necessarily brief. The infectious process must be viewed in terms of both the inflammatory and immune reactions that have been described in detail. Viewing any infection as the result of breakdowns in the integrity of the normal defenses and barriers and under-

standing the specific effects of the causative microorganism, the reader should be able to predict the signs and symptoms of infection, to identify the basic pathophysiologic processes that have produced these signs and symptoms, and to discuss the physiology of treatment appropriate to any given infection.

DISORDERS OF COAGULATION

The process of blood coagulation is a normal defense of the body that functions to confine and contain the blood when the integrity of the cardiovascular system is interfered with. Furthermore, coagulation does not occur independently from the other operating defenses and

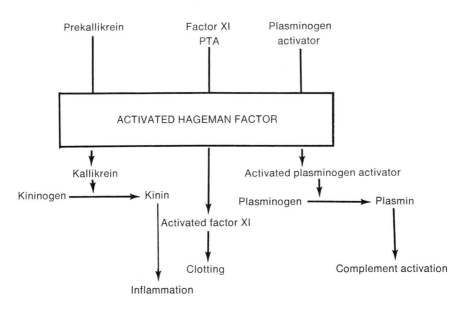

Fig. 5-8. Interrelationships between inflammation, coagulation, and complement. Activated Hageman factor is believed to be involved not only in coagulation cascade but also in formation of kallikrein and activated plasminogen. Thus, kinins, which are involved in inflammation, plasmin, which is involved in fibrinolysis and complement activation, and the coagulation cascade are linked through Hageman factor activation.

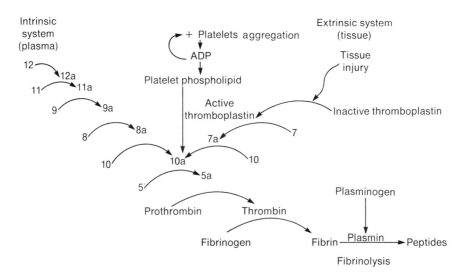

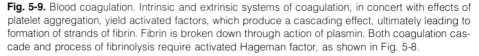

Fig. 5-9. Blood coagulation. Intrinsic and extrinsic systems of coagulation, in concert with effects of platelet aggregation, yield activated factors, which produce a cascading effect, ultimately leading to formation of strands of fibrin. Fibrin is broken down through action of plasmin. Both coagulation cascade and process of fibrinolysis require activated Hageman factor, as shown in Fig. 5-8.

barriers. The activation of Hageman factor by changes in normal surfaces in the body results not only in the blood coagulation cascade by converting PTA to activated PTA (Fig. 5-8) but also sets into play other important responses to injury. Hageman factor initiates the conversion of prekallikrein to kallikrein, which then causes the formation of kinin from kininogen. The importance of kinins in inflammation has been described previously. Contributing also to the inflammatory response is activation of complement by Hageman factor–dependent formation of plasmin from plasminogen. Plasmin also plays a major role in fibrinolysis, or clot dissolution. Thus, it can be seen that there is a tremendous interaction between coagulation, fibrinolysis, and acute inflammation.

Normal coagulation

Blood coagulation is a complex and multifactorial process. A currently plausible scheme is shown in Fig. 5-9, which diagrams the requirements and interactions responsible for coagulation. It can be seen that two major systems operate in coagulation, an intrinsic and an extrinsic system, along with the blood platelets. The ultimate result of these reactions is the formation of strands of fibrin, which form the actual meshwork of a clot. The initiation of coagulation by Hageman factor activation sets off a cascade of events that results eventually in fibrin formation. Once the first event occurs, other events follow as if they were irrevocably "programmed," much like falling dominoes. The factors involved in coagulation are normally present in the blood and tissues as inactive precursors. The initiating event, that of Hageman factor activation, is not well understood. It is believed that this activation is surface dependent. Hageman factor is a protein that becomes activated upon contact with negatively charged materials (kaolin, glass, silicates) and biologic material (e.g., collagen, endotoxin, uric acid, and various crystals). This activation seems to be quite slow but is accelerated by other activated factors as they form and thus is a positive feedback phenomenon.

Arterial and venous thrombi

Changes in the vascular endothelium result in surface activation of Hageman factor. Atherosclerotic plaque formation demonstrates this quite well. Such plaques are often observed to cause localized coagulation, or thrombus formation. The thrombus may obstruct a vessel, causing local tissue ischemia, or may dislodge from the vessel wall and travel through the blood to other sites in the body such as the lungs or brain. Such traveling clots are known as *emboli* and can cause sudden death if they lodge in critical organs such as the lungs (pulmonary embolism), the heart (myocardial infarction), or the brain (cerebrovascular accident). Thrombin formation appears to occur predominantly in the arterial side of the circulation and is mainly caused by roughened endothelium and collagen exposure, resulting in platelet aggregation and activation of the intrinsic and extrinsic coagulation cascades. On the other hand, venous thrombosis appears to represent a different pathophysiology. Most commonly such thromboses develop in the deep veins of the leg and are associated with venous stasis. The veins can hold large quantities of blood in their function as capacitance vessels, but normally the blood moves through these vessels due to the action of muscular contraction, which acts as a pump. Furthermore, the veins contain valves that do not permit backflow of blood distally through the vein. When immobilization of a part of the body occurs with loss of muscle pumping activity, the blood may remain and stagnate in the veins. Increased viscosity of the blood, such as occurs in high hematocrit states, also may result in sluggish flow through all the vessels. It is believed that this stasis creates a local environment in which thrombin is concentrated. Thrombin itself can initiate platelet aggregation and thrombus formation. The intimal endothelium in a thrombosed vein is usually normal, and it is believed that the thrombin is generated elsewhere in the body at sites of arterial injury or microinjury. Normally this endogenously formed thrombin would be removed by the liver and inactivated, but in conditions of venous stasis the thrombin may in a sense be concentrated by the stasis and sequestered from the liver and therefore not destroyed adequately. Thus, it can initiate local venous coagulation, which typically can spread, sometimes the entire length of the involved vein, obstructing blood flow and creating a situation in which multiple emboli may arise. There is also some evidence that fibrinolysis is inadequate in individuals prone to venous thrombosis and may result from impaired plasminogen activation. Thus, in susceptible patients there appears to be a shift toward clot formation rather than dissolution. Some researchers believe that a small amount of natural clotting occurs continuously, but in normal individuals these activated coagulation factors and clots are rapidly removed. In the patient prone to venous thrombosis these control mechanisms may be lost, setting up a situation for thrombus formation whenever venous stasis occurs. Causes of venous stasis include immobility, surgery, childbirth, injury, estrogen-containing oral contraceptives, and systemic illnesses. These factors may interact in very complex ways with other factors in the environment. Of interest, for example, is the finding that patients with blood group A who take oral contraceptives are more at risk for venous thrombosis formation than persons with other blood groups. Furthermore, humans are peculiar among the animal kingdom with regard to the formation of venous thrombosis, and no animal system exists in which to study the process. Thus, the understanding of thrombosis in humans is limited by the lack of experiments on the basic process and the interaction of factors.

Disseminated intravascular coagulation

Disseminated intravascular coagulation (DIC) is a serious major complication of a variety of conditions, including childbirth, abruptio placentae, transfusion reactions, endotoxin shock, infection, surgery, metastatic cancer, necrotizing enterocolitis, snake bite, and severe tissue damage due to trauma. In this condition massive coagulation occurs, mostly in the small vessels, due to activation of the intrinsic coagulation cascade. The process by which this activation occurs is not clear. It is believed that its occurrence in obstetric patients is due to the intravascular invasion of thromboplastic material, perhaps from the placenta. Immune mechanisms are also known to operate, and it is thought that immune generation of tissue thromboplastin may be responsible for

activation of clot formation. Certain malignant tumors may release substances that digest fibrin or otherwise interrupt normal coagulation. DIC may be acute, subacute, or chronic in nature, the subacute being less common and associated with disseminated cancer or retention of a dead fetus in utero for 3 or more weeks, and the rare chronic form occurring in certain vascular deformities.

While the pathogenesis of DIC is not clearly understood, one common characteristic, that of disseminated coagulation resulting in decreased coagulability of the blood appears to result from defibrination. The defibrination, or extremely prolonged clotting time, is thought to be due to the utilization of the coagulation factors in the disseminated coagulation, so that hemorrhage follows, since coagulation is delayed. Fibrinogen levels are usually extremely low, and fibrinolytic digestion products (FDP) are found in the blood. FDPs are formed by the action of plasmin on fibrin and have been shown to inhibit clotting by inhibiting the thrombin-fibrinogen reaction and platelet release of ADP. Thus, the depletion of the coagulation factors and the accumulation of FDPs appear to be responsible for DIC-induced hemorrhage.

The treatment of DIC is complicated by the fact that coagulation and hemorrhage, two opposite phenomena, have occurred in the same patient. The usual treatment is heparin given intravenously at a slow rate. In many patients this will result in cessation of bleeding and be life saving, while in other patients heparin infusion may accentuate the bleeding. Further treatment must also be aimed at the underlying cause of DIC in each individual patient. Attention must be directed to the effects of hypoxia on organs as the result of intravascular fibrin deposition. Gross alteration in function of any organ may result. The reticuloendothelial system's capacity to phagocytose foreign or particulate matter may be overwhelmed, leading to alteration in the body's defenses and barriers.

Effects of increased viscosity on coagulation

Fig. 5-10 illustrates the pathophysiologic effects of high blood viscosity on coagulation. Viscosity is affected by many variables, in-

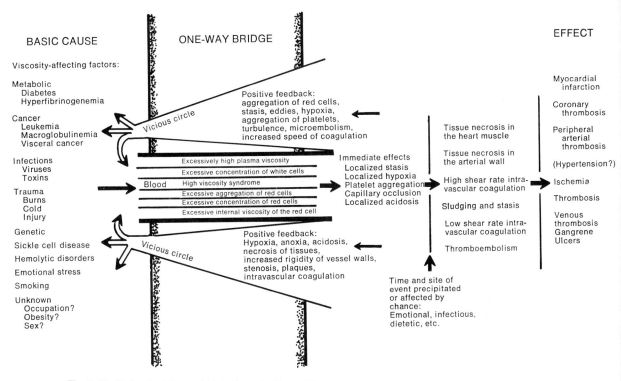

BASIC CAUSE   ONE-WAY BRIDGE   EFFECT

Viscosity-affecting factors:

Metabolic
  Diabetes
  Hyperfibrinogenemia

Cancer
  Leukemia
  Macroglobulinemia
  Visceral cancer

Infections
  Viruses
  Toxins

Trauma
  Burns
  Cold
  Injury

Genetic
  Sickle cell disease
  Hemolytic disorders

Emotional stress

Smoking

Unknown
  Occupation?
  Obesity?
  Sex?

Vicious circle

Positive feedback:
aggregation of red cells,
stasis, eddies, hypoxia,
aggregation of platelets,
turbulence, microembolism,
increased speed of coagulation

Blood — High viscosity syndrome
Excessively high plasma viscosity
Excessive concentration of white cells
Excessive aggregation of red cells
Excessive concentration of red cells
Excessive internal viscosity of the red cell

Vicious circle

Positive feedback:
Hypoxia, anoxia, acidosis,
necrosis of tissues,
increased rigidity of vessel walls,
stenosis, plaques,
intravascular coagulation

Immediate effects
Localized stasis
Localized hypoxia
Platelet aggregation
Capillary occlusion
Localized acidosis

Tissue necrosis in
the heart muscle

Tissue necrosis in
the arterial wall

High shear rate intra-
vascular coagulation

Sludging and stasis

Low shear rate intra-
vascular coagulation

Thromboembolism

Time and site of
event precipitated
or affected by
chance:
Emotional, infectious,
dietetic, etc.

Myocardial
infarction

Coronary
thrombosis

Peripheral
arterial
thrombosis

(Hypertension?)

Ischemia

Thrombosis

Venous
thrombosis
Gangrene
Ulcers

Fig. 5-10. Pathophysiology of high-viscosity blood. When viscosity of blood increases due to factors illustrated, immediate effects in tissue result in long-term alterations that lead to positive-feedback cycles, which may act to further perpetuate initiating factors. (Adapted from Dintenfass, L.: Blood microrheology, New York, 1971, Appleton-Century-Crofts.)

cluding metabolic disease, cancer, infections, trauma, smoking, and blood diseases, all of which may result in the high-viscosity syndrome, leading to aggregation and concentration of blood cells. This, in turn, results in localized vascular stasis and hypoxia, conditions that promote platelet aggregation. These effects set up potent positive feedbacks or vicious cycles, which act to further potentiate the effects of high viscosity. Stress and hypoxia lead to necrosis, intravascular coagulation, and thromboembolism, which may then be overtly manifested as a variety of thrombotic disease states.

High viscosity is usually indicated by a high blood hematocrit (percentage of erythrocytes per 100 ml whole blood). The movement of high-hematocrit blood through capillaries of critical radius leads to sludging and stasis. This always leads to a reduction in the oxygenation of tissues, a phenomenon that may result in damage to the capillary walls such that the per-

meability of the endothelium is increased. Such an effect leads to increased net filtration from the capillary into the tissue space and further hemoconcentration of the blood. This is but one example of the many positive pathophysiologic feedbacks perpetuated in conditions of increased blood viscosity. Hematocrit itself may not always be elevated when blood viscosity is increased. Conditions that cause the erythrocytes to aggregate (viral infections, fever, excess fibrinogen, toxins) may have the same ultimate result as high-hematocrit blood. The red cell aggregation makes the blood more viscous and difficult to transport through the capillaries, and ultimately stasis and hypoxia are produced.

DISORDERS OF PLATELETS
Properties of platelets

Platelets are unique structures formed from giant cells, megakaryocytes, which are normally found only in the bone marrow. Platelets, while not possessing nuclei and therefore not true cells, nevertheless are metabolically active and capable of phenomena such as exocytosis and active transport. They are extremely small bits of megakaryocytes and are surrounded by a true cell membrane. Platelets undergo a process known as viscous metamorphosis when they are activated. Major changes in shape and morphology occur in this process before the platelets undergo ultimate dissolution. Activation of viscous metamorphosis is through contact with foreign surfaces such as exposed collagen, antigen-antibody complexes, thrombin, proteolytic enzymes, endotoxins, ADP, and viruses.

Once the platelet is stimulated through contact via probable receptors on its cell membrane surface, an immediate shape change ensues. This is then followed by a change in the character of the membrane; it becomes sticky, the platelets adhering to surfaces such as collagen and the basement membrane, spreading out pseudopods such that a maximal degree of contact between the platelet and the surface occurs.

The next major phenomenon is platelet aggregation, a process by which platelets adhere to each other, causing a platelet plug, and because of early aggregation, the release phenomenon results. ADP, in particular, is released from platelets at this time, and a positive feedback occurs in which ADP itself causes further platelet aggregation. Aggregation requires Ca^{++} and some fibrinogen to be present. The release of ADP and other factors from platelets is by a process of extrusion of the contents of granules inside the platelet cytoplasm and through the membrane. Substances known to be released by activated platelets include ADP, ATP, serotonin, Ca^{++}, possibly an antiheparin substance, lysosomal enzymes, a permeability factor, fibrinogen, and platelet factor 3, or platelet phospholipid. The latter factor is believed to activate a prothrombin-to-thrombin reaction as does thromboplastin and thus stimulate blood clotting.

It can be seen then that the formation of a plug of platelets is a different process from the actual formation of a blood clot. Although the ultimate result of platelet aggregation is release

of substances that aid in the clotting mechanism, blood clotting can occur without platelets being present, and platelet aggregation can theoretically occur in the absence of blood clotting, although thrombin is required in small amounts for platelet release to occur. Platelets "bridge the gap" between vascular contraction and clotting in an injury. They form a hemostatic plug, which acts to seal the vessel so that the intrinsic and to some degree the extrinsic system can then operate to form fibrin strands.

Vascular contraction, which is the result of many factors (e.g., nervous, mechanical, and myogenic reactions) operating in an injury also is aided by the release of serotonin by the platelets. This amine stimulates the local vessel contraction, which then allows platelets to anchor, aggregate, and form a seal upon which fibrin strands will be laid down. Typically platelets will disappear from a blood clot by 24 hours, to be totally replaced by fibrin. The clot, or thrombus if this is the result of the injury, then is invaded by polymorphonuclear phagocytes and later by monocytes, in an acute inflammatory reaction to the clot. By 11 days after the injury the lesion formed is full of new muscle cells and fibroblasts and is covered with endothelium, and the integrity of the vessel is restored.

Platelet aggregation

The phenomenon of platelet aggregation is interesting in that it is affected by many drugs and disease states and may be fundamental to conditions that were formerly believed to be entirely immune in nature. Platelet aggregation is increased in patients with high triglycerides but not in those with hypercholesterolemia. It is a process that is tremendously enhanced by epinephrine; the possible effects of constant stress in susceptible individuals (which results in increased activity of the sympathetic nervous system) upon coagulation-dependent phenomena (e.g., strokes, myocardial infarctions) are interesting. Platelet aggregation is greatly inhibited by aspirin, and it appears to be the acetyl group that is responsible for this effect. An 0.5 mM blood concentration of aspirin, which could result from the ingestion of two to four tablets, causes a mild bleeding tendency. Furthermore, a single dose of aspirin produces an effect that remains for days, long after the aspirin has been metabolized and excreted. An increased bleeding time can be measured after aspirin ingestion in normal individuals, and in the hemophiliac aspirin can cause severe impairment of hemostasis. The mode of action is believed to result from a surface-active effect of the drug on platelet ADP release. Inhibition of the release will result in loss of positive feedback stimulation of platelet aggregation. Other drugs that are known to inhibit platelet aggregation include PGE_1 (prostaglandin E_1), dipyridamole, and nitroglycerin. Heparin also has some inhibitory effect on platelet aggregation, although this is not its main physiologic action in coagulation disorders.

The interaction of platelet aggregation with immune disorders is of great interest. It has been demonstrated that when antigen-antibody complexes are injected into rabbits they are found in the pulmonary vessels, where they cause obstruction. It has also been shown that the platelet count drops in such an immune reaction, and platelet plugs are also found in the pulmonary vessels. In an important experiment showing the interaction of platelets with immune mechanisms the development of shock in response to the injection of endotoxins in the rabbit did not occur when pretreatment aspirin was given. Thus, the development of platelet plugs was inhibited, and pulmonary vessels did not become obstructed with either immune complexes or platelets. Immune complex disease and the Shwartzman phenomenon then may be intimately involved with activation of platelets by immune complexes, antigens, and microorganisms, and aggregation of platelets in the microvasculature.

Disease models of platelet dysfunction

Idiopathic thrombocytopenic purpura (ITP). Most thrombocytopenia (or decreased production of platelets) is idiopathic in nature, that is, its etiology is unknown. The bone marrow production of megakaryocytes is depressed, sometimes as the result of certain drugs, radiation, or exposure to chemicals. ITP may also have an autoimmune nature, as evidenced by the presence of IgG autoantibodies to platelet proteins. Quinine and quinidine both can cause ITP, and autoantibodies are found in this form as well. Platelet deficiency is manifested by a prolonged bleeding time, ecchymoses, petechiae (minute hemorrhages of the skin and mucous membranes), epistaxis, and low platelet count. In children the disease may undergo spontaneous remission with medical treatment, which nearly always includes the administration of corticosteroids. If the bleeding tendency becomes extremely severe, splenectomy may be done. The spleen is the organ that removes damaged or aged erythrocytes and platelets; it also may be important in the synthesis of autoantibodies. Two thirds of the patients with ITP who undergo splenectomy are cured. There is considerable risk, however, in the surgery itself due to the bleeding dyscrasia.

von Willebrand's disease. This hereditary disorder is manifested by an increased bleeding time and a basic defect in the ability of platelets to aggregate in the presence of a normal platelet count. This condition represents a bleeding dyscrasia that is intermediate between the platelet disorders such as ITP and the disorders of the intrinsic and extrinsic systems of coagulation such as hemophilia. Along with the decreased ability of the platelets to aggregate, there is a deficiency in factor VIII, due to the absence of a plasma factor that normally stimulates the formation of factor VIII. Patients with von Willebrand's disease usually do not bleed into joints as do classic hemophiliacs, can be female, and often improve with age and pregnancy; they are able to produce factor VIII when given transfusions of normal plasma.

Other platelet disorders

Platelet deficiency states may arise in conditions characterized by aplasia or hypoplasia of the bone marrow or in conditions in which platelet survival is decreased, or they can be acquired as the result of transfusions of platelet-poor blood. Platelet function may be impaired in other conditions that are not as yet well characterized. The best example of this is von Willebrand's disease, but other conditions are known to exist (Glanzmann's disease, Bernard-Soulier syndrome, albinism, Wiskott-Aldrich syndrome). These conditions are all hereditary, but acquired disorders of platelet function may be present in uremia, in diseases in which fibrin or fibrinogen degradation products are found (liver disease, DIC, fibrinolysis), in certain myeloproliferative disorders such as polycythemia vera, in scurvy, in glycogen storage disease, and in the presence of certain drugs.

Disease model of coagulation deficiency: hemophilia

At least 11 factors are known to be required for the normal coagulation cascade to proceed. A deficiency of any of nine particular factors (I, II, V, VII, VIII, IX, X, XI, and XIII) results in a bleeding tendency. The type of bleeding tendency associated with various factor deficiencies differs from that associated with platelet abnormalities. In the latter case the bleeding that follows an injury is often profuse, usually immediate, and once it stops, it generally does not recur. With coagulation defects the amount of bleeding after an injury is not usually excessive, but rather it is prolonged and tends to recur. Bleeding into joints, muscle, and subcutaneous tissue characterizes these factor deficiencies, while purpura, ecchymosis, gastrointestinal bleeding, epistaxis, and menorrhagia are the most common forms of bleeding that take place in platelet or hemostatic disorders.

Hemophilia is the most common factor-deficiency disease, although still extremely rare, occurring in 1 out of 25,000 persons in the general population in its severe form. Milder variants are more common. Hemophilia is transmitted as a sex-linked recessive trait (see Fig. 2-10). It is also possible for the hemophilia trait to arise from a mutation, as nearly 30% of the affected males cannot demonstrate the disease in the family tree. Carriers of the trait often show some slight tendency toward bleeding following trauma.

The classic hemophilia is characterized by a qualitative deficiency in factor VIII, seen in 80% of the patients. Factor IX deficiency, or

Christmas disease, clinically resembles hemophilia in every way and is found in 13% of these patients, while factor XI (PTA) deficiency is observed in 6%. Other factor deficiencies make up less than 1% of all hemophilias. Classic hemophilia no longer can be described as an absolute deficiency in factor VIII, as evidence that this factor is present is compelling. It would appear, however, that the factor VIII that is present is abnormal, inactive, and incapable of adequately participating in the coagulation cascade.

The signs and symptoms of classic hemophilia are related to the severity of the disease, but the most common problem is, of course, bleeding with or without trauma, which often occurs into joints. Such joint hemorrhages, which are painful and debilitating, are called hemarthroses. The hemarthrosis itself is damaging to the synovial lining of the joint, but it also causes distension of the joint and resultant ischemia that can progressively result in more and more thickening and scarring of the joint. Ankylosis of the joint may eventually develop with resultant deformity and muscular atrophy due to immobility. Bleeding also may occur in the gastrointestinal tract and into the urine, and the hemophiliac patient may exsanguinate in severe traumatic injury or with major surgery.

The physiology of treatment is based on the qualitative absence of factor VIII. Factor VIII concentrate, which is prepared by cryoprecipitation, is usually given for bleeding episodes, and of course supportive therapy to the joints, muscles, and other involved areas must also be carried out.

SUMMARY

This brief review of normal coagulation and disease models exemplifying defects in the first phase of clotting, that is, the platelet or vascular phase, and in the second or blood coagulation phase is presented in order that the reader will view coagulation as a normal body defense and barrier. It is obvious that when this normal defense is altered by congenital, hereditary, or acquired disease then it is more difficult for a human to maintain the steady state, and indeed, as illustrated, a human being may be threatened by pathophysiologic positive feedbacks, which can greatly aggravate and perpetuate the basic disease process.

SUGGESTED READINGS

Bach, F., and Good, R.: Clinical immunobiology, vol. 1, New York; 1972, Academic Press.

Barrett, J.: Textbook of immunology, ed. 3, St. Louis, 1974, The C. V. Mosby Co.

Bergsma, D., Good, R., Finstad, J., and Paul, N., editors: Immunodeficiency in man and animals, Mass., 1975, Sinauer Associates.

Biggs, R., editor: Human blood, coagulation, haemostasis, and thrombosis, ed. 2, Oxford, Eng., 1976, Blackwell Scientific Publications Ltd.

Burgio, G., and Ugrazio, A.: How infection can trigger autoimmunity, Infection **3**:63, 1975.

Clinics in hematology, vol. 1, no. 2, Philadelphia, 1972, W. B. Saunders Co.

Dintenfass, L.: Blood microrheology, New York, 1971, Appleton-Century-Crofts.

Duckert, F., et al., editors: Immunologic mechanisms in blood coagulation, thrombosis, and hemostasis, Stuttgart, W. Ger., 1971, F. K. Schattauer Verlag.

Ganderton, M., and Frankland, A.: Allergy: 74, New York, 1975, Grune & Stratton.

Goetzl, E., Wasserman, S., and Austen, F.: Eosinophil polymorphonuclear leukocyte function in immediate hypersensitivity, Arch. Pathol. **99**:1-4, 1975.

Haber, E., and Krause, R., editors: Antibodies in human diagnosis and therapy, New York, 1977, Raven Press.

Immunology, its role in health and disease, DHEW publication No. 75-940 (NIH), U.S. Dept. of Health, Education and Welfare.

Johansson, S., Strandberg, K., and Urinas, B.: Molecular and biological aspects of allergy and allergic diseases, New York, 1976, Plenum Publishing Corporation.

Kaplan, A., and Austen, K.: Activation and control mechanisms of Hageman-factor dependent pathways of coagulation, fibrinolysis, and kinin generation and their contribution to the inflammatory response, J. Allergy Clin. Immunol. **56**(6):491-506, 1975.

Litwin, S., Christian, C., and Siskind, G., editors: Clinical evaluation of immune function in man, New York, 1976, Grune & Stratton.

Miescher, P., editor: Immunopathology, New York, 1971, Grune & Stratton.

Mountcastle, V.: Medical physiology, ed. 13, St. Louis, 1974, The C. V. Mosby Co.

Osler, A.: Complement: mechanisms and functions, Englewood Cliffs, N.J., 1976, Prentice-Hall.

Rajka, E., and Korossy, S.: Immunological aspects of allergy and allergic diseases, vols. 6 and 7, New York, 1976, Plenum Publishing Corporation.

Rosenthal, A., Barcinski, M., and Rosenwasser, L.: Function of macrophages in genetic control of immune responsiveness, Fed. Proc. **37**:74-85, 1978.

Schwartz, R. W., editor: Progress in clinical immunology, vols. 1-3, New York, 1972, 1974, 1977, Grune & Stratton.

Shulman, S.: Tissue specificity and autoimmunity, New York, 1974, Springer-Verlag, New York.

Stanvorth, D.: Immediate hypersensitivity, Amsterdam, 1973, North-Holland Publishing Co.

Stutman, O.: Contemporary topics in immunobiology, vol. 7, New York, 1977, Plenum Publishing Corporation.

Top, F. H., and Wehrle, P. F.: Communicable and infectious diseases, ed. 8, St. Louis, 1976, The C. V. Mosby Co.

Webber, A., and Johnson, S.: Platelet participation in blood coagulation aspects of hemostasis, Am. J. Pathol. **60**:19-42, 1970.

Weiss, H. J.: Aspirin, platelets and hemostasis, N. Engl. J. Med. **283**:597, 1970.

Wintrobe, M.: Clinical hematology, Philadelphia, 1967, Lea and Febiger.

Wintrobe, M., editor: Harrison's principles of internal medicine, ed. 7, New York, 1974, McGraw-Hill Book Co.

CHAPTER 6

Response to physical and chemical agents

AT THE COMPLETION OF THIS CHAPTER THE STUDENT WILL BE ABLE TO:

- Discuss the general adaptation syndrome and the relevance of the state of stress to the development of pathophysiology.
- Describe factors that influence the ability of the body to maintain the steady state even during continual stress.
- Discuss general mechanisms by which chemical agents might produce pathophysiology and describe the ways in which the body defends itself against the actions of chemical toxins.
- Describe the nature of the pathophysiology that is produced through the chronic ingestion of ethanol.
- Explain the ways in which ingested lead is a chemical poison and discuss treatment modalities for lead poisoning.
- Describe the general mechanisms by which iatrogenic injury is produced and cite the interacting factors that may predispose an individual to iatrogenic damage.
- Discuss ways in which the organism protects itself from physical injury and describe the general response of the body to trauma.
- Identify the stages of physiologic response to a burn, state the major metabolic alterations that occur, and discuss how these metabolic disruptions act to threaten the steady state.
- Describe the organ system effects of thermal injury and state the signs and symptoms that may arise.
- Compare and contrast the states of hypothermia and hyperthermia in terms of causes, responses, organ system alterations, and physiology of treatment.
- Describe the nature of ionizing radiation and the ways that biologic material may be injured by radiation.
- Discuss the implications of the threshold theory versus the linear theory of radiation damage in terms of pathophysiology.
- Describe the theory of competing risks and detail the implications of this theory for life table morbidity and mortality statistics and disease mechanisms.
- List the organ systems damaged by whole-body radiation, discuss radiation sickness in terms of the pathophysiology of specific radiation syndromes, and describe the late effects of radiation.

The response of the body to environmental toxicants and physical injury is manifold. Both nonspecific and specific reactions can be predicted. For example, the inflammatory reaction is nonspecific and will be elicited in the normal person whenever cell injury and necrosis occur. Another nonspecific response is the stress-adaptation response of organisms to stressors. Stressors in the environment include chemicals, heat, cold, radiation, drugs, anesthesia, infectious agents, trauma, and psychologic factors. The unifying thread among these stressors is that they activate the hypothalamic-hypophyseal-adrenocortical axis, resulting in an out-

146

pouring of adrenocorticosteroids into the blood and body fluids. Each of these stressors also causes a specific response in the body. For example, heat can burn, drugs can sedate, trauma can result in tissue destruction. It can be seen then that nonspecific or specific external factors affecting humans produce many responses superimposed on each other.

STRESS-ADAPTATION RESPONSE

The response of the body to external stressors was first described by Hans Selye, who as a medical student observed that ill patients appeared to have two sets of symptoms, one that characterized the disease process and one that they described as the feeling of "just being sick." Further investigation with animals identified a group of responses that seemed to result whenever the animals were stressed, the responses occurring in a uniform and characteristic manner no matter what the original stressor. Several phenomena were reported. The most prominent result of a stressor was release of adrenocorticosteroids and hypertrophy of the adrenal cortex. This was seen within hours after the stressor was applied. The other aspects of this stereotyped response to stressors were involution of the thymus and other lymphatic tissue, a decrease in the circulating eosinophils,

erosion of the gastric mucosa, and a general anti-inflammatory reaction throughout the body. These characteristics make up what Selye described as the general adaptation syndrome (GAS). An important aspect of the GAS is that either an acute or chronic reaction is possible, and the chronic response, which follows continual and prolonged application of the stressor, leads to the stage of resistance, which allows the organism to adapt to the stressor. However, if the stressor is applied sufficiently long, Selye believes that adaptation diseases will occur. The final stage in the stress response is exhaustion, in which the ability of the organism to respond further to stressors is totally depleted (Fig. 6-1).

One further concept of Selye's theory is the concept of *eustress*. Selye feels that a certain amount of normal stress is necessary for an active, healthy life, and in fact it is eustress that offers protection from disease. Stress as a maladaptive process, causing diseases of maladaptation, is termed *distress*. These responses are considered inappropriate or excessive, and may perhaps eventually lead to peptic ulcers, cardiovascular disease, psychosomatic disease, and allergic disorders.

Superimposed on the acute stress response are the results of sympathetic nervous system

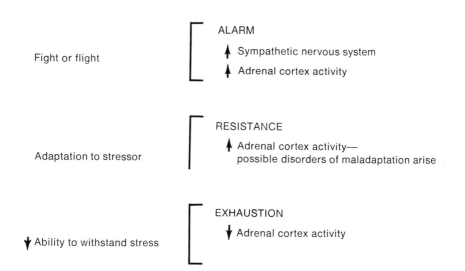

Fig. 6-1. General adaptation syndrome (GAS) consists of three stages: alarm, resistance, and exhaustion.

activation and generalized adrenergic response that are typical of acute stress states in animals. Autonomic nervous system arousal leads to the state of alarm, in which the individual is physiologically prepared to deal with the stressor by "fight or flight." The adrenal cortex activation component leads to a later, more metabolic, adaptive resistant phase. Nevertheless, at the time of acute stress both reactions are occurring in the animal.

The mechanism of action for stress-induced responses is obscure. Whatever the stressor is, some mechanism by which it can activate the nonspecific hypothalamic arousal that ultimately leads to the GAS must exist. This does not appear to be primarily neural, as deafferentation (total severing of the afferent nerves to the area of the hypothalamus that stimulates the hypophysis) does not prevent the stress response, and ACTH release is above normal, as is the plasma corticoid concentration. There-

fore, it is believed that a blood-borne factor must exist, which is liberated by the body whenever stressors act. However, no chemical has yet been identified that acts in this manner. Once the activation of the hypothalamus is achieved, CRF (corticotropin releasing factor) is released into the portal bloodstream, which supplies the adenohypophysis. Activation of the hypothalamus also results in sympathetic nervous system activation and the release of epinephrine from the adrenal medulla; many times ADH is also released. CRF acts on the adenohypophysis, stimulating it to produce and release ACTH (adrenocorticotropic hormone). This hormone then acts to stimulate the release of glucocorticoids and, to a much lesser degree, mineralocorticoids, from the adrenal cortex (Fig. 6-2). Thus, a state of acute stress alarm is typified by an increase in norepinephrine, epinephrine, ACTH, glucocorticoids, and mineralocorticoids. A second effect of stressors ap-

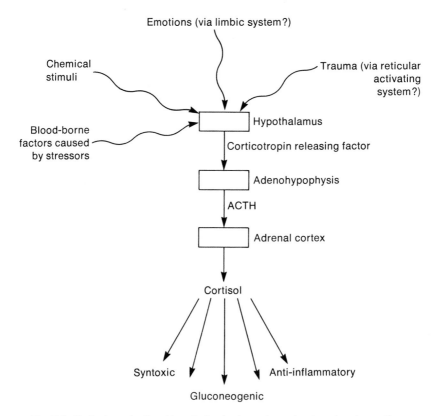

Fig. 6-2. Cortisol production. Hypothalamic–hypophyseal–adrenal cortex pathway.

pears to be an increase in the release of ADH (antidiuretic hormone) from the posterior hypophysis, a phenomenon particularly important after surgical stress (see Chapter 10).

Although high levels of glucocorticoids are typical of the stress response during the alarm stage, a lowering of blood levels characterizes the resistance stage of the GAS. The function of the glucocorticoids during alarm is probably related to their syntoxic effects. A syntoxic hormone is one that allows an individual to adapt to the stressor. Opposed to this are catatoxic hormones such as androgens, which actively "attack" the stressor. The glucocorticoids act in an anti-inflammatory and anti-immune manner (see Chapter 4). These actions essentially permit the individual to coexist with the stressor. These hormones appear to have "permissive" as well as direct effects. They act to produce a favorable environment in which other factors may then act to cause a maximal effect. An example of this permissive action is the enhancement of the arteriolar response to catecholamines, which occurs in the presence of cortisol. An example of a direct effect of glucocorticoids is the inhibition of the enzyme hexokinase, which is required in the catabolism of glucose. Thus, cortisol can inhibit glucose breakdown as it acts in other ways to enhance gluconeogenesis. Cortisol then acts to permit adaptation to the stressor, so that its effects will be minimized.

Another aspect of the stress theory is that certain topical stressors can produce a local adaptation syndrome (LAS), which involves responses at the vicinity of the injury. Selye believes that local stress and general stress are interacting phenomena. They are both characterized by three phases: alarm, resistance, and exhaustion; they are both nonspecific and are sensitive to ACTH, corticoids, and STH; and finally they both may influence each other. Of course, the LAS predominantly involves inflammatory and immune reactions to the local stressor, although local thrombosis, calcification, and necrosis are possible. Selye's work also suggests that the LAS and the GAS are both subject to modification. In particular, "conditioning" an animal by various forms of pretreatment results in a qualitatively different stress response than if no pretreatment is done. From this work has come the idea that certain responses of the body may be caused by a single stressor or by a combination of several stressors distributed through time. For example, necrosis may occur in a tissue as the result of hypoxia and ischemia. Necrosis might also occur if a toxic material that normally does not produce necrosis is applied to tissues pretreated with substances that interefere with vascular absorption of the toxic substance. Thus, the toxic substance is concentrated in the tissue at risk. Another treatment of the tissue with an enzyme that converts the concentrated toxin to an even more potent chemical would eventually result in necrosis. In the living system then it is possible that environmental stressors may act together to produce different local reactions, thus explaining why the lesions produced in different individuals by the same agent may take

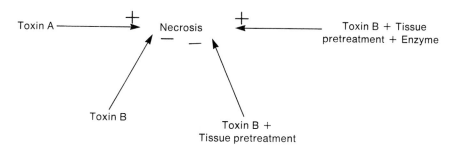

Fig. 6-3. Pathophysiology of necrosis. Necrosis can be caused directly by toxin *A* or by toxin *B* only when the tissue has been altered by pretreatment of a particular type and subsequent application of a particular enzyme. Necrosis is seen as result of many pathogenic processes in this theoretic schema.

many different forms. Disease under these circumstances must be considered multifactorial (Fig. 6-3).

This discussion leads to an important concept, that of *competing risks*. Any given disease process may not occur in an individual because there are at all times in the individual's life span other disease processes "competing" for that individual and causing pathophysiology. Thus, while an individual is afflicted with cancer and may die from the disease process, he may also be at risk for atherosclerosis or diabetes. These processes may not have developed because insufficient time was available, assuming that disease processes are independent. The great complexity of pathophysiology leads us to speculate, however, that a disease process such as carcinogenesis is probably not independent of the effects of hypoxia that may occur in atherosclerotic disease. If both pathogenic mechanisms are occurring together in the same individual, it seems extremely likely that one process will have an effect on the other. Perhaps we may even go so far as to say that one disease process would never develop in a given individual unless the second (or third or fourth, or combination thereof) were also present and contributory.

This idea of dependence of pathophysiologic mechanisms leads us to the realization that morbidity and mortality as usually expressed by public health statistics are entirely misleading. Cause of death may be listed as hypertensive heart disease, but in reality superimposed upon this disease process would be many variables such as the effects of the stress response, hypoxia, inflammation, and calcification, which are widespread throughout the body. The cause of death per se is not sufficient data for us to make a judgment about the true pathophysiology. It has been shown repeatedly in autopsy studies that death from one particular cause is difficult to ascertain. Furthermore, many times one pathophysiologic mechanism is fully developed in the deceased, but evidence of other disease processes can also be found. If the individual had lived long enough, these mechanisms probably would have become pathologic enough to cause severe signs and symptoms or result in his death.

Innate biologic rhythms are another variable superimposed on the response of the body to stressors. Many of these rhythms are circadian (24 hour) in nature. They exist in almost all functions of the body from output of hormones to cellular enzymatic processes. While these circadian rhythms are intrinsic to the organism, they are influenced by environmental variables called *synchronizers,* or Zeitgebers (timekeepers). The most important synchronizer appears to be the daily light-darkness cycle. However, if the predominant synchronizer is removed, other synchronizers can be introduced, which will continue to elicit the circadian rhythm pattern. Mice, for example, are synchronized by the dominant stimulus of the light-dark cycle (which is reversed for humans since mice are nocturnal animals) and secondarily by the modifying synchronizer of the feeding time. The secondary synchronizer may become dominant, however, if the mice are subjected to constant light or constant dark or to a 50% dietary caloric restriction.

Many physiologic rhythms can be reversed if the light-darkness cycle is reversed. The presence of circadian rhythms results in many important physiologic and pathophysiologic phenomena. The time in the cycle in which a drug is introduced to a given individual may play an important role in the efficacy of that drug or its possible toxicity. The response to ionizing radiation is somewhat dependent on the time of day at which it is received. The times at which susceptible individuals usually have brain seizures is also circadian dependent. Indeed, the time of death of terminally ill people appears to be circadian-rhythm dependent as well, commonly occurring between 2 and 3 AM. Fig. 6-4 shows an endogenous circadian rhythm of adrenal cortex activity, as measured by eosinophil count, ACTH, and 17-hydroxysteroid secretion. Thus, the body's ability to maximally withstand stress may be circadian dependent, as the activity of the adrenal cortex has an endogenous rhythm.

Although this chapter deals with the specific effects of chemical and physical agents on the human body, the reader is warned that a separation of specific effects of these agents from other widespread phenomena, such as the state

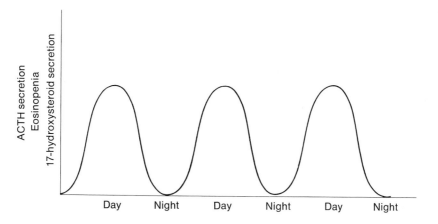

Fig. 6-4. Endogenous circadian rhythms exist at cellular, tissue, and organism level. Shown here are peaks of ACTH, corticosteroid secretion, and eosinopenia, indicating that an endogenous internal rhythm of stress exists.

of stress, that must be occurring at the same time in the body is artificial at best.

CHEMICAL AGENTS
The nature of chemical injuries

Chemicals that are toxic to the body generally have specific effects on certain susceptible cells, which result then in characteristic signs and symptoms. One common underlying result of chemical injury is cellular necrosis, which has been discussed in terms of inflammation. Cell death can result from many pathophysiologic mechanisms. Necrosis that occurs in inflammation may be the result of direct injury to the cells, may be produced by toxins, may result from autocatalytic reactions by which the cell destroys itself, or may occur through hypoxia. The latter cause of necrosis is an important one generally, in that hypoxia may be the result of myriad disease mechanisms. Whenever cell hypoxia occurs, however, a predictable sequence of events ensues. Hypoxic cells are not able to metabolize effectively and must switch to anaerobic glycolysis, which is not an efficient energy-yielding pathway. If the hypoxia does not irreversibly damage the cell, the cell may be able to revert to aerobic metabolism and survive when normal oxygenation is returned. The effects of inefficient anaerobic glycolysis at the cellular level are manifold. Lactic acid is the end product of the Embden-Meyerhof pathway in a hypoxic cell. The lactic acid accumulates, with the result that the pH may become more and more acidic. Furthermore, the lack of ATP generated by anaerobic glycolysis results in inefficient membrane active transport, such that sodium accumulates inside the cell as potassium leaks out. Cellular swelling is the ultimate result of a breakdown in the Na^+-K^+ pump. Cells that have undergone hypoxic changes are characterized as having "cloudy swelling," due to these effects. Osmotic swelling and acid pH changes have many effects on cell function. One important result is interference with various enzyme activities, which can then produce a cascading effect of further derangement until cell function ceases and necrosis appears. Interference with nuclear function seems to be the point at which damage becomes irreversible. Thus, it is difficult to say at what point a dying cell is truly dead!

The process of necrosis takes time and, as we have seen previously, involves the interaction of the tissue in which the cells are found in an acute inflammatory response to necrosis. Progressive functional and structural changes are usually observed unless cell death has been caused by an extremely rapid acting agent (e.g., formaldehyde).

It is also possible for chemical agents to cause reversible changes in the cell that do not always lead to necrosis. These changes are termed degenerative. Degenerative changes usually occur in the cytoplasm and may consist of swelling, formation of cytoplasmic vacuoles, and deposition of lipid in certain tissue cells (e.g., the liver in chronic alcoholism; see Chapter 12).

One important concept to keep in mind is the remarkable ability of cells to adapt to the conditions imposed by the presence of potentially injurious agents. The responses of metaplasia and hyperplasia were discussed in Chapter 3. Other responses include atrophy and hypertrophy of cells in the presence of toxic agents or stressors. Atrophy of cells often leads to pathologic processes. Hypertrophy may be pathologic or physiologic, depending on the degree and tissue involved. For example, the heart hypertrophies in response to the stressor effect of an increased work load, which might occur in hypertensive disease. While this is an adaptive response it will eventually result in pathophysiology, as there is a definite limit to the degree that myocardial fibers can grow and be stretched. At this point the adaptation becomes pathophysiologic. A number of disease models of cell injury caused by chemical agents will be discussed in this chapter. They are intended to illustrate various mechanisms of injury. It would be impossible to describe the effects of all the chemicals that may injure cells or cause damage to the human body. However, the reader is encouraged to consider the basic pathophysiologic concepts that are presented in relation to the disease models and to apply these concepts to the possible damage wrought by other chemical agents.

Pathways of detoxification

The body has elaborated many complicated mechanisms of defense. One defense mechanism that has not yet been described is that of cellular detoxification of environmental chemicals that would normally be extremely toxic to the organism. The study of the human response to these agents is the science of toxicology. Toxicology studies the effect of toxic substances on the body and the cellular response to toxic agents. Such study has become increasingly more important in our time.

The environment is becoming more and more polluted with strange gases and synthetic chemicals to which humans have never before been exposed (xenobiotic substances). Evolutionary mechanisms that would ultimately lead to cellular detoxification processes for these agents cannot operate in the time frame of a 20-year or even a 100-year period. Humans' only hope then is that science will be able to predict the response of the body to these agents and prevent them by manipulation of the environment or medical pretreatment of the population at risk. Of course, the former possibility is much more attractive and reasonable, but is less likely to occur. Therefore, effort must be expended in the area of cellular toxicology, so that a basic understanding of the cellular response can be achieved. Furthermore, the effects of these agents on the biosphere in general and therefore on the ecologic environment cannot be ignored. Thus, humans may be affected directly by toxicants or indirectly through effects on the food chain.

Of course, there are other chemicals in the environment that have been present throughout the course of evolution but to which humans have not evolved adequate detoxification mechanisms. For example, elements such as lead and arsenic were present in humans' early environment but probably not to a degree that they represented any serious threat to their survival as a species. Oxygen, on the other hand, was present in the earliest environment, and all living creatures appear to have evolved from organisms that were able to detoxify oxygen through oxidative processes such as the metabolism of glucose! Clearly this metabolic pathway, which is essential for human survival, may also be viewed as a process that removes oxygen from the cell environment. The effects of high concentrations of oxygen, even in the presence of these detoxification mechanisms, are extremely pathologic. Oxygen can directly damage cells, causing, for example, *retrolental fibroplasia* in the premature infant exposed to high concentrations of oxygen while in the newborn nursery.

The liver is the major organ involved in detoxification of potentially harmful chemicals that are taken into the body. Other tissues

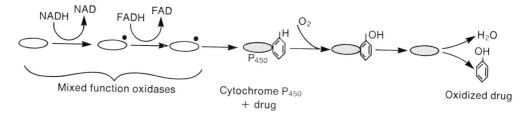

Fig. 6-5. Drug detoxification occurs via an electron transport system comprised of enzymes known as mixed function oxidases. Drug is oxidized and rendered inactive.

also have the capacity to detoxify various substances, but their roles are secondary to that of the liver, at least in mammals. The major site for detoxification in the liver cells is at the cytoplasmic microsomes, which are that subcellular fraction of the cytoplasm obtained by ultracentrifugation containing the endoplasmic reticulum. The membranes of the endoplasmic reticulum contain various enzymes that function in detoxification. Microsomal electron transport chains, similar to those found in the mitochondria (see Chapter 7), appear to play an extremely important role in the detoxification process, involving the introduction of one atom of oxygen into both endogenously produced and xenobiotic toxins, which may be a first step in their ultimate detoxification. By changing the chemical nature of the toxin, the body protects itself against detrimental effects. As in the mitochondria, these electron transport chains involve various types of cytochromes, NADH, NADPH, and flavoproteins. The enzymes that make up these electron transport chains are known as *mixed function oxidases*. The terminal oxidase in the mixed function oxidase chain is *cytochrome P_{450}*, a protein- and heme-containing enzyme that can bind oxygen. Thus, this cytochrome accepts electrons, binds oxygen, and finally delivers the oxygen to the substance that is being detoxified. Along with oxidation of the toxic substance, water is generally produced in this reaction. A general scheme of the reaction sequence is presented in Fig. 6-5. A characteristic of the mixed function oxidase system is that its activity can be induced by many different endogenous and xenobiotic chemicals, which are ultimately oxidized by the reactions of the system. The mixed oxidase system also appears to be linked in many cases to

the conjugation of the toxic substance by glucuronic acid after it has been oxidized. This results in the production of a water-soluble complex, which can then be excreted either into the bile or the bloodstream.

The mixed oxidase system also can be inhibited by certain toxic substances. Lead and other heavy metals in particular exert toxic effects in this manner.

Fig. 6-6 shows various ways in which toxic substances can be converted to harmless substances by the action of liver detoxification mechanisms.

In addition to oxidation of the chemical toxin other possible modes of detoxification include reduction, hydrolysis, and conjugation. All these processes are mediated by microsomal or nonmicrosomal enzymes. The latter process involves the attachment, or conjugation, of the chemical agent to a naturally produced molecule such as glucuronic acid (produced by carbohydrate metabolism), glycine (an amino acid), or acetyl groups, which act to acetylate the chemical agent. The conjugation results in inactivation of the compound, and usually this is then excreted as a waste product from the body. These compounds are excreted primarily through the bile and kidneys.

Certain toxins can induce formation of the appropriate enzymes to detoxify them. This is a major mechanism in developing tolerance to a toxic agent through chronic exposure. Drug tolerance may develop in this manner. The enzymes are induced by low doses of the drug; then more and more of the drug is needed to produce the desired effect, since much of the drug is immediately detoxified when it is taken into the body and thus is inactivated before it can produce the desired effect. This phenom-

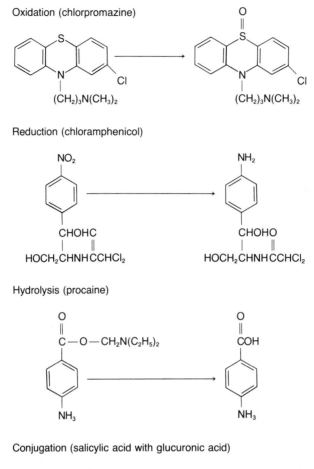

Oxidation (chlorpromazine)

Reduction (chloramphenicol)

Hydrolysis (procaine)

Conjugation (salicylic acid with glucuronic acid)

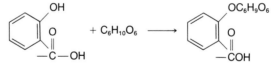

Fig. 6-6. Pathways of detoxification and removal of drugs. Toxic chemicals are either oxidized, reduced, hydrolyzed, or conjugated by liver mechanisms, which act to alter and remove toxic substance.

enon is typified in chronic barbiturate users. The dosage of barbiturates in the chronic user is extremely high, at a level that would kill the unaddicted person. Also, enzyme induction by one chemical may affect the metabolism in the liver of other substances, often detrimentally. Carbon tetrachloride (CCl_4) is an extremely potent toxin; its toxicity is greatly enhanced in the chronic barbiturate user due to its interaction with the barbiturate-induced enzymes.

Much individual tolerance due to the maturity and genetics of the detoxification enzymes is apparent. This effect is most striking in infants. The newborn infant is not capable of the same degree of detoxification as the child or adult and thus is much more susceptible to damage by toxic chemicals than is the older child or adult. This is best exemplified by the toxicity of chloramphenicol in infants. This drug produces the "gray baby syndrome" because liver detoxification and conjugation enzymes are deficient. Thus, the drug accumulates within the tissues and causes hypoxia, leading to dyspnea, cyanosis, and shock. Certain drugs (barbiturates and morphine) can also pass through the placenta and affect the fetus, accumulating there and causing respiratory depression.

Genetic influences may also be important in the ability of one individual to withstand a drug or chemical that would have extremely adverse effects on another person.

Pathophysiology caused by chemical agents

Those agents that cause the most profound effects on the human physiology are agents against which the body has not evolved elaborate defenses. Naturally, synthetic compounds in particular would be most likely to disturb normal physiology. Drugs are common examples of substances that can cause serious side effects due to pathophysiologic mechanisms they promote. Such effects are usually entirely apart from the therapeutic aspects of drug treatment. There is a definite difference among individuals in the manner in which they respond to a particular drug and the degree to which specific side effects may be manifested.

Other chemicals that cause serious effects in humans include heavy metals and metallic salts. These include lead, mercury, ferrous sulfate, cobalt, cadmium, nickel, thallium, uranium, and platinum. A general pattern of heavy metal poisoning is the deposition of the metal or salt in various tissues such that with continued exposure, large concentrations of the substance accumulate in the body, causing chronic disease. Lead poisoning will be discussed later in this chapter as a disease model of heavy metal poisoning.

Gases may also be considered chemical poisons. Many gases are produced by industrial and automobile pollution of the environment, for example, carbon monoxide and ozone. Other hazardous pollutants include acids, polycyclic hydrocarbons, insecticides, and pesticides.

Many people have occupations that expose them to substances not normally found in the environment, for example, asbestos workers and silica workers. Both asbestos and silica dust cause chronic pulmonary disease; exposure to asbestos may result in mesothelioma (see Chapter 3). Other dusts that can cause disease include coal dust, iron oxide, soot, and kaolin. Accumulation of dust in the lungs of exposed workers results in pneumoconiosis. The disease process involves a chronic inflammatory response by the lungs to the inhaled and deposited dust, ultimately resulting in decreased lung function, which may progress to severe, chronic, obstructive lung disease. Certain chemicals may irritate the lungs, resulting in chemical pneumonia. This condition predisposes the individual to pulmonary edema, which develops as a direct result of damage by the chemical to the alveolocapillary epithelium. Such a situation sets up pathophysiologic mechanisms, leading to the development of right-sided heart failure due to pulmonary hypertension (see Chapter 9).

Other chemical poisons include various alcohols. Ethyl alcohol (ethanol) and methyl alcohol (methanol) are the two most commonly ingested alcohols that result in serious disease in humans.

DISEASE MODELS OF CHEMICAL INJURY
Alcohol

Ethanol is a unique chemical poison in that it is purposefully ingested and may lead of course to addiction. It is a direct hepatotoxin but also causes damage to other organs. Chronic alcohol ingestion may lead to cirrhosis of the liver in the susceptible person (see Chapter 13).

While many organ and tissue changes are often present in the alcoholic, the effects of ethanol itself must be separated from the effects of various contaminants that are commonly found in liquor. These include toxic substances such as lead, cobalt, ethylene glycol, and methanol. The major effects of ethanol include fatty infiltration of the liver, which proceeds in the chronic alcoholic to Laennec's cirrhosis. The cirrhotic process involves necrosis of liver parenchymal cells, which eventually results in fibrotic changes throughout the liver and loss of liver function. To understand the gross morphologic evidence of liver cell damage the effects of alcohol on liver cell metabolism and function must be examined.

Ethanol is a calorie-yielding substance (7 calories/g) that is readily absorbed through the stomach and intestinal wall. Once absorbed into the bloodstream, almost all the ethanol is removed by the liver, 5% being excreted by the lungs, kidney, and skin. In the liver, ethanol is metabolically degraded to acetaldehyde, which then forms CO_2 and H_2O. In many alcoholics this metabolism is the major source of calories. Since alcohol directly decreases appetite by causing gastritis, and also may interfere with the activation of vitamins in the liver, and since many alcoholics have a poor diet due to the cost of their habit, malnutrition is commonly seen in the alcoholic. Therefore for many years it was assumed that the development of liver disease in the alcoholic was the direct result of this malnutrition. However, much recent work indicates that ethanol can cause direct damage to liver cells. The leading researcher in this field of inquiry is Charles Lieber. Some of his work in this regard is discussed in Chapter 12.

Cellular metabolism of ethanol. There are three pathways for the oxidation of ethanol in liver cells: the alcohol dehydrogenase system, the microsomal oxidizing system, and the enzyme catalase. The first pathway appears to be the most significant involving the enzymatic breakdown of ethanol in the presence of NAD to acetaldehyde.

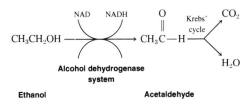

The alcohol dehydrogenase system requires NAD and zinc to function. Thus, NADH must be oxidized to NAD before the reaction can proceed. In the chronic alcoholic the NAD → NADH reaction is speeded up tremendously, so that the metabolism of ethanol to acetaldehyde is also increased, evidence of an adaptive response to the ethanol. The NADH generated by the reaction shown above is then utilized by the liver cell in the mitochondrial electron transport chain. The excess NADH levels achieved by ethanol metabolism block the utilization of

fatty acids, so that these accumulate and are not used for energy. Because the general metabolism of alcohol is so active, many alcoholics (when they are sober) are able to tolerate large doses of drugs such as barbiturates and sedatives, since the enzymatic detoxification machinery is available. However, this does not occur when the alcoholic is drinking. Ingestion of sedatives at this time may produce a lethal depression of the brain because the sedative is poorly detoxified due to competition between the sedative and the alcohol. This action of alcohol and sedatives is termed *synergistic*.

While the NADH produced by the oxidation of alcohol is utilized for energy, there appears to be a qualitative difference between the calories generated by alcohol and those generated by carbohydrate metabolism. Lieber has shown that diets supplemented with equivalent amounts of calories, one from ethanol and the other from carbohydrates, produced entirely different patterns of weight gain. Chocolate supplementation causes a fairly linear increase in weight over time, whereas alcohol supplementation shows an irregular pattern of weight gain and loss with little or no net gain over time. An explanation for this phenomenon might be related to the fact that the microsomal oxidizing system, which is induced in chronic alcoholism, does not generate ATP but rather results in heat production, which is essentially wasted energy in terms of the body's needs. Thus, the calories in ethanol are to a large degree ''wasted'' calories, or incomplete calories.

The effects of alcohol on physiologic function are related to dosage. Thus, ethanol intoxication severe enough to cause the classic signs (stupor, sensory and motor disturbance, slurred speech, etc.) is caused by a 100 to 150 mg/100 ml blood level. A fatal level of ethanol is about 500 mg/100 ml blood. This is rarely achieved, however, because most people lapse into a deep stupor before being able to imbibe enough to reach this blood level!

Both ethanol and acetaldehyde are considered toxic to many tissues, such as the heart, the bone marrow, and the brain. The difficulty in definitively ascribing the noted changes to a direct effect of alcohol is related to the fact that

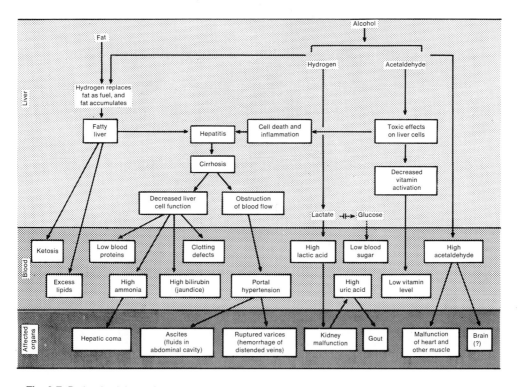

Fig. 6-7. Pathophysiology of alcohol toxicity. Excessive consumption of ethanol leads to development of fatty liver, which in turn causes severe impairment of liver and other organs as indicated. (From The metabolism of alcohol by Charles S. Lieber. Copyright © 1976 by Scientific American, Inc. All rights reserved.)

malnutrition so commonly accompanies chronic alcoholism. In the liver cells it has been reported that both ethanol and acetaldehyde can injure mitochondria. Ethanol easily traverses the placental barrier, and there is an increased incidence of skeletal abnormalities in the offspring of alcoholic mothers. Acetaldehyde also may be involved in the phenomenon of addiction at the level of brain metabolism, interfering in such ways that psychogenic compounds are formed, or forming compounds with neurotransmitters in the brain, which have chemical structures similar to morphine. Persons with defective acetaldehyde metabolism might be prone to alcohol addiction when these compounds build up in the blood and tissues. The brain appears less sensitive to the effects of alcohol in the chronic alcoholic.

Whatever mechanisms are involved in chronic alcoholism, the pattern of pathophysiology once it appears is fairly uniform (Fig. 6-7). Excess alcohol causes a variety of liver abnor-malities such as fat accumulation, hepatitis, necrosis, and decreased liver function, blood flow, and vitamin activation. Profound changes in the blood are indicative of chronic alcoholism, and the effect of these changes on various organs produces the symptoms typically seen in this disease process. These include hepatic coma, ascites, esophageal varices, kidney disease, gout, heart and muscle disturbances, and brain disruption. Many of these effects are related to Laennec's cirrhosis, which has a complex pathophysiology (see Chapter 13).

Lead poisoning

Another disease model that illustrates the concept of chemical injury is lead poisoning. Lead poisoning is common among children exposed to lead-base-painted furniture and walls. Children with pica (the eating of nonfood substances) are particularly at risk to develop lead poisoning. Small children are more likely to become poisoned than adults, even by low environmental concentrations of lead, because gastrointestinal absorption of lead is much more efficient in the very young. Present statistics still indicate the possible hazard of lead poisoning; as many as 10% of all children in the United States under the age of 6 have abnormally elevated levels of lead in their blood. Once lead is ingested it is stored in the body and thus exerts its toxic actions for many months or even years after its ingestion. Thus, lead poisoning is a chronic environmental disease.

Lead is absorbed into the blood through both the respiratory and digestive tracts. Then it may either be excreted or deposited in various tissues. Sources of environmental lead are manifold. Lead has been used by humans since about 250 BC, when large stockpiles of it began to accumulate as humans separated out the valuable silver contained in lead sulfide ore. The lead was used in many ways as it is today. Pipes, cisterns, eating and drinking vessels, salves, ointments, and paints were but a few of the early uses for lead. Thus, lead is the oldest environmental pollutant to which human beings as a species have been exposed. More than 3.5 million tons of lead are produced industrially every year. This lead pollutes oceans and the atmosphere. Drastic increases in atmospheric lead have recently occurred because of the increased utilization of lead-burning automobile fuel. Lead is concentrated in the urban areas, which are centers of industrialization. People living in these contaminated atmospheres have higher blood lead levels, one third of which is derived from leaded gasoline exhausts that have entered their bodies. Some workers are occupationally exposed to high levels of lead (e.g., traffic policemen, automobile inspectors, garage workers, and Boston Sumner Tunnel workers) and thus show the highest blood levels (25 to 31 μg/100 ml). Most of the lead stored in the body is found in bone, where it acts as a bone seeker, replacing calcium in the apatite crystalline structure of mineralized bony tissue. Some of this lead contacts and is freely exchangeable with the hematopoietic tissue and bloodstream. Large deposits are present in the epiphysis and may be seen radiographically. Tissues most affected

by lead poisoning are those of the hematopoietic, gastrointestinal, and nervous systems.

Lead has marked effects on the erythropoietic process and on the circulating cells. It appears that lead is a specific inhibitor of the enzyme δ-aminolevulinate dehydrase as well as other enzymes. This enzyme is required in the biosynthesis of hemoglobin by precursor cells of the erythrocyte series. The enzyme catalyzes the conversion of δ-aminolevulinic acid into porphobilinogen. When the enzyme is inhibited, aminolevulinic acid accumulates in the body and may be excreted in the urine. One test for determining lead poisoning is the excretion of this acid. Erythrocytes are often smaller than normal, and their hemoglobin concentration is also less than normal. Thus, anemia is often present in lead poisoning. The red blood cells also show an unusual basophilic stippling, which is thought to be due to agglutination of ribosomes in the precursor cells. The cells may also appear to be coated with lead salts, which are present in the blood. Thus, the fragility of these cells is increased, leading to hemolysis, which also may contribute to anemia.

Other cellular effects of lead appear to be related to damage to cytoplasmic organelles such as mitochondria. Lead is bound by mitochondria and can actually be actively transported by mitochondria. It appears that lead competes with calcium on the ion carrier in these organelles, thus inhibiting the uptake of calcium and causing, in this manner or in other more direct ways, swelling and interruptions in the normal ionic distribution across the mitochondrial membrane. Lead is also known to enter the cell nucleus and accumulate there in inclusions.

Lead poisoning involves the gastrointestinal tract, causing nausea, vomiting, diarrhea, distension, and wandering abdominal pain. Gastritis and peptic ulceration are common in lead poisoning. Although the etiology of these effects is unknown, it has been suggested that lead may cause spasms of the capillaries of the pyloric and upper duodenal area. Lead has been reported to cause vascular spasm throughout the body. This could result in ischemia and atrophic or ulcerative changes. Lead has also been reported to decrease acid secretion in the stomach. One characteristic of chronic lead poisoning in adults is the presence of the "lead line," a dark line of accumulated lead sulfide in the gingiva lining the teeth.

In chronic lead poisoning the central nervous system is the most dramatically affected of all the systems. The major effects appear to be deposition of lead with resultant degeneration and necrosis of the neurons of the brain and demyelination of the peripheral nerves. Edema usually occurs extensively throughout the brain as well and may cause acute life-threatening symptoms from increased intracranial pressure. The signs and symptoms are related to the degree of involvement. Children manifest central nervous system signs more frequently than do adults. Convulsions, delirium, and coma may occur, or changes in behavior may be the only signs. Lead encephalopathy is associated with a high mortality rate in children and may often be followed by retardation in the child who survives. Peripheral nerves that become involved may have impaired function. Thus, neuritis is a frequent sign in the adult; footdrop, wristdrop, and paralysis may be present.

Other organs susceptible to damage in long-term lead poisoning include the kidney, the liver, and the myocardium. Lead sulfide may also be deposited in the retina, where it is often found even in early cases.

Physiology of treatment. Obviously the best form of treatment is to remove the individual from the source of lead. A disturbing factor in our times is that many children may have subacute forms of chronic lead poisoning due to environmental pollutants, the effects of which may be considered minor and insidious but are not without significance. Lead has been shown to cause developmental anomalies, particularly growth retardation in the fetus, and the young child appears to be generally more susceptible to the effects of lead. Thus, body burdens of lead of a certain level may cause inapparent cumulative damage in the child but be without effect in the adult.

When lead poisoning has been identified, one approach to the treatment is aimed at removal of the lead by chelating agents. These chemicals act to bind metals such as lead. However, most lead is found in the bone, and chelating agents are not able to reach this site. Thus, chelating agents such as calcium disodium edetate (Calcium Disodium Versene) may be administered to remove the lead from soft tissue, but removal from the bone is more or less a time-dependent process, which can be speeded up by vitamin D administration, increased body temperature, and acidosis. An important observation is that in the presence of an increased body burden of lead in the bone, an infection, fever, or other stress may cause increasing amounts of lead to essentially demineralize from the bone, enter the soft tissues and bloodstream, and cause acute signs and symptoms of lead poisoning.

IATROGENIC CHEMICAL POISONING

Iatrogenic chemical poisoning results from the use and abuse of drugs. Some general principles regarding iatrogenic effects are that many drugs have known and expected toxicity, that some individuals manifest allergic reactions or are more susceptible to toxicity, and that overdosage and polypharmacy (the combining of many drugs) are important contributing factors. Some systems are extremely susceptible to the toxic action of drugs. The blood, for example, is a sensitive tissue and may often manifest signs of disturbance. Aplastic anemia is caused by many drugs and continues after the drug is discontinued. Leukopenia (a decrease in the white blood cell count) is the result of drugs such as the sulfonamides, thiouracil, barbiturates, and phenothiazide derivatives. Hemolytic anemia can be caused by penicillin, and thrombocytopenia (a fall in the platelet count) is seen after administration of streptomycin, meprobamate, and barbiturates. These are only a few examples of drugs that affect the hematopoietic system.

The liver is also a sensitive organ, as it is the major site of drug detoxification and can be directly injured by certain drugs. The kidney is the major organ involved in drug excretion and thus is also at risk. Other organs that often show signs of drug toxicity are the gastrointestinal tract (peptic ulcers after chronic aspirin ingestion), the respiratory tract (alveolar damage caused by high concentration of oxygen), and the nervous system (extrapyramidal tract damage after phenothiazines).

Many factors appear to interact within any given individual to determine the response to a drug and the possibility of toxicity of the drug. The very young and the very old both appear most likely to develop toxic drug reactions, perhaps for the same reason. In the infant various detoxification enzyme systems may not have reached an appropriate level of efficacy, whereas in the aged a decline in absolute amounts and activities of these enzymes renders them susceptible to drug toxicity. Deficient excretory function may also contribute to increased drug toxicity in both the young and the old.

Drugs and degenerative changes due to old age may act together to cause toxic reactions. The use of young animals for the vast majority of toxicologic testing may provide results that are not applicable to the treatment of the geriatric patient.

The effect of temperature on drug toxicity has also not been determined for humans. The sympathomimetic amines in particular have been shown to have increased acute toxicity with increased ambient temperature. It has also been reported that treatment with the phenothiazines can result in hyperthermia if the ambient temperature is high. Any drug that affects thermoregulation may have toxic effects if the ambient temperature is changed and perhaps even if it is not.

The phenomenon of polypharmacy also deserves mention in relation to the iatrogenic effects of drugs. The administration of many different drugs to a patient at one time is common, particularly in the aged, a group least able to tolerate it. In most cases the combination of drugs is used to treat many different symptoms, although drug combination may be used to treat one symptom. The degree of adverse drug reactions in patients treated by polypharmacy is not as high as one would expect. In one study 6.9% of the adverse reactions to drugs in a large group of individuals were due to the actual combining of the drugs. Nevertheless, the problem among certain groups is probably significant. Those who are having great difficulty maintaining a steady state because of disease- or age-related deterioration may suffer further loss when certain drug combinations produce toxic effects. An individual with reduced renal function will obviously be more affected when treated with a drug combination of a cephalosporin and furosemide. Furosemide enhances the nephrotoxicity of cephalosporin; if a patient with kidney damage combines these two drugs, renal failure can result.

The disease model chosen to illustrate iatrogenic toxicity demonstrates one important concept. A drug may occasionally be administered to a wide population for many years before its iatrogenic effects are discovered.

Disease model of iatrogenic toxicity: hexachlorophene poisoning

Hexachlorophene is an antiseptic agent that was used in many different products such as soaps, baby powders, and deodorants. Its use had been widespread for nearly 30 years when it was discovered in 1971 by toxicologic experiments (which were done to study a possible use of the chemical in foods) that there was a direct neurotoxic effect. The compound caused cerebral edema and an encephalopathy of the white matter, which led to the development of a multitude of large cysts throughout the brain in experimental animals.

One year after these studies were done, several infants in France developed severe encephalopathy. It was discovered that they all had been exposed to baby talc containing 5% hexachlorophene (soap containing hexachlorophene may have as much as 3%). Several infants died as a result of the effects, which included convulsions, vomiting, spasms, and coma. The damage wrought by the drug in the central nervous system appears to be reversible over a long period of time. Nevertheless, continued exposure to rather high concentrations of hexachlorophene in soap leads to high blood levels, as it is readily absorbed through the skin. Use of the drug on burned skin especially leads to high blood levels. Neurotoxic effects, while not observed in the population exposed at large, may nevertheless have occurred at a subclinical level.

Hexachlorophene's mechanism of action is

unknown, but it has been reported that mitochondrial metabolism is disturbed in its presence. In rats the white matter and the peripheral nerves are the tissues chiefly affected.

Hexachlorophene is available only in prescription products in the United States now, and these products are not recommended for babies or for use on burned or broken skin. This drug is one example of a chemical with potentially lethal effects that was present in many products and in fact was highly recommended for disinfection purposes in hospitals. The sophistication of toxicologic testing has improved tremendously since the first appearance of the drug on the market. Potentially toxic agents with a similar background may be in use today.

SUMMARY

Chemical toxins are ubiquitous, having many environmental and endogenous sources. Exposure to these agents is increasing at a tremendous rate yearly, and evolution has not provided humans with effective mechanisms to deal with many of these chemicals. A human being's detoxification mechanisms are mainly hepatic and generally are fairly nonspecific. Many abnormal metabolites, drugs, and chemicals can be detoxified by these enzymatic processes. Many agents on the other hand are not efficiently detoxified and can cause serious pathyphysiologic effects. It is a continual challenge to discover the cellular actions of these agents in order to devise ways that they may either be made safe in the environment or inactivated in the body. The signs of toxicity are multitudinous and often specific to the agent. Many factors enter into the response of any given individual to a potentially toxic chemical agent.

PHYSICAL AGENTS

Human defenses to stressors that injure the body through their physical properties are not as finely regulated and complex as those that protect us against chemical agents. Obviously the sheer mass of the body helps to prevent physical injury from trauma, but this protection is not particularly effective when severe forces are applied to the body!

The skin functions as a major thermoregulatory organ and as a protective coating against extremes of heat and cold. Nevertheless, humans are easily injuried by such extremes, and thus the defenses are not very effective even when variation is small.

Radiation is another physical force that can greatly damage human cells and tissues. Carcinogenesis is but one subtle effect of radiation. Radiation also can have gross effects such as burns, necrosis, ischemia, vascular damage, and systemic sickness.

This section of the chapter will describe various forms of physical insults to the body's normal physiology and the pathophysiologic mechanisms that may result from such interferences.

Thermal injury

Thermal injury to living tissue is one of the most acute physical injuries that humans can suffer. Burns not only produce traumatic cutaneous wounds of varying thickness but also set the stage for many other disruptions of the steady state. Destruction of large areas of the skin results in the loss of one of the major body defenses—the integrity of the skin. Thus, body fluids can be easily lost through the broken barrier, and microorganisms can enter. Furthermore, a burn represents an acute stressor, causing the typical alarm stress reaction of sympathetic nervous system activation and hypothalamic-adenohypophyseal-adrenocortical axis activation. Due in part to these responses and to other as yet unknown mechanisms a unique metabolic state exists in the postburn patient.

The body of a patient who has sustained a thermal injury has been subjected to an insult that ultimately affects every system. The early effects of extreme heat range from physical carbonization of cells to lesser degrees of cellular injury, such that enzyme systems are disrupted, mainly through protein denaturation. Change in the metabolic activity of the cells begins to occur with heat exposure of approximately 42 C (107.6 F). The temperature and length of exposure to the heat source are the major determinants of the degree of cellular injury. The cell may essentially burn away, the cellular machinery may be greatly interrupted

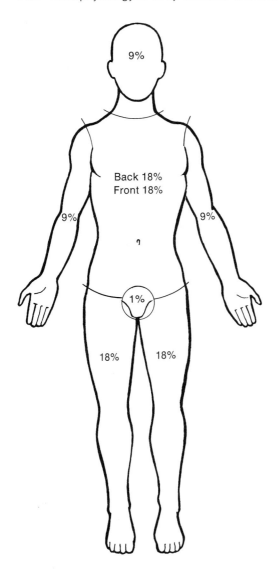

Fig. 6-8. Rule of nines for estimating percentage of body surface areas burned.

The former classification of burns as first, second, and third degree has been replaced with the classification of partial- and full-thickness burns. The new classification is based upon the presence or absence of epithelializing elements. In partial-thickness burns (Fig. 6-9) there is a possibility of reepithialization of the burned area without skin grafting. This is true for burns in which even the stratum germinativum, the innermost layer of dividing epithelial cells, is destroyed, as other epithelial structures lie deeper in the dermis (e.g., hair follicles and sweat glands). These structures can then supply epithelial cells to heal the burned area. In full-thickness burns this is not possible, as even the dermal epithelial elements have been destroyed. Such burns usually require skin grafting to achieve some degree of normal structure and function. It is also possible that a partial-thickness burn of a deep dermal nature may become a full-thickness burn through infection. Infection can cause necrosis of the epidermal elements that had originally survived the burn, resulting in the development of a full-thickness injury. Such responses of partial-thickness burns are now often avoided through the use of topical antibacterial ointments.

Full-thickness burns, which involve the epidermis, dermis, and subcutaneous tissue, result in the formation of a tough, dark, dry eschar, which often contains thrombosed veins. The eschar is usually without sensation, as the sensory nerve endings in the dermis are destroyed by the burn. Sensation may never return or may return gradually over a long period of time. The total burned area often consists of patches of burns of varying depths. Diagnosis of the total depth is then based on the physical examination and the cause of the burn. For example, electrical burns are usually deeper than first suspected, and substances not readily washed off, such as grease, oil, and certain chemicals, will remain on the skin, continuing to cause damage until adequately diluted or removed.

The anatomic area burned must also be considered. Burns of the head and neck region may be accompanied by respiratory distress due to damage of the upper airways. Inhalation of smoke and hot gases alone (even without actual

such that necrosis develops, or the cell may be less affected, with recovery possible. The extent of the burn is the single criterion upon which prognosis is based. This is determined by various computations of the percentage of the total body surface area that has been burned. The most frequently used assessment is based on the "rule of nines" (Fig. 6-8), in which the body surface is divided into areas of 9% or multiples of 9%. The rule of nines is modified for infants and children.

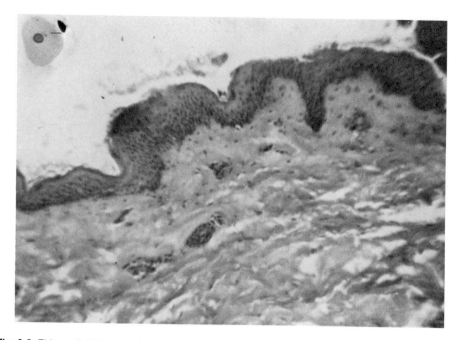

Fig. 6-9. This partial-thickness burn affected epithelium, causing some epithelial damage, but stratification of cells and integrity of epithelium are preserved. Edema is present as sign of inflammatory response. (From Department of Pathology, University of Tennessee, Memphis.)

surface burns) may result in laryngeal edema and obstruction of the airway, which requires that a tracheostomy be performed. Respiratory damage is most likely when the individual was exposed to fire in an enclosed space. Because of its nonresilient nature, eschar on the chest and trunk may also aggravate respiratory burns by restricting expansion of the chest cavity. When this occurs a procedure known as an escharotomy is performed to relieve constriction. Other anatomic sites to consider are the perineum and hands and feet. Burns around the perineal area are more susceptible to contamination by fecal material. Burns of the hands and feet restrict mobility and the patient's ability to care for himself.

Preexisting disease states may present special problems in terms of management and recovery during the postburn period. For example, underlying cardiac or renal diseases will complicate fluid management. The diabetic is more susceptible to the development of infection and is more prone to problems with wound healing. The stress of the burn may aggravate an underlying endocrine problem.

The fluid and electrolyte problems and treatment of the severely burned patient are complex (see Chapter 10). This chapter will deal with thermal injury as a stressor that affects many systems of the body, causing a variety of pathophysiologic mechanisms to develop. We will therefore consider the acute stage of the burn and the stages after the burn during which many responses and complications can arise that may aggravate these pathophysiologic mechanisms.

The first 24 hours. The acutely burned patient is nearly always alert, anxious, and talkative. While the burned area may appear white, yellow, or red, or even black if there has been significant tissue carbonization, the usual pattern is of an immediate blanching followed by reddening as the arterioles dilate. This is a typical inflammatory response, and within 24 hours after the burn, cellular infiltration and inflammatory exudate move into the burned area. Thus, by 24 hours the burned area becomes grossly edematous, and blisters may be obvious. Erythrocytes in skin vessels are destroyed by the burn, and this destruction may be massive enough to cause hemolysis and anemia. Other tissue elements may also be destroyed, and the blood vessels may be grossly visible in the burned skin as darkened, thrombosed structures.

Due to the massive shift of fluid from the vascular compartment into the interstitial space, a major problem in the acute stage is hypovolemic "burn" shock. Thus, fluid therapy (see Chapter 10) is absolutely essential.

While the respiratory complications associated with severe burns usually do not develop immediately, many patients hyperventilate during the acute postburn stage because of fear and anxiety. Many times true respiratory complications, if they do appear, will be noticeable by about 24 hours, when edema becomes significant. Aspiration is a potential complication in burn patients, as vomiting is a frequent problem and when combined with respiratory obstruction and distress can lead to aspiration.

The initial endocrine response to injury is widespread sympathetic nervous system arousal. This, combined with fluid shift from the vascular space, may be severe enough to cause a drop in glomerular filtration rate and decreased renal output with kidney failure a possibility. ADH is also released, as are the adrenal corticoids in a typical stress response. These reactions can lead to other long-term problems.

Burn patients often do not complain of pain until several hours after the injury. Then increasing tissue pressure as fluid accumulates is probably the most significant factor causing pain. Many times in acute traumatic injury of all types no sensation of pain is recalled during the early stage. This may be due to a selective blocking of afferent pain fiber messages by the nervous system.

Shock may develop in the first 24 hours after the burn due either to fluid shift from the plasma to the interstitial fluid, or to the trauma itself, which causes neurogenic shock. Septic shock may develop later in the postburn period. Accurate measurement of blood pressure and pulse pressure is critical in determining which type of shock is present. In neurogenic shock a complete loss of vascular tone results in tremendous vasodilation throughout tissues such as the splanchnic bed and muscles. In hypovo-

lemic shock due to fluid shift the mean arterial pressure falls, the pulse pressure is usually decreased because of the effects of the sympathetic nervous system on pulse rate and arteriolar diameter, and central venous pressure is low.

Second stage. We have arbitrarily divided the response of a patient to thermal injury into an acute stage and a second stage, which occurs after the first 24 hours. Nevertheless, the burn patient will experience many acute problems for many days and even weeks after the initial injury.

The burn patient's general metabolic state is altered greatly from the normal, a factor that must be considered at all times. While the response of many organs and systems to a burn is unique, superimposed on these responses is the change in metabolism, which may then act synergistically with specific responses to cause pathophysiology.

Hypermetabolism. The BMR increases dramatically in the postburn patient. Increases to 100% of normal may be sustained for long periods of time. It was always assumed that this increase resulted from the demand due to increased evaporation of water from the surface of the burned tissue. For every gram of water that evaporates from the human body, 0.58 kcal of heat is produced. This is the normal response of the body to heat stress: an increased evaporative rate and heat loss due to perspiration. Even under normal conditions, 25% of the heat lost from the body is in the form of evaporative water lost through the skin and lungs. It has recently been shown, however, that the burn patient's hypermetabolism is not a response to heat loss through evaporation. When a waterproof film was applied to burns a decrease in evaporation and weight loss was observed, but no change in the BMR occurred.

This state of hypermetabolism may result from other effects of the burn on the normal physiology. One theory of hypermetabolism in burns implicates catecholamine release. Catecholamines are released when the sympathetic nervous system is aroused. The release of catecholamines appears to be sustained at a high level even during the second stage of the burn injury. Blockade of both alpha and beta receptors in the hypermetabolic burn state causes a drop in the BMR, whereas administration of exogenous epinephrine increases it. In Wilmore and associates' studies of the hypermetabolism of burn patients, they noted that the BMR increased with the size of the burn, and that the ambient temperature when increased to a warm environment of 32 C results in a decrease in the metabolic rate. However, the patients' core temperature and skin temperature were both increased above normal levels at all ambient temperatures studied. Research indicates that the burned human being has a normal physiologic response to a warm environment but an adverse and pathophysiologic response to a cold environment, in that cold appears to augment the hypermetabolic state.

Temperature regulation is further disturbed in burn patients because of the normal inflammatory hyperemia that occurs in the burned skin. Large amounts of blood are shunted into the skin as a result. Thus, the burn patient cannot reduce his skin temperature in response to cooling as adequately as can the normal individual, and the skin stays warmer at all ambient temperatures. This suggests that a burn victim is not capable of thermoregulation with the same efficiency as is a normal person, and that evaporative losses to the environment do not account for the state of hypermetabolism. Evaporative loss that does occur is simply a route of heat loss produced by the increased metabolism. It is conjectured that this state is due to an alteration in metabolism caused by catecholamine release. Catecholamines, which have a direct effect on cellular heat production, are increased in burn patients; thus, they are the most likely agents of hypermetabolism. Catecholamines are, of course, released in many stress situations, and thus the hypermetabolic state they produce, with its associated increase in heat production, may be an underlying survival mechanism common to many stress states, including burns. The beta receptors are those receptors stimulated by catecholamines to cause calorigenic (heat-producing) activity. Glucose metabolism, oxygen consumption, and catabolism are all increased through the effects of catecholamines.

The hypermetabolic response requires that adequate amounts of catecholamines be available. Depletion of these stores or tissue refractoriness to them is a possibility in severe burns. The severely burned patient may not be able to elaborate additional catecholamines in response to further stressors in his environment. Thus, the effects of all types of stressors may be greatly aggravated by his potential catecholamine depletion. Infection, a serious problem in the burn patient, can be viewed as a stressor to which the patient is unable to adequately respond. The burn patient who is not able to maintain the hypermetabolic state, due to infection or other stressors, undergoes a progressive hypothermia and appears to have a tissue refractoriness to catecholamines.

The hypermetabolic state of the burn patient is associated with great demands on the cardiovascular and pulmonary systems. Exercise, even so mild as limited ambulation, may cause severe stress in patients with preexisting circulatory or ventilatory problems. The caloric demands of the burn patient are obviously very high, and weight loss is common. Often there will be nausea, vomiting, or anorexia, which make adequate caloric intake impossible. Hyperalimentation therefore may be required in order to meet the excessive body demands for calories.

The net increase in catabolism that is associated with catecholamines and with the state of postburn hypermetabolism leads to a state of *negative nitrogen balance*. All types of traumatic injury can produce this response. The cause of the negative nitrogen balance is cell breakdown and net increases in proteolysis, gluconeogenesis, and ureagenesis. It appears that the catecholamines and the insulin:glucagon (I:G) ratio are the major agents producing this state. Catecholamines stimulate glucagon production and inhibit insulin release. Thus, the I:G ratio is decreased. The normal I:G ratio is 3.27 ± 0.2. This can drop to values as low as 1.1 ± 0.4 during catabolic states associated with severe stressors such as burns, infections, starvation, or trauma. A low ratio means that more amino acids are being utilized for gluconeogenesis and urea production at the expense of protein synthesis. It is possible that the amino acids released through the process of tissue breakdown stimulate the pancreatic alpha cells directly, resulting in the production and release of glucagon. Nondiabetic humans who were studied in the postburn stage showed an increase in circulating glucagon, even when exogenous intravenous administration of glucose was carried on. Therapeutic measures for treatment of the catabolic state might therefore be aimed at the production of an anabolic state by the administration of exogenous insulin and glucose when necessary. This might become particularly important in the individual with either overt or latent diabetes. These people are susceptible to infection and are deficient in wound healing. Furthermore, the catabolic state that follows severe injury such as trauma or burns can produce a pathophysiologic aggravation of the diabetes, leading to severe symptoms.

Infection and physiology of treatment. Hypovolemic shock must be avoided if the patient is to survive the immediate postburn period. Prevention of infection is the major need of the patient during healing, as infection is still the major cause of death. Infection not only can interrupt the healing process but also can result in massive tissue destruction, septicemia, and septic shock. The organisms that commonly infect burns are microbes that make up the normal flora; they are gram-negative organisms such as *Pseudomonas* and *Escherichia coli,* which tend to invade blood vessels. Another factor in the high incidence of infection in burn patients appears to be a general immunodepression, which therefore makes infection more likely to occur. The inflammatory reaction that occurs immediately after the burn appears to be less effective in burn wounds than in other forms of injury. When sepsis does occur, organisms often invade other portals of entry, such as through catheters and tracheostomies.

Infection is prevented in part by maintenance of either a sterile or a clean environment. While the philosophy of care varies from one burn center to another, a major goal is to reduce the possibility of infection. Environmental cleanliness is but one means. Care of the skin, eschar, and graft are all essential

measures. Removal of the eschar presents the greatest problem in this regard. As the eschar dries and sloughs away, debridement of the dead tissues can be done. Escharotomy may also be necessary; dermabrasion, which abrades the surface of the eschar, thus removing necrotic debris, is another possible approach. The eschar must be kept dry during the healing process. Open exposure treatment of the burn, which is most commonly done today, appears to accelerate the drying and eventual cracking and sloughing of the eschar. Most burns are also treated with antibacterial ointment application. The major ointment in use is Sulfamylon Cream. This drug is a carbonic anhydrase inhibitor, and thus a possible side effect, especially in the patient with respiratory disease, is acidosis. A major problem in the use of this most effective cream is the pain that many patients experience upon its application. Since the drug inhibits bacterial growth, the inflammatory response is retarded, and the eschar takes longer to slough away than in the untreated patient.

Organ and organ system effects of burns. Virtually every organ and organ system is affected by a severe burn. Much of this effect may be due to sympathetic nervous system activation, which over a prolonged period of time can lead to hypoxia and ischemia of various organs due to vasoconstriction of the major blood supplies. Other effects of burns on organ structure and function are most likely related to the hypermetabolic state of the postburn patient and to specific mediators released from the burned necrotic tissue.

The respiratory system is often affected by the direct effects of heat on the tissues or by the inhalation of smoke and other toxic fumes during exposure to the fire. Respiratory disease aggravates any effects that the burn might have on pulmonary function. Of course, if shock has occurred, the possibility of shock lung must also be considered. Another complication that may occur in the lungs or elsewhere is embolism, due to the thrombosis of vessels in the burned tissue. Most burn victims are immobilized for long periods of time, and this factor can contribute to the formation of pulmonary embolism.

The cardiovascular system is also often compromised in the burn patient. Some of the changes that have been observed are probably due to fluid overhydration in the treatment of the burn.

The high incidence of stress or Curling's ulcers in acutely burned individuals is probably related to the effect of sympathetic nervous system–induced gut ischemia. The detailed pathophysiology of this condition is described in Chapter 13. Other effects of burns include paralytic ileus, which may be the result of splanchnic vasoconstriction, infection and sepsis, fear, pain, and hypokalemia.

There is also a high incidence of osteoporosis in burn patients. This is probably related to the catabolic, hypermetabolic state and the patient's immobility. Both calcium and phosphorus are depleted in these patients, and replacement therapy is usually ineffective. Thus, renal calculi are a possible result of therapy.

Renal changes are extremely common in burn patients and may be due to renal ischemia caused by prolonged sympathetic nervous system activation. Another possible cause is the hemoconcentration observed in burn patients as the result of fluid shifts from the vascular space. The sludging of blood leads to occlusion of minute vessels, and hypoxia. It also predisposes the patient to coagulation, which can lead to thrombi and emboli formation in any organ. Another possible factor contributing to renal damage in the burn patient is the nephrotoxic effect of some common systemic antibiotics. Also important can be the effects of hemoglobin released from lysed erythrocytes, which may clump in the tubule, causing obstruction. Acute tubular necrosis can lead to renal failure, which presents grave problems for the burn patient who has a limited ability to respond to any stress.

The blood is also affected by a thermal injury. All circulating elements may be harmed, but the erythrocytes and platelets in particular are subject to heat-induced lysis. Thus, coagulation deficiencies and anemia are common in the burn patient. One interesting phenomenon is the increased fragility of surviving erythrocytes, which may be due either to heat damage to the membranes or to the catabolic state of the burn patient. There is high intracellular sodium and low potassium in the circulating erythrocytes, which return to normal values within 3 to 5 days after a diet of 6,000 cal per day. Thus, it would seem that these alterations in erythrocyte cations reflect the patient's nutritional status and catabolic state and indicate that erythrocyte active transport is inhibited.

The liver is often described as undergoing necrotic changes in burn patients. While these changes had previously been thought to be due to ischemia, it now appears that they are primarily iatrogenic effects of treatment of the burn patient with tannic acid.

Summary. The thermally injured patient is subject to many possible pathophysiologic interactions due to the injury itself, the metabolic state, and the normal stress response. Treatment must therefore be aimed at the conditions manifested in the patient, and those that can be anticipated should be prevented if possible. The burn patient who survives the first few days following the injury is nevertheless continuously subject to further pathophysiologic mechanisms, which develop through the interaction of many systems that become disordered as the result of the burn, the patient's response, or even occasionally the treatment. The major needs of the patient throughout the postburn period are related to fluid and electrolyte balance, infection, metabolism, and maintenance of the steady state in the presence of many possible decompensating pathophysiologic effects.

The effects of temperature extremes

Heat. Humans are exposed to great swings in ambient temperature in accordance with climatic, seasonal changes. Evolution has provided humans with mechanisms with which to adjust to sudden changes in temperature and to adapt over longer periods of time to temperature extremes. The degree of compensation and adaptation is limited, however, and various pathophysiologic mechanisms can occur when humans are exposed to environmental temperature extremes. Thus, states of hyperthermia and hypothermia can result when the ability to adequately adjust to heat and cold stressors is insufficient.

Hyperthermia. The hyperthermic state is characterized by an elevation in core temperature. Humans respond to many infections by hyperpyrexia, or fever. In most situations the fever is not believed to aid the response of the organisms to infection; it is considered to be pathophysiologic rather than physiologic, in that fever causes more stress than benefit. The details of fever production are described in Chapter 5. Humans also may respond to other conditions or situations by hyperthermia. It will be recalled that heat is normally produced in the body through metabolism of food, and the major organ sources of heat are the liver and the skeletal muscles. The heat is used to maintain the body core temperature at a species-specific, genetically determined set point, which appears to be regulated by the hypothalamus. Various thermoreceptors throughout the body "inform" the hypothalamic heat-regulating center of the temperature, and the hypothalamus, through a variety of negative-feedback mechanisms, acts to either activate heat-gaining or heat-losing mechanisms. In states of hyperthermia either these mechanisms are impaired, or the hypothalamus itself is not responding to the elevation in temperature. Thermoreceptors must, of course, also be intact and functional if the hypothalamus is to receive temperature information from various parts of the body.

Heat stroke. While other responses to heat produce symptoms, for example, heat cramps and heat exhaustion, these are not characterized by an elevation in body temperature. Heat stroke, or heat pyrexia, is associated with a greatly elevated core temperature. Heat stroke develops in people in humid, hot environments in which cooling by evaporation cannot be accomplished due to the absence of an evaporation gradient from the skin to the air. Thus, the temperature cannot be regulated and increases to the point that collapse occurs. It occurs more readily in patients who are already debilitated due to preexisting disease or in the elderly. Hyperpyrexia can result in generalized vasodilation, which will cause the diastolic pressure to fall, and the end diastolic pressure and cardiac output may be significantly reduced, such that shock ensues. Initially the pulse and the respiratory rate are rapid, but both fall as the patient deteriorates. The erythrocytes may be affected by heat, and their increased permeability leads to increased leakage of potassium into the extracellular fluid, causing a state of hyperkalemia. The effects of heat are in a sense similar to those observed in cells that have been mildly burned. The metabolism and enzyme functions are impaired, and cells may swell and undergo necrosis. Wide degenerative changes occur throughout the tissue in patients surviving prolonged periods of hyperthermia. The incidence of myocardial infarction and other acute ischemic or hemorrhagic processes is high following recovery from heat stroke.

The condition is to be contrasted with the effects of heat in healthy individuals. Sweating may be accomplished by these people, but often the water and electrolytes that are lost through sweating are not replaced adequately. Ingestion of water alone further dilutes the extracellular fluid, leading to signs of hyponatremia. These individuals are able to maintain their core temperature but suffer signs of salt depletion, a condition known as *heat exhaustion*. Stoker's cramps may develop in muscles due to salt depletion, but the collapse, weakness, dizziness, and headaches that are found in heat exhaustion are related to excessive sweating that leads to hypovolemia. Thus, these patients show the signs of widespread sympathetic nervous system activation that characterizes hypovolemic shock. The skin is cold and moist, the pupils are dilated, the heart rate and blood pressure are increased, and the pulse pressure is narrow. Nevertheless, the core temperature is maintained. The physiology of treatment is aimed at the restoration of electrolytes and water and treatment of shock. In the case of hyperpyrexia, treatment is aimed initially at restoration of the body temperature by cooling the individual rapidly (an ice water immersion is the best treatment). The skin should be vigorously massaged following the drop in temperature to stimulate the return of the cooler peripheral blood to the hotter internal organs. Close observation of the patient is essential, as the dangers of a return to a hyperthermic state, cardiac failure, and hemorrhage are imminent in the acute stage of the disease process.

Hypothermia. Hypothermia may be a pathophysiologic response of the body to cold stress or may occasionally be accomplished therapeutically during surgery. A decrease in body temperature to values ranging from 35 to 25 C (95 to 77 F) constitutes hypothermia. The effects of temperature drop on the human physiology are manifold. Both local and systemic effects may occur. Metabolism in general is temperature dependent and will be greatly depressed in hypothermia. Cell ischemia and necrosis in various organs may also occur. An important effect of hypothermia appears to be cold-induced injury to the capillary endothelium, which in turn results in increased capillary permeability and loss of plasma into the interstitial space. Hypovolemia may thus result. If chilling of the tissues is accomplished very rapidly, edema may not occur until after the individual is rewarmed. The degree of vascular injury is related to the extent and length of the exposure to cold. In frostbite, for example, the vascular effects are so profound as to cause first occlusion and then ischemia leading to necrosis and gangrene of the affected part. In systemic hypothermia there is tissue ischemia, but it is usually not as profound. Systemic hypothermia is most commonly due to exposure. Particularly susceptible are mountain climbers at high altitudes and the elderly at normal altitude during the winter months. The hypothermic individual has an extremely low rectal temperature (usually off the scale of the thermometers commonly used in the hospital) and appears pale, cold, and stiff. Respiratory rate, heart rate, and blood pressure are all usually decreased markedly. Edema is also often present. There may be signs of cardiac failure, and usually the patient is either extremely lethargic or unconscious. Treatment is not rapid rewarming, as this will act to dilate only peripheral vessels and thus decrease the blood supply to the critical internal organs. The plasma volume must be expanded to aid cardiac function and prevent the effects of hemoconcentration and resultant ischemia. The administration of warm fluids and the utilization of either hemodialysis or peritoneal dialysis with

warmed blood or dialyzing fluid acts to restore core temperature. Even after recovery from the acute hypothermic episode, there are generally pathologic changes throughout the tissues, which may lead to further disease.

Adaptation to a chronic cold environment is necessary for a person to maintain a normal body temperature and not suffer the effects of hypothermia. While humans usually respond to a cold ambient temperature by heat production through shivering, and heat containment by peripheral vasoconstriction, the cold-adapted person produces required extra heat through a process called *nonshivering thermogenesis,* which is characterized by increased oxygen consumption, BMR, and caloric requirements. The mechanism for nonshivering thermogenesis may be uncoupling of ADP from the electron transport chain in the cellular mitochondria. Thus, if the constraint of the ADP concentration, which limits the speed of the electron transport, is removed, electron movement can be increased, and heat production would also increase. The thyroid gland activity is also increased in the cold-adapted animal, and there are increased concentrations of circulating catecholamines. Humans with decreased function of the endocrine system thus would be less able to adapt to a cold environment. Exposure of infants to either acute or chronic cold will lead to deterioration. Newborns are unable to shiver and thus must rely on their supply of *brown fat,* which is present in significant amounts in humans only during fetal and neonatal life. Brown fat is found normally in hibernating mammals and is rich in mitochondria. Its particular biochemistry allows it to participate in nonshivering thermogenesis. It allows therefore some degree of cold adaptation in the infant, but it is not able to keep up with the heat requirements of the small, nonshivering infant who is suddenly exposed to a cold ambient temperature.

It is conceivable that inability to adapt to cold may lead to significant pathophysiology among the human population in the future, as humans slowly and purposefully change their environment and deplete it of all available heat-producing fuel. Therefore, an understanding of this process is necessary in order to develop

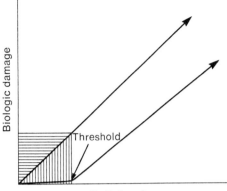

Fig. 6-10. Linear and threshold dose–response curve theories of radiation damage. Linear theory holds that some damage occurs at all doses, whereas threshold theory states that a threshold dose exists below which no damage occurs and above which damage of a linear nature with dose occurs.

possible biochemical means for manipulating the response of humans to cold.

Radiation

Ionizing radiation has been present in the environment since life began. Many believe that without it no life could have evolved, since mutation is necessary in order for diversity to exist, and ionizing radiation is a powerful mutagen. As our technology becomes more and more complex, the peaceful utilization of radioactivity for energy production, treatment of disease, and food preparation is becoming increasingly widespread. Questions are continually being raised as to what is a "safe" level of radiation in the environment and what are the dangers of accidental exposure to human physiology.

Some basic questions in radiation biology are related to the effects of low doses of radiation on humans. The most scientifically acceptable concept of low-dose effects is that of a threshold to radiation. This is in contrast to the linear hypothesis, which basically implies that there is damage to living organisms from all exposures to radiation, down to even the most infinitesimal amount. The threshold theory, on the other hand, suggests that there is a threshold

dose, below which no damage occurs and above which damage dependent on dosage occurs. These two theories are illustrated in Fig. 6-10.

Research into the cellular mechanisms of repair is a basic approach to studying the effects of low doses of radiation. These enzymatic processes appear to be highly efficient at low doses of radiation but may be "swamped" by the damage caused by larger doses. Large doses may also produce irreparable damage. Implicit in the threshold concept is the idea of accumulated damage in the cell, which eventually results in disturbances in cellular function. As discussed in Chapter 3, radiation-induced carcinogenesis is a process that appears to require certain events to happen over time (the latent period) before the cell becomes malignant. These events do not necessarily have to be the result of radioactivity. They could be due to the effects of chemicals, viruses, or immune phenomena. Thus, radiation as an agent that can cause damage to living cells must be viewed in perspective. Many other phenomena are interacting with each other and competing with each other to cause damage to the cell. The effects of radiation may not be manifested in certain cells until other events occur, which disrupt the cell. On the other hand, a cell exposed to radiation may never develop damage due either to efficient repair such that no deleterious effects of the radiation remain or to competing risks, which damage or kill the cell before radiation-induced damage can be manifested. It is a major task of scientific research to sort out the interactions among agents that compromise cell function and to determine the extent of competing risks. Are competing risks independent of each other, or do they themselves interact with each other? In view of the complexity of pathophysiologic mechanisms the latter possibility seems most likely and thus presents us with an almost insurmountable task in terms of describing the true etiology and pathogenesis of various disease states.

Ionizing radiation exists in three basic forms: alpha particles, which are helium nuclei; beta particles, which are highly reactive electrons formed from the nucleus of an atom; and

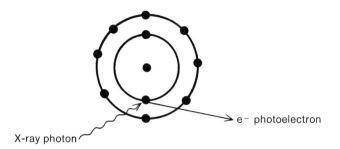

X-ray photon

e− photoelectron

Fig. 6-11. Ionization is a process by which orbital electrons are ejected. A low-energy x-ray photon, which is a "packet" of x-ray energy "hits" an atom and interacts with an orbital electron, transferring its energy to electron and knocking it out of orbit. This produces a photoelectron, which can cause further ionization, and leaves behind a charged atom, or ion.

gamma rays, which are basically identical to x-rays. Alpha particles are heavy and slow and can be stopped by the skin. Beta particles can move through the skin and tissue, and gamma rays can move through all biologic material; lead shielding must be used to protect humans who are exposed to gamma or x-rays. Other particles can be made highly energetic in accelerators. The term *ionizing* implies that these forms of radiation can cause the ejection of electrons from the outer shells of an atom, thus forming an ion. The electrons so produced are of sufficient energy to cause further ionization (Fig. 6-11). The energy of these particles or waves can result in direct damage to molecules that they impinge upon. For example, if a radioactive particle strikes a DNA molecule, the energy transferred by the reaction may be sufficient to cause abnormal structural configurations of the DNA. Thus, mutations may be formed in the DNA. If the mutation is not repaired, it may kill the cell, or be lethal. If it is sublethal, then the mutation may cause abnormal coding for proteins, and it may also be passed on to daughter cells if the damaged cell divides. The presence of oxygen permits ionizing radiation to do more damage to biologic material because free radicals can be formed through the interaction of ionizing radiation and water. Since water is present in high concentrations inside cells and tissue, this interaction assumes great importance because the free radical formation results in molecules that can produce secondary effects. Free radicals, for example, can peroxidate biologic molecules such as membrane lipids. Sulfhydryl groups can be

oxidized so that disulfide bonds may ultimately form between adjacent molecules. Large molecules may be degraded into smaller fragments, thus losing their chemical specificity. Cross-linking of molecules can also result, such that two or more molecules will be held in a rigid configuration. These effects are all produced by the free radicals formed by the radiation in the aqueous solution and thus are termed *secondary effects. Primary effects* of radiation are direct hits of molecules with damage produced by this interaction.

When biologic molecules are damaged either directly or indirectly by ionizing radiation, the cell may protect itself against the effects of the damage in a variety of ways. Certain enzymes such as catalase or peroxidases act to protect the cell, in that peroxides that are formed are removed through the action of these enzymes. Nuclear damage to DNA molecules is also repaired through enzymatic reactions. When ionizing radiation breaks a single DNA strand, repair enzymes exist to patch the DNA together. When both strands of DNA are broken by the radiation, repair is less likely to occur. Radiation can produce minute point mutations in DNA or can result in gross structural damage to the chromosome, which is observable upon microscopic examination of the cell. Radiation can also interrupt the normal division patterns of the cell and can affect cells in various ways, depending on which stage of the cell cycle the cell is in at the time of the radiation. If the genetic damage is in germ cells, there exists a possibility that the DNA damage will be handed down to subsequent generations. When the damage occurs in a somatic cell, there is no possibility of its becoming part of the gene pool. As we have previously discussed, the more immature or undifferentiated a cell, the more radiosensitive it is. The germ cells are generally more sensitive to the effects of radiation than are most somatic cells.

So far we have described the effects of radiation on specific cells. The teratogenic and carcinogenic properties of radiation have been described in previous chapters. The therapeutic aspects of radiation have been discussed in terms of cancer radiotherapy. Another effect of radiation occurs with exposure of the whole body, either intentionally or by accident. There are groups of individuals who have been exposed to large doses of whole-body radiation,

and it is from these people that we have learned the most about the effects of radiation on humans. These include the survivors of the atomic bombings of Hiroshima and Nagasaki, the radium–watch dial painters, early radiologists, people treated for a variety of conditions with either large doses of radiation or radium, and more recently workers in contact with radioactivity who have been accidentally exposed. Confirmation of the effect of whole-body radiation on animals has been obtained in humans.

Radiation sickness is the acute result of large doses (greater than 50 rads) of whole-body radiation and consists of changes in three major organ systems: the hematopoietic, the gastrointestinal, and the central nervous systems. Of

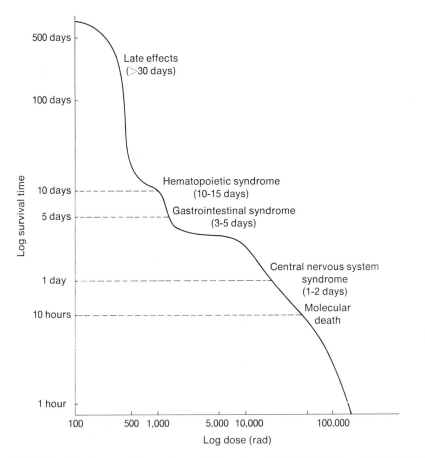

Fig. 6-12. Relationship between dose and survival time for adult rats following a single total-body exposure of x-rays. Radiation damage produces many alterations, leading to breakdown of steady state. (From Casarett, A. P., Radiation biology, © 1968, pp. 222 and 223. Reprinted by permission of Prentice-Hall, Inc., Englewood Cliffs, N.J.)

course, alterations in any of these systems will have effects on other systems as well. The effects of radiation on these three systems is related to dose. While radiation sickness may occur after exposures greater than 50 rads, specific central nervous system damage is not seen unless the exposure has been to a very high dose. The central nervous system syndrome is an early effect of very high doses of radiation. When exposures high enough to cause signs of central nervous system damage have occurred, death is inevitable. With doses of radiation between 500 and 2,000 rads the signs and symptoms are related to damage in the gastrointestinal tract. Symptoms begin to appear 3 to 5 days after the exposure and consist of nausea, vomiting, anorexia, and diarrhea. These can then progress to gastrointestinal hemorrhage, which may lead to severe anemia. The body becomes extremely susceptible to infection

under these circumstances. With radiation doses under 500 rads, or in individuals surviving the effects of the gastrointestinal syndrome, the hematopoietic syndrome appears within 10 to 15 days after the exposure. This is caused by the effects of radiation on sensitive blood-forming elements, and once there is depletion of the red cells, white cells, and platelets, signs appear in the patient. Due to blood cell depletion there is great susceptibility to infectious disease at this time. Fig. 6-12 illustrates this process. If recovery from the hematopoietic syndrome occurs, diseases may develop later in the individual's lifetime as the direct result of the radiation. Cancer is, of course, a major risk. There may be disorders of growth, and hair loss that occurs during the hematopoietic syndrome may be permanent. The aging process may appear to be accelerated (see Chapter 18). Permanent sterility may result, and radiation-in-

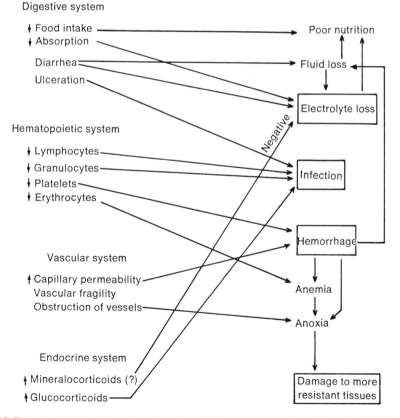

Fig. 6-13. Pathophysiologic interactions in acute radiation syndrome. (From Casarett, A. P., Radiation biology, © 1968, pp. 222 and 223. Reprinted by permission of Prentice-Hall, Inc., Englewood Cliffs, N.J.)

duced cataracts may appear many months or even years after the exposure.

The treatment of an individual with radiation sickness is aimed at prevention of infection, hemorrhage, and fluid and electrolyte imbalances. Each case of radiation exposure must be handled on an individual basis. Transfusions, antibiotics, and bone marrow transplantation are all possible modes of treatment. Fig. 6-13 shows the pathophysiologic interactions of the systems most affected by radiation.

While radiation sickness of the degree just described is rarely encountered clinically, many patients receiving radiation therapy do experience minor variants of the radiation sickness syndrome. Nausea, vomiting, and hematopoietic depletion are all commonly experienced. Furthermore, the target tissue of the radiotherapy may be damaged significantly, and if the tissue is radiosensitive, the patient will show signs and symptoms related to this damage.

Various chemicals and drugs have been described as radioprotective, in that they may diminish some of the damage caused by radiation when administered before and sometimes after the radiation exposure. These include sulfhydryl-containing compounds such as cysteine, a naturally occurring amino acid. These compounds may act as free radical "scavenger" molecules, thus removing these highly reactive compounds before they can damage biologic molecules. Radioprotective drugs include those that produce tissue hypoxia, such as histamine, epinephrine, and carbon monoxide. Pentobarbital, morphine, heroin, and central nervous system depressants also protect against radiation damage to some degree.

SUMMARY

This chapter has described the pathophysiologic effects of chemical and physical agents. It has related the specific effects of various agents to the general, nonspecific effects of stressors of all types in the body. The agents that can cause pathophysiologic processes are agents that have penetrated, overcome, and overwhelmed the normal body defenses and barriers. All of the defenses and barriers act in cooperation with each other to protect the normal steady state. While we have separated these defenses and barriers in the preceding chapters, nevertheless they are mutually interactive at all times in the healthy person. When pathophysiology of one defense system develops, often the structural and functional integrity of the other defenses also breaks down. All pathophysiology can be viewed in some sense as a breakdown in the normal body defenses and barriers. While we will discuss various disease mechanisms in the organ systems of the body in the following chapters it is well for the reader to keep this concept in mind: no matter what disease mechanism is perpetuated in the heart, the kidneys, or the gut, necrosis, regardless of where it occurs will always provoke defense reactions such as inflammation and immune responsiveness. When studying the process of peptic ulceration, for example, we must keep in mind not only the effects of peptic ulceration on normal gastrointestinal physiology. Peptic ulceration must also be viewed as an inflammatory, necrotic, ulcerative process, which has both resulted from a breakdown in normal barriers and has further perpetuated a state in which the normal defenses are depressed. This example typifies pathophysiology, for it is important not only to understand a disease mechanism but also to relate the disease process to normal physiology as a whole, and always in relationship to the individual's ability to maintain the steady state.

SUGGESTED READINGS

Aldridge, W. N., editor: Mechanisms of toxicity, New York, 1971, St. Martin's Press.

Anderson, W. A. D., and Kissane, J. M., editors: Pathology, ed. 7, St. Louis, 1977, The C. V. Mosby Co.

Bernstein, I. A., editor: Biochemical responses to environmental stress, New York, 1971, Plenum Publishing Corporation.

Cassaret, A.: Radiation biology, Englewood Cliffs, N.J., 1968, Prentice-Hall.

Curreri, P., et al.: Intracellular cation alterations following major trauma: effect of supranormal caloric intake, J. Trauma **11**:391-396, 1971.

Gump, F., Martin, P., and Kinney, J.: Oxygen consumption in surgical patients, Surg. Gynecol. Obstet. **173:** 499-512, 1973.

Hayes, W., editor: Essays in toxicology, vol. 7, New York, 1976, Academic Press.

Ingram, D. L., and Mount, L. E.: Man and animals in

hot environments, New York, 1975, Springer-Verlag New York.

Jacoby, F. G.: Nursing care of the patient with burns, ed. 2, St. Louis, 1976, The C. V. Mosby Co.

Jernigan, E., editor: Lead poisoning in man and animals, New York, 1973, MSS Information Corporation.

Kappas, A., and Alvares, A.: How the liver metabolizes foreign substances, Sci. Am. **232:**22-31, 1975.

Khan, M. A. Q., and Bederka, J., editors: Survival in toxic environments, New York, 1974, Academic Press.

Lieber, C. S.: The metabolism of alcohol, Sci. Am. **234:**24-33, 1976.

Magalhaes, H., editor: Environmental variables in animal experimentation, Lewisburg, Pa., 1974, Bucknell University Press.

Millis, J., editor: Biological aspects of circadian rhythms, London, 1973, Plenum Publishing Corporation.

Robbins, S., and Angell, M.: Basic pathology, Philadelphia, 1976, W. B. Saunders Co.

Rocha, D., Santeusandio, F., Faloona, G., and Unger, R.: Abnormal pancreatic alpha-cell function in bacterial functions, N. Engl. J. Med. **288:**700-703, 1973.

Selye, H.: Forty years of stress research: principal remaining problems and misconceptions, Can. Med. Assoc. J. **115:**53-56, 1976.

Selye, H., Somogyi, A., and Vegh, P.: Inflammation, topical stress and the concept of pluricausal diseases. In Chemical biology of inflammation. Brook Lodge conference on inflammation, Oxford, Eng., 1968, Pergamon Press Ltd.

Stein, M., Schiavi, R., and Camerino, M.: Influence of brain and behavior on the immune system, Science **191:**435-440, 1976.

Wilmore, D. W., Lindsey, C. A., Moyland, J. A., et al.: Hyperglucagonaemia after burns, Lancet **1:**73-75, 1974.

Wilmore, D. W., Long, J. M., Mason, A. D., Jr., et al.: Catecholamines: mediator of the hypermetabolic response to thermal injury, Ann. Surg. **180:**653-668, 1974.

Wintrobe, M., editor: Harrison's principles of internal medicine, ed. 7, New York, 1974, McGraw-Hill Book Co.

Zawacki, B., Spitzer, K., Mason, A., and Johns, L.: Does increased evaporative water loss cause hypermetabolism in burned patients? Ann. Surg. **171:**236-240, 1970.

Zbinden, G.: Progress in toxicology, vols. 1 and 2, New York, 1973, 1976, Springer-Verlag New York.

PART FOUR

Pathophysiology of physical and chemical equilibria

CHAPTER 7

Oxygenation and cellular metabolism

AT THE COMPLETION OF THIS CHAPTER THE STUDENT WILL BE ABLE TO:

- Discuss the role of oxygen in energy production.
- Describe the effects of a lack of oxygen on cellular energy production.
- Differentiate between aerobic and anaerobic cellular metabolism.
- Identify four causes of tissue hypoxia.
- Describe the cellular and systemic effects (clinical manifestations) of hypoxia.
- Relate principles of the gas laws to blood gas determination.
- Discuss the significance of blood gas determination and pulmonary function studies in evaluating oxygenation status.

NORMAL OXYGENATION PROCESSES

The term *oxygenation* denotes those processes by which oxygen is delivered to the cell and carbon dioxide (CO_2) is removed from the cell. These processes include ventilation, exchange, and transport or circulation. Ventilation refers to the mechanics of drawing oxygen from the atmosphere into the alveoli of the lungs and expelling carbon dioxide from the alveoli of the lungs into the atmosphere. Ventilation consists of two phases: inspiration and expiration. Exchange refers to the diffusion of oxygen from the alveoli into the blood and subsequently into the body tissues, replacing carbon dioxide, which is removed in the same manner. Transport refers to the process by which oxygen and carbon dioxide are carried between the lungs and body tissues. Disruption of these processes can lead to an oxygen deficiency or to disruption of normal levels of carbon dioxide at the cellular level.

The production of energy in the form of adenosine triphosphate (ATP) is essential for the cell to carry on metabolic activities. In the mitochondria of the cell, hydrogen atoms, released from glucose molecules, combine with oxygen in a series of oxidative reactions from which energy is generated to convert adenosine diphosphate (ADP) to ATP, the form of energy that can be utilized by the cell. The role of oxygen in ATP production is summarized in the following equation:

$$CHO + O_2 \rightarrow CO_2 + H_2O + ATP$$
Simple sugars

Hypoxia is an important concept in the study of pathophysiology because it can be produced by a variety of disease mechanisms. Cellular hypoxia seriously impairs the process of cellular energy production and thus limits the cell's ability to carry on normal cellular functions. This chapter will examine the effects of hypoxia on cellular metabolism and function. Cellular and systemic manifestations will also be discussed in terms of the disruption in normal structure and function and the compensatory mechanisms that occur in response to hypoxia. An introduction to the methods of clinical evaluation of the tissue oxygenation status is included in this chapter in order that the correlation between the assessment data thus obtained and the underlying pathophysiologic

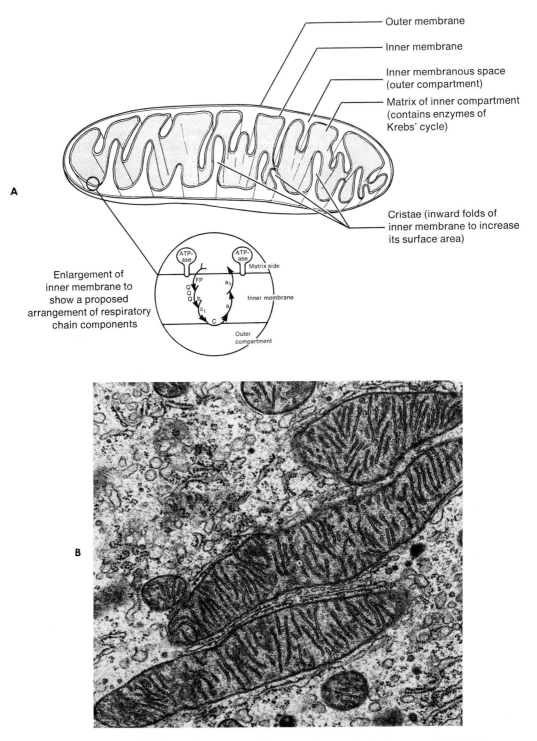

A

Outer membrane

Inner membrane

Inner membranous space
(outer compartment)

Matrix of inner compartment
(contains enzymes of
Krebs' cycle)

Cristae (inward folds of
inner membrane to increase
its surface area)

Enlargement of
inner membrane to
show a proposed
arrangement of respiratory
chain components

ATP-ase

ATP-ase

Matrix side

FP

Q
Q
Q

b

c_1

C

a_3

a

Inner membrane

Outer
compartment

B

Fig. 7-1. A, Mitochondrion with enlargement of inner membrane, showing proposed structural arrangement of respiratory chain components. **B,** Mitochondria sectioned both longitudinally and across. (×25,000.) (**B** from Anderson, W. A. D., and Kissane, J. M.: Pathology, ed. 7, St. Louis, 1977, The C. V. Mosby Co.)

mechanisms be less ambiguous to the student. This discussion is also intended to aid the student in evaluating the reliability of various assessment factors as indicators of the tissue oxygenation status. With this ability the student will be able to interpret assessment data in a more meaningful and valid manner.

CELLULAR OXYGEN UTILIZATION

The cell requires energy for the transport of substances across the cell membrane and for the synthesis of substances within the cell. Additionally, specialized cells require energy in order to perform mechanical and electrical work functions. The form of energy utilized by the cell is ATP, a nucleotide composed of adenine, a nitrogen base, ribose, a sugar, and three phosphate radicals. Two of the phosphate radicals are connected by a high-energy bond. When energy is needed by the cell, a phosphate radical is enzymatically hydrolyzed, releasing the energy from the bond (approximately 8,000 calories per mole of ATP) and leaving ADP.

The formation of ATP from nutrients depends on a series of chemical reactions. Enzymes in the cytoplasm of the cell convert glucose into pyruvic acid and fatty acids, and most amino acids into acetoacetic acid. The pyruvic and acetoacetic acids are converted into acetylcoenzyme A, which is then transported into the mitochondria of the cell. Located within the mitochondria are the enzymes of the Krebs cycle and the enzymes and respiratory pigments that form the electron transport chain.

The mitochondria are active organelles of the cell, which are constantly changing shape. They are especially active and numerous in highly metabolic tissue such as the liver. The outer membrane separates the mitochondrion from the cytoplasm of the cell. The inner membrane has deep folds within itself, which are called cristae and which are lined with spherical particles. It is thought that the enzymes and respiratory pigments of the electron transport chain are arranged along the inner membrane so that the sequential occurrence of reactions and the orderly flow of electrons from one assembly to another are enhanced. Fig. 7-1 illustrates the normal mitochondrion schematically

and in an electron micrograph and the proposed arrangement of the components of the electron transport chain.

In the mitochondria, hydrogen and carbon dioxide are released from the acetyl portion of acetylcoenzyme A through the sequence of chemical reactions of the Krebs cycle (Fig. 7-2). Some ATP is formed as a result of the reactions occurring within the Krebs cycle; however, approximately 90% of the ATP needed by the cell is formed during the subsequent oxidation of the released hydrogen. Hydrogen atoms and electrons are transferred via a series of oxidation-reduction reactions along the electron transport chain to oxygen, the final acceptor, to form water. During these reactions, at different points along the chain, inorganic phosphate becomes coupled with ADP to form ATP. This process of electron transfer from donor to acceptor with the resultant phosphorylation of ADP to form ATP is called *oxidative phosphorylation* (Fig. 7-2).

Oxidative phosphorylation is dependent on both a supply of oxygen adequate to meet the cell's requirements and on the cell's ability to utilize the delivered oxygen. Cellular oxygen requirements are determined by the rate of the cell's metabolic reactions. These energy-producing metabolic reactions occur in response to the availability of ADP, and its presence acts as a feedback mechanism to initiate the glycolytic reactions. As the end products of the metabolic reactions accumulate, the hydrogen ion concentration increases (pH decreases), and the respiratory center is stimulated to increase the rate of respiration to make more oxygen available for oxidative phosphorylation. The respiratory rate and depth, the arterial oxygen and carbon dioxide content, and the total blood flow and oxygen-carrying capacity will determine the amount of oxygen delivered to the cell each minute. The intactness of the mitochondria and the enzymes and respiratory pigments of the electron transport chain will determine the cell's ability to utilize the oxygen effectively.

Disruption of cellular oxygen supply and utilization

The term *hypoxia* refers to a condition of inadequate cellular oxygenation, which can be

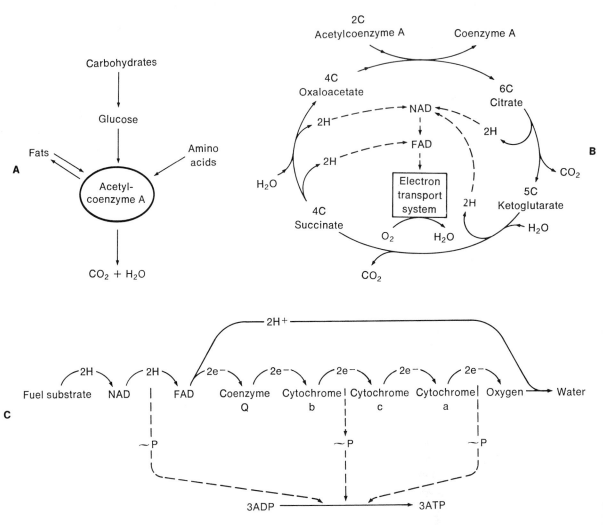

Fig. 7-2. A, Acetylcoenzyme A is an important intermediate in oxidation of carbohydrates, proteins (amino acids), and fats. **B,** Citric acid cycle. **C,** Electron transport system. Electrons are transferred from one carrier to next, terminating with molecular oxygen to form water. A carrier is reduced by accepting electrons and then is reoxidized by donating its electrons to next carrier. ATP is generated at three points in the chain. These electron carriers are located on inner membrane spheres of mitochondria. (From Hickman, C. P., Hickman, F. M., and Hickman, C. P., Jr.: Integrated principles of zoology, ed. 5, St. Louis, 1974, The C. V. Mosby Co.)

the result of a deficiency in either the delivery or the utilization of oxygen at the cellular level. When hypoxia develops, oxidative phosphorylation is impaired, and cellular energy production is severely reduced; 1 minute of anoxia results in a tenfold decrease in the ATP:ADP ratio. Glycolysis, the series of chemical reactions in which glucose is broken down into pyruvic acid and hydrogen, does not require oxygen and can continue in the presence of hypoxia but will yield only a relatively small amount of ATP. Under aerobic conditions the accumulation of greater than normal quantities of the products of glycolysis, pyruvic acid and hydrogen, would cause the glycolytic reactions to stop due to feedback inhibition. Under anaerobic conditions, however, the pyruvic acid and hydrogen are converted to lactic acid, which allows glycolysis to continue since there is no accumulation of the normal end

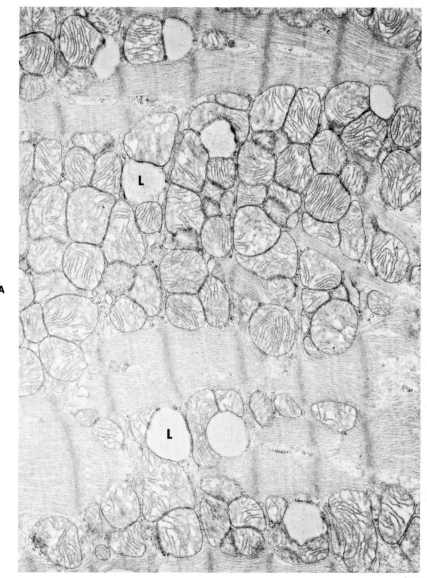

A

Continued.

Fig. 7-3. A, Ischemic injury of myocardium in a patient who died of severe irreversible shock. Mitochondria are swollen and numerous droplets of neutral lipid, *L,* are present. **B,** Various factors responsible for control of cell volume. High intracellular concentration of protein requires continuous active pumping of ions (largely sodium and potassium ions) and passive outward diffusion of water to counteract tendency for water to enter cells because intracellular osmolality is higher than that in extracellular space. Control is mediated by vectorial transport enzymes associated with cell membranes, particularly plasma membrane, that are driven by dephosphorylation of high-energy compounds like adenosine triphosphate (ATP). *Upper left,* Extracellular and intracellular concentration of various ions in "normal" cells are shown; maintenance of intracellular concentration of various ions requires expenditure of considerable work against a chemical gradient. Energy in form of ATP is supplied by aerobic glycolysis and mitochondrial phosphorylation (oxidative phosphorylation). Latter reaction or reactions are highly sensitive to alterations of substrate and oxygen concentration and are interrupted by ischemia. When pump is effective, it pumps Na^+ ions at a rate to balance their entry into cell by passive leak, which in turn regulates inward passive diffusion of water and thus cell volume. Note that active transport of Na^+ and K^+ ions also occurs in intracellular membrane systems such as endoplasmic reticulum. (From Scarpelli, D., and Trump, B. F.: Cell injury, Bethesda, Md., 1974, Universities Associated for Research and Education in Pathology, Inc.)

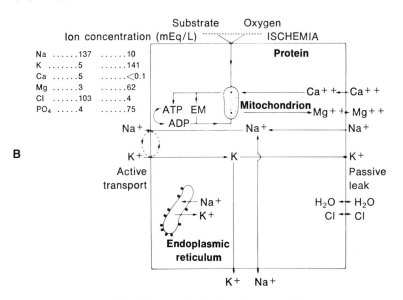

Fig. 7-3, cont'd. For legend see p. 183.

products of glycolysis. Anaerobic glycolysis via the Embden-Meyerhof pathway provides an energy source in the absence of oxygen, but it is an inefficient energy source, and the long-term effects are potentially detrimental to the functioning of most cells.

The presence of increased quantities of lactic acid under hypoxic conditions shifts the pH of the cellular environment to the acid side. A state of metabolic acidosis rapidly develops as the lactic acid is produced and diffuses out of the cell into the extracellular fluids. The Na^+-K^+ pump breaks down due to a decrease in the energy available for this active-transport process. Na^+ ions move into the cell, and K^+ ions leak out. This results in osmotic swelling of the mitochondria and cell, which gives the cell a swollen, cloudy appearance (Fig. 7-3). This cloudy swelling is especially prevalent in metabolically active tissue and is reversible. Mitochondrial function can be restored with a return of adequate oxygenation even after permanent changes have occurred elsewhere in the cell. The reduction in energy production and shift in pH further inhibit the chemical reactions of the cell, and the cell becomes unable to perform any of its functions (homeostatic control, motility, uptake of materials, synthesis, export, and reproduction) and is considered dead. The cellular effects of hypoxia then are the shift to

anaerobic metabolic pathways and the production of lactic acid, a reduction in ATP production, and a shift in the pH of the body fluids to an acidotic state, with eventual cell death if oxygen does not become available before irreversible cell death occurs.

Hypoxia can be classified according to cause:

anemic hypoxia hypoxia caused by a reduction in the amount of hemoglobin or blood available for oxygen transport.

histotoxic hypoxia hypoxia that results from the cell's inability to utilize the oxygen being delivered to it due to impairment of the cell's enzyme systems and the electron transport chain.

hypoxemic hypoxia hypoxia caused by a reduction in the total amount of oxygen available in the blood.

stagnant (ischemic) hypoxia hypoxia caused by poor tissue perfusion; the hemoglobin and oxygen content of the blood is normal, but oxygen is not being delivered to the cells.

Disorders of ventilation and exchange will lead to the condition of reduced arterial oxygen content, ultimately causing hypoxemic hypoxia. Disorders of oxygen transport will lead to alterations in the volume, oxygen-carrying capacity, and circulation of the blood, ultimately causing either anemic or stagnant hypoxia. Diseases that impair the processes of ventilation, exchange, and oxygen transport will be discussed in the following chapters.

Disorders of chemical equilibrium and the presence of poisonous chemical substances such as cyanide or arsenic lead to disruption of the cell's enzyme systems and inhibition of electron transport and the oxidation-reduction reactions of oxidative phosphorylation, ultimately causing histotoxic hypoxia.

In some disease states the body is able to meet normal cellular oxygen requirements but is unable to increase the supply of oxygen to the cell when oxygen requirements become greater than normal. In the presence of such a disease state any condition that would increase the metabolic rate would also enhance the development of hypoxia. Examples of conditions that increase the metabolic rate include exercise, fever, anxiety, stress, and an increase in the work load or energy expenditure of any organ system. Infectious processes and increased muscular activity due to seizures and shivering also increase the metabolic rate. Regulation of the metabolic rate is under the control of the thyroid hormones, which exert a calorigenic action. An increased amount of thyroid hormone has the effect of increasing the metabolic rate and oxygen consumption. The "normal" oxygen requirement for patients with hyperthyroidism is grossly increased, and therefore these patients are more susceptible to the development of hypoxia.

Manifestations of hypoxia may appear locally, the result of hypoxia affecting one particular organ, or systemically, the result of hypoxia affecting all the body tissues. Localized hypoxia is usually the result of a condition obstructing the delivery of oxygen to one particular area. The obstruction may be of the blood supply to the area or of the exchange process (the diffusion of oxygen out of the blood) at the cellular level. Generalized hypoxia can result from a variety of conditions affecting ventilation, exchange, and oxygen transport.

Manifestations of hypoxia vary. Some conditions cause only a slight reduction in the amount of oxygen delivered to the cell; other conditions result in a major reduction in the amount of oxygen; while still other conditions result in a total lack of oxygen (anoxia) in the tissues. Manifestations of hypoxia in some conditions may progressively worsen over a period of time. In these conditions physiologic mechanisms develop that help the body compensate for the chronic hypoxia. Manifestations of hypoxia may also indicate that the degree of hypoxia present is so severe that it poses a grave and immediate threat to the patient's survival.

Clinically detectable hypoxia results from functional impairment or death of the hypoxic cells in the various organ systems and tissues. A state of tissue ischemia is said to exist when the oxygen and substrate requirements of the tissue exceed the supply being delivered to and utilized by the cells. The ultimate effects of prolonged ischemia include cell death and necrosis (Fig. 7-4). Different tissues and organ systems respond to hypoxia in specific ways. Some are much more susceptible to the effects of ischemia than others. Nerve cells, for example, die after a few minutes of anoxia due to impaired blood flow. In contrast, fibroblasts can survive for a much longer period in the presence of anoxia.

An example of an extreme response to hypoxia is mesenteric ischemic disease, a life-threatening condition for which the prognosis is poor. Certain physiologic characteristics of the mesenteric circulation make it more susceptible to ischemic damage when blood flow is reduced due to a preexisting cardiovascular condition or circulatory problem. For this reason mesenteric ischemic disease is most frequently seen in aged patients with preexisting cardiovascular disease.

In the small vessels of the villi there is a countercurrent exchange mechanism, which allows shunting of oxygen from arteriole to venule. Normally the distal villi do not experience significant oxygen deprivation. However, when mesenteric blood flow is reduced, tissue hypoxia may become marked with subsequent necrosis of the mucosal villous tips. Blood viscosity increases, and microthrombi develop due to the reduced blood flow. In response to hypotension, sympathetic activity increases and the renin-angiotensin system is activated. This causes the release of vasoactive substances such as norepinephrine, dopamine, angiotensin II, and vasopressin, all of which act to constrict

Injury induced by ischemia

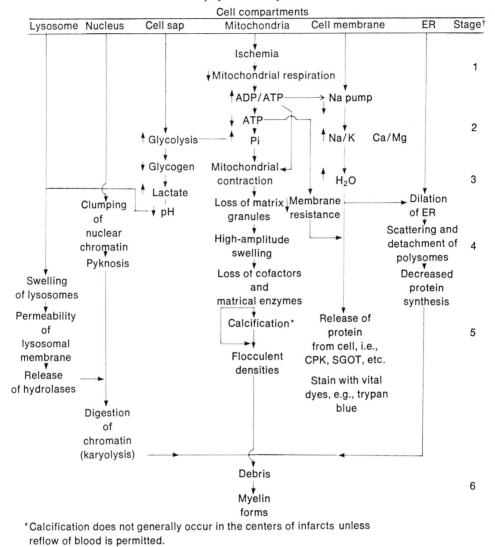

Fig. 7-4. Flow sheet of sequential events that occur in ischemic injury. (From Scarpelli, D., and Trump, B. F.: Cell injury, Bethesda, Md., 1974, Universities Associated for Research and Education in Pathology, Inc.)

the precapillary sphincters in the mesenteric circulation. Resistance to blood flow is further increased as the critical closing pressure in the small vessels is reached. Necrosis of the bowel leads to acute obstruction and allows the release of toxic substances into the general circulation, and toxemia and death rapidly ensue. Fig. 7-5 illustrates the sequence of events just described. Cardiac glycoside drugs may contribute to this

condition because of their tendency to constrict the mesenteric arterioles.

The cells of the central nervous system are particularly sensitive to hypoxia, as the metabolism of simple sugars is the usual source of energy for central nervous system cell function. Oxygen is rapidly utilized by cerebral tissue, and oxygen consumption by the brain accounts for 20% of the basal oxygen con-

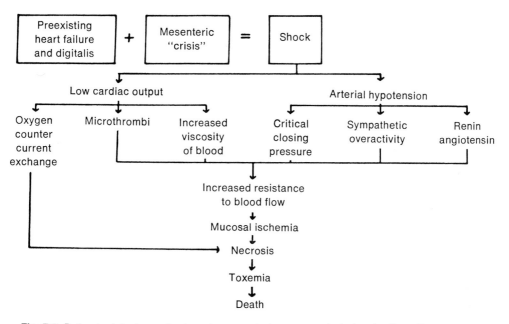

Fig. 7-5. Pathophysiologic mechanisms in nonocclusive mesenteric ischemia. (From Frohlich, E. D.: Pathophysiology, ed. 2, Philadelphia, 1976, J. B. Lippincott Co.)

sumption. Increased permeability of the cerebral capillaries is a response to hypoxia that contributes to the formation of cerebral edema. The subsequent disruption of the normal function of the cells of the central nervous system due to hypoxia results in a wide variety of clinically observable signs and symptoms, reflecting physiologic dysfunction of that system. Changes in behavior such as an increase in restlessness or uncooperativeness, inability to concentrate, apprehension, or any change in the level of consciousness from lethargy or mild confusion to unconsciousness may be indicative of hypoxia. None of these signs are specific for hypoxia, however, and all possible causes of central nervous system dysfunction must be ruled out.

Tachycardia, or increased cardiac rate, is a response to the direct effect of hypoxia on the automaticity of cardiac cells. Cardiac conducting tissue has a high oxygen consumption rate, and this may account for the increased irritability of cardiac tissue under hypoxic conditions. Oxygen extraction in myocardial tissue is extremely efficient, and increased coronary blood flow is the only mechanism that can increase oxygen delivery to the myocardium. Irreversible injury and death of the cardiac muscle cells will occur quickly in the absence of oxygen because of the extreme dependence of these cells on aerobic metabolism for ATP production. Anaerobic glycolysis will also fail to supply ATP as myocardial glycogen stores become depleted.

Hypoxia causes vasoconstriction of the precapillary vessels in the pulmonary vascular bed, which increases pulmonary vascular resistance. When hypoxia is chronic, the normal function of the right side of the heart is impaired because its work load is chronically increased as a result of the increased pulmonary vascular resistance. Renal tubular absorption is dependent on renal oxygen consumption and will be altered in hypoxic states. Renal ischemia is a known etiologic factor in the development of acute renal failure, the most extreme manifestation of disrupted renal function. The centrilobular cells of the liver receive a greatly diminished oxygen supply under normal conditions due to the low oxygen concentration of the blood in the portal system and the anatomic structure of the supplying blood vessels. Therefore, these cells are particularly susceptible to the effects of hypoxia. Liver dysfunction, cell death, and centrilobular fibrosis may result.

Hypoxia also alters the blood flow to the tissues and results in a shunting of the blood to the major organs. Blood flow through the tissues is determined by the availability of oxygen; the lower the concentration of oxygen in the tissues, the greater the blood flow to those tissues. Two theories attempt to explain this phenomenon. The *oxygen demand theory* is based on the fact that smooth muscle requires oxygen to remain contracted. According to this theory the oxygen concentration in the tissues regulates the contractile state of the precapillary sphincters in the arterioles. When the oxygen concentration in the tissues increases, the precapillary sphincters close and remain closed until oxygen concentrations decrease, causing the sphincters to reopen.

The second theory is the *vasodilator theory;* according to this theory vasodilator substances affect the precapillary sphincters and arterioles directly, causing vasodilation and increasing the blood flow and oxygen concentration in the tissues. An increase in the metabolic rate or a decrease in the availability of nutrients or oxygen would cause an increase in the rate of formation of the vasodilator substances. One of the postulated vasodilator substances is lactic acid, the product of anaerobic metabolism.

Pain is often the primary manifestation of tissue ischemia. In conditions where tissue perfusion is decreased, the removal of the products of metabolism, as well as the delivery of oxygen, becomes a problem. The pain is thought to occur in response to the stimulation of neural receptors by the lactic acid remaining as a result of anaerobic metabolism. The effects of stagnant hypoxia are usually local and in peripheral areas may also include abnormal sensations such as numbness and tingling as nerve endings are affected.

When tissue hypoxia is extreme due to either hypoxemic or stagnant hypoxia, cyanosis may be present. Cyanosis is a dusky bluish or grayish discoloration of the skin and mucous membranes that occurs when increased amounts of reduced hemoglobin are present in the blood. It is not a reliable sign of oxygenation status, however. First of all, cyanosis is a subjective observation dependent on many factors; for example, lighting, skin thickness and pigmentation, and the observer's perception. Second,

hemoglobin must be present in normal amounts in order for cyanosis to be interpreted meaningfully. Cyanosis is apparent when 5 g of hemoglobin per 100 ml of blood has been reduced and has reached the superficial capillaries. A person with a hemoglobin deficiency may be extremely hypoxic before cyanosis becomes apparent. A person who has an overabundance of hemoglobin might appear cyanotic, even though oxygen continues to be delivered in sufficient quantities to the cells. The absence or presence of cyanosis is not an absolute indicator of oxygenation status and must be interpreted in light of all other data.

Dyspnea is defined as air hunger accompanied by difficult or labored breathing. The manifestation of dyspnea varies from merely the subjective sensation of breathlessness to a visible, extremely exaggerated respiratory effort characterized by use of the accessory muscles of respiration, flaring of the nares, and an extreme increase in the rate and depth of respiration. Dyspnea is not directly related to the state of tissue oxygenation but rather indicates a discrepancy between the need for ventilation and the ability to meet that need. The development of dyspnea is dependent on three factors:

1. The state of the patient's mind
2. The relative concentrations of oxygen and carbon dioxide in the blood
3. The amount of work necessary to maintain normal blood gas relationships and ultimately oxygenation status (work of breathing)

As with cyanosis, the presence of dyspnea must be carefully evaluated. It is a subjective sensation that often accompanies anxiety states. Indeed, anxiety over real or imagined cardiopulmonary disease may cause a person to become acutely aware of his own respiratory pattern. A person may apply the label "shortness of breath" to other subjective complaints and symptoms such as pain on breathing, difficult expectoration of secretions, and severe coughing fits during which the breath is lost.

It was mentioned earlier that the symptom of dyspnea represents an imbalance between the need for ventilation and the ability to meet that need. The relative concentrations of oxygen and carbon dioxide in the blood determine the ventilatory requirement. They provide the stimulus for and determine the level of ventilation needed to meet the body's metabolic requirements through the following mechanisms.

Under normal conditions the carbon dioxide level provides the primary stimulus to ventilation. The hydrogen ion concentration is directly related to the carbon dioxide level since an increase in carbon dioxide causes increased formation of carbonic acid, which readily dissociates to free the hydrogen ions. The respiratory center in the medulla and pons of the brain stem responds to an increase in the hydrogen ion concentration by increasing the rate and depth of respiration. When the hydrogen ion concentration decreases, the respiratory center inhibits respiration so that carbon dioxide can be retained to maintain the balance between the bicarbonate and carbonic acid content of the body fluids.

The hypoxic drive provides a secondary stimulus to ventilation under normal conditions. Peripheral chemoreceptors in the aortic and carotid bodies are responsive to low arterial oxygen levels or hypoxemia. The peripheral chemoreceptors are also sensitive to carbon dioxide and hydrogen ion levels but not to the extent of the central respiratory centers. The peripheral chemoreceptors are stimulated by either a decreased partial pressure of oxygen in the blood or by a reduction in the flow of blood since they are sensitive to oxygen levels over a period of time. A reduction in oxygen content or flow stimulates the chemoreceptors, which in turn reflexly stimulate the respiratory centers to increase the rate and depth of ventilation.

In patients experiencing chronic carbon dioxide retention, the hypoxic drive becomes the main stimulus for respiration as the central respiratory centers become nonresponsive to the high carbon dioxide levels. This is seen in emphysema where airway obstruction results in chronic hypoventilation and chronically elevated arterial carbon dioxide levels. The hydrogen ion concentration normally increases with a rise in carbon dioxide levels; however, in chronic carbon dioxide retention the change in pH is slight because of the compensatory mechanisms of bicarbonate ion retention and hydrogen ion excretion by the kidneys.

Administration of high levels of oxygen to these patients will remove the stimulus of low oxygen levels that causes respiration. As CO_2 levels increase in response to the depressed respirations, a condition referred to as *carbon dioxide narcosis* develops. The effects of this condition vary from a headache and drowsiness to complete disorientation, extreme lethargy, and eventually coma and death.

In an acute condition the inability to respond to the stimulus provided by the blood gases in a manner that returns them to normal will cause dyspnea. This is related to the ventilatory pattern, which the altered blood gases stimulate, and the corresponding amount of work involved. There is an optimal ventilatory frequency at which the work of breathing is at a minimum. A slow, deep ventilatory pattern, for example, that seen when carbon dioxide levels are low, or a shallow, rapid pattern, for example, that seen with high carbon dioxide levels, has the effect of increasing the total work of breathing.

There is a high correlation between an increase in the work of breathing and the occurrence of dyspnea. A change in ventilatory pattern is only one factor that may affect the work of breathing and produce dyspnea. The work of breathing is also determined by the degree of compliance of the lung tissue, the resistance of the airway, the presence of active expiration (normally a passive process), and use of the accessory muscles of respiration. Decreased pulmonary compliance, increased airway resistance, active expiration, or use of accessory muscles will increase the work of breathing and thus dyspnea. The actual sensation of dyspnea is thought to be the result of stimulation of nerve endings in the muscles and lungs. The neural pathways involved are not completely understood.

Certain compensatory mechanisms will develop in response to chronic hypoxia so that cellular needs can continue to be met. Hypoxia of renal tissue and possibly of other organs stimulates the kidneys to release the enzyme renal erythropoietin factor (REF) into the plasma, where it reacts with a plasma protein pro-

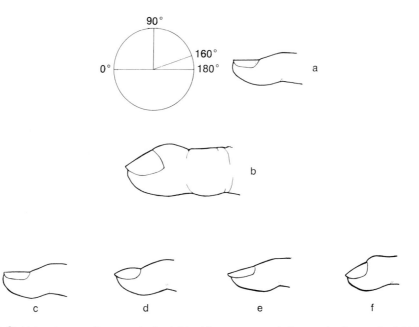

Fig. 7-6. Clubbing: *a*, normal base angle; *b*, clubbed finger; *c*, normal; *d*, curved nail; *e*, early clubbing (loss of base angle); *f*, advanced clubbing.

duced by the liver to form erythropoietin. Erythropoietin stimulates the bone marrow to increase red blood cell production. Formation of erythropoietin begins immediately in response to the hypoxia, but the peak of its effects is reached after 5 or more days. This mechanism increases the oxygen-carrying capacity of the blood and is demonstrated in persons who live in high altitudes and develop high-altitude polycythemia. Polycythemia is often seen in patients with severe emphysema and congenital heart disease who experience chronic hypoxemia and tissue hypoxia.

Another compensatory response to chronic hypoxia is the development of collateral circulation to areas where the flow of blood and hence oxygen delivery are obstructed. An increase in the vascularity of chronically hypoxic peripheral tissue results in a phenomenon called clubbing (Fig. 7-6). This is an increase in the size of the terminal digits with a loss of the normal nail bed angle.

CLINICAL INDICES OF OXYGENATION STATUS

It is not clinically feasible to measure the state of oxygenation of tissues directly. There are various clinical diagnostic studies that yield information relative to the adequacy of the various processes of oxygenation and thereby allow an approximate determination of the oxygenation status of the cells. The study of arterial blood samples to determine the amounts of oxygen and carbon dioxide present is called *arterial blood gas analysis* and indicates the effectiveness of the ventilatory exchange and, to a limited extent, the oxygen transport processes. Pulmonary function studies measure various lung volumes and capacities and the rate of air flow during ventilation. Measurement of pressures within the cardiovascular system and determination of the presence and rate of pulses throughout the body provide information on the adequacy of circulation and the oxygen transport process. Measurement of the hematocrit and hemoglobin content of the blood indicates the oxygen-carrying capacity of the blood. Observation of the patient's respiratory rate and rhythm, color, and various body characteristics as well as careful attention to and interpretation of the patient's subjective complaints can provide important information as to the oxygenation status of the tissues. Subjective as well as objective data must be considered; often subjective data provide the only means for valid and meaningful interpretation of objective data. This points up the necessity of complete and continual assessment of the patient's condition. Changes in the oxygenation status are frequently reflected in subjective data or data that can be interpreted subjectively. Changes may occur quickly and may require rapid action if the patient is to survive, or they may be insidious and thus difficult to detect.

Arterial blood gas analysis provides information about the tension or pressure being exerted by the gases in the blood. The pressures being measured are actually partial pressures since each gas exerts a particular amount of pressure. This is based on Dalton's law of partial pressures, which states that the total pressure of a given volume of a gas mixture is equal to the sum of the separate or partial pressures that each gas would exert if it alone occupied the entire volume. Partial pressure can be calculated using the total amount of pressure exerted by the gas mixture and multiplying it by the percent concentration of the particular gas being evaluated although electrodes are used that measure blood gas concentrations directly and accurately. The following data can be obtained through arterial blood gas analysis:

PO$_2$ the partial pressure or oxygen tension in the arterial blood. This reflects the amount of oxygen dissolved in the blood. Hypoxemia is the term used to describe a decrease in the partial pressure of oxygen in the blood.

PCO$_2$ the partial pressure of carbon dioxide in arterial blood. This value is directly affected by the rate of alveolar ventilation.

pH the negative logarithm of the hydrogen ion concentration. It is an indicator of the relative acidity and alkalinity of the body fluids.

O$_2$ saturation the amount of oxygen combined with hemoglobin and expressed as a percentage. This reflects the amount of oxygen being carried in combination with hemoglobin as oxyhemoglobin in the blood.

Blood gas values are interrelated. For this reason, interpretation of the results requires analysis of each value in relation to the others rather than in isolation. The box above contains the normal values obtained through blood gas analysis.

NORMAL ARTERIAL BLOOD GAS VALUES	
pH	7.35-7.45
PCO$_2$	38-42 mm Hg
PO$_2$	95-100 mm Hg
O$_2$ saturation	97%

Pulmonary function studies primarily provide information about the level of ventilation. The box (p. 192) presents the normal lung volumes, capacities, and flow rates. Alterations in these values can be expected in the presence of conditions that cause hypoventilation or hyperventilation. The diagnosis of these conditions is often made on the basis of the degree and type of alteration that is demonstrated.

DISEASE MODEL: ISCHEMIC HEART DISEASE

The nature of ischemic tissue injury in the heart and kidneys has been studied extensively. The disease model chosen for this chapter is ischemic heart disease because it so aptly illustrates a variety of pathophysiologic mechanisms that may evoke hypoxia in myocardial tissue.

The factors that determine myocardial oxygen consumption include the cardiac rate, left-sided ventricular wall tension, and the contractile state of the myocardial fibers. The cardiac rate depends on intrinsic and autonomic control. Left-sided ventricular wall tension is a function of the arterial blood pressure, ventricular volume, and the size of the ventricular muscle. The contractile state of the myocardium can be altered by catecholamines or sympathetic stimulation. Increases in the cardiac rate, wall tension, or contractility all have the effect of increasing myocardial oxygen consumption.

The factors that determine the supply of oxygen to the myocardium are the oxygen content of the blood, coronary blood flow, and coronary vascular resistance, the latter two factors being the most important. The distribution of the flow is as important as the total flow in providing oxygen to the myocardium. Any disease state that alters coronary vascular resistance, total

RESPIRATORY PARAMETERS

Lung volumes

Tidal volume (V_T)	Volume of air inspired and expired with a normal breath (400-500 ml or 5 ml/kg body weight)
Inspiratory reserve volume (IRV)	Maximal volume that can be inspired from the end of a normal inspiration
Expiratory reserve volume (ERV)	Maximal volume that can be exhaled by a forced expiration after a normal expiration
Residual volume (RV)	Volume of gas left in lung after maximal expiration
Minute volume (MV)	Amount of air inspired per minute

Lung capacities

Vital capacity (VC)	Maximal amount of air that can be expired after a maximal inspiratory effort (70 ml/kg body weight)
Inspiratory capacity (IC)	Maximal volume that can be inspired after a normal expiration (V_T + IRV)
Functional residual capacity (FRC)	Volume of air left in lungs after a normal expiration (ERV + RV)
Total lung capacity (TLC)	Total volume of gas in lungs after maximal inspiration (IRV + V_T + ERV + RV) (Men: 3.6-9.4 liters; women: 2.5-6.9 liters)

Flow rates

Forced expiratory volume (FEV, FEV_1, FEV_2, FEV_3)	Volume of air forcibly exhaled after a maximal inspiration in 1-, 2-, and 3-second intervals
Maximal expiratory flow (MEF)	Total amount of air expired per minute, breathing as rapidly as possible (approx. 400 liters/min)
Maximal inspiratory flow (MIF)	Total amount of air inspired per minute, breathing as rapidly as possible (approx. 300 liters/min)
Peak expiratory flow rate (PEFR)	Highest rate of flow sustained for 10 msec or more at which air can be expelled from the lungs

flow, or the distribution of the supplying vessels has the potential for reducing the oxygen supply. Additionally, diseases that decrease the oxygen-carrying capacity of the blood or the amount of oxygen available to combine with hemoglobin in the blood also have the capacity for reducing the oxygen supply to the myocardium, although not to the same extent as the other factors previously mentioned due to the extremely efficient oxygen extraction ability of the myocardium.

Ischemic cardiac disease can be produced by a variety of mechanisms that interrupt the delivery to (supply) or use of (consumption)

oxygen by the myocardium. Fig. 7-7 schematically illustrates the various sites at which myocardial ischemia might originate.

The most common cause of interrupted delivery of oxygen to the myocardium is occlusion of a coronary artery by an atherosclerotic plaque. This process usually involves the larger coronary arteries; however, small vessel or arteriolar disease may affect the coronary circulation. The microangiopathy of diabetes mellitus illustrates this mechanism. As muscle mass increases or hypertrophies, the blood supply to it does not increase to a comparable degree; for this reason hypertrophied myocardial tissue

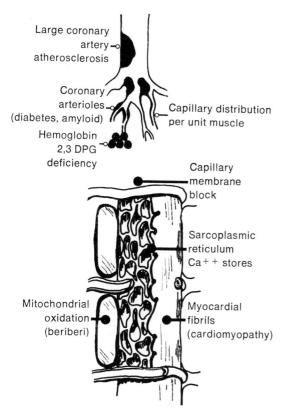

Large coronary
artery
atherosclerosis

Coronary
arterioles
(diabetes, amyloid)

Hemoglobin
2,3 DPG
deficiency

Capillary distribution
per unit muscle

Capillary
membrane
block

Sarcoplasmic
reticulum
Ca^{++} stores

Mitochondrial
oxidation
(beriberi)

Myocardial
fibrils
(cardiomyopathy)

Fig. 7-7. Circulatory and cellular sites where myocardial ischemia might arise. (From Frohlich, E. D.: Pathophysiology, ed. 2, Philadelphia, 1975, J. B. Lippincott Co.)

tion of intracellular enzyme systems may decrease the cell's ability to utilize oxygen. A thiamine deficiency (also known as beriberi) will cause a reduction in ATP production since thiamine is an essential component of the enzymes of the Krebs cycle.

The problem may lie in the utilization of ATP. In the disease condition known as thyrotoxicosis, where thyroid hormone is secreted in excess, much energy is lost in the form of heat rather than being coupled to high-energy phosphate compounds. A state of hypermetabolism exists due to the effects of the excess thyroid hormone, which normally controls the metabolic rate. As a result the oxygen demands of all the tissues are increased, and the work load of the heart is increased as it attempts to meet those demands. ATP production is already impaired by the uncoupling of oxidative phosphorylation, and "high output" heart failure may occur when the heart is no longer able to meet those demands in spite of a normal or possibly even increased cardiac output. Fatigue will occur more rapidly due to the reduction in ATP production.

No matter what the causative mechanism, the clinical manifestations of ischemic heart disease will be the same: pain, myocardial failure, arrhythmias, and possible necrosis or infarction of the tissue. Underlying these manifestations is the cellular hypoxia, which can be detected as a concentration of lactate in the blood of the coronary sinus, exceeding that of the arterial blood. Anginal pain is thought to be due to neural stimulation by the products of anaerobic metabolism. Arrhythmias reflect dysfunction of the highly oxygen-dependent conduction tissue. Contraction of the ischemic myocardial muscle weakens and eventually fails due to lack of ATP for energy and failure of Ca^{++} transport for activation of muscle myosin. Impairment of ventricular function sets up a feedback loop, which perpetuates the ischemia. Left-sided ventricular dysfunction creates a vicious cycle that perpetuates ischemia via three distinct mechanisms, one of which increases myocardial oxygen consumption while the other two act to reduce coronary flow. As the ventricle fails, it dilates, which increases wall tension and thus oxygen

lacks the necessary distribution of vessels to supply oxygen in an amount sufficient to prevent hypoxia. This is especially true for conditions in which myocardial oxygen demand is increased. Cardiac hypertrophy occurs in conditions in which the work load of the heart is chronically increased; for example, congestive heart failure and hypertensive vascular disease.

Blood and oxygen may be delivered to the myocardial tissue in sufficient amount, but an increase in the affinity of hemoglobin for oxygen may prevent gas exchange at the tissue level. This increased affinity occurs when red cell glycolysis is inhibited and less than normal 2,3-diphosphoglycerate (2,3-DPG) concentrations are being formed. Various physiologic situations are known to inhibit red cell glycolysis and therefore decrease 2,3-DPG. A low pH of the blood has this effect, and therefore in acidotic states an increased affinity between hemoglobin and oxygen exists. Disrup-

consumption, aggravating the ischemic condition. Ventricular dysfunction will lower cardiac output and arterial pressure, thus decreasing coronary perfusion and further aggravating the ischemic condition. The increase in end-diastolic pressure that accompanies ventricular failure also reduces blood flow in this endocardium during diastole, and this tissue becomes extremely susceptible to the effects of ischemia.

SUMMARY

A review of the role of oxygen in cellular metabolism is presented in this chapter. Hypoxia, or inadequate cellular oxygenation, results in a shift to anaerobic metabolic pathways, causing acidosis, decreased energy production, and inhibition of function at the cellular levels. A state of ischemia is said to exist when the tissue demands for oxygen exceed the ability to meet those demands; if ischemia is prolonged, it may cause necrosis of the affected tissues. Clinical manifestations of hypoxia depend on the degree and extent of the hypoxia. Hypoxia may be systemic or local.

Various compensatory mechanisms come into play in the presence of chronic hypoxia.

The diagnostic studies used clinically to indirectly evaluate the state of cellular oxygenation are also reviewed briefly. These diagnostic studies must be interpreted in light of all other signs and symptoms exhibited by the patient.

SUGGESTED READINGS

De Robertis, E. D. P., et al.: Cell biology, ed. 6, Philadelphia, 1975, W. B. Saunders Co.

Ditzel, J.: Impaired oxygen transport in diabetes, Metab. Ther. 6(4):1-4, 1977.

Keyes, J.: Blood-gases and blood-gas transport, Heart Lung 3(6):945-954, 1974.

Montgomery, R. Dryer, R. L., Conway, T. W., and Spector, A. A.: Biochemistry: A case-oriented approach, ed. 2, St. Louis, 1977, The C. V. Mosby Co.

Nadel, J.: Pulmonary function testing, Basics R. D. vol. 1, no. 4, 1973.

Rose, S.: The chemistry of life, Baltimore, 1970, Penguin Books.

Shapiro, B., et al.: Clinical application of blood gases, ed. 2, Chicago, 1977, Year Book Medical Publishers.

Weber, K., et al.: Myocardial oxygen consumption; the role of wall force and shortening, Am. J. Physiol. 233(4):21-31, 1977.

CHAPTER 8

Disorders of ventilation and exchange

AT THE COMPLETION OF THIS CHAPTER THE STUDENT WILL BE ABLE TO:

- Explain the pathophysiologic mechanisms of disorders of ventilation and exchange.
  - Describe the alterations in normal function, dynamics, and regulation that occur in response to disruption of the normal ventilatory and exchange processes.
  - Identify compensatory and adaptive mechanisms that occur in response to disruption of the normal ventilatory and exchange processes.
  - Describe the clinical manifestations of altered dynamics and resultant adaptation.
- Cite the etiology of disorders of ventilation and exchange.
- Cite predisposing factors to the development of disorders of ventilation and exchange.
- Explain the treatment of disorders of ventilation and exchange.
  - Identify treatment measures.
  - Describe the physiologic basis of treatment.

Ventilation is the process by which oxygen is drawn into the lungs and carbon dioxide is expelled from the lungs. The two phases of ventilation are inspiration and expiration. Tidal volume is the measurement used to represent the volume of air inspired and expired with each breath. The physiologically significant portion of ventilation is the alveolar or effective ventilation, which is the portion that actually participates in the exchange process. Assessment of the adequacy of alveolar ventilation is not possible through clinical observation of the patient alone. The physiologic parameter that most directly and accurately reflects the adequacy of alveolar ventilation in relation to the metabolic rate is the partial pressure of carbon dioxide in arterial blood (Pco_2). Adequate ventilatory function depends on an intact thoracic musculoskeletal system, patent conducting airways, and functioning neurochemical regulatory controls, as well as the patency and integrity of the lung tissue itself.

Exchange is the process by which oxygen diffuses from the alveoli into the blood and from the blood into the tissues. Carbon dioxide is removed in a reversal of the same process. Exchange depends on adequate alveolar ventilation and pressure gradients and intact membranes between the areas where the exchange occurs.

NORMAL VENTILATORY FUNCTION, DYNAMICS, AND REGULATION

With an increase in the chest cavity size, air is drawn into the alveoli through the conducting airways. The conducting airways (nose, nasopharynx, trachea, bronchi, and bronchioles) warm, humidify, and filter the air. Approximately 150 ml of air remains in the conducting airways and is considered nonfunctional for gas exchange. Any portion of the ventilation that does not participate in gas exchange is termed *dead space ventilation*. Changes in the amount of dead space ventilation require a compensatory change in the rate of alveolar ventilation in order to maintain a normal level of alveolar ventilation. The ratio of dead space volume to tidal volume is an important measure of the efficiency of ventilation. A departure from the normal ratio, if uncorrected, will result in abnormal concentrations of blood gases.

Enlargement of the chest cavity is accomplished through muscular contraction. Contraction of the diaphragm causes the diaphragm to descend, and the downward movement causes the chest cavity to lengthen. Elevation of the sternum and ribs causes an increase in the anteroposterior chest size. The abdominal muscles can also be utilized to further increase chest expansion. While inspiration is an active process, expiration is achieved through passive relaxation of the muscles, which allows the elastic recoil of the thorax and lungs, causing chest cavity size to decrease.

The thorax and lungs have a continuous tendency to collapse, which is referred to as recoil tendency. Intrapleural pressure is the amount of negative pressure in the intrapleural spaces necessary to keep the lungs from collapsing and is considered a measure of the recoil tendency. As the lungs expand and the recoil tendency becomes greater, intrapleural pressure increases. This recoil tendency is due to the presence of elastic fibers throughout the lung tissue, which are constantly attempting to shorten, and the surface tension of the fluid lining the alveoli, which causes the sides of the alveoli to be attracted to one another and therefore causes the alveoli to tend to collapse. Specialized secretory cells in the alveolar epithelium secrete *surfactant,* a lipoprotein containing dipalmitoyl lecithin, which reduces the surface tension and prevents the collapse of the alveoli.

The movement of air in and out of the lungs is ultimately the result of pressure changes that occur as the lungs are alternately compressed and distended. During inspiration as the lung volumes increase, the intra-alveolar pressure becomes less than atmospheric pressure, and air is pulled into the expanded lungs. During expiration as lung volumes decrease, the intra-alveolar pressure becomes greater than atmospheric pressure, and air is forced out of the lungs.

During normal tidal respiration when the lungs return to a resting position at the end of expiration, some alveoli do collapse as a result of the recoil tendency and the volume and pressure changes in the lung. The pressures and volumes associated with tidal respiration are insufficient to reexpand the already collapsed alveoli and to prevent the collapse of others. Higher pressures and volumes than normal are needed. The highest intra-alveolar pressure is reached while coughing. In normal respiration very deep breaths and sighs also provide such pressures and volumes, promoting reexpansion of the alveoli.

The inherent ability of the lungs and thorax to expand in response to an increase in intra-alveolar pressure is referred to as *compliance.* Pulmonary compliance is expressed as the volume increase in the lungs for each unit increase in the intra-alveolar pressure. For each centimeter increase in pressure the normal lungs can increase in size by approximately 130 ml. Pulmonary compliance is decreased in the presence of any condition that limits the ability of the lungs to expand.

In addition to the energy expended by contraction of the respiratory muscles, energy must be expended to overcome resistance to air flow and lung expansion. Both the airway and the viscosity of the pulmonary tissues offer resistance to air flow. The resistance caused by the pulmonary tissue is also called nonelastic tissue resistance. The *work of breathing* is the total amount of effort required to expand and contract the lungs. Any condition that results in an energy expenditure above that normal for respiration is said to increase the work of breathing. This includes conditions that decrease pulmonary compliance and increase resistance to air flow. An increase in energy expenditure accelerates metabolic activity, and consequently the need for oxygen is also increased. In conditions where the work of breathing is increased a vicious cycle has been set up: an increased need for oxygen in the presence of a reduced ability to meet even normal oxygen demands (Fig. 8-1).

Control of the rate and rhythm of respiration is highly developed, maintaining alveolar ventilation at a level sufficient to meet the oxygen needs of the body even during periods of extreme demand. Control is maintained through both neural and chemical mechanisms.

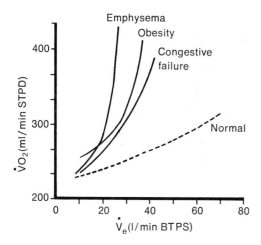

Fig. 8-1. Changes in oxygen consumption ($\dot{V}O_2$) associated with increasing ventilation in a normal person and in patients with congestive heart failure, obesity, and emphysema. (From Cherniack, R. M., Cherniack, L., and Naimark, A.: Respiration in health and disease, ed. 2, Philadelphia, 1972, W. B. Saunders Co.)

The respiratory center is located in the medulla oblongata and pons of the brain stem. The rate, rhythm, and depth of the respiration and subsequently the level of alveolar ventilation are controlled by this center. In response to signals from inspiratory and expiratory neurons in this center the respiratory muscles are alternately stimulated and inhibited. Efferent fibers carry impulses away from the center to the respiratory muscles via the phrenic and intercostal nerves.

The respiratory center responds to afferent nerve impulses from pulmonary stretch receptors, central and peripheral chemoreceptors, the cortex and thalamus of the brain, and arterial and venous baroreceptors. Stretch receptors, located throughout lung tissue and especially in the bronchi and bronchioles, are stimulated by inflation of the lungs. Upon stimulation, these receptors transmit impulses via the vagal afferent fibers to the respiratory center. The respiratory center responds, causing reflex inhibition of inspiration to prevent further inflation. This is called the Hering-Breuer reflex and serves to prevent overdistension of the lungs.

The central chemosensitive areas are located in the anterior medulla and are responsive to changes in the carbon dioxide levels and hydrogen ion concentration of the surrounding fluid. An increase in carbon dioxide levels causes a corresponding increase in the hydrogen ion concentration. This is because carbon dioxide in combination with water yields carbonic acid, which dissociates into hydrogen and bicarbonate ions. This is summarized in the following equation:

$$CO_2 + H_2O \leftrightarrow H_2CO_3 \leftrightarrow H^+ + HCO_3^-$$

A rise in carbon dioxide levels and hydrogen ion concentration directly stimulates the neurons of the respiratory center, and the rate of respiration and ultimately alveolar ventilation are increased.

Peripheral chemoreceptors located in the carotid and aortic bodies have afferent nerve fibers leading to the respiratory center. In response to both low arterial oxygen levels and to a lesser extent high carbon dioxide levels impulses from these chemoreceptors stimulate the respiratory center.

Arterial oxygen levels do not exert the major control over respiration and alveolar ventilation, however. This is because changes in alveolar ventilation have little effect on the degree of oxygen saturation of the blood. Alveolar ventilation can decrease to one half the normal rate, and the oxygen saturation of the blood can remain within 10% of normal. However, changes in alveolar ventilation have a profound effect on the level of carbon dioxide in the blood and interstitial fluids. Carbon dioxide is an end product of the metabolic reactions occurring in the cells, and accumulation of carbon dioxide and the resultant change in the hydrogen ion concentration (pH) will adversely affect the course of the metabolic reactions. For this reason it is important that the carbon dioxide level be regulated precisely and that it serve as the major feedback mechanism for alveolar ventilation.

The respiratory center is also stimulated by impulses from both the cortex for conscious hyperventilation and the thalamus in response to emotions. Additionally baroreceptors in the aortic and carotid sinuses respond to an increase in blood pressure by inhibition of the respiratory center.

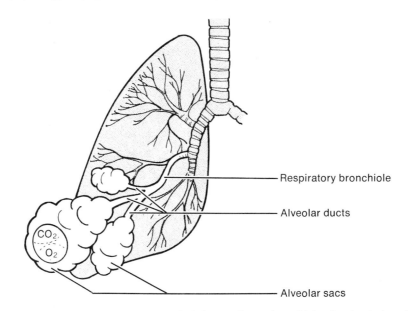

Fig. 8-2. Primary respiratory unit, the acinus, includes respiratory bronchiole, alveolar duct, and terminal alveolar sac.

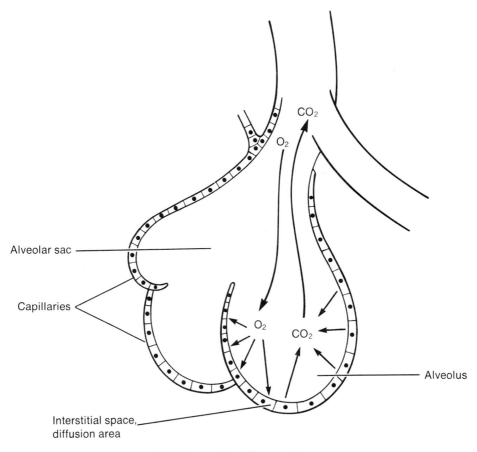

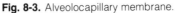

Fig. 8-3. Alveolocapillary membrane.

NORMAL EXCHANGE PROCESSES

The primary respiratory unit, or *acinus,* is that portion of the lung distal to the terminal nonrespiratory bronchiole. It is composed of the respiratory bronchiole, the alveolar duct, and the terminal alveolar sac (Fig. 8-2). In the lungs there is an extensive network of capillaries, which are in close proximity to the thin alveolar walls. The capillary and alveolar walls are separated by a thin interstitial space. This approximation constitutes the alveolocapillary membrane (Fig. 8-3). Diffusion of oxygen and carbon dioxide is continually taking place across the alveolocapillary membrane. Exchange across the membrane depends on several factors:

1. Adequate ventilation to maintain normal gas concentrations and volumes in the alveoli
2. Normal flow of blood through the pulmonary capillary bed (perfusion)
3. The thickness of the membrane itself
4. The surface area of the membrane
5. The relative pressure gradients and solubility of the gases on each side of the membrane (Diffusion is the movement of molecules or atoms from an area of higher concentration to one of lower concentration.)

Disruption of ventilation, pulmonary blood flow, the intactness and permeability of the alveolocapillary membrane, or the normal pressures of the gases in the alveoli and the blood will alter the exchange process. For effective gas exchange to occur, the ventilation and perfusion of alveoli must take place in a fairly uniform way. The ratio of ventilation to perfusion controls the concentration of oxygen and carbon dioxide in the alveolar air and in the blood. In other words, perfusion of poorly ventilated alveoli will result in low oxygen and high carbon dioxide tensions in the blood. This is termed a low ventilation-perfusion ratio. A high ventilation-perfusion ratio occurs when ventilation of alveoli is relatively greater than blood flow around them. This has the effect of increasing dead space ventilation.

Various conditions can affect either ventilation or perfusion in the lungs, resulting in a ventilation-perfusion mismatch. Even in normal lungs there is a certain degree of ventilation-perfusion mismatch. When a person is in an upright position, the apices of the lungs are well ventilated but, because of the effects of gravity, poorly perfused. In the bases of the lung the opposite effect is true; perfusion is greater than ventilation.

The units with high ventilation-perfusion ratios can compensate for those with low ratios to a limited extent. The amount of oxygen that can combine with hemoglobin is limited so the low oxygen concentrations will remain. The carbon dioxide level, however, can be adjusted. In the alveoli with the high ventilation-perfusion ratios more carbon dioxide will be removed from the blood, resulting in a lowered P_{CO_2}. When this blood mixes with the blood from alveolar units having low ventilation-perfusion ratios, the overall effect will be a normal arterial P_{CO_2}.

ALTERATIONS OF VENTILATION

Abnormalities of ventilation that can occur include hyperventilation and hypoventilation of the alveoli. Since the rate of removal of carbon dioxide from the alveoli is directly dependent on the rate of alveolar ventilation, measurement of the pressure exerted by carbon dioxide in the blood (P_{CO_2}) yields information on the adequacy of alveolar ventilation. Normal alveolar ventilation is defined as that level of alveolar ventilation sufficient to maintain a normal arterial carbon dioxide pressure of approximately 40 mm Hg.

Hyperventilation

Pathophysiologic mechanisms and clinical manifestations. The term *alveolar hyperventilation* refers to ventilation in excess of that required to maintain normal carbon dioxide levels in the body tissues. The pressure exerted by the carbon dioxide in the blood will fall below normal levels, as carbon dioxide is expired in greater than normal amounts by the lungs. As a result there is less carbon dioxide available to combine with water and form carbonic acid. There is a deficit of carbonic acid with a subsequent decrease in the hydrogen ion concentration.

The plasma pH (a measure of hydrogen ion

concentration) will be alkaline, and the normal ratio of 1 part carbonic acid to 20 parts bicarbonate is decreased on the carbonic acid side. Other terms used to describe this condition include respiratory alkalosis, primary carbonic acid deficit, hypocapnea, and nonmetabolic alkalosis.

The renal system attempts to compensate for this abnormality in acid-base balance by excreting bicarbonate ions and retaining hydrogen ions and nonbicarbonate anions. As a result of this homeostatic mechanism the pH (an expression of the hydrogen ion concentration) of the urine will be on the alkaline side, plasma bicarbonate levels will fall below normal, and the normal carbonic acid–base bicarbonate ratio of 1:20 will be restored.

In the presence of alkalosis, calcium ionization is decreased, which causes muscular irritability since the muscle becomes more responsive due to the altered membrane potential. The decrease in ionized Ca^{++} is due to the fact that protein-bound Ca^{++} is in equilibrium with H^+ according to the following formula:

$$CaPr + H^+ \rightleftharpoons HPr + Ca^{++}$$

When H^+ decreases, as in alkalosis, the reaction is driven toward the production of bound Ca (CaPr), thus reducing the amount of Ca^{++}. Muscular stiffness, aching, and cramps may be the only symptoms experienced; however, twitching, convulsions, and tetany may also occur. Tetany is more likely to occur only if the alkalosis developed rapidly. Signs that indicate abnormal muscular irritability can be elicited in the presence of respiratory alkalosis. Contraction of the muscles around the mouth in response to tapping the facial nerve in front of the ear is referred to as a *positive Chvostek's sign*. Muscular spasms of the hand and wrist as a result of compression of the brachial artery for 1 to 5 minutes is called a *positive Trousseau's sign*.

Blood flow to the vital organs is decreased as a result of both the vasoconstrictor effect of the low carbon dioxide concentration and the reduced cardiac output. Increased respiratory effort causes an increase in the intrathoracic pressure, which in turn impedes cardiac return, a major determinant of cardiac output. Subjec-

tive feelings of shortness of breath and chest pain due to the increased thoracic pressure and respiratory effort may be experienced. The alkalotic condition of the plasma inhibits the release of oxygen from oxyhemoglobin. The combination of vasoconstriction, reduced cardiac output, and inhibition of the release of oxygen from oxyhemoglobin results in tissue hypoxia.

The brain, because it utilizes approximately 20% of the total oxygen supply, is extremely sensitive to hypoxia, and symptoms such as dizziness, light-headedness, inability to concentrate, tinnitus, blurred vision, and disorientation may develop; ultimately unconsciousness may occur. Alkalosis also causes increased neuronal excitability. Convulsions are probably partially due to the cerebral ischemia, as well as to the muscular and neuronal irritability.

Etiology and treatment. Alveolar hyperventilation leads to respiratory alkalosis because of the excessive loss of carbon dioxide through the lungs with a resultant decrease in the arterial carbon dioxide concentration. One of the most common causes of alveolar hyperventilation and respiratory alkalosis is the abnormally rapid rate of respiration that accompanies anxiety and extreme emotional states. These persons sometimes hyperventilate to the point of unconsciousness. Treatment is aimed at promoting the accumulation of carbon dioxide by breath holding and rebreathing expired air. Reoccurrence is prevented by making the person aware of the effects of his breathing patterns and helping him understand and overcome the cause of his anxiety.

Another primary cause of alveolar hyperventilation is increased respiratory drive. High fever and infections such as encephalitis and meningitis cause irritability of the brain tissue, including the tissue of the respiratory center, causing it to become more sensitive than normal to stimuli. The result is an exaggerated respiratory response to even normal stimuli. Salicylate poisoning causes excessive stimulation of the respiratory center. Central nervous system lesions can also alter the sensitivity and response of the respiratory center, causing alveolar hyperventilation.

Mechanical overventilation with a respirator

will cause the loss of excessive amounts of carbon dioxide. Readjustment of the rate or addition of dead space to allow the patient to rebreathe greater amounts of his own air will correct the problem.

Alveolar hyperventilation can also occur as a compensatory homeostatic mechanism. In the presence of metabolic acidosis, pulmonary ventilation increases in order to reduce the amount of carbon dioxide available to form carbonic acid. Treatment is directed toward resolving the underlying metabolic acidosis. Alveolar hyperventilation can be caused by hypoxemia. A low arterial oxygen concentration stimulates peripheral chemoreceptors, which in turn stimulate the respiratory center to increase the respiratory effort. Administration of supplemental oxygen will usually increase oxygen saturation and eliminate the stimulus to increased respiratory effort.

Exposure to increased environmental temperatures causes hyperventilation as the lungs attempt to help maintain the normal body temperature. The same mechanism is partially true for the hyperventilation that occurs as a result of fever. Increased body temperature causes a 7% increase in the metabolic rate per degree Fahrenheit increase in body temperature. Any condition that increases the body's metabolic rate will also increase production of carbon dioxide, an end product of metabolism and the primary stimulus to respiration.

Hypoventilation

Pathophysiologic mechanisms and clinical manifestations. Alveolar hypoventilation is ventilation at a level insufficient to prevent retention of carbon dioxide. The result of alveolar hypoventilation is carbon dioxide retention, which is accompanied by hypoxemia. As the carbon dioxide concentration increases, oxygen concentrations decrease and carbonic acid levels rise, causing the ratio of 1:20 to increase on the carbonic acid side. Terms used to describe this condition include respiratory acidosis, primary carbon dioxide excess, nonmetabolic acidosis, hypercarbia, and hypercapnia.

The renal system attempts to compensate for the increase in extracellular carbonic acid by conserving base bicarbonate and excreting hydrogen ions and nonbicarbonate anions. This results in excretion of an acid urine and an increase in plasma bicarbonate levels. Before compensation occurs, the plasma pH will decrease. When carbon dioxide retention is chronic, the compensatory action of the kidney will keep changes in plasma pH minimal. Elevated arterial carbon dioxide and decreased arterial oxygen levels stimulate the carotid and aortic chemoreceptors to cause an increase in the rate and force of cardiac contraction, with a corresponding increase in pulse rate, strength, and blood pressure. Palpitations or a subjective awareness of the heart beat may be experienced due to the increase in the rate and strength of cardiac contraction.

Elevated carbon dioxide levels also cause cerebral vasodilation and an increase in cerebral blood flow. This causes both an increase in cerebrospinal fluid (CSF) pressure and cerebral edema. Dizziness, headache, confusion, and a feeling of pressure in the head are symptoms. Papilledema, or swelling of the optic nerve, may also result. The headache is usually in the occipital area, is throbbing, and is of greatest intensity when the patient first awakens.

As the extracellular hydrogen ion concentration increases, hydrogen ions begin to enter the cell. Potassium ions leave the cell in order to maintain the normal electrical gradient. Serum potassium levels will be increased at first but will decrease as a deficit in the total body potassium stores develops. Symptoms of low potassium levels (hypokalemia) include generalized muscle weakness and cramping. Long-term potassium loss causes degenerative changes in myocardial cells: loss of striation, nuclear disintegration, and eventually fibrosis. Life-threatening cardiac arrhythmias may occur since potassium is necessary for normal myocardial performance. These arrhythmias may also be attributed to the direct effects of hypoxia and hypercapnia on myocardial cells.

Changes in behavior in the presence of hypercapnia and hypoxemia are to be expected. Lethargy, disorientation, confusion, and uncooperativeness may occur in varying degrees. *Asterixis,* a flapping motion of the wrist when the hand is extended, may also be present. If the carbon dioxide concentration increases rapidly, convulsions and unconsciousness may result.

In response to the hypoxemia and acidosis, vasoconstriction of the pulmonary vessels and elevation of the pulmonary artery pressure occur as compensatory mechanisms to improve perfusion in the pulmonary vascular bed. This increases the work load of the right side of the heart, causing hypertrophy and a predisposition in the patient to the development of right-sided heart failure, or *cor pulmonale*. This is a constant threat to patients with chronic conditions that cause hypoventilation.

Another effect of chronic carbon dioxide retention is the nonresponsiveness of the respiratory centers to arterial carbon dioxide levels. The hypoxic drive becomes the primary stimulus to respiration. *Carbon dioxide narcosis* will develop if this stimulus is removed. The effects of this condition vary from a headache and drowsiness to complete disorientation, extreme lethargy, and eventually coma and death. Compensatory responses to chronic hypoxia (see Chapter 7), including erythropoiesis and increased vascularity of peripheral tissues, will also occur in the presence of chronic conditions causing hypoventilation.

Collapse of the alveoli is referred to as *atelectasis* and is the result of inadequate expansion of lung tissue. The tendency to develop atelectasis is enhanced in conditons that cause alveolar hypoventilation. Alveolar collapse occurs in obstructive disorders where the flow of inspired air is partially or completely obstructed with the subsequent reabsorption of alveolar air (absorption atelectasis) and as a result of space-occupying lesions or fluid accumulation in the chest, which compresses lung tissue (compression atelectasis). Microatelectasis is the result of "inspiratory failure" or respiration at a constant or reduced tidal volume. Microatelectasis can also occur as a result of increased surface tension within the alveoli due to surfactant deficiency. The collapsed alveoli are no longer functional for gas exchange, and the immediate result of atelectasis is disruption of normal blood gas values. A later result may be superimposed infection and broncho-pneumonia due to the anaerobic conditions existing in the collapsed lung tissue.

Etiology and treatment. Alveolar hypoventilation causes respiratory acidosis through retention of carbon dioxide and hypoxemia. Conditions that lead to alveolar hypoventilation and respiratory acidosis can be grouped under two major headings: those that decrease respiratory drive or the sensitivity and function of the respiratory center and those that decrease the ventilatory response through impairment of the mechanics of respiration. Another term used to describe varying degrees of alveolar hypoventilation is *ventilatory failure*. Ventilatory failure can be either acute or chronic with superimposed acute ventilatory failure accompanying chronic ventilatory failure. Acute ventilatory failure is characterized by a high arterial Pco_2 and a low arterial pH (acidemia). Ventilatory failure is considered chronic when compensation for the acidemia has occurred. Chronic ventilatory failure is characterized by a high arterial Pco_2 and a near normal pH.

Various drugs and anesthetic agents inhibit the sensitivity and function of the respiratory center. Sedatives, narcotics, and certain analgesics and anesthetics depress the sensitivity and function of the respiratory center, which in turn depresses respiration and leads to alveolar hypoventilation. Judicious use of such agents will prevent the development of alveolar hypoventilation.

Oxygen is a drug that can have toxic effects, and it should always be administered accordingly. For patients in whom the hypoxic drive provides the main stimulus for respiration, administration of high concentrations of oxygen will remove the sole stimulus for respiration. Alveolar hypoventilation is already present, and elimination of the stimulus to breathe will further depress ventilatory functions. In these patients the sensitivity of the respiratory center is altered since it is nonresponsive or refractory to chronically elevated levels of carbon dioxide.

The function of the respiratory center may also be depressed as a result of disease processes and direct damage to it. The respiratory center can be damaged by a reduction or loss of its blood supply, trauma (surgical or accidental), or increased intracranial pressure.

Blood supply to the medulla can be reduced or "lost" as a result of hemorrhage, narrowing, or obstruction of an artery by clot formation or arteriosclerotic processes. Increased intracranial pressure is the result of an increase in the volume of the intracranial matter and fluids. The volume increase can be due to a variety of causes: abnormal tissue growth of a tumor, hemorrhage, overproduction of cerebrospinal fluid, obstruction of the circulation of the cerebrospinal fluid, or the edematous swelling of brain tissue. *Primary ideopathic alveolar hypoventilation* is a disease condition in which there appears to be a primary defect in the functioning of the respiratory centers, leading to hypoventilation.

The goals of treatment of alveolar hypoventilation include

1. Restoring or maintaining optimal ventilatory function
2. Improving cellular oxygenation
3. Restoring or maintaining normal acid-base balance

Obviously the second and third goals depend on successful achievement of the first. To improve impaired ventilatory function the cause of the impairment must be considered. Where the cause of the impairment is decreased respiratory drive, the patient can be ventilated using an artificial respirator set on automatic so it "breathes" for him. This is a temporary, emergency measure. To permanently correct hypoventilation the cause of the decreased respiratory drive must also be treated. When decreased respiratory drive is the result of drugs, dosage or use should be decreased. An antagonist can be given in some cases, and in other cases various procedures to remove the drug from the body will have to be utilized. When the decreased respiratory drive is the result of disease or trauma, surgery to reduce intracranial pressure, restore blood supply, or repair damage might be done. Various drugs can be used to reduce cerebral edema and consequently intracranial pressure. Where severe damage to the medullary centers has occurred, restoration of normal respiratory function is highly improbable.

Alveolar hypoventilation can also occur in conditions where the ventilatory response is decreased due to disruption of the normal mechanics of respiration. These conditions can be classified according to the type of impairment that occurs:

1. Obstructive disorders
2. Restrictive disorders
3. Surfactant deficiency

Airway obstruction may be chronic or acute. Acute obstruction may result from aspiration of a foreign object, swelling of the trachea and pharyngeal area, spasm of the larynx or bronchi, or accumulation of respiratory tract secretions. Swelling or edema of the airway is an inflammatory response that can be evoked by physical or chemical trauma (e.g., airway obstruction following a burn with smoke inhalation), a hypersensitivity response (e.g., a severe anaphylactic reaction), or an infectious process (e.g., acute epiglottitis or tracheobronchitis).

The development of airway occlusion due to accumulated secretions is enhanced in conditions where a greater than normal amount of secretions is produced, where the secretions are thicker than normal, or where the normal protective cough mechanism is depressed. Alteration in the amount and character of the respiratory tract secretions occurs in the chronic obstructive disorders to be discussed later in this chapter.

Cystic fibrosis is a hereditary disease characterized by abnormal secretions of the exocrine glands. It is inherited as an autosomal recessive trait. When the lung is affected a thick, viscoid mucus is secreted, which can plug bronchioles and bronchi. The development of secondary infection and permanent fibrotic changes in the lungs also results from this disease process. The cough mechanism may be depressed or nonexistent in an altered state of consciousness such as coma or as a result of the direct action of drugs that depress cerebral function.

After surgery the expectoration of respiratory tract secretions becomes more difficult than it is normally. This is due to the increased viscosity of the secretions, inhibition of ciliary action, and the depression of the cough mechanism. Prior to surgery, anticholinergic drugs are administered to promote smooth muscle relaxation and to decrease body secretions. The mucous membranes of the respiratory tract, nasopharynx, and mouth become very dry, and mucus secretion is reduced. Endotracheal intubation bypasses the normal humidifying mechanisms of the upper airways. Ciliary action is inhibited because of damage to the cilia during endotracheal intubation and lack of proper humidity, and by the direct drug action of narcotic and anesthetic agents. Depression of the cough mechanism after surgery is the result of a combination of direct drug action (i.e., of anesthetic, narcotic, and sedative agents) and the altered level of consciousness. If secretions are allowed to accumulate, crusting and eventually occlusion may occur.

The signs and symptoms accompanying total acute obstruction are choking and gasping, severe dyspnea (air hunger), extreme anxiety, cyanosis, and eventually loss of consciousness. Arterial hypoxemia rapidly ensues, and the tissues are subjected to extreme hypoxia. Partial airway obstruction may also occur, and manifestations will be somewhat less extreme. Any degree of acute airway obstruction is serious and requires immediate treatment.

The first concern in treating acute obstruction is reestablishing the airway by removing or bypassing the obstruction. A foreign body can sometimes be forced out of the airway using the Heimlich maneuver. Compression of the abdomen causes residual air from the lungs to be pushed out, dislodging the foreign body. Bypassing an obstruction requires insertion of an endotracheal tube or the creation of an external opening to the trachea (tracheostomy). Removal of accumulated secretions can be done by inserting a catheter attached to suction into the airway to remove the secretions. The airway must be open for ventilation to occur at all.

Chronic airway obstruction is the result of a group of diseases that have the ultimate effect of obstructing the flow of air from the lungs, leading to hypercapnia and hypoxemia. This group of diseases is classified as chronic obstructive lung disease (COLD) or chronic obstructive pulmonary disease (COPD). Included in this group of diseases are asthma, bronchitis, and emphysema. Chronic obstructive pulmonary disease is the most common cause of alveolar hypoventilation with associated hyp-

oxemia, chronic hypercapnia, and compensated respiratory acidosis (Table 8-1).

The obstruction that occurs in asthma, which is intermittent in nature, is caused by narrowing of the bronchioles and bronchi, edema of the mucous membrane, and excessive production of abnormally viscous mucus. Asthma can be classified as either extrinsic (allergic) or intrinsic (ideopathic). Extrinsic asthma occurs as an anaphylactic type of hypersensitivity reaction. An inhaled antigen (allergen) combines with a specific antibody of the IgE immunoglobulin class on an effector cell membrane (usually basophils and mast cells), causing the cell to degranulate and release mediating substances, which stimulate the responses described above. Histamine, as a mediator, seems to be of less importance in asthma than SRS-A (slow-reacting substance of anaphylaxis). Extrinsic or allergic asthma is characterized by childhood onset and a positive family history of allergy; a positive wheal and flare skin reaction is obtained upon injection of antigens, and high levels of IgE are present.

The stimulus for asthmatic attacks in persons with intrinsic or ideopathic asthma is nonspecific. This type of asthma is characterized by a negative family history for allergy, normal IgE levels, onset later than childhood, and a negative skin test for allergens. Many factors can precipitate an attack, including changes in temperature and humidity, worry and stress, exercise, fatigue, exposure to pollutants and smoke, infections, and pollens.

Histologic changes that occur in asthma include the following: an increase in the size and number of the mucosal goblet cells and submucosal mucous glands, thickening of the bronchial basement membrane, hypertrophy of smooth bronchiolar and bronchial muscle, submucosal infiltration of mononuclear inflammatory cells, and usually eosinophils and plugs of mucus blocking small airways.

Treatment of asthma includes the administration of bronchodilating drugs in nebulized form, steroids to decrease swelling, and good bronchial hygiene measures to prevent superimposed infection. The alteration in blood gases that will occur depends on the extent and length of the attack. Hypoxemia will show up first as

Table 8-1. Differential features of COPD*

Feature	Emphysema	Chronic bronchitis	Asthma
Family history	Occasional (α_1-antitrypsin deficiency)	Occasional (cystic fibrosis)	Frequent
Atopy	Absent	Absent	Frequent
Smoking history	Usual	Usual	Infrequent
Sputum character	Absent or mucoid	Predominantly neutrophilic	Predominantly eosinophilic
Chest x-ray film	Useful if bullae, hyperinflation, or loss of peripheral vascular markings is present	Often normal; occasional hyperinflation	Often normal; hyperinflation during acute attack
Spirometry	Obstructive pattern unimproved with bronchodilator	Obstructive pattern improved with bronchodilator	Obstructive pattern usually shows good response to bronchodilator

*From American Lung Association: Chronic obstructive pulmonary disease, ed. 5, New York, 1977, The Association.

a decrease in Po_2, and as the attack persists oxygen saturation will also decrease. The Pco_2 may remain normal or even decrease as a result of the hyperventilation response in mild to moderate attacks. In severe attacks of long duration Pco_2 levels will increase as carbon dioxide is retained. An attack of more than 24 hours in duration is referred to as *status asthmaticus* and is considered a threat to the person's life. Increased respiratory effort increases intrathoracic pressure and reduces venous return to the heart. This effect, along with the vasoconstriction and increased resistance in the pulmonary vascular bed, increases the predisposition to right-sided heart failure.

The morphologic changes that occur in bronchitis include hypertrophy and hyperplasia of mucus-secreting bronchial glands and mucosal goblet cells, loss of cilia, and permanent inflammatory changes in the bronchial epithelium and wall. The enlargement and overactivity of the mucus-secreting glands constitute the primary defect. The airway lumen can be significantly narrowed as a result of hypertrophy and hyperplasia of the mucus-secreting glands and goblet cells since mucus glands form a large proportion of the bronchial wall (Fig. 8-4). Clinically the manifestations of bronchitis include excessive sputum production and coughing. Chronic bronchitis commonly precedes and sometimes accompanies emphysema.

In emphysema the acinus, or that portion of the lung distal to the terminal nonrespiratory bronchiole, is involved. The acinus includes the respiratory bronchiole composed of alveoli and nonalveolated epithelium, the alveolar duct, which is completely alveolated, and the terminal alveolar sac, or blind end of the airway, which is also entirely alveolated. Classification of emphysema depends on the area of the acinus involved. *Centrilobular emphysema* affects the respiratory bronchioles and is also called *centriacinar emphysema*. Involvement of the entire acinus is termed *panlobular* or *panacinar emphysema*. Involvement of the alveolar ducts and sacs is termed *periacinar* or *distal acinar emphysema*. The two principal types of emphysema are centrilobular and panlobular (Fig. 8-5).

Centrilobular emphysema is more prevalent in men than in women and is rarely seen in nonsmokers. The incidence of panlobular emphysema is related to a hereditary deficiency of a normal serum α_1-globulin, α_1-antitrypsin. This deficiency is genetically transmitted by a single, autosomal, recessive gene. Homozygotes develop panlobular emphysema, which is sometimes called *familial emphysema*. Panlobular emphysema has also been found in the lungs of aged persons, in persons with bronchitis who also smoke, and in persons with some degree of preexisting bronchial or bronchiolar obstruction. It is as common in women as it is in men. Air pollution and industrial pollutants do not appear to directly cause chronic obstructive pulmonary disease (Fig. 8-6) to the ex-

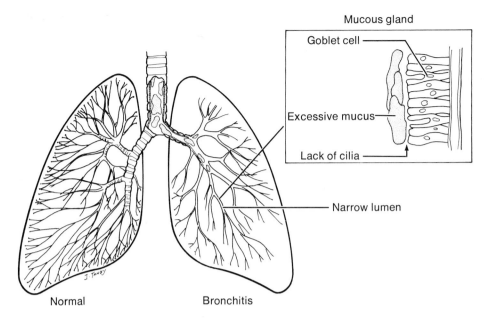

Fig. 8-4. Characteristic defect of bronchitis is hyperplasia and overactivity of mucus-secreting bronchial glands. Airway lumen can be significantly narrowed as a result of this.

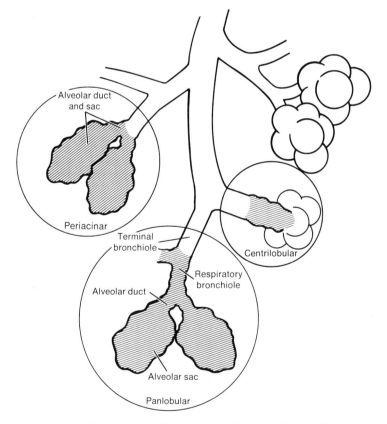

Fig. 8-5. Two types of emphysema: atrophic and destructive. Atrophic centrilobular emphysema is asymptomatic because peripheral alveoli are available. As centrilobular emphysema advances, periphery of acinus will also be destroyed, and condition becomes similar to panlobular emphysema and is symptomatic.

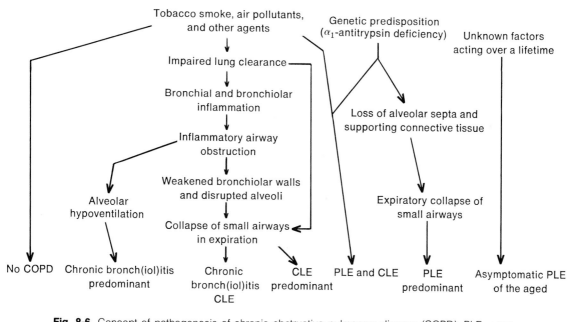

Fig. 8-6. Concept of pathogenesis of chronic obstructive pulmonary disease (COPD). PLE = panlobular emphysema; CLE = centrilobular emphysema. (From American Lung Association: Chronic obstructive pulmonary disease, ed. 5, New York, 1977, The Association.)

tent that they cause some other respiratory problems. Exposure to pollutants, noxious gases, fumes, and dust and the presence of infection will aggravate any preexisting cardiopulmonary problem. Smoking appears to be the leading etiologic factor in the development of emphysema and bronchitis.

The morphologic changes of lung tissue that occur in emphysema include thickening of the bronchiolar walls due to submucosal edema and cellular infiltration as well as hyperplasia of the mucus-secreting glands and goblet cells and dilation of the distal air spaces with destruction of the alveolar septa. Obstruction occurs because of the narrowing of the bronchiolar lumen, loss of the elastic recoil of the lung tissue, and secretion of excessive amounts of thick, tenacious mucus. This obstruction is greater during expiration than during inspiration and is irreversible, in contrast to the obstruction that accompanies asthma and bronchitis and that is potentially treatable.

In normal lungs expiration is passively achieved through relaxation of the diaphragm and chest muscles, which allows the elastic recoil of the thorax and lungs to reduce the size of the chest cavity. As the lung tissue is compressed, intra-alveolar pressure becomes greater than the pressure in the airways, and air is forced out of the alveoli into the airways and into the atmosphere. In emphysemic individuals expiration becomes an active process that increases the work of breathing and the energy expenditure of the body. The airway diameter is already reduced as a result of changes described above, and during expiration the increased pressure of the surrounding tissue causes further compression and collapse of the airway due to loss of the supporting tissue (Fig. 8-7). Air becomes trapped, causing distension of the distal airways. This airway distension leads to further destruction of the alveolar parenchyma. The elastic recoil of the tissue is reduced as the elastic fibers are destroyed, and surface tension decreases due to the reduction in alveolar surface area (Fig. 8-8). According to Poiseuille's law, as airway diameter decreases, the resistance to air flow increases. Pursed-lip breathing with use of accessory muscles will develop as the patient tries to exhale more completely and forcefully. In emphysemic individuals, then, the work of breathing

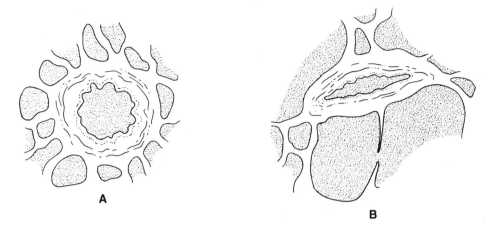

Fig. 8-7. A, Normal terminal bronchiole in cross section. **B,** Emphysematous terminal bronchiole in cross section. Loss of alveolar surface in emphysematous tissue surrounding lung results in partial bronchiolar collapse. (Adapted from American Lung Association: Chronic obstructive pulmonary disease, ed. 5, New York, 1977, The Association.)

is increased as a result of decreased compliance, increased resistance to air flow, and active expiration. The trapped air causes the lung tissue to become hyperresonant on percussion. Eventually the anteroposterior diameter of the chest will increase due to the airway distension and respiratory pattern. This causes the chest to become barrel shaped. Patients with emphysema can assume the supine position with no discomfort since this position increases the total vital capacity in this type of patient.

The onset of emphysema is insidious. Much damage may occur before dyspnea becomes bothersome or flow rates are measurably impaired. The clinical manifestations of emphysema depend on the severity of the obstructive processes. In mild obstructive disease the arterial oxygen level and oxygen saturation are slightly below normal. The Pco_2 may be normal or slightly below normal because of hyperventilation occurring as a result of stimulation of the hypoxic drive by low oxygen levels. Arterial pH is within normal limits due to renal compensatory mechanisms, which cause selective excretion of bicarbonate ions and retention of hydrogen ions. As a result the serum bicarbonate levels may fall below normal.

In moderately severe obstructive disorders the reduction in Po_2 and O_2 saturation is more severe, and mild hypercapnia results due to the alveolar hypoventilation. Because the hydrogen ion concentration normally increases with a rise in carbon dioxide levels, the arterial pH becomes slightly acidotic. With chronic carbon dioxide retention, however, arterial pH changes are minimal because of the compensatory mechanisms of selective bicarbonate ion retention and hydrogen ion excretion by the kidneys. Serum bicarbonate levels may be elevated as a result.

In severe obstruction, severe hypoxemia and hypercapnia are present. Severe acidosis is a result of both the greatly increased carbon dioxide levels and the accumulation of lactic acid as metabolism shifts to anaerobic pathways. Table 8-2 summarizes the blood gas changes that occur in varying degrees of obstructive disease. Fig. 8-9 shows the blood gas changes as the obstructive process proceeds to cause ventilatory failure.

The secondary polycythemia that occurs as a compensatory mechanism favors reduction of hypoxemia but causes increased blood volume and viscosity. The increased blood volume will increase the work load of the heart. The increased viscosity increases resistance to blood flow in the lungs and heart and thus also contributes to the increased cardiac work load as well as predisposing the patient to thrombus formation (see Chapter 5). The increased car-

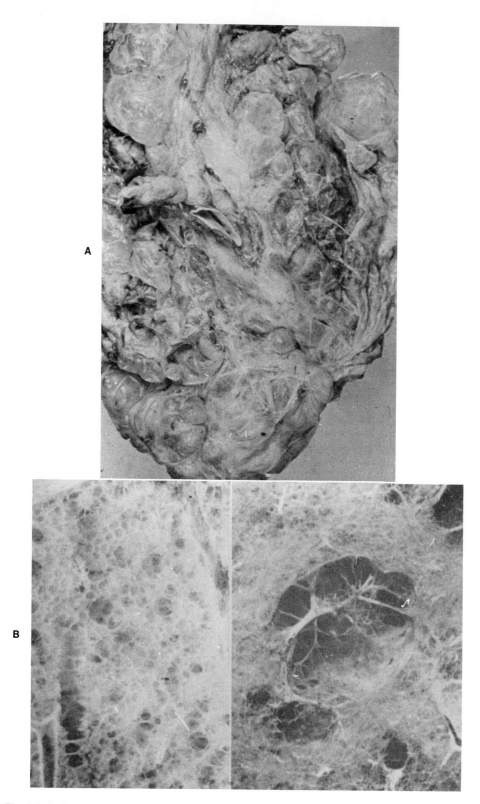

Fig. 8-8. A, Gross pathology of emphysemic lung. **B,** Microscopic view of alveolar tissue in panlobular and centrilobular emphysema. (Courtesy Department of Pathology, University of Tennessee, Memphis.)

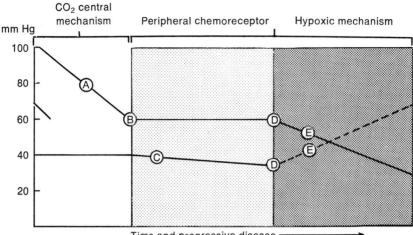

Fig. 8-9. A theory on pathogenesis of ventilatory failure in chronic obstructive pulmonary disease. *A,* Decreasing arterial Po_2 due to early disease process. *B,* Peripheral chemoreceptor stimulation begins and becomes primary drive to breath. *C,* Arterial Po_2 level remains fairly constant while arterial Pco_2 level may decrease to some degree. *D,* Theoretic points at which work of breathing is so costly that a decreased arterial Po_2 is unavoidable. *E,* Arterial Po_2 begins to decrease, and arterial Pco_2 begins to increase. (From Shapiro, B. A., Harrison, R. A., and Walton, J. R.: Clinical application of blood gases, ed. 2. Copyright © 1977 by Year Book Medical Publishers, Inc., Chicago. Used by permission.)

Table 8-2. Arterial blood gases in obstructive disease

	Normal	Mild	Moderately severe	Severe
Po_2	8-100 mm Hg	60-80 mm Hg	50-60 mm Hg	50 mm Hg
O_2 sat.	97%	88%-95%	75%-87%	75%
Pco_2	38-42 mm Hg	32-38 mm Hg	45-55 mm Hg	55 (may be as high as 80) mm Hg
pH	7.35-7.45	7.35-7.45	7.30-7.35	7.25
HCO_3	22-26 mEq/liter	20-24 mEq/liter	26-35 mEq/liter	20 mEq/liter

diac work load will contribute to the development of cor pulmonale in the hypoxic emphysemic patient.

The degree of hypoxemia and the adequacy of the compensatory mechanisms will determine the type and severity of the clinical signs and symptoms. Two syndromes describing emphysema have been identified: the "pink puffer fighter" and the "blue bloater nonfighter." The pink puffers maintain relatively normal blood gas values and show progressive dyspnea and weight loss, no cyanosis, little cardiac enlargement or sputum production, and a large increase in residual volume. They are able to hyperventilate, and therefore hypoxemia is not extreme, and cyanosis does not result, hence the name. The pink puffers show an increase in lung capacity. The blue bloaters show marked cyanosis and the edema of right-sided heart failure, hence their name. Arterial hypoxemia is marked, and compensatory mechanisms are not as effective as in the other group. The heart is hypertrophied, the hematocrit is increased, lung capacity is decreased, and sputum production is increased. These patients experience

Table 8-3. Physical signs in COPD*

Stage	Signs
Early	Examination may be negative or show only slight prolongation of forced expiration (which can be timed while auscultating over the trachea—normally 3 seconds or less), slight diminution of breath sounds at the apices or bases, scattered rhonchi or wheezes, especially on expiration, often best heard over the hila anteriorly (the rhonchi often clear after cough)
Moderate	Above signs are usually present and more pronounced, often with decreased rib expansion, use of the accessory muscles of respiration, retraction of the supraclavicular fossae in inspiration, generalized hyperresonance, decreased area of cardiac dullness, diminished heart sounds at base, increased anteroposterior distance of the chest†
Advanced	Examination usually shows the above findings to a greater degree, and often shows evidence of weight loss, depression of the liver, hyperpnea and tachycardia with mild exertion, low and relatively immobile diaphragm, contraction of abdominal muscles on inspiration, inaudible heart sounds except in the xiphoid area, cyanosis
Cor pulmonale	Increased intensity and splitting of pulmonic second sound, right-sided diastolic gallop, left parasternal heave (right ventricular overactivity), early systolic pulmonary ejection click with or without systolic ejection murmur
	With failure: distended neck veins, functional tricuspid insufficiency, v waves and hepatojugular reflux, hepatomegaly, peripheral edema

*From American Lung Association: Chronic obstructive pulmonary disease, ed. 5, New York, 1977, The Association.
†Physicians may put misplaced confidence in relating the shape of the thorax to the presence or absence of obstructive lung disease. It has been shown that the classic "barrel chest" with poor rib separation may be due solely or largely to dorsal kyphosis. In such patients ventilatory function may nonetheless be normal because of good diaphragmatic motion.

frequent episodes of right-sided heart failure (Table 8-3).

Treatment of obstructive disorders such as bronchitis and emphysema is aimed at maximizing ventilatory function. Clearing the airways of mucus is of primary importance. Teaching bronchial hygiene measures that help clear the airway and breathing exercises that decrease the work of breathing is also important. Oxygen can be administered to correct hypoxemia but only at low flow rates. Administration of high levels of oxygen will remove the stimulus to breathe and cause further respiratory depression. Correction of hypoxemia will also reduce the stimulus for erythrocytosis.

Encouraging the patient to stop smoking is important not only because further tissue damage may occur but also because carbon monoxide is inhaled in the smoke. Carbon monoxide competes with oxygen for combination with the hemoglobin molecule and increases the affinity of the remaining hemoglobin for oxygen, which impairs its release from hemoglobin to the tissues. Smoking directly increases both hypoxemia and hypoxia of the tissues.

Intermittent positive pressure breathing treatments may also improve ventilation. Fluid intake should be maintained to reduce the possibility of dehydration (due to exaggerated respiratory effort) and to thin secretions. The patient should also be taught the signs of infection and methods to avoid it since infection increases the metabolic rate and need for oxygen. A severe respiratory infection can intensify the hypoventilation and cause acute ventilatory failure superimposed on the already present chronic ventilatory failure. Infections must be treated promptly and aggressively.

Restrictive disorders are those in which the mobility or size of the thoracic cavity is decreased for some reason. Hypoventilation results because the full expansion of the thoracic cage is impossible. Because expansion is impaired, functional lung volume is reduced, and this results in a decrease in pulmonary compliance and an increase in the work of breathing. These disorders include musculoskeletal defects and neuromuscular impairment. Additionally many other conditions may impair ventilation by causing restriction of the size and movement of the thoracic cage. Kyphoscoliosis and muscular dystrophy are examples of disorders in which musculoskeletal function is impaired, causing restricted movement and expansion of the thoracic cage. Weakness and paralysis of respiratory muscles are possible complications of Guillain-Barré syndrome and myasthenia gravis, neuromuscular diseases. Respiratory muscle paralysis can also be caused by certain drugs that are used to promote skeletal muscle relaxation, for example, curare and succinylcholine.

Other conditions that can lead to restricted expansion of the thoracic cage and hypoventilation include obesity, abdominal distension (with gas or fluid), pain, immobility, and tightly applied bandages. When the volume of the abdominal cavity increases, the downward movement of the diaphragm is restricted. Grossly obese individuals may experience the *pickwickian syndrome,* which is characterized by dyspnea, hypoventilation, and hypoxemia with the compensatory mechanism of increased pulmonary artery pressure leading to hypertrophy and failure of the right side of the heart (cor pulmonale).

Severe abdominal or chest pain results in ''splinting'' of respirations in order to avoid any movement that may increase the pain. ''Splinting'' refers to a shallow type of respiratory effort with tidal volume at a constant and reduced level. Lung compliance and lung volume will decrease continuously during ventilation at a constant tidal volume since the pressures and volumes associated with tidal respiration are insufficient to reexpand the already collapsed alveoli and to prevent the collapse of others. This pattern of respiration is seen most frequently after abdominal surgery.

Conditions that affect the pleurae may also cause restricted thoracic movement. The pleurae are a double-layered serous membrane covering the lungs. The parietal pleura adheres to the chest wall surrounding the lungs. The visceral pleura covers the lungs. The parietal pleura is well supplied with nerve endings. A layer of serous fluid between the two membranes allows them to glide over each other as the lungs expand and contract. *Pleurisy,* or inflammation of the lungs, impairs this movement. Pleuritic pain can be quite severe. It is usually described as a stabbing, acute pain felt on breathing or moving. Pleuritic pain is referred to the chest wall because of the nervous innervation that exists. Pleuritic pain in the costal or cervical regions is referred to the chest wall and causes tenderness to the touch, while pain in the diaphragm is referred to the shoulder and abdomen. Pleurisy associated with a decrease in the amount of serous fluid between the pleura is called dry, or fibrinous, pleurisy. A pleural friction rub can be heard on auscultation of the chest. Pleurisy associated with an abnormal accumulation of fluid in the pleural space is called wet, or serofibrinous, pleurisy. The accumulation of fluid is called a pleural effusion and can be the result of an exudate or a transudate. A transudate is the result of conditions affecting tissue other than lung tissue, such as heart failure, kidney disease, malnutrition, and immune disorders. An exudate is the result of an infectious or inflammatory process involving the lung tissue. Accumulation of large amounts of fluid restricts the amount of space in which the lung has to expand and may even cause collapse of the lung. The introduction of air into the pleural space will also cause collapse of the lungs, or *pneumothorax.* Dysfunction of the pleurae causes hypoventilation due to restriction of respiratory movement secondary to pain and to decreased volume.

Pulmonary function studies will reflect both obstructive and restrictive disorders. In obstructive disorders residual volume will be increased, and expiratory flow rates will decrease. In restrictive disease the vital capacity will be reduced, and flow rates will be normal. Tumor growth can cause obstruction to air flow as well as restriction through a decrease in the size of the thoracic cavity.

Surfactant deficiency can also cause a disruption in the mechanics of breathing, which will eventually cause hypoventilation. Surfactant is secreted by cells in the alveolar epithelium and reduces the surface tension of the alveoli, thus reducing the tendency of the alveoli to collapse. In conditions where there is a deficiency in the amount of surfactant being secreted, the alveoli will have a greater than normal tendency to collapse. When alveoli collapse they become nonfunctional for gas exchange, and lung expansion becomes extremely difficult. There is a decrease in pulmonary compliance and an increase in the work of breathing. Respiratory distress syndrome (RDS) of the newborn, or *hyaline membrane disease,* is thought to be caused by a lack of adequate amounts of surfactant in the lungs of premature infants. Surfactant deficiency is also thought to play a partial role in the development of *adult respiratory distress syndrome (ARDS),* sometimes called *shock lung* or *stiff lung;* evidence is inconclusive on this point, however. Surfactant has a half-life of 14 hours, and replacement is dependent on normal ventilation of the alveoli. Surfactant production will be adversely affected in those conditions in which ventilation is impaired, thus setting up a vicious cycle to perpetuate ventilatory impairment.

Treatment of these conditions is aimed at reexpanding collapsed alveoli to improve ventilation in spite of the surfactant deficiency. Continuous positive airway pressure (C-PAP) and positive end expiratory pressure (PEEP) are two techniques that help reexpand alveoli by providing increased airway pressure and preventing the normal collapse of alveoli at the end of expiration.

ALTERATIONS OF EXCHANGE

Extrapulmonary as well as pulmonary conditions can result in a disruption of the normal gas exchange process. Conditions that alter the normal ventilatory process and the relative concentrations of gases on either side of the alveolocapillary membrane, the perfusion of alveoli with arterial blood, or the permeability of the membrane itself will ultimately disrupt the exchange process.

Gas exchange between the atmosphere and the blood is the result of both ventilation and perfusion of the alveoli. Alterations in the normal relationship between these two processes will result in disruption of the normal exchange

of gases and consequently of the blood gas concentrations. Aside from the altered lung volumes and capacities, the clinical manifestations of disorders of ventilation that were previously discussed are a direct reflection of the concomitant disruption of the exchange process since exchange is dependent on ventilation.

Because the gases diffuse across the alveolocapillary membrane space, changes in the cellular integrity of and fluid pressures around the membrane must also be considered when evaluating alterations of exchange. Alterations of exchange can be caused by both disruption of the normal ventilation-perfusion ratios as well as changes in the functional capacity of the alveolocapillary membrane space.

Ventilation-perfusion abnormalities

The alveolus with its associated pulmonary capillary is the basic functional respiratory unit in which gas exchange takes place. Shapiro (1977) states that this unit can theoretically exist in any of four different types of ventilation-perfusion relationships (Figs. 8-10 and 8-11) that affect gas exchange:

1. Normal unit: ventilation and perfusion are relatively equal
2. Dead space unit: alveolus is ventilated, but blood flow through capillary is reduced or nonexistent
3. Shunt unit: alveolus is not ventilated, or ventilation is reduced, but perfusion continues
4. Silent unit: both alveolus and capillary are nonfunctional

Shapiro goes on to say that an infinite number of ventilation-perfusion relationships may exist on the spectrum between the two extremes of dead space and shunt.

Dead space ventilation is that portion of the total ventilation (tidal volume) that does not participate in gas exchange. There are three possible components of dead space ventilation:

1. Anatomic dead space: the portion of the total ventilation that remains in the conducting airways
2. Alveolar dead space: ventilation in an alveolus that is not being perfused with blood
3. Dead space effect: effect that occurs when

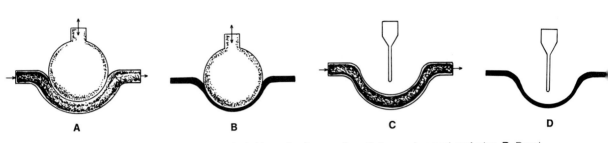

Fig. 8-10. Theoretic respiratory unit. **A,** Normal unit: normal ventilation and normal perfusion. **B,** Dead space unit: normal ventilation and no perfusion. **C,** Shunt unit: no ventilation and no perfusion. **D,** Silent unit: no ventilation and no perfusion. (From Shapiro, B. A., Harrison, R. A., and Walton, J. R.: Clinical application of blood gases, ed. 2. Copyright © 1977 by Year Book Medical Publishers, Inc., Chicago. Used by permission.)

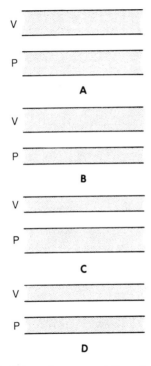

Fig. 8-11. Schematic representation of relationship between ventilation, *V,* and perfusion, *P,* which exists normally, **A,** and in dead space, **B,** shunt, **C,** and silent, **D,** respiratory units.

ventilation is relatively greater than perfusion, and the excess ventilation does not participate in gas exchange (this can result from either overventilation or underperfusion).

A shunt is that portion of the cardiac output that does not participate in gas exchange. The physiologic or total shunt can be divided into three components:

1. Anatomic shunt: approximately 2% to 5% of the cardiac output that normally bypasses the pulmonary circulation and returns to the left side of the heart unoxygenated; this is the blood return from the bronchial, pleural, and part of the coronary circulations.

2. Capillary shunt: blood that perfuses totally unventilated alveoli; the sum of the anatomic and capillary shunts is called the true, or absolute, shunt; this is refractory or unresponsive to any form of oxygen therapy.

3. Shunt effect: effect that occurs when perfusion is relatively greater than ventilation; this can be the result of either poor ventilation of the alveoli or an excessive rate of blood flow; this results in *venous admixture,* and it is responsive to oxygen therapy.

Conditions that contribute to dead space or shunting will result in a disruption of the exchange process. The extent of the disruption and the degree to which normal blood gas values are altered will depend on the severity and persistence of the underlying defect. The maldistribution and mismatching of ventilation and perfusion that occur in chronic diffuse bronchopulmonary disease result in an increase in both the dead space and shunting effects throughout the lungs. Initially hypoxemia alone will be present. The carbon dioxide level of the mixed arterial blood will remain normal because alveolar units with high or normal ventilation-perfusion ratios can compensate for the increased carbon dioxide level in the blood coming from alveolar units with low ventilation-perfusion ratios by "blowing off" greater amounts of carbon dioxide. The exchange of oxygen differs from that of carbon dioxide in that it is much more limited. Oxygen is far less soluble than carbon dioxide, and its saturation level in the blood is limited by the amount of hemoglobin available. The compensatory increase in the rate of alveolar ventilation in response to the resultant hypoxemia also helps keep arterial carbon dioxide levels within normal limits. As the disease progresses, however, carbon dioxide retention will also occur as increasingly greater numbers of alveolar units are affected by the disease process (see Fig. 8-9).

An increase in dead space ventilation is the result of disrupted perfusion or overventilation that does not participate in the exchange process. Perfusion can be disrupted by a variety of causes. An embolism in a major vessel, numerous microemboli in smaller vessels, a decrease in cardiac output, or increased pulmonary vascular resistance can all have the effect of increasing dead space ventilation.

Alveolar septal destruction reduces the amount of alveolar surface area available for gas exchange, so that the overall effect is ventilation in excess of perfusion, or dead space effect. Use of a volume ventilator without a simultaneous increase in the amount and distribution of the pulmonary blood flow will also enhance the dead space effect. Anatomic dead space increases with a rapid, shallow respiratory pattern. Alveolar gas is never completely renewed, and the work of breathing is increased.

Anatomic shunting is a direct flow of blood between the right and left sides of the heart without passing through the pulmonary capillaries to be made available for gas exchange. Congenital heart defects such as septal defects and patent ductus arteriosus are examples of conditions in which a direct anatomic communication exists between the pulmonic and systemic circulations, completely bypassing the lungs. Blood flow through vascular pulmonary tumors may also result in an anatomic shunt as blood flows through the tumor into the pul-

monary veins. Blood flowing past collapsed, fluid-filled, or pus-filled alveoli results in a capillary shunt. Underventilation of alveoli due to hypoventilation of alveoli and uneven distribution of ventilation within the lungs results in venous admixture because of the shunt effect.

Alveolocapillary membrane alterations

A reduction in functional membrane space through a loss of total surface area will result in disruption of the exchange process. The destruction of the alveolar septa that occurs in emphysema is one example of this. Tuberculosis and pneumoconiosis are others. The rate of exchange will be reduced as a result of fluid in the interstitial, alveolar spaces such as that which occurs in pulmonary edema. Changes in the cellular structure of the membrane itself can also adversely affect exchange. This is the primary functional abnormality in conditions such as sarcoidosis, systemic sclerosis, berylliosis, and bronchioloalveolar cell carcinoma, where there is a progressive granulomatous process, and in interstitial fibrosing pneumonitis.

SUMMARY

An overview of the process of ventilation and exchange and the normal dynamics and compensatory mechanisms that are evoked in response to disruptions is presented in this chapter. The terms *hyperventilation* and *hypoventilation* are used in reference to the adequacy of alveolar ventilation as measured by the removal or retention of carbon dioxide in the arterial blood. These terms are not used to describe a pattern of respiration demonstrated by a patient. A person who is breathing very rapidly may still be retaining carbon dioxide and would therefore be considered to be hypoventilating. The following terms would be more appropriately used when describing a pattern of respiration:

tachypnea a rapid, shallow pattern of respiration.

hyperpnea a rapid, deep pattern of respiration, which is usually seen after exercise.

eupnea quiet, ordinary respiration with no exaggerated effort or awareness of the sensation of breathing, usually 16 to 20 respirations per minute.

bradypnea a pattern of slow breathing, usually less than ten respirations per minute.

apnea cessation of respiration.

Cheyne-Stokes a pattern of periodic respiration characterized by initial shallow respirations, which increase in depth, reach a peak, and then decline, and are followed by a period of apnea.

The relatively equal distribution of ventilation in relation to perfusion of the alveoli is essential for the exchange of gases to occur normally. Disorders of ventilation will subsequently disrupt exchange since normal ventilation is a prerequisite for exchange. Arterial blood gas values reflect the altered exchange process while pulmonary function studies reflect more accurately the altered ventilatory process.

SUGGESTED READINGS

American Lung Association: Chronic obstructive pulmonary disease, ed. 5, New York, 1977, The Association.

Caughlin, G. P., et al.: Alpha 1-antitrypsin deficiency. A literature review and a case report of a patient with chronic obstructive airways and cirrhosis, Aust. N.Z. J. Med. 7(4):400-403, 1977.

Cook, W.: Shock lung: etiology, prevention and treatment, Heart Lung, 3(6):933-938, 1974.

Hensley, M., et al.: A test of the ventilatory response to hypoxia and hypercapnia for clinical use, Aust. N.Z. J. Med 7(4):362-367, 1977.

Johnson, R.: The lung as an organ of oxygen transport, Basics R.D. vol. 2, no. 1, 1973.

Ribon, A., et al.: Air pollution: its effects on health and respiratory disease—a review, Allergy 39(4):279-283, 1977.

Richerson, H.: Immunology of the respiratory system, Basics R.D. vol. 2, no. 5, 1974.

Shapiro, B., et al.: Clinical application of blood gases, ed. 2, Chicago, 1977, Year Book Medical Publishers.

Stockby, T. A.: The estimation of the resting reflex hypoxic drive to respiration in normal man, Respir. Physiol. 31(2):217-230, 1977.

Talamo, R. C.: Alpha-1 antitrypsin deficiency and emphysema, Chest 72(4):421, 1977.

Terry, P. B., et al.: Collateral ventilation in man, N. Engl. J. Med. 298(1):10-55, 1978.

Thurlbech, W.: Chronic bronchitis and emphysema. The pathophysiology of chronic obstructive lung disease, Basics R.D., vol. 3, no. 1, 1974.

CHAPTER 9

Disorders of circulation

- Explain the pathophysiologic mechanisms of disorders of circulation.
  Describe the alterations in normal function, dynamics, and regulation in response to disruption of normal circulation.
  Identify compensatory and adaptive mechanisms in response to disruption of circulation.
  Describe the clinical manifestations of the altered dynamics and resultant adaptation.
- Cite the etiology of disorders of circulation.
- Cite predisposing factors to the development of disorders of circulation.
- Explain the treatment of disorders of circulation.
  State the goals of treatment.
  Identify the treatment measures.
  Describe the physiologic bases of treatment.

Transport of oxygen and carbon dioxide between the lungs and body tissues depends on both an intact transport system and an intact transport medium. The transport system is the body's cardiovascular system, whose components are the heart, blood vessels, and lymphatic system. The transport medium is the blood. Alterations in the function of the heart or blood vessels and in the volume or composition of the blood affect the oxygenation status of the cells. Additionally the delivery of nutrients and other substances to the cells or various parts of the body is also impaired.

REVIEW OF NORMAL FUNCTION, DYNAMICS, AND REGULATION

Under normal conditions in a healthy adult the human heart functions as a pump. With each contraction, blood is ejected into the pulmonary and general circulations with a regular rate, rhythm, force, and volume. The normal rate, force, and volume of blood pumped into the circulation are maintained in a resting state and increased when metabolic demands increase.

The cardiac muscle, valves, conduction system, blood supply, and regulatory (neural) mechanisms must be intact and operating for the heart to perform its pumping function efficiently.

The cardiac cycle is divided into two stages: a period of relaxation, diastole, and a period of contraction, systole. During the cardiac cycle, blood continually enters the atria of the heart. The right atrium receives the blood returning from the general circulation via the great veins. The left atrium receives the blood returning from the lungs via the pulmonary veins. During the first part of diastole, approximately 70% of the blood entering the atria flows directly into the ventricles. In the latter part of diastole, atrial contraction forces more blood to flow into the ventricles. As ventricular contraction begins, pressures rises quickly in the ventricles and causes the AV valves (mitral and tricuspid) to close and the aortic and pulmonic valves to open. Closure of the AV valves prevents a backflow of blood to the atria during systole. With the opening of the pulmonic and

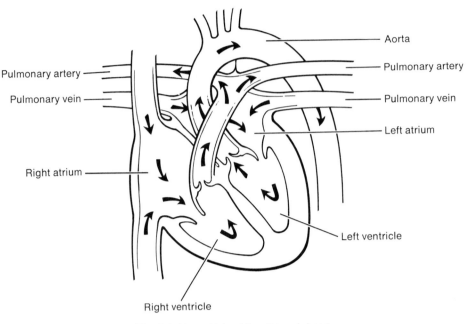

Fig. 9-1. Normal blood flow through heart.

aortic valves, blood in the right ventricle enters the pulmonary artery and is carried to the lungs, and blood in the left ventricle enters the aorta and is carried to the organs and tissues throughout the body. At the end of systole the ventricular muscle relaxes, and intraventricular pressures decrease. During systole the AV valves remain closed, and blood is allowed to accumulate in the atria, causing increased atrial pressures. As a result of the decreased ventricular pressures and increased atrial pressures the AV valves reopen, allowing blood to flow between the atria and ventricles (Fig. 9-1).

The cardiac cycle is initiated by the spontaneous generation of an electrical impulse in the sinoatrial (SA) node, the heart's pacemaker. *Automaticity* is the property of the cardiac cells that allows their spontaneous, repetitive self-stimulation. This is a result of a gradual change in the electronegativity of the cell. The cell membrane actively transports sodium into the extracellular compartment and potassium into the intracellular compartment. The presence of sodium ions in the extracellular fluid and potassium ions in the intracellular compartment results in a relative difference in the electric charge on either side of the cell membrane. This electrical difference creates what is called

the *resting-membrane potential*. The interior of the cell is negatively charged relative to the exterior of the cell. A state of *polarization* is said to exist. When the cell is depolarized, the change in the electric potential is called the *action potential*. Depolarization is the result of stimulation, which causes sodium to rush into the cell and the charge of the interior of the cell to become positive. Noncardiac cells depend on an outside stimulus to initiate the action potential. In cardiac cells there is a gradual reentry of sodium ions into the cell during phase 4 of the action potential. The intracellular charge becomes more electropositive, finally reaching the threshold level, causing spontaneous depolarization and initiation of the action potential. The automaticity of cardiac cells can be directly affected by any abnormal cellular conditions, that is, lack of oxygen, electrolyte imbalance, change in pH, or damage to the cell.

The cardiac action potential has five phases. Phase 0 is the depolarization with an influx of sodium. Phase 1 is a brief change in electric potential toward repolarization. Phase 2 is a stabilization of the repolarization, or a plateau period with calcium entering and potassium leaving the cell. Phase 3 is active repolarization as the cell membrane actively transports the sodium back into the extracellular compartment and retains potassium. Phase 4 is the resting phase.

The various phases of the action potential correspond to the refractory periods of the cardiac muscle. During depolarization and the beginning of repolarization (phases 0, 1, 2, and the beginning of phase 3) the cell cannot respond to a stimulus because there is essentially no electrical difference between the two sides of the cell membrane. This is called the *absolute refractory* period. During phase 3 the cell again becomes electronegative, and a stronger than threshold stimulus can initiate an action potential. This is called the *relative refractory period*. As phase 4 begins, the cell enters a vulnerable period during which a lower than threshold stimulus can initiate an action potential. During this time a single stimulus can initiate a repetitive series of action potentials, causing the cardiac muscle to contract in a rapid, repetitive, nonfunctional pattern.

The rate and rhythm of cardiac contraction is primarily determined by the self-generated impulse. The pacemaker cells of the sinoatrial node have the fastest rate of spontaneous depolarization and therefore are the primary pacemaker cells of the heart. The impulse or action potential spreads throughout the heart muscle via the conduction system. Cells in this system are highly specialized and provide for rapid excitation and conduction of impulses in the heart. Conduction of the action potential should be differentiated from transmission. Transmission refers to the perpetuation of the action potential across the neuroeffector junctions. This process requires the presence of a neurohumoral substance. Conduction refers to a wave of sequential ionic changes that precede the action potential and follow its passage along the nerve fiber. It does not require the presence of a neurohumoral substance but only integrity of the tissue and normal concentrations of electrolytes. Cardiac muscle is a form of striated muscle fiber that responds to an impulse by contracting or shortening its fibers in the same manner as skeletal muscle.

Regulation of the heart's pumping effectiveness is also provided by the autonomic ner-

vous system and through intrinsic autoregulation in response to increased venous return. The autonomic nervous system affects cardiac function by altering the strength and rate of the heart's contraction. Parasympathetic stimulation slows the rate and slightly decreases the strength of cardiac contraction. Sympathetic stimulation markedly increases the rate and strength of cardiac contraction. Autonomic control is maintained through reflex action, allowing the heart to respond to constantly changing body conditions.

Intrinsic autoregulation refers to the heart's ability to increase cardiac output in response to an increased amount of blood returning to it. The basis of this adaptive ability is *Starling's law of the heart*. This law states that cardiac output increases as cardiac filling increases because striated muscle fiber responds to the increased stretch with an increase in the force of its contraction. In other words, the normally functioning heart will pump out all of the blood (minus the end-systolic volume) returned to it without any increase in the right atrial pressure. Venous return is the primary factor determining cardiac output as the heart itself plays a permissive role in cardiac output regulation.

Blood is pumped by the right side of the heart into the pulmonary circulation, where it is oxygenated, and by the left side of the heart into the systemic circulation, where it delivers oxygen and nutrients to the tissues, removes the metabolic waste products, and carries various substances throughout the body. The blood vessels must be intact and functioning for this to occur.

The vascular system is a series of distensible conduits that can be subdivided into arterial, venous, and capillary components. Additionally the lymphatic system performs a complementary function to the circulatory system and therefore must also be considered in a discussion of the circulatory system.

Large-diameter arteries such as the aorta and its main branches have a high elastic fiber content, which allows them to accommodate cardiac stroke volume and convert the intermittent flow of blood to a more even, steady flow. These vessels are often called *Windkessel* vessels after the air compression chambers on old-fashioned, hand-operated fire engines. They are distensible, thus allowing them to accommodate large volumes of blood. This distensibility along with the high resistance offered by the terminal arterioles constitutes a *hydraulic filtering* system, which converts intermittent blood flow to a continuous blood flow to the capillaries. Blood flow during systole is the result of cardiac contraction. Blood flow during diastole is the result of the elastic recoil of the arteries as they discharge the blood that had caused their distension during systole. Reduced distensibility of the arteries results in less efficient hydraulic filtering, reduced capillary blood flow during diastole, and increased cardiac work load (Fig. 9-2).

The nutrient arteries arise from the aorta and its main branches, forming parallel systems

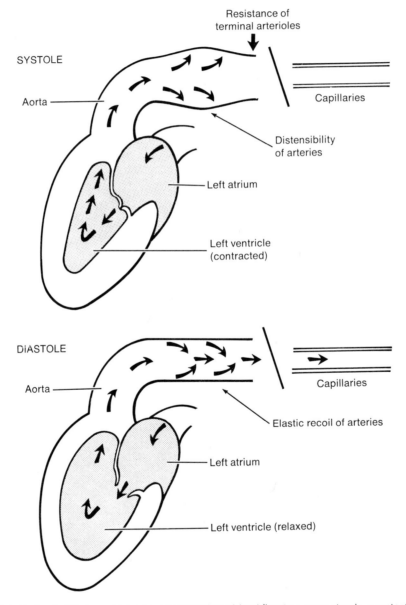

Fig. 9-2. Hydraulic filtering, which converts intermittent blood flow to a more steady, constant flow to capillaries.

that supply various organs and vascular beds (Fig. 9-3). As a result of sympathetic innervation, the vascular tone of the arterioles can be altered to increase or decrease their diameter and hence resistance to blood flow. For this reason these vessels are called *resistance vessels;* they regulate volume and pressure in the arterial system and blood flow to the capillary bed. The arterioles, capillaries, and venules constitute what is called the *microcirculation* (Fig. 9-4).

Capillary distribution varies among the different types of tissues present in the body. Metabolically active tissue such as skeletal tissue will have a relatively greater concentration of capillaries than does metabolically inactive tissue such as cartilage. The exchange of nutrients and oxygen between the blood and tissues occurs in the capillary bed. Some capillary

beds have arteriovenous connections that allow blood to pass directly between the arterial and venous systems. This mechanism allows heat exchange from these vessels. Capillary blood flow throughout the body is not uniform. True capillaries have no smooth muscle tissue, and changes in capillary diameter are passive and caused by changes in precapillary and post-capillary resistance. Capillary flow is under neural as well as local and humoral control. The arterioles and precapillary sphincters are sympathetically innervated and respond to sympathetic stimulation. Additionally, local factors such as pH, oxygen, and reduction of available nutrients also affect local blood flow. Humoral control refers to the effect various body substances, hormones, ions, and so on have on local blood flow. *Vasomotion,* rhythmic constriction and relaxation of the precapillary sphinc-

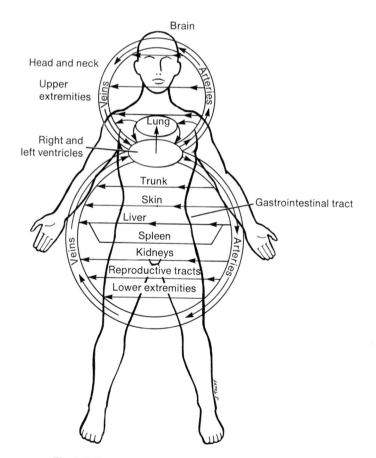

Fig. 9-3. Parallel system of nutrient artery supply routes.

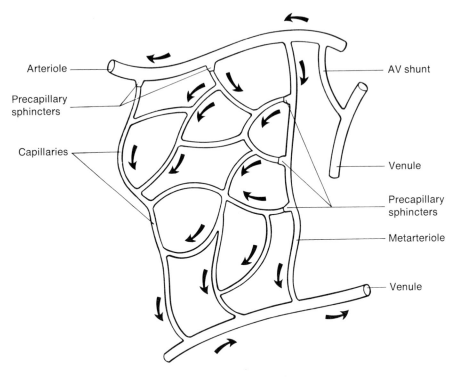

Fig. 9-4. The microcirculation.

ters, results in an intermittent pulsatile flow of blood through the capillaries.

The capillary membrane is highly permeable to the various substances dissolved in the plasma and tissue fluids with the exception of relatively large particles such as the plasma proteins. Permeability of the capillary membrane is not uniform throughout the body tissues either. The liver capillaries are relatively more permeable than are any other capillaries, and the venous ends of the capillaries are more permeable than are the arterial ends.

The exchange of gases, nutrients, and waste products between the capillaries and tissues is dependent on the processes of diffusion, filtration, and absorption. Some transfer occurs as a result of *cytopemphis,* or movement across the cell membrane within a pinocytotic vessel. Filtration and absorption within the capillary bed depend on the balance between hydrostatic and osmotic forces. A summary of these Starling forces is presented in Chapter 10 in the discussion of fluid equilibrium between compartments.

Similar in appearance and closely aligned to the capillaries and tissue cells are the terminal lymphatic vessels. The surface areas of the two capillary systems are almost equal. These vessels are more permeable to large particles than are the capillaries, due to absence of a basement membrane and looser junctions between endothelial cells. The lymphatics remove excess fluid and larger-size particles from the interstitial space and return them to the venous circulation. The lymph vessels have valves to prevent reflux, and movement of fluid within them is the result of the milking action transmitted from neighboring arteries and muscles. The lymphatics also constitute a defense mechanism. In the lymph nodes, foreign materials and bacteria are phagocytized and thus removed from the body. The lymph system is the only means by which proteins that have left the intravascular compartment can be returned to it.

The venules are formed as the capillary network coalesces. The venules are considered exchange vessels because it is felt that there is exchange across the venule wall. The venules converge to form veins of progressively larger diameters. Like the lymphatics, veins also have valves to prevent reflux, and the action of the muscles exerts a milking action to help promote venous return. The veins are referred to as *capacitance vessels* because approximately 75% of the total blood volume can be stored within them. Muscular tissue in the venules and small veins, which is innervated by sympathetic fibers, can, through constriction, cause the return of large amounts of "stored" blood to the circulating blood volume.

Blood flow through the vessels depends on a *pressure difference* between the two ends of the vessel. Blood will flow from an area of high pressure to an area of low pressure. Arterial blood pressure is a measurement of the force that is exerted by the blood against the artery wall. Pressure (P) is dependent on the cardiac output (CO), or volume, and the resistance (R). This relationship is summarized by the following equation:

$$P = CO \times R$$

From this equation it is apparent that arterial pressure will increase as either cardiac output or resistance increases. A change in any one of these factors will necessitate a change in the others to maintain homeostasis.

Arterial pressure is maintained through various compensatory mechanisms. Cardiac output and total peripheral resistance can be adjusted to maintain a fairly constant arterial pressure despite constantly changing body conditions. A persistent or exaggerated increase in either, however, will result in an elevated arterial pressure, *hypertension*. A persistent or exaggerated decrease in either will result in a reduced arterial pressure, *hypotension*.

Arterial pressure is regulated by reflex action of the sympathetic nervous system to cause changes in peripheral resistance and by hormonal and renal control of the total blood volume. Total peripheral resistance is determined by the vasomotor tone, the diameter of the blood vessels, and the viscosity of the blood. Blood viscosity will increase as the solid constituents of the blood increase or the liquid portion of the blood decreases. Although many factors are involved, the arterioles are responsible for most of the peripheral resistance to blood flow. The arterioles and venules are innervated by the sympathetic nervous system. Sympathetic control is the most important single factor related to peripheral resistance.

Sympathetic control of peripheral resistance is mediated through baroreceptor reflexes, which constitute a negative-feedback mechanism. The blood vessels are in a state of constant partial contraction as a result of the continued transmission of vasoconstrictor impulses from the vasomotor center. This is referred to as *vasomotor tone*. The baroreceptor cells in the carotid and aortic bodies are sensitive to stretch and send inhibitory impulses to the vasomotor center when stimulated by increased pressure. As a result vasodilation occurs. Additionally impulses are sent via the vagus nerve to slow the rate and decrease the contractility of the heart, resulting in decreased cardiac output. As peripheral resistance decreases and cardiac output drops, arterial pressure will also be reduced.

The baroreceptors become relatively inactive in the presence of normal or reduced arterial pressure. Baroreceptors will no longer be stretched, and the inhibitory effect on the vasomotor center is decreased. This allows vasomotor activity to increase, and vasoconstriction results. Additionally heart rate increases as a result of decreased stimulation of the cardioinhibitory center and decreased inhibition of the cardioaccelerator center. As peripheral resistance and cardiac output increase, arterial pressure rises. Sympathetic stimulation also causes the adrenal medullae to secrete epinephrine and norepinephrine into the general circulation.

The response of the local vessel systems is determined by the presence of adrenoceptors, or target sites, on the cell membrane. Activation of alpha receptor sites results in vasoconstriction, and activation of beta receptor sites results in vasodilation. Norepinephrine binds with alpha sites, while epinephrine can bind with both alpha or beta receptors. Alpha receptors predominate in the precapillary sphincters of most of the arterioles. Beta receptors predominate in the heart, coronary arteries, brain, and liver. When epinephrine and norepinephrine are secreted, blood is shunted preferentially from the vascular beds where alpha receptors and vasoconstriction predominate to those vascular beds with both alpha and beta receptors and consequently vasodilation. The parasympathetic system promotes vasodilation, although the mechanism for this action is unclear at this time. The neurotransmitter is acetylcholine, which by itself has a vasodilatory effect.

Other humoral and hormonal substances have vasoactive properties. For example, angiotensin II is an extremely potent vasoconstrictor, and histamine has potent vasodilatory properties.

The blood is the transport medium. It helps to maintain homeostasis not only through its various transport functions but also through its role in maintaining the body defenses, acid-base balance, and normal body temperature.

Components of the blood include plasma, the liquid portion, and the blood cells, erythrocytes (red blood cells), leukocytes (white blood cells), and thrombocytes (platelets). The various blood cells are suspended within the plasma portion of the blood. The plasma and the erythrocytes play the greatest role in terms of oxygenation of the tissues.

Plasma is 90% water and 10% solutes. In solution are proteins, which represent the greatest quantity of the solutes, nutrient substances (glucose, amino acids, lipids, fatty acids, etc.), products of metabolism (lactic and pyruvic acids, creatinine, etc.), other humoral substances (hormones, enzymes, etc.), and inorganic chemicals (electrolytes, minerals, etc.). Also in solution in the plasma are the respiratory gases, oxygen and carbon dioxide.

The erythrocytes are cells shaped like biconcave disks. This shape can change readily as the erythrocytes pass through the capillaries. There are approximately 5 million red blood cells per cubic millimeter of blood. Women have fewer red blood cells than men. Red blood cells are produced in the bone marrow. Newly formed erythrocytes, which still contain small amounts of basophilic reticulum interspersed among the hemoglobin, are called *reticulocytes*. Normally only 1% of the blood is composed of reticulocytes.

The hormone erythropoietin stimulates bone marrow to produce erythrocytes. Hypoxia stimulates the kidneys to release renal erythropoietic factor (REF), which reacts with a plasma protein produced by the liver to form erythropoietin. Androgenic hormones also stimulate erythropoietin production. Red blood cell maturation can be inhibited by lack of either vitamin B_{12} or folic acid.

The major function of the erythrocytes is the transport of hemoglobin. There are two portions to the hemoglobin molecule. The heme portion is made up of an iron atom in the ferrous state in the center of a protoporphyrin ring. Four heme groups are contained within one molecule of hemoglobin. The heme groups give the blood its red color and its ability to combine with oxygen since they contain the oxygen-binding sites. The globin, or protein portion of the hemoglobin molecule, contains two alpha and two beta polypeptide chains. Each of the alpha chains contains 141 amino acid residues, and each of the beta chains contains 146 amino acid residues. The various chains are held together by noncovalent forces to form a three-dimensional, globular protein. Each of the four heme groups is associated with a polypeptide chain.

There is a known structural change that occurs within the hemoglobin molecule when it reacts with oxygen. Of this structural change Perutz (1964) has said, "Hemoglobin's change of shape makes me think of it as a breathing molecule, but paradoxically it expands not when oxygen is taken up but when it is released." When oxygenation of the hemoglobin molecule occurs, the beta chains move approximately 0.7 nm closer to each other and will move apart by the same distance when deoxygenation occurs.

Each iron in the heme portions of the molecule has six potential covalent bonds. Four of the bonds are attached to the pyrrole nitrogens, and the fifth is attached to the globin. The sixth available bond is a weak one that allows oxygen to combine with hemoglobin in a reversible manner. There are four potential oxygen-binding sites on the hemoglobin molecules.

Oxygen is transported in the blood both in chemical combination with hemoglobin and dissolved in the plasma. Normally the amount of oxygen carried in the dissolved state is negligible, only about 3% of the total amount of oxygen being transported. The term *oxygen content* refers to the total amount of oxygen in combination with the blood, that is, the sum of the oxygen in combination with hemoglobin and that dissolved in plasma.

In the normal adult there is 12 to 16 g of hemoglobin per 100 ml of blood. Hemoglobin normally exists as either *oxyhemoglobin* (in combination with oxygen: HbO_2) or as reduced hemoglobin (Hb). A pressure gradient between the alveoli and the blood causes oxygen molecules to move into the blood. These molecules immediately bind with oxygen. The ability of hemoglobin to bind with oxygen at different oxygen tensions is expressed graphically by the hemoglobin dissociation curve. This curve shows the percent saturation of hemoglobin that can be expected at different partial pressures of

oxygen in the blood. The nonlinear shape of the curve demonstrates that oxygen saturation of the blood can be relatively high in spite of low partial pressures of oxygen. For instance, with a Po_2 of 40 mm Hg the hemoglobin saturation would be approximately 75% (Fig. 9-5).

Carbon dioxide is also transported in the blood both in clinical combination with hemoglobin as carbaminohemoglobin and dissolved in plasma. Carbon dioxide is also carried by the red blood cells through the bicarbonate ion mechanism. Approximately 25% of the carbon dioxide in the blood is carried as carbaminohemoglobin. Approximately 7% is dissolved in plasma. The rest of the CO_2 is transported through the bicarbonate ion mechanism. Dissolved CO_2 readily diffuses into the red blood cell where it reacts with water to form carbonic acid. This reaction is catalyzed by the enzyme *carbonic anhydrase*. Carbonic acid readily dis-

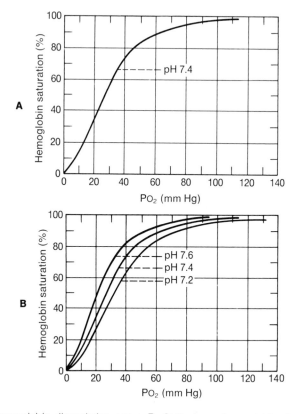

Fig. 9-5. A, Oxyhemoglobin dissociation curve. **B,** Shifts in oxyhemoglobin dissociation curve at various pH levels (Bohr effect).

sociates into hydrogen and bicarbonate ions. This reaction is summarized in the following equation:

$$CO_2 + H_2O \xrightarrow[CA]{} H_2CO_3 \longrightarrow H^+ + HCO_3^-$$

Bicarbonate ions then move out of the red blood cell into the plasma to reestablish equal concentrations of bicarbonate ions on either side of the cell membrane. Chloride ions must diffuse from the plasma into the erythrocyte to maintain chemical neutrality. This movement of chloride ions from the extracellular to the intracellular compartment is called the *chloride shift*.

Disruption of the circulation can occur at any of the levels described previously. It may result from failure of the pump (heart), altered pressure or flow within the vessels, disrupted vessel patency or integrity, or altered oxygen-carrying capacity of the blood. Pathophysiologic mechanisms that come into play, the precipitating disease states, and the physiology of treatment for each type of disruption will be discussed later.

PUMP FAILURE

Pathophysiologic mechanisms. The heart's ability to perform its pumping function effectively may become impaired as a result of various disease states to be discussed later in this chapter. Impairment of the heart's pumping function causes a decrease in cardiac output as well as an increase in systemic venous pressure since the heart is unable to pump all of the blood being returned to it. *Heart failure* and *pump failure* are terms used to describe the condition that exists when cardiac output becomes inadequate to meet the body's needs.

When cardiac output becomes less than normal for any reason, some acute adjustments are made by the body. Reflex stimulation of the sympathetic nervous system causes vasoconstriction of the blood vessels, which helps raise blood pressure as well as redistribute blood flow to those organs requiring the most oxygen (heart, brain, and kidneys). Sympathetic stimulation also results in an increase in the rate and force of cardiac contraction. An increase in heart rate above normal is called *tachycardia*. Stimulation of the sympathetic

nervous system is primarily through baroreceptor reflexes, although some response through chemoreceptor reflexes is also thought to occur as the decreased blood supply causes local tissue hypoxia. Baroreceptors located in the vessels respond to decreased arterial pressure (carotid sinus and aortic reflexes) and increased venous pressure (Bainbridge reflex). In response to the increased venous pressure, cardiac filling is increased, and the cardiac muscle fibers are stretched. This stretching of the muscle fibers causes an increase in the force of their contraction (Starling's law of the heart).

These acute responses of vasoconstriction, increased heart rate (tachycardia), and increased force of contraction are short-term adjustments that cannot totally compensate for the effects of heart failure over an extended period. In fact, the long-term effects of these adjustments are detrimental to the heart's pumping action. Vasoconstriction promotes blood return to the heart, further increasing venous pressure, and increases the resistance against which the heart must pump. The cardiac muscle fibers can be stretched beyond their physiologic limits. An increase in the rate of contraction shortens the diastolic period of the cardiac cycle. This shortens filling time for both the ventricles and coronary arteries. As a result of the reduced ventricular filling time, cardiac output per contraction is actually decreased. As a result of reduced coronary artery filling time, the oxygen requirement of the myocardium cannot be completely met. The increased rate and force of contraction further increase myocardial oxygen requirements. This increased demand for oxygen in the presence of reduced ability to meet the demand further impairs cardiac function and contributes to fatigue of the myocardium. For a short period of time, however, cardiac output can be maintained through these mechanisms.

Expansion of the extracellular fluid volume is another compensatory mechanism evoked by reduced cardiac output. Expansion of extracellular fluid volume occurs as a result of depression of kidney function, the activation of the renin-angiotensin system, and the action of antidiuretic hormone (ADH).

Renal function is depressed in the presence of

heart failure due to the negative effect that reduced arterial pressure and sympathetic vasoconstriction of the afferent arterioles in the kidney have on glomerular pressure. Formation of dilute urine is inhibited since the glomerular filtration rate drops as a result of the decreased glomerular pressure.

When blood flow in the kidneys is below normal, the juxtaglomerular cells of the kidneys are stimulated to release the enzyme renin. Renin catalyzes the conversion of a plasma protein polypeptide, angiotensinogen or renin substrate, into a peptide, angiotensin I. Angiotensin I is converted into angiotensin II by a converting enzyme. Angiotensin II raises arterial pressure directly by causing vasoconstriction of arterioles and veins, which increases peripheral resistance. Angiotensin II indirectly elevates arterial pressure through expansion of extracellular fluid volume. It directly affects the kidneys to retain sodium and subsequently water, and it stimulates the adrenal cortex to release aldosterone, a mineralocorticoid that also causes retention of sodium and subsequently water by the kidneys.

Secretion of ADH is the body's response to stimulation of the volume receptors in the great vessels and decreased cerebral blood flow and stimulation of osmoreceptors. ADH acts on the distal tubules of the kidneys to cause reabsorption of water. These three mechanisms (Fig. 9-6) raise arterial pressure through expansion of extracellular fluid volume, but they also increase venous return to the heart from the systemic circulation. Thus, a vicious cycle has been set up, further stressing an overburdened heart.

Initially only one side of the heart may be considered in failure. Failure of the right and left sides may occur independently of one an-

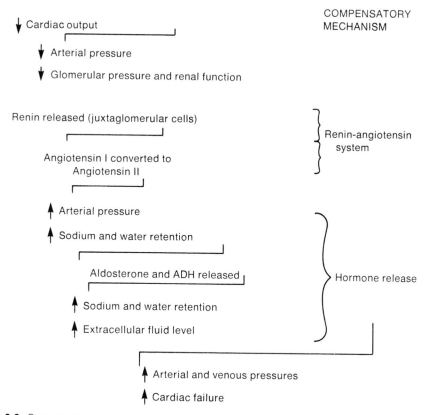

Fig. 9-6. Compensatory mechanisms in cardiac failure that promote volume expansion, which increases venous return, thus contributing to further cardiac decompensation and failure.

Table 9-1. Effects of heart failure*

Backward effects	Forward effects
FAILURE OF THE LEFT VENTRICLE	
Decreased emptying of left ventricle	Decreased cardiac output
Increased volume and pressure in left ventricle	Decreased perfusion of body tissues
Increased volume and pressure in left atrium	Decreased blood flow to kidneys and glands
Increased volume in pulmonary veins	Increased secretion of sodium- and water- retaining hormones
Increased volume in pulmonary capillary bed	Increased reabsorption of sodium and water
Transudation of fluid from capillaries to alveoli	Increased extracellular fluid volume
Rapid filling of alveolar spaces	Increased total blood volume
Pulmonary edema	
Decreased emptying of right ventricle	
Sometimes referred to as congestive theory or backward theory of heart failure	Sometimes referred to as low output theory or forward theory of heart failure
FAILURE OF THE RIGHT VENTRICLE	
Decreased emptying of right ventricle	Decreased volume from right ventricle to lungs
Increased volume and increased end-diastolic pressure in right ventricle	Decreased return to left atrium and subsequent decreased cardiac output
Increased volume (pressure) in right atrium	All forward effects of left-sided heart failure
Increased volume and pressure in great veins	Expansion of blood volume
Increased volume in systemic venous circulation	
Increased volume in distensible organs (liver, spleen)	
Increased pressure at capillary line	
Hepatomegaly, splenomegaly	
Dependent edema and serous effusion	

*From Kernicki, J., et al.: Cardiovascular nursing: rationale for therapy and nursing approach, New York, 1970, G. P. Putnam's Sons.

other, but as the failure progressively worsens, the function of the unaffected side will be compromised since both sides are part of the same closed system. Most often, heart failure begins with failure of the left side of the heart, which progressively worsens until the backward effects of left-sided failure cause such intense tension in the pulmonary circulation that the function of the right side is impaired due to the increased resistance it is pumping against. The backward and forward effects of right- and left-sided heart failure are summarized in Table 9-1.

Clinical manifestations. Pump failure can occur as an acute or a chronic condition. When cardiac damage has occurred slowly over a long period of time, the heart is able to maintain cardiac output at a normal level except during periods of stress and activity. The heart does this through the adaptive mechanisms of dilation and hypertrophy.

Cardiac output of the damaged heart is maintained chiefly through the retention of fluid in the body. In the presence of heart disease an increase in the volume of blood entering the ventricles results in a sustained lengthening of their muscle fibers, or *dilatation*. This dilatation allows the heart to contract more forcefully; however, there is increased tension on individual muscle fibers rather than on cardiac muscle as a whole. This results in increased myocardial oxygen consumption. As dilatation increases, cardiac reserve, the maximum percentage that cardiac output can increase above normal, is decreased. This mechanism is related to Starling's principle of autoregulation, and as stated previously, it has a physiologic limit. At a critical point, further lengthening of cardiac muscle fibers is no longer physiologic, and contraction becomes weak.

Dilatation is usually associated with hypertrophy or enlargement of the muscle mass of the heart. There is disagreement as to which condition appears first. Hypertrophy occurs in response to the increased cardiac work load and does result in augmented pumping ability due to the increase in the muscle wall size. However, as muscle mass increases, the blood supply to it does not increase to a comparable degree. As a result of this, cardiac function in a hypertrophied heart will be severely compromised by even a slight reduction in coronary blood flow.

During periods of stress and activity the damaged heart is unable to increase cardiac output because the compensatory mechanisms normally utilized to increase cardiac output are already being utilized to maintain a cardiac output adequate for meeting normal cellular oxygen requirements. A term used to describe this chronic type of heart failure is *compensated heart failure.* Under normal conditions, in a resting state or with limited activity, the weakened heart is able to compensate for the weakness and maintain a normal cardiac output.

Other terms used to describe heart failure include *cardiac failure, myocardial failure, power failure, low output failure, high output failure, right* or *left ventricular failure,* and *decompensated failure.* The term *congestive heart failure* is usually used to describe chronic, combined failure of the right and left sides of the heart.

For the purpose of discussion, the effects of right- and left-sided heart failure will be examined separately. Keep in mind, however, that in a closed system, such as the heart, a totally isolated condition cannot exist for any length of time.

Left-sided heart failure occurs when the output of the left side of the heart is less than the total volume of blood received from the right side of the heart. More blood is being received from the pulmonary circulation than the left side of the heart can pump out. As a result pulmonary filling pressure rises while systemic filling pressure falls. Signs and symptom of left-sided failure result from decreased cardiac output and pulmonary congestion.

Shortness of breath or difficult breathing during strenuous activity, exercise, or stress is referred to as *dyspnea on exertion.* In response to increased cellular demands for oxygen, the normal heart increases the cardiac output. As blood flow through the lungs increases, the rate of oxygenation of the blood increases. The failing or failure-prone heart is unable to increase cardiac output during exercise, and the rate of oxygen saturation of the blood cannot increase. Exercise increases venous return, and the right side of the heart pumps the total increased volume of returning blood to the left side. The failing left side of the heart is unable to pump the total amount of blood received to the systemic circulation. As a result blood accumulates in the pulmonary vascular bed, and pulmonary vascular pressure rises. When pulmonary capillary pressure rises above 28 mm Hg, the colloid osmotic pressure of plasma fluid will filter out of the capillaries and into the interstitial spaces and alveoli of the lungs. This portion of the alveolocapillary membrane becomes nonfunctional for gas exchange, and oxygen saturation of the blood falls further below normal levels. In response to the ensuing hypoxia the work of breathing accelerates due to the stimulation of chemoreceptors and the respiratory center of the brain. As the failure worsens and functional vital capacity is further decreased, dyspnea occurs, not only during periods of exercise or stress but also during periods of rest.

Hypoxia of the body tissues occurs in response to the minimal cardiac output and decreased oxygen saturation of the blood. Easy fatigability, weakness, and dizziness are indicative of hypoxic tissues. The brain responds rapidly to hypoxia, hence the dizziness; and as failure and the resultant hypoxia worsen, disorientation, confusion, and ultimately unconsciousness can occur. The muscle weakness is a response to the loss of potassium, as well as hypoxia of muscle tissue. Aldosterone, secreted to expand fluid volume, causes the kidneys to excrete excessive amounts of potassium in addition to retaining sodium and water. Unless potassium is replaced, muscle function, including that of cardiac muscle, will be adversely affected. Increased fatigue and weakness are often the earliest symptoms of left-sided heart failure.

Orthopnea, or the inability to breathe in a lying position, is also a symptom of left-sided heart failure. In the supine position, blood that has pooled in the lower extremities returns to the heart due to the effects of hydrostatic pressure and gravity. This sudden increase in venous return cannot be handled by the left side of the heart, and blood accumulates in the pulmonary circulation. The effect is the same as that following exercise. Also the movement of the diaphragm is mechanically restricted by the abdominal organs pushing against it, and this further contributes to the shortness of breath.

Orthopnea is relieved by sitting because venous blood again pools in the lower extremities, venous return decreases, and vascular pressure in the pulmonary circulation decreases. Pressure on the diaphragm is relieved as the abdominal organs move downward in the abdominal cavity. The onset and increase in severity of orthopnea can be insidious. A person experiencing orthopnea may not realize he is actually having trouble breathing while lying down but knows he feels more comfortable when using several pillows for sleeping. The degree of severity of orthopnea is measured by the number of pillows needed by a person for comfortable sleep. A person who uses four pillows for sleeping is said to be experiencing "four-pillow orthopnea."

Paroxysmal nocturnal dyspnea is another symptom of left-sided heart failure. Periods of difficult breathing or air hunger (dyspnea) occur intermittently during the night. The person experiencing left-sided heart failure will awaken suddenly with severe shortness of breath and coughing spasms. He may open a window and gulp for air in an attempt to catch his breath. It is thought that paroxysmal nocturnal dyspnea (PND) occurs in response to a sudden increase in right ventricular output or a sudden increase in the body's need for oxygen. Possible triggering events include dreams, nightmares, or a full bladder. The attack is self-limiting and usually lasts only a short time. The change in position from lying to standing or sitting probably aids in decreasing the venous return in the same way as relief for orthopnea is achieved.

The most extreme form of left-sided failure is *pulmonary edema*. Pulmonary edema is an acute, life-threatening condition that occurs when serum transudation into the pulmonary interstitial space and alveoli becomes rapid and extreme. Functional vital capacity is severely reduced, and arterial hypoxemia results. Cardiac output and consequently systemic arterial pressure are severely decreased also. Signs and symptoms of acute pulmonary edema include intense dyspnea of sudden onset; rapid, gasping, gurgling respirations; extreme anxiety and restlessness; a rapid, weak irregular pulse; increased venous pressure; and decreased urinary output. The skin feels cool and damp to the touch and appears ashen gray and cyanotic. Auscultation of the heart reveals the presence of a third heart sound and a very rapid atrial rate called a *gallop rhythm*. Auscultation of the lungs reveals rales in the basilar segments. The patient seems to be unable to catch his breath and resists lying flat. A cough accompanied by expectoration of frothy, pink-tinged sputum may be present also. The pallor, sweating, rapid pulse rate, and cold skin are due to the sympathetic stimulation that occurs in response to the decreased cardiac output. Kidney function is depressed due to the decreased cardiac output and the resultant decrease in arterial pressure in the kidneys. Pulmonary symptoms are the result of pulmonary congestion.

Treatment of pulmonary edema must be rapid if the patient is to survive. Treatment goals include increasing the cardiac output, decreasing venous return, and improving oxygenation. Cardiac output is increased through the use of rapid-acting cardiotonic drugs that improve the function of the failing left side of the heart. These drugs are classified as cardiac glycosides and have positive inotropic and negative chronotropic effects. The positive inotropic effect is the increased contractility of the muscle fibers, which augments the strength of contraction and increases stroke volume. The negative chronotropic effect is the slowing of the myocardial contraction rate through an increase in vagal sensitivity and the refractory period of the AV conduction tissue. The net result is an increase in cardiac output, better utilization of available energy (oxygen) by the myocardium, and a lengthening of the period of diastole, which allows the myocardium to rest and increases the filling time for the coronary arteries. The use of the cardiac glycosides must be closely monitored in the presence of low potassium levels as this enhances the action of these drugs, and alterations in the heart's normal rhythm may occur.

Intravascular blood volume is reduced through the use of rapid-acting diuretic drugs, which increase urinary output; rotating tourniquets, which trap blood in the extremities; and phlebotomy, or the physical removal of blood. Reduced intravascular blood volume results in a decreased venous return and, concomitantly, decreased venous pressure. Because less blood is returning to the heart, the output of the right ventricle decreases, and as a result pulmonary vascular pressure also drops. The reduced pulmonary vascular pressure allows the serous fluid in the pulmonary interstitial space and alveoli to filter back (be reabsorbed) into the intravascular compartment.

Oxygenation of the blood is improved by administration of (1) high concentrations of oxygen under positive pressure and (2) the drugs aminophylline and morphine sulfate. Oxygen administered under pressure promotes the rapid formation of oxyhemoglobin, prevents further fluid transudation out of the capillaries, and helps move fluid already in the lung tissue back into the capillaries. Alcohol in a nebulized form can be administered with the oxygen to decrease the frothing of the serous fluid in the lung tissue, which is caused by the inspired air passing through it.

Aminophylline promotes dilation of the bronchioles. Morphine sulfate decreases the work of breathing and reduces metabolic demands for oxygen through two mechanisms. First, it acts as a sedative to relieve feelings of apprehension and anxiety and promote relaxation. Second, morphine directly depresses the respiratory center in the medulla, decreasing the respiratory rate and the work of breathing. Additionally it has a peripheral vasodilating effect, which probably also contributes to the relief of acute pulmonary edema.

The improved oxygenation and decreased venous return reduce the work load of the heart. Cardiac function is enhanced by both the reduced cardiac work load and the direct effect of the cardiac glycosides. As the circulation improves, the function of the body's various organ systems also improves and potentiates the effects of the treatments just described. As circulation to the kidneys improves, urinary output increases, and renin will no longer be secreted. As liver function improves, aldosterone and ADH are deactivated more rapidly.

Failure of the right side of the heart occurs when the output of the right ventricle becomes less than the total volume of blood being returned to the heart from the systemic circulation. Right-sided failure can occur independently, but it most often occurs as the sequela to left-sided heart failure. Isolated right-sided failure is usually the result of pulmonary disease (cor pulmonale) or congenital defects that increase pulmonary vascular resistance or pressure in the pulmonary artery. Defective functioning of the tricuspid valve will also cause isolated right-sided heart failure.

Signs and symptoms of right-sided failure result from decreased cardiac output and increased venous pressure. In response to the decreased cardiac output, urinary output drops, and hypoxia of the tissues causes weakness and fatigue with little exertion. Compensatory mechanisms, namely, fluid retention and an increase in the heart rate, occur. Systemic venous pressure rises as a result of the expansion of the intravascular fluid volume and the accumulation of blood in the systemic circulation due to the inability of the right side of the heart to pump it into the pulmonary circulation. The resultant rise in systemic capillary pressure causes filtration of serous fluid into the interstitial spaces. In the early stages of right-sided heart failure, edema (Fig. 9-7) or the presence of fluid in the interstitial spaces is visible as the swelling of dependent parts of the body, that is, the lower extremities where hydrostatic pressure is the greatest. As the heart failure worsens, edema occurs in the upper body tissues and affects various organ systems (see Chapter 10 for discussion of edema).

The distensible sinusoids of the liver and spleen expand to act as reservoirs for the excess blood. This results in an enlargement of both these organs, which is referred to as hepatomegaly (liver enlargement) and splenomegaly (spleen enlargement). Palpation of the

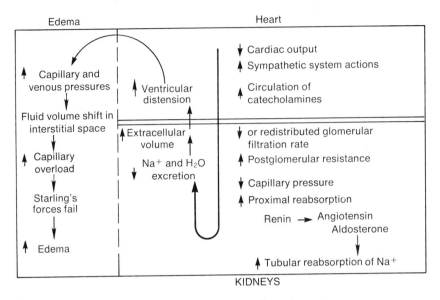

Fig. 9-7. Pathogenesis of cardiac edema.

abdomen reveals tenderness in the right and left upper quadrants where these organs lie and definition of their borders. Inadequate deactivation of aldosterone and ADH because of poor liver function will lead to further fluid volume expansion, contributing to the vicious cycle already set up.

Ascites, or free fluid in the abdominal cavity, occurs as serous fluid filters out of the portal system because of the increased vascular pressure. The function of the gastrointestinal system is adversely affected by the edema and depressed functioning of the intestines and other abdominal organs. Ascites leaves little room for expansion of the stomach and intestines. These conditions lead to such symptoms as anorexia (loss of appetite), indigestion, nausea, and vomiting. The presence of any electrolyte imbalances, drug interactions, or toxicity will further aggravate these symptoms.

Peripheral vein distension allows direct observation of the results of increased venous pressure. With increased venous pressure the jugular vein appears distended or bulging, even with elevation of the head, a state in which the vein is normally flat and unobservable. When the jugular vein is compressed and emptied it should fill from the top; however, in the presence of increased venous pressure it will fill from the bottom. Distension, or bulg-

ing, of the hand veins with the hands raised to heart level is also a sign of increased venous pressure. The severity of the increase in venous pressure can be directly measured by means of a catheter inserted into the right atrium and attached externally to a manometer. The measurement thus obtained is called *central venous pressure.* Normal central venous pressure is between 0 and 10 cm of water pressure. This value will be elevated in the presence of increased venous pressure.

Physiology of treatment. Heart failure seen clinically is usually a combination of left- and right-sided failure; it is usually referred to as congestive heart failure. Treatment goals are similar to those for pulmonary edema; they include

1. Improvement of cardiac output and circulation throughout the body
2. A decrease in the work load of the heart
3. Prevention of potential complications
4. Promotion of an optimal level of function

Cardiac output is increased through the use of the cardiac glycoside drugs. These drugs cause an increase in the contractility and a decrease in the rate of contraction of the myocardium. With increased cardiac output and better circulation to all parts of the body, many of the signs and symptoms of heart failure disappear. Organ function throughout the body improves as tissues once again receive the oxygen and nutrients necessary for metabolism. As blood supply to the brain is increased, the sensorium improves. Edematous fluid will begin to be mobilized as a result of improved circulatory dynamics.

Cardiac work load is decreased by keeping venous return within normal limits (or at a level that the failure-prone heart can manage) and by reducing tissue demands for oxygen. Venous return is reduced through the use of diuretic drugs to increase urine output and through restriction of the amount of fluid and sodium allowed in the diet. After the acute phase of heart failure when the heart has begun to compensate, venous return from the peripheral, dependent areas of the body is facilitated through the use of elastic support stockings. These also help prevent any further formation of edema in the tissues and assist circulation to prevent clot formation.

Tissue demands for oxygen are reduced through frequent rest periods, avoidance of fatiguing activities and becoming overtired, and spacing activities to avoid doing too much at one time. Positioning the patient with his head elevated helps reduce the work of breathing, which also helps reduce tissue demands for oxygen. Because of the effects of gravity, the head-elevated position also decreases venous return to the heart. Blood will remain in the lower extremities and pelvic region.

Complications can occur as a result of the disease process or as a result of the treatment. Edematous tissue is easily injured and is prone to the development of infection. Once injured, it heals more slowly than normal tissue. Special skin care and protection should be given to edematous areas to avoid injury. Venous stasis occurs in the presence of a sluggish circulation and predisposes the individual to intravascular clot formation and thrombophlebitis. Bed rest as a treatment measure also contributes to venous stasis. The feet and legs should never be massaged as a clot may be jarred loose into the circulation. Diet and drug therapy can lead to severe fluid and electrolyte imbalances, which in turn can lead to dehydration or cardiac arrhythmias.

An optimal level of functioning is promoted through rehabilitation and teaching. Increasing the patient's understanding of the disease and its treatment may promote cooperation and consistent compliance with the regimen in the treatment of chronic heart failure. The patient requires information about the disease process in order to assume responsibility for the management of it and to prevent recurrent episodes.

Etiology. Heart failure is not a disease entity in itself but rather the result of other disease processes that affect the entire transport system: the heart, the connecting vessels, and the blood. Alteration in the heart's ability to pump or its pumping effectiveness can result from many problems:

1. An overwhelming increase in extracellular fluid volume (e.g., too rapid administration of IV fluids)
2. Damage to or loss of functional myocardial muscle tissue (e.g., myocardial infarction)
3. Aberrations in the rate and rhythm of the heart (e.g., bradycardia and tachycardia arrhythmias)
4. Incompetence of the cardiac valves (e.g., mitral stenosis)
5. Inflammatory or infectious processes that result in the weakening of myocardial muscle tissue (e.g., myocarditis, endocarditis, pericarditis)
6. Increased resistance to the heart's pumping action (e.g., hypertensive vascular disease)
7. Congenital defects (e.g., patent ductus arteriosus)
8. Constriction of heart tissue resulting in mechanical limitation of the heart's pumping action (e.g., constrictive pericarditis, cardiac tamponade)
9. Conditions in which cardiac output is normal or even high but metabolic requirements of the body are greatly increased, *high output failure* (e.g., hyperthyroidism)
10. Conditions in which the oxygen-carrying capacity of the blood is decreased accompanied by compromised cardiac function (e.g., anemia coexisting with coronary artery disease)

11. Cardiomyopathies: a heterogeneous group of chronic myocardial disorders not due to ischemia, hypertension, valve disease, or shunts, and which appear to be noninflammatory in nature (e.g., endomyocardial fibrosis)

A complete analysis of aberrations of cardiac rate and rhythm and valvular and congenital defects is beyond the scope of this book. However, a descriptive survey will be presented so that the reader can better understand the effect these disorders have on oxygen transport processes.

A cardiac rate that is extremely rapid or slow or a cardiac rhythm that is grossly abnormal results in a decrease in cardiac output. Furthermore, it is indicative of some underlying abnormality in the cardiac tissue, interfering with the normal spontaneous generation or conduction of the cardiac impulse. Changes in the cardiac cell itself and in its environment can result in disruption of normal electrical activity. Examples of these changes include electrolyte imbalance, hypoxia with resultant ischemia or infarction of tissue, abnormal temperature, and effects of drugs. The type of arrhythmia that occurs depends on the area of the heart affected. For example, conduction will be affected if the tissue in the conduction system is damaged. Pacemaker activity will be affected by damage to the cells of the SA node, altered SA node function (sick sinus syndrome), or by ectopic areas of irritable tissue that are generating impulses.

Fig. 9-8 diagrams the normal electrocardiogram and the electrical sequence of events it represents. Arrhythmias are detected through changes in the electrocardiogram. Arrhythmias are classified according to the site of origin (sinus if in the SA node, atrial if in the atria, junctional if in the AV node, and ventricular if in the ventricles), the rate, if abnormal (bradycardia for a rate below 60 beats per minute and tachycardia for a rate above 100 beats per minute), and the rhythm.

Congenital heart disease refers to structural defects of the heart that developed in embryo. The exact cause of these disorders has not been elucidated; however, maternal viral infections, especially rubella, during the first 3 months of

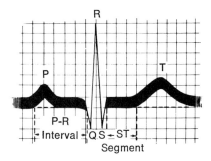

Fig. 9-8. Normal electrocardiographic tracing. The P wave represents atrial depolarization; the QRS complex, ventricular depolarization; and the T wave, ventricular repolarization. (From Burke, S. R.: The composition and function of body fluids, ed. 2, St. Louis, 1976, The C. V. Mosby Co.)

pregnancy are known to result in disorders of fetal development. The reader is referred to Chapter 2 for a more complete discussion of disorders of embryonic development and teratogenic mechanisms.

Congenital heart defects can affect oxygenation by causing a reduction in effective cardiac output or by increasing the resistance against which the heart must pump. "Effective" cardiac output is reduced because of the mixing of arterial and venous blood (anatomic shunting) that occurs in many of these defects. The direction of the shunt will determine the severity of the manifestations.

Valvular disease is most often the result of rheumatic fever; however, it can be caused by some other conditions as well: syphilis, bacterial endocarditis, and calcific atherosclerosis. Chronic valve deformities result in hemodynamic changes that increase the work load of the heart.

Valvular disorders are of two types. In the first type, *stenosis,* blood flow is obstructed. The valve cusps become thickened and fibrotic and may even become calcified and fused with one another. They cannot open completely. The second type of valvular disorder, referred to as *insufficiency* or *regurgitation* (Fig. 9-9), occurs when the valve cusps retract and no longer close completely; hence, leaking of blood occurs during systole.

With stenosis, pressure in the cardiac chamber antecedent to the affected valve increases because of the resistance against which it is

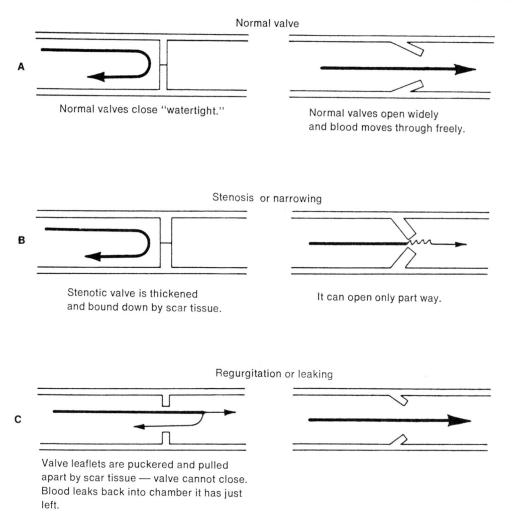

Normal valve

A

Normal valves close "watertight."

Normal valves open widely
and blood moves through freely.

Stenosis or narrowing

B

Stenotic valve is thickened
and bound down by scar tissue.

It can open only part way.

Regurgitation or leaking

C

Valve leaflets are puckered and pulled
apart by scar tissue — valve cannot close.
Blood leaks back into chamber it has just
left.

Fig. 9-9. Diseases of heart valves. (From Phibbs, B.: The human heart: a guide to heart disease, ed. 3,
St. Louis, 1975, The C. V. Mosby Co.)

pumping. This increase in pressure is reflected
backward throughout the heart, increasing the
work load of the heart. The sequelae of events
in mitral stenosis illustrate this point. When the
mitral valve creates an obstruction to blood
flow, cardiac output falls, and pressure increases in the left atrium, which in turn creates
increased pressure in the pulmonary veins. As
pressure increases in the pulmonary veins, it
also increases in the pulmonary vascular bed
with resultant congestion of that vessel system
and decreased exchange of oxygen and carbon
dioxide. With aortic stenosis there is an additional problem. Blood flow to the coronary ar-

teries is reduced due to decreased pressure in
the aorta.

Regurgitation, or leaking of blood, has similar effects. Cardiac work is increased because
the heart never empties completely and must
work harder to pump an adequate amount of
blood to meet tissue demands. The severity of
these effects depends on the extent to which the
valve can still function.

Rheumatic fever, the major cause of valvular
disease, is an inflammatory condition that in
itself is not an infection but the aftermath of an
infection of the group A beta-hemolytic streptococci. The course of rheumatic fever is simi-

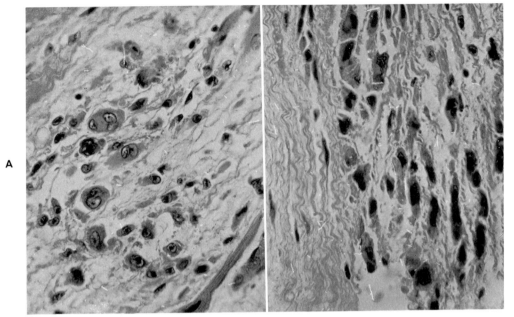

Fig. 9-10. Aschoff bodies in myocardium in 15-year-old boy. **A,** Intermediate phase with distinct Aschoff cells. **B,** More advanced lesion with elongation of cells, pyknosis, and smudging of nuclei. (From Anderson, W. A. D., and Kissane, J. M.: Pathology, ed. 7, St. Louis, 1977, The C. V. Mosby Co.)

Table 9-2. Major and minor criteria for the diagnosis of rheumatic fever

Major	Minor
Migratory polyarthritis: swelling, pain, redness, tenderness, heat in one or more joints (not all joints are affected at once, and pain may move from joint to joint)	Malaise
	Arthralgia
	Fever
	Leukocytosis
Carditis	Increased ESR (erythrocyte sedimentation rate)
Myocarditis, muscle inflamed and dilated	Increased CRP (C-reactive protein)
Endocarditis, valves and inner lining affected	Increased P-R interval (ECG)
Pericarditis, outer lining inflamed	Previous infection of group A beta-hemolytic
Pancarditis, all layers affected	streptococci
Chorea (St. Vitus' dance): purposeless, non-repetitive movements with grimacing of face	Previous episodes of rheumatic fever
	Presence of rheumatic heart disease
Erythema marginatum (rash)	
Subcutaneous nodules	

lar to serum sickness and occurs in three phases:

Phase I   Streptococcal infection
Phase II   Latent period (1 to 5 weeks)
Phase III Acute rheumatic fever

The characteristic lesion is the *Aschoff body* (Fig. 9-10), a collection of reticuloendothelial cells mixed with plasma cells and lymphocytes, surrounding a necrotic, collagenous center. It is actually a "point of inflammation," and many of these points can be found in the heart, lungs, joints, and brain.

Diagnosis of rheumatic fever is made on the basis of major and minor criteria (Table 9-2). At least one of the major criteria must be present along with minor criteria. The complica-

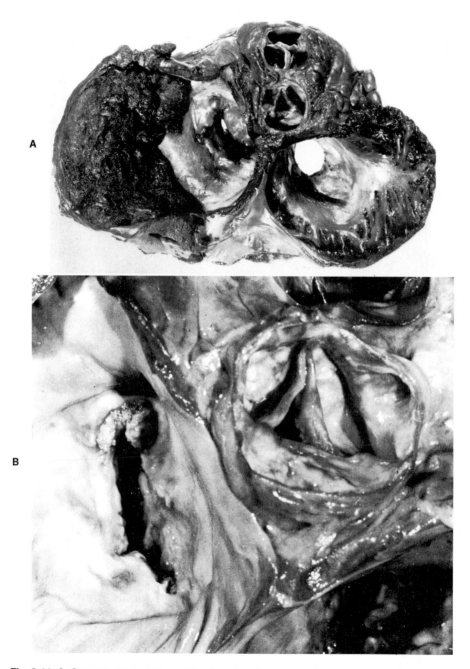

Fig. 9-11. A, Stenosis of mitral tricuspid and aortic valves caused by chronic rheumatic endocarditis. Mitral orifice is mere slit. Note large thrombus in dilated left atrium. **B,** Mitral and aortic stenosis with calcification of both valves. (From Anderson, W. A. D., and Kissane, J. M.: Pathology, ed. 7, St. Louis, 1977, The C. V. Mosby Co.)

tions of rheumatic fever include congestive heart failure due to valvulitis and rheumatic heart disease. Whether permanent heart damage will occur depends on the area of the heart involved and whether there have been previous episodes of rheumatic fever. Acute carditis occurs in 40% to 50% of patients experiencing their first attack. Permanent scarring of the valves may result from the first episode, but in most instances the first attack does not leave permanent damage.

Valve damage occurs through inflammation and scar tissue formation. During acute rheumatic fever, valvulitis may occur and cause the valves to become thickened with edema. Aschoff bodies cover the valves, especially the free margins (leaflets). As healing takes place, scar tissue forms and causes fusion of the valve cusps and chordae tendineae. Calcification of the affected areas may also occur (Fig. 9-11). The mitral valve is most frequently affected. Persons with valvular damage are more susceptible to the development of subacute bacterial endocarditis (SBE) as the scars of rheumatic heart disease provide crevices in which bacteria can lodge and multiply. Even bacteria normally present in the body are potentially virulent to these patients. Special precautions for even minor surgical procedures and dental work must be taken to avoid an acute episode of SBE.

The relationship between rheumatic fever and the group A beta-hemolytic streptococci is not certain, but evidence suggests that it is a hypersensitivity or autoimmune disorder. Other areas of research have examined whether rheumatic fever results from persistence of viable streptococci or variants of the organism and whether the lesions of rheumatic fever are the result of toxins or enzymes. These areas of research have not produced positive results.

Studies have shown that many of the factors which seem to predispose a person to the development of rheumatic fever are the same as those factors predisposing a person to the development of a streptococcal infection, including positive familial tendency, worldwide occurrence but a tendency to predominate in temperate zones and to follow the same seasonal variations, environment and life-style (crowded substandard living conditions, poor hygiene, inadequate medical care, inadequate dietary habits), and age (6 to 15 years is the range in most cases, and 8 years seems to be the peak). Since there is a higher incidence of streptococcal infections in families living under acute and chronic stress, this group would appear to be at risk for the development of rheumatic fever.

Approximately 2% of persons with streptococcal infections will develop rheumatic fever. Half this group will acquire rheumatic heart disease.

Primary prevention of rheumatic fever and rheumatic heart disease involves treating all streptococcal infections with antibiotics. A throat culture should be performed on all patients presenting with the complaint of "sore throat" in order to determine the causative organism. Secondary prevention involves preventing the reoccurrence of streptococcal infections after rheumatic heart disease has occurred. Antibiotics are administered prophylactically on a regular basis throughout the patient's life.

ALTERATIONS IN PRESSURE, FLOW, AND PATENCY

An intact vessel system must be functioning for blood to be carried to the various body organs and tissues. Changes in the normal pressure and flow within the system require that compensatory mechanisms come into play so that the transport process can continue. The patency of the vessels themselves is also important. Conditions in which there is an alteration in pressure, flow, or patency include circulatory failure, hypertension, occlusive disorders, peripheral vascular disease, and disease of the lymphatic system.

Circulatory failure

Etiology. Circulatory failure, or *shock*, is a pathophysiologic state in which tissue perfusion is totally inadequate to meet the oxygen or nutritional needs of the cells. Shock has been described as "a momentary pause in the act of death" (Warren, 1895). Shock, like cardiac failure, is not a disease entity in itself but a response to some assault or injury the body has experienced. No matter what the initiating event, the cause of death in irreversible shock is microcirculatory failure and the subsequent depression of cellular metabolism. Conditions in which cardiac output is reduced predispose the patient to the development of shock. Hence, any condition that reduces the heart's ability to pump effectively or decreases venous return has the potential of causing shock. Factors that decrease venous return include diminished blood volume (hypovolemia) and decreased vasomotor tone (increased venous capacity).

Shock has been classified according to the physiologic event that evokes it. The differentiation is not in terms of pathophysiology (which is the same for all types of shock) but in terms of etiology.

Hypovolemic shock is the result of diminished blood volume. Blood volume loss leads to diminished venous return, reduced cardiac output, and poor tissue perfusion. Volume loss can be the result of either (1) excessive bleeding, or hemorrhage, where all the components of the blood are lost, or (2) the loss of plasma only. Hemorrhage can occur as a result of trauma (accidental or surgical), coagulation disorders, delivery of a baby, or carcinoma. With the exception of intracranial bleeding, internal bleeding, or bleeding into a body cavity, can also lead to hypovolemic shock. This is because the amount of blood loss into the cranium is limited due to the relatively small size of the cranium. Crushing injuries may also result in hypovolemic shock. When the pressure is removed, whole blood and plasma leak into the interstitial space as a result of the capillary endothelial damage and the subsequent change in capillary permeability that occurs. Other conditions that may ultimately lead to hypovolemic shock include burns, intestinal obstruction, and dehydration.

Plasma loss due to a burn can be quite extensive. Where plasma alone is lost, blood viscosity becomes markedly increased and enhances the development of venous stasis in the presence of the already compromised blood flow. Where a thermal injury has occurred, both capillary damage and increased capillary permeability are present and lead to disruption of the normal capillary equilibrium. Plasma shifts from the intravascular compartment to the interstitial space. The loss of plasma pro-tein from the intravascular compartment reduces the plasma colloid osmotic pressure, which limits the return of fluid to the capillary. Intestinal obstruction and the resultant intestinal distension cause plasma loss into the intestinal walls and lumen. This plasma shift may result from capillary damage or from increased hydrostatic pressure in the intestinal capillary bed. The venules are collapsed, and as a result resistance and consequently hydrostatic pressure are both increased, tending to force fluid from the intravascular compartment.

Dehydration, or a decrease in total body fluid volume, can also cause reduced blood volume and hypovolemic shock. Vomiting, diarrhea, sweating, diuresis, adrenal insufficiency, inadequate consumption of fluid, or heat exhaustion can lead to depletion of total body fluid volume. When this occurs, plasma will shift from the intravascular compartment to the interstitial space.

Relative hypovolemia occurs in conditions where venous return is diminished although total blood volume is not. Venous return is reduced in the presence of increased thoracic or abdominal pressure because of the compression of the vena cava that occurs. For example, with the pregnant patient in the supine position, the pregnant uterus can exert enough pressure on the vena cava to cause obstruction to such a degree that venous return is severely reduced.

Neurogenic shock is the result of generalized vasodilation due to decreased vasomotor tone. Blood volume remains within normal limits; however, the capacity of the blood vessels themselves is increased. Consequently venous return is diminished, leading to a reduced cardiac output that is inadequate to maintain tissue perfusion. The reduction in vasomotor tone can occur at the level of the vasomotor center or at the level of the blood vessels themselves. Shock caused by vasodilation due to factors affecting the blood vessels locally is called *vasogenic shock*.

The predisposition to develop neurogenic shock is enhanced in conditions where vasomotor tone is reduced or lost. Examples of these conditions include spinal anesthesia, spinal cord injury, direct damage to the vasomotor center of the medulla or altered function of the vasomotor center in response to low blood glucose levels (insulin shock), severe pain, or the action of tranquilizer, narcotic, or sedative drugs.

The most common form of vasogenic shock is *anaphylactic shock,* which is the result of an antigen-antibody reaction. The release of histamine, serotonin, and bradykinin directly affects local blood vessels, causing vasodilation and increased capillary permeability. Slow reacting substances (SRS) is also released and causes constriction of the bronchioles.

Cardiogenic shock, or low output syndrome, occurs when cardiac function is severely compromised, and cardiac output becomes extremely low. Cardiogenic shock can result from extensive myocardial damage due to infarction or open heart surgery, as a sequela to heart failure, or as a result of prolonged arrhythmias. The extent of myocardial damage can be correlated with the incidence of cardiogenic shock after myocardial infarction. Cardiogenic shock is more likely to be a complication of myocardial infarction when 40% or more of the myocardium is damaged. The mortality rate of patients developing cardiogenic shock continues to be high (approximately 80%) in spite of new methods of treatment. It is considered a grave complication of myocardial infarction.

It is not known whether cardiogenic shock is related to heart failure or whether they are two entirely different clinical entities. However, therapy to correct heart failure is ineffective in the treatment of cardiogenic shock, indicating that they are different entities.

Septic shock is also endotoxic shock. It results from widespread, overwhelming infection. Infections due to gram-positive organisms such as staphylococci, streptococci, and pneumococci result in approximately one third of the cases of septic shock. The mortality rate in cases of septic shock as a sequela to infections caused by the gram-positive organisms is 50%. The mortality rate in cases of septic shock occurring with infections caused by gram-negative organisms is 75%. The enteric coli are responsible for the majority of gram-negative infections that result in septic shock. The incidence of septic shock caused by gram-negative organisms is increasing. This is pos-

sibly related to the widespread and sometimes indiscriminate use of antibiotic therapy, leading to ever increasing numbers of antibiotic-resistant organisms.

Patients at risk for the development of septic shock include persons with indwelling catheters, peritonitis, burns, chronic, debilitating disease, or postpartum infection. Additionally patients who have had gastrointestinal or genitourinary tract surgery or a septic abortion, as well as those patients on immunosuppressant therapy or with defects in the function of the immune system, are at risk.

At the present time, two theories have been postulated for the inception of septic shock. One theory implicates the toxins released from the bacteria, and the other implicates the bacteria themselves as the causative factor. Present in the cell wall of all gram-negative bacteria is endotoxin lipopolysaccharide, which is released upon cell death. Experimental studies with animals have demonstrated that administration of this substance results in manifestations similar to those seen in bacteremic, or septic, shock. The value of these studies is questionable, however, because septic shock may result from infection due to gram-positive organisms, which do not contain endotoxin. Through these studies gram-negative bacteria and endotoxin have been shown to bind and activate Hageman factor, which in turn activates the fibrinolytic, clotting, complement, and kinin-generating pathways.

Pathophysiologic mechanisms and clinical manifestations. As a result of diminished cardiac output, arterial pressure falls. This hypotension is the most immediate antecedent of hypovolemic, cardiogenic, and neurogenic shock. In response to the generalized arterial hypotension, various negative-feedback control mechanisms come into play to return arterial pressure and tissue perfusion to normal limits.

Sympathetic stimulation through baroreceptor reflexes provides immediate compensation and results in tachycardia, vasoconstriction, redistribution of blood flow, and increased cardiac contractility. Vasoconstriction of the capacitance vessels results in increased venous return as the blood from these vessels is added to the circulating blood volume. Arteriolar constriction increases total peripheral resistance to help raise arterial pressure but does not occur uniformly in all tissues. Blood flow is shifted to those organ systems in which arteriolar constriction is minimal, such as the heart and brain. Arteriolar constriction is very great in the peripheral tissues and is manifested by cool, pale skin as blood flow is diverted from those areas because of the high resistance.

The increased rate and force of cardiac contraction improves cardiac output. The augmented contractile force results in more complete cardiac emptying, reducing end systolic ventricular volume. The mobilization of this blood and that previously stored in the capacitance vessels prior to their constriction is called *autotransfusion* or *intravascular fluid mobilization*.

There is a reduction in capillary filtration pressure as a result of both the decreased arterial pressure and the subsequent constriction of the resistance vessels. Because some arterioles constrict more than venules the ratio between precapillary and postcapillary resistance increases. As a result of these changes in capillary dynamics there is a net movement of fluid from the interstitial space into the vascular compartment, further augmenting venous return and subsequently cardiac output. This movement of fluid is limited because of the dilution of the plasma proteins, which reduces plasma oncotic pressure. This phenomenon is termed *autoinfusion* or *extravascular fluid mobilization*.

Urine output is reduced due to the negative effect that reduced arterial pressure and vasoconstriction of the kidney arterioles have on glomerular filtration. The reduction in renal afferent arteriolar pressure activates the renin-angiotensin system previously described, which results in the selective retention of sodium and subsequently water by the kidneys. ADH is also secreted, and the thirst mechanism is stimulated in response to a relative decrease in the size of the extracellular volume. These mechanisms act to restore lost fluid volume.

Most of the clinical manifestations to this point are the result of the sympathetic stimulation that has occurred: rapid, thready pulse, decreased pulse pressure, cool, pale skin, oliguria, and increased sweat gland activity. In the presence of dehydration the skin turgor will be reduced, features may appear sunken, eyeballs may feel "soft," the mouth will be dry, and there will be extreme thirst. Respiratory activity increases as chemoreceptors are activated by reduced arterial pressure.

The mechanisms delineated thus far are negative-feedback control mechanisms; that is, the drop in arterial pressure serves to stimulate the compensatory mechanisms by which arterial pressure is restored and maintained. This stage is termed *compensated shock*. If the underlying cause of the shock has not been corrected or if the cause is not self-limiting, continued sympathetic stimulation becomes detrimental to the body. Shock at this point is referred to as *progressive*. The response of the body to poor tissue perfusion becomes one of positive feedback, which sets up a vicious cycle in which cardiac output and tissue perfusion will continually decrease until a point is reached where death becomes inevitable. At this point the shock is said to be *irreversible* or *decompensated*.

Vasoconstriction of the arterioles and venules results in decreased blood flow to and through the microcirculation. The surrounding tissues experience ischemic hypoxia. The pH of the tissue fluid becomes acidotic as the products of metabolism accumulate. As a result of the local stimulation provided by the hypoxia and altered pH the arterioles dilate. The venules, however, remain constricted. Blood can enter the microcirculation but becomes trapped within due to constriction of the venule. Pressures in the capillary bed are altered so that the net movement of fluid is out of the intravascular compartment and into the interstitial space. Plasma proteins are also lost from the intravascular compartment because the permeability of the capillary membrane is altered due to the adverse conditions in the surrounding tissue. The reduction in the flow of blood enhances intravascular clot formation. In fact, thrombosis of minute vessels has been postulated as one of the causes of progressive shock.

Cellular metabolism becomes anaerobic,

leading to formation of increased quantities of lactic acid in addition to the normally produced quantities of organic acids. As progressively greater amounts of acidotic metabolic products form and accumulate, the buffer systems and other compensatory mechanisms that serve to maintain normal acid-base balance become ineffective. Cellular energy production is progressively depressed, and if shock is not corrected, energy production eventually ceases. The cells are unable to perform even the most vital functions. When cellular function is severely depressed or totally stopped, the organ systems fail.

As the myocardium becomes weaker, cardiac output diminishes even further. In addition to the lack of oxygen and energy, a substance that has a direct depressant effect on the myocardium has been isolated, namely, myocardial depressant factor (MDF), or myocardial toxic factor (MTF). This substance is thought to interfere with the function of calcium ions in the excitation-contraction coupling mechanism, and as a result cardiac contractility is reduced. It is thought that pancreatic ischemia causes the release of proteolytic enzymes, which serve to either stimulate the release of the toxic factor or alter the plasma proteins to form a new substance with toxic properties.

Also implicated in the progression of shock are various vasoactive substances, including histamine, serotonin, and bradykinin. The plasma kinins act directly on smooth muscle to cause dilation. The prostaglandins are also being investigated for vasodilatory action.

The progression of septic shock in terms of metabolic effects and decompensation is the same as for all other types of shock. However, since the initiating events are quite different from reduced venous return or reduced cardiac output, a discussion of it at this time is appropriate. Two syndromes related to septic shock have been described. One is characterized by high cardiac output, high central venous pressure, a normal urine output, low peripheral resistance, and warm, dry extremities. This is referred to as the *hyperdynamic* type of septic shock. The other is characterized by low cardiac output, high peripheral resistance, and decreased urine output. This is referred to as the *hypodynamic* type of septic shock.

This differentiation has implications in terms of the potential development of shock. Patients experiencing the hyperdynamic type of septic shock will not exhibit the classic signs of shock: decreased arterial blood pressure, cold, clammy, cyanotic skin (which may also appear blotchy or mottled), oliguria (possibly even anuria), increased respiratory rate (compensatory response to metabolic acidosis), and a weak, rapid (thready) pulse. As cerebral perfusion is diminished, restlessness, coma, convulsion, or other disturbances of behavior may occur.

Measurement of blood pressure is not useful in the diagnosis of shock. The initiating hypotension is rapidly corrected via reflex control, and when hypotension becomes clinically detectable through use of a sphygmomanometer, compensation is no longer effective, and shock has become progressive. To more accurately monitor cardiac function, placement of a flow-directed, balloon-tipped catheter (Swan-Ganz) into a branch of the pulmonary artery becomes necessary. Through this catheter the pulmonary pressure can be measured. This parameter is a reflection of left atrial pressure and, in the absence of mitral valve disease, of left ventricular diastolic pressure and thus serves as an indicator of left ventricular function.

Physiology of treatment. The goals of treatment include

1. Correction of the underlying cause
2. Improvement of tissue perfusion
3. Correction of acid-base imbalance
4. Prevention of complications

Correction of the underlying cause in septic shock requires intensive antibiotic therapy; in hypovolemic shock, replacement of the effective circulating volume; in neurogenic shock, restoration of vasomotor tone; and in cardiogenic shock, augmentation of cardiac performance. Cardiac function in cardiogenic shock can sometimes be improved by administration of drugs with positive inotropic and chronotropic actions, as well as drugs to counteract peripheral vasoconstriction to reduce resistance to flow and thus reduce cardiac work load. If these fail, mechanical circulatory assistance becomes necessary by means of insertion of a balloon into the aorta (intra-aortic balloon counterpulsation). The intra-aortic balloon, as it is called, is alternately inflated and deflated, controlling the capacity of the aorta for blood.

Normally correction of the underlying cause of the shock syndrome will also help to increase perfusion as it takes effect. Immediate pharmacologic intervention often is necessary as these effects take time. Drugs that promote vasodilation and increased cerebral and renal perfusion (isoproterenol and dopamine) may be indicated. The corticosteroid drugs are utilized for their positive inotropic effect. The steroids are also thought to help overcome peripheral resistance, as well as to counteract the effects of endotoxin in septic shock.

Complications of shock include disseminated intravascular coagulation, gastric ulceration, renal insufficiency leading to acute tubular necrosis, and adult respiratory distress syndrome (ARDS, or shock lung).

Hypertension

More than 20 million people in the United States suffer from systemic hypertension. Over one half of these cases are undiagnosed and untreated. Systemic hypertension increases in frequency and severity with age and occurs more frequently in blacks than in whites. It has a very insidious course, which the patient often refuses to recognize because he "feels good," hence, the nickname the "silent killer." It is the leading cause of strokes and congestive heart failure.

Blood pressure varies between individuals so it is hard to define high blood pressure as a specific number of units over normal. Generally an elevation of the diastolic pressure above 95 mm Hg and of the systolic pressure above 160 mm Hg is considered to be high blood pressure. The diastolic pressure reflects the total peripheral resistance.

Common findings in patients with elevated blood pressure include a positive family history, obesity, a smoking history, increased lipid levels, and excessive salt intake. Hypertension is predictably more severe in patients who smoke.

Classification and etiology. The commonly used classifications include primary, secondary, benign, and malignant. The classifications of primary and secondary refer to etiology. Hypertension in which the cause is unknown is referred to as primary, essential, or idiopathic hypertension. Secondary hypertension is elevation of the blood pressure as a result of some other primary disease process. In terms of this classification the most common type of hypertension is primary, which accounts for 85% of all cases. The remaining 15% can be classified as secondary. Examples of diseases that cause an elevation of the arterial pressure as part of the disease process include renal disease and pheochromocytoma, a tumor of the adrenal medulla. Treating the primary cause can resolve the elevated blood pressure.

The other two classifications refer to the course of the disease process. Malignant, or accelerated, hypertension is characterized by a rapid and severe increase in blood pressure. Complications occur more frequently and develop more rapidly in malignant hypertension. Benign, or chronic, hypertension refers to a more moderate rise in blood pressure, which occurs over a longer period of time. The term *benign* is somewhat of a misnomer because the blood pressure elevation can be quite significant and if left uncontrolled can cause complications. In 10% of all cases malignant hypertension occurs as a sequel to benign hypertension. Malignant hypertension also occurs without any evidence of preexisting benign hypertension.

Pathophysiologic mechanisms and clinical manifestations. The major defect in primary hypertension is a persistent increase in the total peripheral resistance. Without a compensatory decrease in cardiac output this will result in an elevated blood pressure. The increased resistance to blood flow increases the cardiac work load, which in turn causes left-sided ventricular hypertrophy. Hypertrophy makes the myocardium more susceptible to ischemia as blood supply does not increase to the same degree that muscle mass does. Congestive heart failure occurs when the heart can no longer pump against the increasing resistance. Angina pectoris, the characteristic pain resulting from cardiac ischemia, may occur. Other complications include arteriosclerotic vessel changes, cerebral hemorrhage, cerebral encephalopathy, renal damage, papilledema (swelling of the optic disk), and other retinal changes. The arteriosclerotic process results in thickening of the vessel walls and replacement of smooth muscle and elastic tissue with fibrous tissue. As a result the vessel becomes more rigid. The vessel itself is weakened by this process and tends to rupture more easily (Fig. 9-12). The organ damage that occurs, causing the complications of hypertension, is the result of hemorrhages within the various organs affected. The incidence and severity of the complications increase with the duration and severity of the hypertension.

The cause of essential hypertension is unknown; however, many factors are thought to be related to its development. Genetic factors are indicated because of observed familial, sexual, and racial predispositions. The incidence of hypertension among blacks is approximately double that found in the white population. Women have been found to tolerate hypertension better. Age is a factor in that age-related vessel changes may contribute to the hypertensive process. The cause of the persistent increased peripheral resistance is also thought to be multifactorial, with the following mechanisms postulated as having possible contributory roles: (1) increased sympathetic stimulation; (2) abnormal Na^+ metabolism leading to increased Na^+ and H_2O retention and expansion of extracellular volume (the arterial walls of some hypertensive patients have been found to have an abnormally high Na^+ content); (3) excessive renin secretion and generation of angiotensin II, a potent vasoconstrictor (hyperplasia of the juxtaglomerular cells has been found in severe hypertension); (4) excessive arterial responses; and (5) possible humoral vasoconstrictive substances.

Physiology of treatment. The goals of treatment include

1. Reduction of the elevated blood pressure and maintenance of normal blood pressure levels
2. Prevention of complications of both the treatment and the disease process

Treatment depends on the degree of hypertension. Mild hypertension is defined as a diastolic

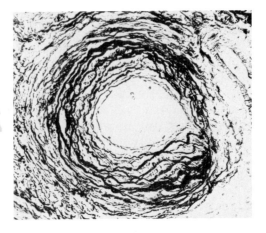

Fig. 9-12. Elastosis in branch of renal artery from case of essential hypertension. (From Anderson, W. A. D., and Kissane, J. M.: Pathology, ed. 7, St. Louis, 1977, The C. V. Mosby Co.)

pressure of 90 to 109 mm Hg and is treated by a low-sodium diet and a diuretic drug. Moderate hypertension is defined as a diastolic pressure of 109 to 129 mm Hg and is treated by a diuretic drug in combination with a milder antihypertensive drug. Severe hypertension is defined as a diastolic pressure over 130 mm Hg and is treated by a diuretic drug and a combination of antihypertensive drugs.

Physiologically the disease process can be managed by a combination of diet, diuretic, and antihypertensive drugs. The low-sodium diet and the use of diuretic drugs promotes the excretion of fluid from the body. This helps to lower blood pressure because venous return and consequently cardiac output are reduced. Antihypertensive drugs block sympathetic innervation and thus prevent or reduce vasoconstriction in decreasing peripheral resistance. Sedation may also be helpful in terms of reducing the level of sympathetic stimulation.

The greatest problem in management of the disease process lies in patient compliance with the treatment regimen. The patient must realize that there is no cure for high blood pressure. At best it is controlled. The problem is that once the patient begins to feel better and no longer can identify the effects of the disease process, he stops taking the prescribed medication. Careful teaching about the side effects of the medication he is receiving and about the disease process will allow the patient to actively participate in his care.

The peripheral vascular diseases are a group of diseases in which vessel patency and thus flow are disrupted. The peripheral circulation may be disrupted by disease processes outside of the vascular system, as well as by those disease processes primarily considered vascular in origin. Diseases such as diabetes, lupus erythematosus, and endocrine disorders may involve the peripheral vasculature.

Arterial disorders may be the result of two basic mechanisms: obstruction and generalized constriction or dilation of the vessels. Exposure to freezing temperatures may also impair arterial circulation through the mechanisms of vasoconstriction and thrombosis (see Chapter 6).

The absence of palpable pulses, coldness to the touch, a chalk-white pallor alternating with cyanosis, anesthesia or paresthesia, and collapse of superficial veins in the affected extremity are manifestations of an occlusive process. These signs and symptoms will appear suddenly if an embolism is the cause. Complete occlusion, which is the result of a progressive thrombotic phenomenon, may be preceded by intermittent claudication or pain in the legs with exercise. The skin becomes extremely vulnerable to even minor trauma, as healing will be impaired due to the lack of nutrient and oxygen supply.

Venous disorders may be the result of obstructive or nonobstructive processes. The condition of varicose veins falls into the latter category. The manifestations of venous obstruction depend on how deep the affected vein lies. Thrombosis of a superficial vein may be observed as a red streak that is tender and palpable. Thrombosis of the deeper veins usually results in swelling of the extremity. The danger of venous thrombosis is that it can dislodge and migrate to a vital organ, causing occlusion of its blood supply.

Varicose veins are tortuous, palpable, distended veins that are usually observable in the lower extremities. An increase in the venous pressure of the lower extremities as a result of nonvascular conditions (pregnancy, a job that requires sitting or standing with the legs in a dependent position for long periods of time) may cause the initial distension and pooling of blood. As veins are stretched, further pooling results, and the valves become incompetent. A vicious cycle is set up that perpetuates the development and progression of varicosities. Dependent edema will form as pressure increases. Pain may be intense and is usually relieved by elevating the affected extremity. The pain is usually of a dull, achy character.

Varicose veins and chronic venous insufficiency (the sequela of obstruction and the resultant valvular incompetence) may both result in serious damage to the skin and soft tissue. Venous insufficiency is characterized by hyperpigmentation and brown indurated skin. Venous stasis or pooling of venous blood occurs in both disorders and can lead to progressive edema and hypersensitivity, or *stasis dermatitis*. Itching and scratching may cause an infectious process to develop, and the subsequent inflammatory response may result in extensive interstitial fibrosis and cellulitis. Ulceration may be the sequela to even the most minor trauma (Fig. 9-13).

Reduced vessel patency and flow: occlusive processes

Flow through a vessel depends on the force with which it is propelled and the size and integrity of the lumen it is passing through. Various occlusive disorders serve to reduce the lumen diameter. These include arteriosclerosis, atherosclerosis, thrombus formation, and embolism. When vessel flow is obstructed, signs of insufficiency depend on the vessel system in which the alteration took place. Obstruction of the flow of arterial blood with its resulting hypoxia has two possible effects: creation of a state of *ischemia* or actual *infarction* of tissue. Ischemia refers to a state of tissue hypoxia that is reversible when oxygen is again supplied to the tissues. Infarction refers to cell death or necrosis that occurs as a result of oxygen lack.

Arteriosclerosis refers to a thickening and hardening of the arteries. Muscles and elastic tissue are replaced with fibrous tissue. Calcification may occur. The ability of the arteries to change the lumen size is reduced. Atherosclerosis refers to a process in which there is deposi-

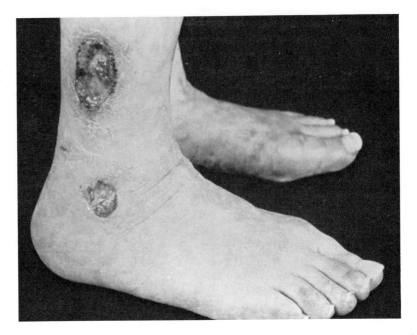

Fig. 9-13. Ulcer formation in patient with venous insufficiency. (From Beyers, M., and Dudas, S.: The clinical practice of medical surgical nursing, Boston, 1977, Little, Brown & Co.)

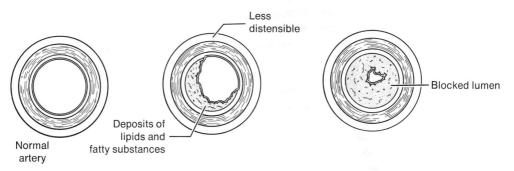

Fig. 9-14. Atherosclerotic vessel changes.

tion of lipids and possibly fibrin in the intimal linings of the arteries. Subsequent calcification may also occur. This makes the arteries less distensible and physically occludes the lumen. ''Atherosclerotic plaques'' in these arteries often give rise to thrombus formation (Figs. 9-14 to 9-16).

A thrombus is an abnormal clot that develops in and is attached to a blood vessel. An embolus is a clot that has broken loose and is circulating throughout the vascular system. The danger from an embolus is that it can lodge in the vascular beds of vital organs, occluding blood flow and possibly causing infarction. Thrombus for-

mation is enhanced in the presence of a roughened endothelial surface of a vessel. The rough surface serves to activate the clotting process. Inflammation of the vessel lining can cause clotting. Stasis of the blood flow also predisposes to thrombus formation as red blood cells settle out of solution and become ''sludged.'' Products of metabolism also accumulate to a greater degree in the presence of stasis of the blood flow, and the presence of these substances causes agglutination of blood cells. Thrombus and embolism formation are discussed more completely in Chapters 5 and 17. Embolization may also be the result of other

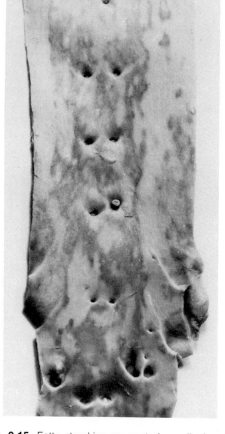

Fig. 9-15. Fatty streaking on posterior wall of aorta from boy aged 11. (From Anderson, W. A. D., and Kissane, J. M.: Pathology, ed. 7, St. Louis, 1977, The C. V. Mosby Co.)

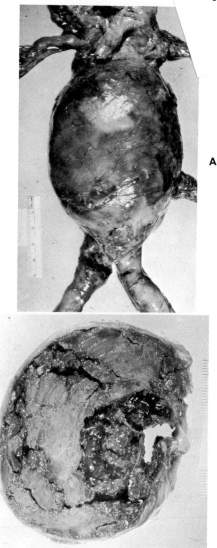

Fig. 9-16. A, Fusiform atherosclerotic aneurysm occupying infrarenal segment of abdominal aorta. **B,** Cross section of aneurysm, showing its lumen mostly occupied by laminated thrombus, but a small blood channel is preserved. (From Anderson, W. A. D., and Kissane, J. M.: Pathology, ed. 7, St. Louis, 1977, The C. V. Mosby Co.)

foreign material circulating in the bloodstream in addition to a loose thrombus. Air, bacteria, fat globules, and amniotic fluid may all have the same effects as a dislodged thrombus. Air introduced into the arterial system may be fatal if it reaches the heart or the cerebral circulation. Clumps of bacteria sometimes become dislodged from the primary site of infection. This sometimes is a complication of subacute bacterial endocarditis, in which vegetative colonies of bacteria grow on the valve cusps and are constantly subjected to the flow of blood and the movement of the valves. Amniotic fluid can be introduced into the maternal circulation via the placental circulation. This can occur during the labor and delivery period in normal childbirth but is usually seen only in the presence of obstetric complications.

After severe trauma, usually involving multiple skeletal fractures, a syndrome known as *fat embolism syndrome* may develop. The presence of these microscopic fat emboli is not completely understood, but two theories have been advanced in an attempt to explain this phenomenon. The metabolic theory asserts that fat globules, formed at the time of the injury, combine with platelets to form emboli. The mechanical theory asserts that fat globules are released from the marrow of the injured bones and enter the vascular system through damaged vessels at the injury site. The fat emboli travel throughout the body, resulting in the appearance of signs and symptoms within a few hours to days after the original injury. The real danger of fat emboli is their effect in the pulmonary vascular bed, where they lodge in capillaries, blocking perfusion and causing an interstitial pneumonitis to develop. Gaseous exchange at the alveolocapillary membrane is impaired, and a ventilation-perfusion abnormality develops (see Chapter 8). Adult respiratory distress syndrome (ARDS) may develop as the interstitial damage worsens.

Most of the clinical manifestations are related to the effects on the respiratory system and the resulting hypoxia. Restlessness and disorientation may be the first signs to appear. The significance of these and other subtle signs and symptoms, such as tachycardia, a temperature elevation, or a feeling of uneasiness or anxiety expressed by the patient, may easily be missed. The presence of dyspnea, wheezing, and rales indicates more extreme respiratory distress. Petechiae may appear on the anterior trunk and axillae and on the soft palate and conjunctiva. These petechiae are thought to be the result of either thrombocytopenia or involvement of the dermal vessels, although the reason for the particular localization is unknown.

Coronary artery disease: a model of occlusion. Atherosclerosis causes 90% of all cases of coronary artery disease (Figs. 9-17 and 9-18) or ischemic heart disease. It occurs six times more frequently in white men than in white women.

Various factors that predispose a person to coronary artery disease have been identified. Presence of these conditions indicates that an individual is at risk for the development of coronary artery disease. These risk factors include family history of cardiovascular disease, a sedentary, stressful occupation, obesity,

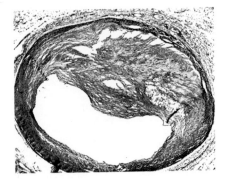

Fig. 9-17. Atherosclerosis of small branch of anterior descending coronary artery. Patient, 47-year-old woman, died of myocardial infarction. (From Anderson, W. A. D., and Kissane, J. M.: Pathology, ed. 7, St. Louis, 1977, The C. V. Mosby Co.)

smoking, hypertension, and the presence of various metabolic influences such as diabetes, increased amounts of circulating catecholamines, increased levels of blood cholesterol, and hyperlipidemia.

The progression of the disease and manifestation of complications depends on the portion of the coronary circulation that is obstructed and the degree of the obstruction. The mildest complication is myocardial ischemia, which is manifested by chest pain of a fairly typical nature, angina pectoris. Anginal pain can also occur in any condition that can cause myocardial ischemia. Typically angina is triggered by exercise, cold, or anything that increases the work of the heart and consequently myocardial oxygen utilization. The pain is described as a heaviness or fullness, sharp and stabbing. It usually radiates down the left arm from the chest and intrascapular regions. It goes away spontaneously with rest, usually after 2 to 3 minutes or at the maximum 10 minutes. It frightens the patient so that he stops what he is doing.

Treatment of angina pectoris involves avoidance of precipitating factors, rest, and the use of vasodilating drugs, which increase blood flow to the myocardium. The patient is counseled to stop smoking since nicotine is a vasoconstrictor. He will also be counseled in the prophylactic use of vasodilator drugs prior to performing some physically stressful activity.

Myocardial infarction (Figs. 9-19 and 9-20)

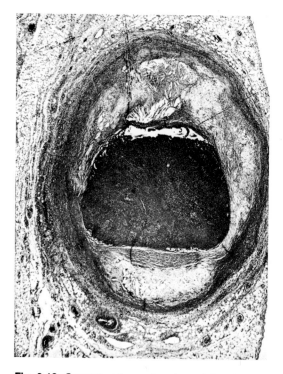

Fig. 9-18. Coronary atherosclerosis and thrombosis. Intima irregularly thickened and media thinned because of advanced atheromatosis. (From Anderson, W. A. D., and Kissane, J. M.: Pathology, ed. 7, St. Louis, 1977, The C. V. Mosby Co.)

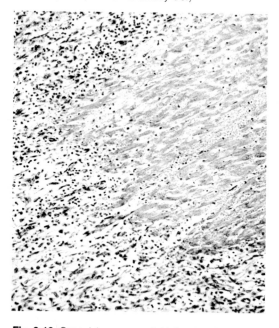

Fig. 9-19. Organizing myocardial infarction. (From Anderson, W. A. D., and Kissane, J. M.: Pathology, ed. 7, St. Louis, 1977, The C. V. Mosby Co.)

is a more severe complication of coronary artery disease. It indicates a severe occlusion, either partial or complete, resulting in tissue necrosis of the myocardium.

A severe, crushing pain that radiates through the chest, to the neck and jaw, down the left arm, and sometimes even to the right arm is the classic type of chest pain. It is not relieved by rest and is accompanied by other symptoms such as nausea, sweating, tachycardia, a drop in blood pressure, and dyspnea. When tissue becomes damaged, cellular substances are released into the blood. When cardiac cells are damaged, enzymes are released into the blood and can be used to make a diagnosis. Table 9-3 summarizes the serum enzymes and their typical responses in myocardial infarction and in other diseases. Changes in the electrocardiogram can also help in the diagnosis of myocardial infarction as electrical activity is altered in the presence of tissue damage.

Complications that can occur include cardiogenic shock, arrhythmias, heart failure, embolism, ventricular aneurysm, and ventricular rupture. Additionally postmyocardial infarction syndrome may occur. This syndrome is characterized by increased white blood cell count and fever and is self-limiting. The shoulder-hand syndrome, which is characterized by aching pain in the left arm and shoulder, may also occur. This is sometimes treated with cortisone to reduce the inflammation.

The treatment goals of acute myocardial infarction include

1. Relief of pain
2. Promotion of oxygenation of the tissues
3. Prevention of further occlusion and improvement of coronary circulation
4. Prevention of complications

Analgesic drugs such as meperidine hydrochloride (Demerol) or morphine sulfate are administered for relief of pain. Anticoagulant therapy is begun to decrease the tendency to develop thromboembolism. Supplemental oxygen is administered to improve tissue oxygenation, especially of the myocardium. With improved oxygenation of the body tissues, the cardiac work load is decreased.

Activity levels should be kept at a minimum to allow the myocardium to rest. Gradual return

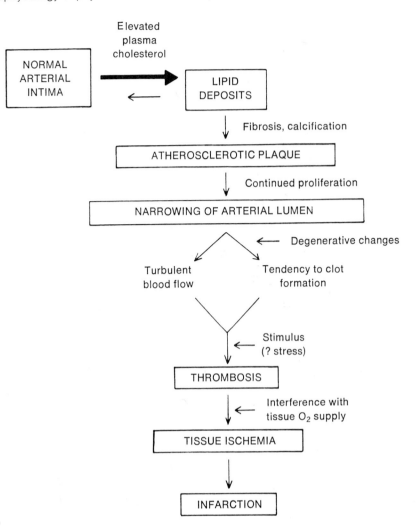

Fig. 9-20. Mechanism producing atherosclerosis and tissue infarction. (From Montgomery, R., Dryer, R. L., Conway, T. W., and Spector, A. A.: Biochemistry: a case-oriented approach, ed. 2, St. Louis, 1977, The C. V. Mosby Co.)

to complete levels of activity promotes the regenerative processes. Rehabilitation programs designed to increase activity and exercise tolerance in carefully measured gradients are structured according to the stage of cardiac tissue regeneration that can be expected at given time frames within the convalescent period.

ALTERATIONS IN OXYGEN-CARRYING CAPACITY

Oxygen-carrying capacity refers to the blood's ability to bind with oxygen. Since the greatest amount of oxygen is transported in chemical combination with hemoglobin in the erythrocyte, the oxygen-carrying capacity is altered in any condition that affects the red blood cells or hemoglobin. These include changes in the volume and in the physical and chemical characteristics of the red blood cells and the hemoglobin molecules.

Anemia

Classification and etiology. Anemia is defined as a significant decrease in the red blood cell or hemoglobin concentration in the circulating blood. This is detected through measurement of the hemoglobin concentration and the relative concentration of the solid constituents

Table 9-3. Enzymes in myocardial infarction*

Enzyme	Normal value per milliliter †	Elevation in myocardial infarction	Elevation in other diseases
SGOT (serum glutamic-oxaloacetic transaminase)	12 to 40 units	Occurs about 6 hours after infarction; in 24 to 48 hours reaches peak that is 2 to 15 times normal value; usually returns to normal after 3 to 4 days	Occurs in acute pericarditis, congestive heart failure, coronary insufficiency, and hepatocellular disease
LDH (serum lactic dehydrogenase)	150 to 300 units	Occurs 6 to 12 hours after infarction; in 48 to 72 hours reaches a peak that is two to eight times normal; usually returns to normal 5 to 6 days later, but may persist to tenth day	Occurs in variety of muscle, renal, neoplastic, hepatic, and hemolytic diseases as well as in number of pulmonary conditions simulating myocardial infarction
SHBD (serum alpha-hydroxy-butyrate dehydrogenase)	50 to 250 units	Increases within 12 hours after acute MI; reaches peak values of four or five times normal after 48 to 72 hours; remains abnormal for 1 to 3 weeks	Elevated in liver disease, megaloblastic anemia, other blood dyscrasias, and hemolysis
CPK (creatine phosphokinase)	6 to 30 units	Increases within 2 to 5 hours after acute MI; peak value during first 24 hours; 5 to 15 times normal; returns to normal by second or third day	Elevated in muscle disease, brain damage, and hypothyroidism

*From Andreoli, K., Hunn, V. K., Zipes, D. P., and Wallace, A. G.: Comprehensive cardiac care, ed. 3, St. Louis, 1975, The C. V. Mosby Co.
†May vary with different laboratory determinations.

of the blood. The latter measurement is called the *hematocrit*. There are three types of functional disturbances that lead to anemia:

1. Proliferative disorders, in which production of red blood cells is decreased
2. Maturational disorders with ineffective erythropoiesis
3. Increased red blood cell breakdown or loss

Hypoproliferative anemias can be the result of bone marrow failure, reduced production of erythropoietin, or iron deficiency. Bone marrow failure can result from the effects of myelotoxic drugs or the replacement of marrow with malignant cells. Depressed erythropoietin production accompanies chronic renal disease and certain endocrine disorders.

Erythropoiesis becomes self-limiting in the presence of reduced amounts of iron. The primary defect in the anemia that accompanies inflammation is a decreased supply of iron to the bone marrow due to a block in release of iron by the reticuloendothelial cells. Another factor in this type of anemia is moderately increased destruction of red blood cells, which is sometimes accompanied by fragmentation due to vasculitis or intravascular clotting. There is also thought to be a relative decrease in the amount of erythropoietin available.

Other iron deficiency anemias are the result of depleted iron stores. The sequence in which an iron deficiency occurs involves first the depletion of body stores accompanied by normal hemoglobin and hematocrit levels. When there is no longer an adequate amount of iron for hemoglobin synthesis, the hemoglobin and hematocrit levels drop. Dietary intake of iron may be insufficient during periods of increased need such as pregnancy and infancy, and dietary supplements become necessary during this time. Iron deficiency anemias can be the result of physiologic losses such as menstruation or pathologic losses such as hemorrhage. They can also be the result of malabsorption states such as sprue or postgastrectomy.

Anemias due to maturational disorders are

characterized by normal marrow proliferation not accompanied by a corresponding increase in the concentration of the reticulocytes. This indicates destruction of the red cells due to some abnormality. There are two types of disorders in this category, and they are differentiated by the changes in the red blood cell and hemoglobin that occur. Macrocytic anemias include those in which there is some defect in the nucleus of the maturing red cell. The ratio of cellular DNA to RNA is reduced due to enzymatic abnormalities in the pathway of DNA synthesis, which in turn are due to deficiency of either vitamin B_{12} or folic acid. A deficiency of vitamin B_{12} is usually not dietary in origin but the result of a disorder in its absorption because of either a lack of the intrinsic factor (pernicious anemia) or disease of the terminal ileum where absorption usually occurs.

Folic acid deficiency may be the result of a dietary deficiency, increased need (pregnancy or infection), or some interference with folate metabolism. Drugs, especially alcohol, are usually responsible for the latter.

Hypochromic microcytic anemias reflect some defect in hemoglobin synthesis. Genetically transmitted hemoglobinopathies are included in this group. In the thalassemia and sickle cell disorders the defect is in the globin portion of the hemoglobin molecule. Abnormal porphyrin synthesis results in defects in the heme portion of the hemoglobin molecule.

The hemolytic anemias are characterized by increased destruction of red blood cells. This destruction may be due to abnormal phagocytic activity or increased fragmentation, intravascular lysis, or increased breakdown in the tissues. This classification includes the anemias that occur as a result of increased splenic activity and also those that occur in conjunction with the autoimmune and complement-immune disease.

Clinical manifestations. The signs and symptoms of anemia are those of oxygen lack and hypoxia of the tissues: easy fatigability, weakness, dyspnea, pallor, syncope, headache, insomnia, and palpitations. Pallor is observable in the conjunctivae, nail beds, and oral mucosa. In the elderly, local vascular disease may sensitize certain tissues to the effects of anemia. In the presence of preexisting coronary

artery disease, anemia may precipitate heart failure or angina. In the presence of central nervous system vascular disease, anemia may produce disturbances in mentation and orthostatic hypotension (a drop in blood pressure when going from a lying to a standing position).

Alterations in hemoglobin affinity

Fig. 9-5 illustrates the normal oxyhemoglobin dissociation curve and the effect of pH changes on this curve. Table 9-4 lists various conditions associated with alterations in the af-

Table 9-4. Conditions associated with alterations of O_2-Hb affinity (O_2 = Hb dissociation curve)*

Shift to left	Shift to right
Increased pH	Decreased pH
Decreased P_{CO_2}	Increased P_{CO_2}
Decreased temperature	Increased temperature
Decreased 2,3-DPG	Increased 2,3-DPG
Decreased pH	Increased pH
Stored blood	Hypoxemia
Increased ADP	Anemia
Phosphate depletion	Phosphate retention
Red cell pyruvate kinase excess	Red cell pyruvate kinase deficiency
Red cell hexokinase deficiency	
Chemical inhibition of glycolysis (e.g., monoiodoacetate)	
Decreased 2,3-DPG binding to Hb	
Fetal hemoglobin	
Diabetes mellitus	

Abnormal hereditary hemoglobins

Hb Ranier	Hb Kansas
Hb Barts	Hb Seattle
Hb H	Hb S
Hb Yakima	
Hb J Capetown	
Hb Chesapeake	
Hb Kempsey	
Hb Hiroshima	
Hb Little Rock	

Abnormal acquired hemoglobins

Carboxyhemoglobin
Methemoglobin

*Adapted from Frohlich, E. D.: Pathophysiology: altered regulatory mechanisms in disease, ed. 2, Philadelphia, 1972, J. B. Lippincott Co.

finity of hemoglobin for oxygen. A shift to the right of the curve indicates a decreased affinity of hemoglobin for oxygen. A shift to the left of the curve indicates an increased affinity of hemoglobin for oxygen. The Bohr effect (the effect of pH on hemoglobin affinity) serves to promote the uptake of oxygen in the lung and to promote the release of oxygen in the tissue, where pH is relatively low. It is obvious from the curve that acid-base imbalance may compromise normal oxygen uptake and release.

Polycythemia

Absolute polycythemia is defined as an increase in the number of red blood cells. Polycythemia is determined by an increase in the hematocrit. Absolute polycythemia represents a normal compensatory response to hypoxia, or it can be the result of some disorder in the regulation of erythropoiesis. An elevated hematocrit can also be the result of a decrease in plasma volume; this is called relative polycythemia. Relative polycythemia can occur as a result of the frank loss of plasma fluid as in burns or a shift in fluid from the intravascular to the interstitial space. Clinically polycythemia is significant in that it increases the blood viscosity, which predisposes the patient to intravascular clot formation (see Chapter 5). Polycythemia as a response to chronic hypoxia is discussed in Chapter 7. An example of polycythemia in response to chronic hypoxia is that seen in the emphysemic patient.

SUMMARY

This chapter has presented an overview of the various pathophysiologic mechanisms by which oxygen transport to the body tissues may be disrupted. In many instances these mechanisms can be compensated for during acute episodes as a direct result of medical and nursing intervention. It is therefore important to understand the physiologic basis of restoring normal function as these disease processes may represent a grave threat to the patient's survival.

SUGGESTED READINGS

Adams, C.: Recognition and evaluation of cardiogenic shock, Heart Lung 2:893-895, 1973.

Ahanies, H. M.: Noncardiogenic pulmonary edema, Med. Clin. North Am. 61(6):1319-1337, 1977.

Artz, C. P.: Shock and trauma, Postgrad. Med. 48:81-210, 1970.

Beirman, E. L.: Fat metabolism, atherosclerosis, and aging in man: a review, Mech. Ageing Dev. 2:315, 1973.

Benditt, E.: The origin of atherosclerosis, Sci. Am. 236 (6):74, 1975.

Ditzel, J.: Impaired oxygen transport in diabetes, Metab. Ther. 6(4):1-4, 1977.

Gulford, M.: Medical management of angina pectoris, Primary Cardiology, pp. 29-31, Aug. 1975.

Hultgren, H. M.: Medical management of unstable angina, Practical Cardiology, pp. 29-32, fall 1975.

Kottke, B., and Subbiah, M.: Pathogenesis of atherosclerosis. Concepts based on animal models, Mayo. Clin. Proc. 53:35-48, 1978.

McFarland, M. M.: Fat embolism syndrome, Am. J. Nurs. 76(12):1942-1944, 1976.

McLaughlin, J. S.: Physiologic consideration of hypoxemia in shock and trauma, Ann. Surg. 173:667-677, 1971.

Matsumoto, T., and Hayes, M.: Septic shock—what to do and when, Consultant 13:163-165, 1973.

Papahadjopoulas, D.: Cholesterol and cell membrane function. A hypothesis concerning etiology of atherosclerosis, J. Theor. Biol. 43:329, 1974.

Perutz, M. F.: The hemoglobin molecule, Sci. Am. 211: 64-76, 1964.

Raab, W.: Pleuricausal pathogenesis and preventability of ischemic heart disease, Dis. Chest 53(5):629-631, 1968.

Reid, J. M., et al.: Plasma noradrenalin and hypertension Postgrad. Med. 53(suppl. 3):40-42, 1977.

Ross, R., et al.: A platelet dependent serum factor that stimulates the proliferation of arterial smooth muscle cells in vitro, Proc. Natl. Acad. Sci. U.S.A. 7(4):1207-1210, 1974.

Ross, R. M., and Glomset, J. M.: Atherosclerosis and arterial smooth muscle cell, Science 180:1331, 1973.

Sacksteder, S., et al.: Common congenital cardiac defects, Am. J. Nurs. 78(2): 266-272, 1978.

Subbiah, M.: Prostaglandins and the arterial wall: an avenue for research in the pathogenesis of atherosclerosis, Mayo Clin. Proc. 53(1), 1978.

Warren, J. C.: Surgical pathology and therapeutics, Philadelphia, 1895, W. B. Saunders Co.

Weil, M., et al.: Colloid osmotic pressure and pulmonary edema, Chest 72(6):692-693, 1977.

Wright, I.: Thromboembolism and the aged heart, Primary Cardiology, pp. 20-22, Oct. 1975.

CHAPTER 10

Mechanisms of chemical disequilibrium

AT THE COMPLETION OF THIS CHAPTER THE STUDENT WILL BE ABLE TO:

- Explain the pathophysiologic mechanisms of chemical disequilibrium in terms of the disruption of fluid, electrolyte, and acid-base balance and the resultant compensatory mechanisms.
- Identify factors and conditions that may precipitate fluid, electrolyte, and acid-base imbalance.
- Describe the clinical manifestations of fluid, electrolyte, and acid-base imbalance.
- Describe the effects of fluid, electrolyte, and acid-base imbalance on various systems and organs of the body.
- Relate principles of fluid, electrolyte, and acid-base balance to therapeutic measures designed to correct the pathophysiologic state.

The chemical equilibrium achieved through fluid, electrolyte, and acid-base balance within the body is fundamental to the maintenance of homeostasis. This chemical equilibrium is reflected in the normal volume, distribution, composition, and pH of the body fluid. The body fluid constitutes both the external and internal environments of the cell and as such serves many important functions. It serves as the medium for transport of substances to and from the cell and across its membrane. It also serves as the medium in which most metabolic reactions occur, as well as being a necessity for these reactions to occur at all since chemicals must come into contact within a solution to react with one another. The body fluid provides lubrication for moving body parts and assists in heat regulation through evaporation of perspiration. Alterations in the composition, volume, distribution, or pH of the body fluid will disrupt homeostasis and impair cellular function.

CHARACTERISTICS OF BODY FLUID
Composition

The body fluid is composed of water with various substances in solution (solutes). These solutes are of two major types: electrolytes and nonelectrolytes. Nonelectrolytes are substances that do not dissociate in solution but remain intact and uncharged, for example, dextrose, urea, and creatinine. Electrolytes are substances that dissociate and that carry an electric charge. These charged particles are called *ions* and in solution will conduct an electric current. An ion carrying a positive charge is called a *cation*, and an ion carrying a negative charge is called an *anion*. Chemical-combining activity is dependent on the relative concentrations of anions and cations, which are measured using milliequivalents per liter of solution.

The major body electrolytes are sodium, potassium, calcium, and chloride. Other electrolytes found in the body fluid include magnesium, phosphorate, sulfate, bicarbonate, and other trace elements such as zinc.

Regulation. Regulation of electrolyte levels is normally provided by the kidneys (which excrete excesses) and hormones. Hormones of the adrenal cortex (aldosterone, cortisone) promote reabsorption of sodium and chloride and increase excretion of potassium, calcium, and magnesium. The parathyroid hormone functions in promoting the absorption of calcium in the intestine and the movement of calcium

Table 10-1. Normal concentrations and functions of the major body electrolytes

Electrolyte	Serum concentration	Functions
Sodium (Na)	137-142 mEq/liter in plasma	Retention of fluid in body Generation and transmission of nerve impulses Maintenance of acid-base balance Replacement of potassium in cell Enzyme activities Regulation of osmolarity and electroneutrality of cell
Potassium (K)	3.5-4.5 mEq/liter in plasma	Maintenance of regular cardiac rhythm Deposition of glycogen in liver cells Function of enzyme systems necessary for cell energy production Transmission and conduction of nerve impulses Regulation of osmolarity and electroneutrality of cell
Calcium (Ca)	5 mEq/liter in plasma	Formation of bone and teeth (calcium phosphate) Transmission of nerve impulse Muscular contraction Clotting of blood Maintenance of cell membrane permeability
Chloride (Cl)	97-103 mEq/liter in plasma	Transport of CO_2 (chloride shift) Formation of hydrochloric acid in stomach Retention of potassium Maintenance of osmolarity of cell

from bone cells. The latter action is accomplished through synergistic action with a metabolite of vitamin D and is activated by low serum calcium levels. Parathyroid hormone also decreases renal reabsorption of phosphate by the kidney tubules. Thyrocalcitonin is a hormone secreted by the thyroid, which acts synergistically with phosphate to inhibit movement of calcium from bone to blood. This is stimulated by high levels of serum calcium.

The three sources of body water are fluids, solid food, and the water released from oxidation of foodstuffs. To maintain overall fluid balance, intake should approximately equal output. The box (see opposite column) summarizes the average amounts of fluid intake and output for a 24-hour period.

If all intake stops, the body still continues to lose water. This is called _obligatory loss_. This loss occurs through the lungs, skin, and urine; the amount of loss for a 24-hour period is given in the box below.

Intake	
Fluids	1,500 ml
Solid food	800 ml
Water of oxidation	300 ml
TOTAL	2,600 ml

Output	
Urine	1,500 ml
Perspiration	600 ml
Lungs (vapor) (insensible)	400 ml
Feces	100 ml
TOTAL	2,600 ml

Obligatory loss	
Lungs	500 ml
Skin	500 ml
Urine	500 ml
TOTAL	1,500 ml

Regulation of the total amount of water in the body is the result of the action of two hormones: antidiuretic hormone (ADH) and aldosterone. ADH increases the permeability of the distal and collecting tubules of the kidneys to water, which results in the reabsorption of water. The posterior pituitary gland releases ADH in response to impulses from osmoreceptors in the

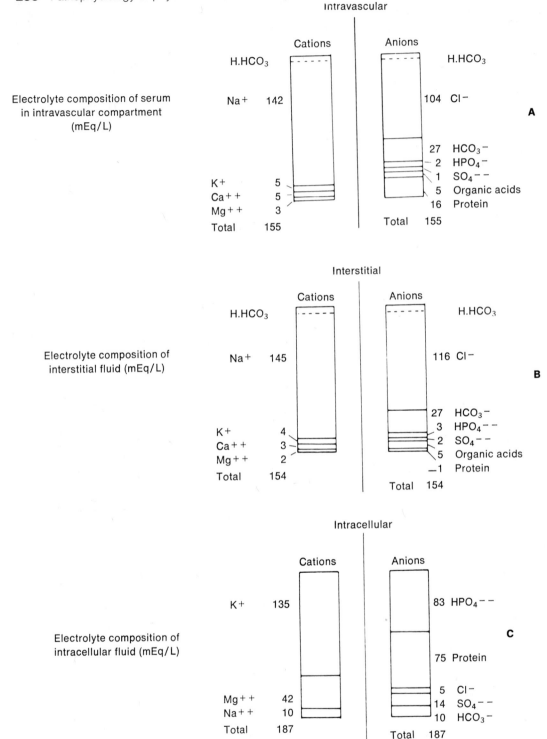

Fig. 10-1. A, Electrolyte composition of serum in intravascular compartment (mEq per liter); **B,** electrolyte composition in interstitial fluid (mEq per liter); **C,** electrolyte composition of intracellular fluid (mEq per liter). (From Weldy, N. J.: Body fluids and electrolytes, ed. 2, St. Louis, 1976, The C. V. Mosby Co.)

hypothalamus. When osmolarity of the body fluid increases, fluid leaves the cells, causing them to shrink, which stimulates the hypothalamus to signal the posterior pituitary gland to release the hormone, and subsequently reabsorption of water by the kidneys occurs. Conversely, when the osmolarity of the body fluid decreases, the osmoreceptor cells swell, which inhibits secretion of ADH, causing the excretion of water through the kidneys.

The volume of extracellular water is also controlled by the adrenocortical hormone, aldosterone, which is secreted in response to decreased renal blood flow and the subsequent activation of the renin-angiotensin system. Aldosterone causes the retention of sodium by the kidneys, and when sodium is retained, water is also retained. Another substance, possibly a hormone, is also thought to participate in extracellular water balance. This substance may be responsible for the observed loss of sodium that sometimes occurs when salt-retaining hormones (e.g., aldosterone) remain elevated for prolonged periods.

Compartmental distribution

Sixty percent of the total body weight in a lean man is fluid. It is not only the quantity but the relative distribution of the body fluid throughout the different compartments that is important in the maintenance of homeostasis. The fluid contained in the intracellular compartment accounts for 40% of the total body weight. The remaining 20% of the total body weight is the fluid contained in the extracellular compartment, which can be further subdivided into the interstitial and intravascular compartments. The interstitial compartment, the body fluid that bathes the tissue cells, is 15% of the total body weight. The intravascular compartment, that portion of the total body fluid contained in the blood, is 5% of the total body weight.

The fluid in each compartment has a distinctive electrolyte pattern. In the intracellular fluid, potassium is the major cation, and phosphate and protein are the major anions. In the extracellular fluid, sodium is the major cation, and chloride is the major anion. Most of the body sodium is outside of the cell, while most

of the body potassium is insid
important difference between
of the intravascular and inter
greater concentration of the a
intravascular fluid. Fig. 10-1
ferences.

The intracellular and extracellular compartments are separated from each other by a cell membrane. Cell membranes are freely permeable to water and selectively permeable to most electrolytes while relatively impermeable to the plasma proteins and other colloids under normal conditions. The movement of water and electrolytes between compartments is accomplished through both active and passive processes. The passive processes include osmosis, diffusion, and filtration.

Concentration of constituents. Osmosis is defined as the diffusion of a solvent through a selectively permeable membrane to an area where the concentration of solutes is relatively greater (Fig. 10-2). Osmotic pressure is the force needed to draw the solvent across the membrane. It is determined by the relative number of particles in solution on either side of the membrane and is sometimes referred to as *pull pressure,* although this term is technically incorrect. The osmolality of the fluid in the intravascular compartment (plasma) is slightly greater than in the other compartments due to the presence of plasma proteins. The osmotic pressure exerted by the plasma proteins is also referred to as *oncotic pressure* and is very important in the maintenance of fluid homeostasis. Once an osmotic gradient is established, water will move from the compartment of low osmolality to the compartment of high osmolality until the osmotic pressures are equalized.

When the osmotic pressure is relatively equal on both sides of the membrane (concentrations of solutes are equal) the solutions are *isosmotic* to one another. They are also considered to be isosmotic if no volume change occurs between them. A solution that contains a lesser concentration of solutes than another solution is *hypotonic* in relation to the other. Water is hypotonic in relation to the body fluids. If a red blood cell is placed in a container of fresh water, water will move into the cell by the pro-

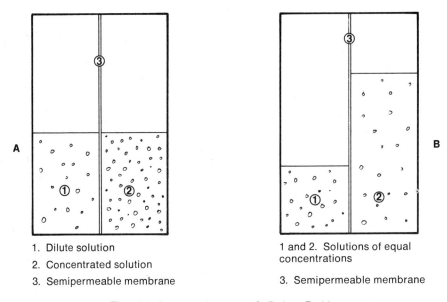

A

1. Dilute solution
2. Concentrated solution
3. Semipermeable membrane

B

1 and 2. Solutions of equal concentrations
3. Semipermeable membrane

Fig. 10-2. Process of osmosis. **A,** Before. **B,** After.

cess of osmosis, causing the cell to swell and diluting the body fluid inside it. Eventually the cell would burst. A solution that has a higher concentration of solutes than another is *hypertonic* in relation to the other. A cell placed in a hypertonic solution would have the water drawn out of it by the process of osmosis, causing it to become crenated (wrinkled and shrunken).

Osmotic forces are the prime determinant of water distribution in the body and depend on the relative permeabilities of solutes on either side of a membrane. In other words, the relative numbers of osmotically active ions in each compartment determine the distribution of fluid between the extracellular and intracellular compartments. For example, sodium ions are partly responsible for extracellular osmolality, while potassium ions are partly responsible for intracellular osmolality. The osmotic activity of these ions is effective because of the Na^+-K^+ pump in the cell membrane, which restricts the movement of these ions between compartments. The activity of this pump appears to be regulated by sodium-potassium-activated ATP (Na-K-ATPase), an enzyme that hydrolyzes ATP into ADP. The released energy is then utilized to actively transport Na^+ out of the cell and K^+ into the cell. The mechanism by which this energy is coupled to the work is

not understood at this time. A solute able to cross the cell membrane freely and reach equal concentrations on either side is ineffective in generating an osmotic pressure and therefore cannot affect fluid distribution, for example, urea. However, when the cell membrane, due to some pathologic process, becomes permeable to a solute to which it is normally impermeable, serious alterations in fluid distribution may occur.

The plasma sodium concentration is considered to be a fairly accurate indicator of the plasma osmolality. Since the body fluids normally exist in a state of osmotic equilibrium, plasma sodium concentrations also reflect the osmolality of the total body water (TBW). This relationship is expressed in the following series of equations:

$$\text{Plasma osmolality} = 2 \times \text{plasma } [Na^+]$$

$$\text{Osmolality of TBW} = \frac{(2\,[Na^+]) + (2\,[K^+])}{\text{TBW}}$$

$$\text{Plasma osmolality} = \text{TBW osmolality}$$

$$\text{Plasma } [Na^+] = \frac{[Na^+] + [K^+]}{\text{TBW}}$$

From these equations it becomes apparent that a low plasma sodium concentration represents a hypo-osmolar (hypotonic) state, while an in-

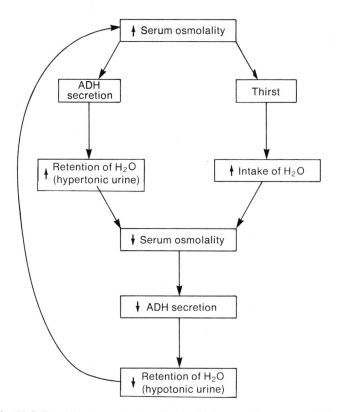

Fig. 10-3. Physiologic mechanisms that maintain normal serum osmolality.

creased plasma sodium concentration represents a hyperosmolar (hypertonic) state. A low serum Na$^+$ concentration (hypo-osmolality) can be the result of either Na$^+$ loss or water retention. Even potassium loss will lower the serum sodium concentration because the loss of K$^+$ from the plasma favors movement of K$^+$ out of the cells into the extracellular fluid. To maintain electroneutrality, Na$^+$ will then move out of the extracellular fluid into the cell. A high serum sodium concentration (hyperosmolality) can be the result of a Na$^+$ gain or water loss. The loss of Na$^+$ and water in isotonic proportions will cause no change in the osmolality or sodium concentration of the plasma. The hematocrit will be elevated, however, reflecting the isotonic volume loss. Plasma osmolality is maintained through variations in water intake and excretion, which are mediated by changes in thirst and ADH secretion. The usual mechanisms by which plasma osmolality is maintained within normal limits are illustrated in Fig. 10-3.

Exchange between compartments. Diffusion is the passive movement of particles from an area of higher concentration to an area of lower concentration, specifically, the movement of permeable solutes and water across the membrane. Permeable solutes and gases diffuse between the intravascular and interstitial fluid at the capillary membrane. The process of diffusion is passive; that is, it requires no energy expenditure by the body. Osmosis has already been referred to as diffusion of water. Water moves from an area of higher concentration of water molecules (solutes will be less concentrated) to an area of lesser concentration of water molecules (solutes will be more concentrated).

Filtration is the process by which water and diffusible substances move out of the solution with the greater hydrostatic pressure when a difference in hydrostatic pressure exists on two sides of a membrane. Filtration results from the interaction of forces that serve to promote net fluid movement across a membrane. In the capillary beds of the body these forces include the hydrostatic pressure, the interstitial fluid pressure, and osmotic pressure. The hydrostatic pressure is the force with which the fluid presses against the vessel wall. It is the result not only of the weight of the blood against the vessel wall but also of the force with which the blood is propelled by the heart. Hydrostatic pressure is higher at the arterial end of the capillary bed than at the venous end. Interstitial fluid pressure is exerted against the outside of the blood vessel wall by the interstitial fluid. Also to be considered is the osmotic force exerted by the plasma proteins, which is called *oncotic pressure*. This is the only effective osmotic pressure in the capillary bed since the capillary membrane, unlike the cell membrane, is freely permeable to Na^+. As a result of the various pressure and concentration differences on either side of the membrane, fluid moves out of the capillary into the interstitium at the arterial end and is reabsorbed carrying cellular waste products into the intravascular compartment at the venous end. The filtration-ab-

sorption relationships (Fig. 10-4) that are a result of these forces were first described by Starling in 1896. Alterations in any of the forces described will result in abnormal filtration-absorption relationships and disrupt this movement of fluid.

Passive diffusion of large polar molecules such as amino acids and sugars would occur slowly if at all. Experimental evidence suggests that the movement of such molecules must occur in some manner requiring special mechanisms built into the cell structure. It is thought that these molecules bind to specific sites on the cell membrane where their movement across the membrane is facilitated. This process is called *mediated transport* and can be further subdivided to include facilitated diffusion and active transport. Facilitated diffusion allows the movement of substances down their concentration gradients much more quickly than could normally be expected. Active transport mechanisms can move substances against their concentration gradients at the expense of cellular energy. Carrier models have been proposed to

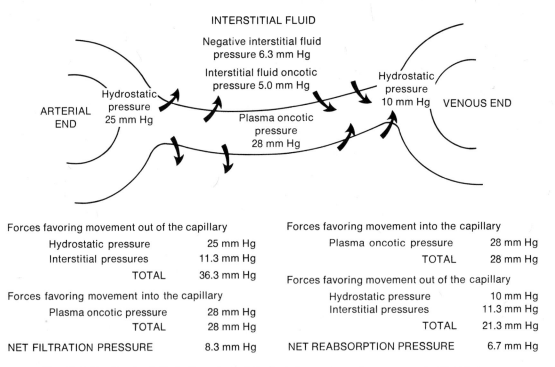

INTERSTITIAL FLUID

Negative interstitial fluid pressure 6.3 mm Hg

Interstitial fluid oncotic pressure 5.0 mm Hg

Hydrostatic pressure 25 mm Hg

ARTERIAL END

Plasma oncotic pressure 28 mm Hg

Hydrostatic pressure 10 mm Hg   VENOUS END

Forces favoring movement out of the capillary	
Hydrostatic pressure	25 mm Hg
Interstitial pressures	11.3 mm Hg
TOTAL	36.3 mm Hg

Forces favoring movement into the capillary	
Plasma oncotic pressure	28 mm Hg
TOTAL	28 mm Hg

NET FILTRATION PRESSURE	8.3 mm Hg

Forces favoring movement into the capillary	
Plasma oncotic pressure	28 mm Hg
TOTAL	28 mm Hg

Forces favoring movement out of the capillary	
Hydrostatic pressure	10 mm Hg
Interstitial pressures	11.3 mm Hg
TOTAL	21.3 mm Hg

NET REABSORPTION PRESSURE	6.7 mm Hg

Fig. 10-4. Capillary bed, illustrating effect of Starling's forces governing movement of fluid between intravascular and interstitial compartments (values shown are arbitrary).

explain both types of mediated transport, but as yet no carrier molecule has been identified. The mechanism by which energy is linked to active transport remains a matter of speculation also.

Hydrogen ion concentration (pH)

The pH is an expression of the relative acidity and alkalinity of the body fluid. More specifically it is the negative logarithm of the hydrogen ion concentration. The pH is arrived at using the Henderson-Hasselbalch equation:

$$pH = pK + \log \frac{BHCO_3}{H_2CO_3 + CO_2}$$

where $pK = 6.1$, $B =$ any cation, $HCO_3 =$ bicarbonate, and $H_2CO_3 + CO_2 =$ carbonic acid and dissolved CO_2. Normal pH should be in the range of 7.35 to 7.45. When the bicarbonate concentration of the blood rises or the carbonic acid concentration falls, the bicarbonate–carbonic acid ratio increases, and the pH becomes greater than 7.45, reflecting a decrease in the hydrogen ion concentration. This state is called *alkalosis*. When bicarbonate concentration of the blood falls or carbonic acid contration increases, the bicarbonate–carbonic acid ratio decreases, and the pH becomes less than 6.35, reflecting an increase in the hydrogen ion concentration. This is called *acidosis*. Cellular metabolism cannot proceed at excessively high or low pH levels. Fig. 10-5 schematically illustrates the normal range of pH and the effects of alterations in the bicarbonate–carbonic acid ratio and thus abnormal pH values. The clinical manifestations of alkalotic and acidotic states are discussed in Chapter 8.

With the constant addition of the products of metabolism, the maintenance of acid-base balance within normal limits is a constant, dynamic process. The body has three mechanisms by which it can maintain acid-base balance: the buffer systems, the respiratory system, and the renal system. The buffer systems function immediately to prevent drastic changes in hydrogen ion concentration. The respiratory system acts within minutes to correct a sudden change, while the kidneys require a longer period of time in which to readjust the pH.

An acid-base buffer is a solution of two or more chemical compounds that prevents excessive changes in the hydrogen ion concentration when either an acid or a base is added to the solution. A buffer system is made up of a weak acid and its conjugate base. The acid component can neutralize a strong base; however, this will not prevent a departure from the

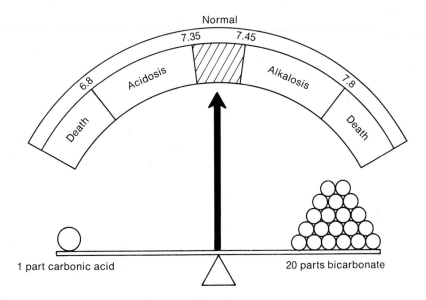

Fig. 10-5. The pH and its relationship to bicarbonate–carbonic acid ratio.

normal acid-base ratio. To illustrate this point, a strong acid added to a buffer system is converted into the weaker buffer acid through interaction with the buffer base, thereby increasing the concentration of the acid component and decreasing the buffer base component. This results in a pH change but not to the extreme that would have occurred in the absence of a buffer system. The pH varies directly with the buffer base component: as the buffer base increases, pH also increases, and as the buffer base decreases, pH also decreases.

There are several buffer systems in the body, but the bicarbonate–carbonic acid buffer system is the most important physiologically. The components of this system can also be regulated by the lungs and kidneys, which ultimately determine the pH status of the blood. The various buffer systems also work together to minimize pH changes: a change in the base-acid ratio of one system will cause a corresponding change in the other systems.

The respiratory system acts as a feedback system with the carbon dioxide concentration. When increased amounts of carbon dioxide are present, the respiratory system becomes more active and ''blows off'' the excess carbon dioxide, making less available to form carbonic acid. When decreased amounts of carbon dioxide are present, the respiratory system becomes less active and retains carbon dioxide, making more available to form carbonic acid.

The kidneys regulate the plasma bicarbonate concentration through excretion of hydrogen ions in the urine and reabsorption of bicarbonate ions. The kidneys normally excrete an acid urine since the products of metabolism are acid. When there is an excess of bicarbonate ions the kidneys will excrete an alkaline urine.

DISRUPTION OF CHEMICAL EQUILIBRIUM

Chemical disequilibrium occurs when the volume, distribution, composition, or pH of the body fluid is altered. These alterations can occur as a result of primary disorders in the intake, excretion, or regulation of the components of the body fluid or secondarily as part of the pathophysiologic response to other disease states impinging on homeostasis. Chemi-cal disequilibrium can also be iatrogenically caused; various treatment modalities have as an inadvertent side effect the loss of fluid, electrolyte, and acid-base equilibrium. Disorders of elimination and its regulation that lead to chemical disequilibrium are discussed in Chapter 11. Disorders of nutrition and the gastrointestinal tract that lead to chemical disequilibrium are discussed in Chapters 12 and 13.

Changes in volume and composition of body fluid

Disruption of homeostasis may be the result of changes in the volume and composition of the body fluid. Of particular importance are volume changes in infants, obese individuals, and aged persons. The fluid volume in the infant represents approximately 75% to 80% of the body weight. Although this amount of fluid is relatively greater than that of the adult, the infant has a proportionally greater surface area and a higher metabolic rate. The combination of these factors creates the potential for much greater insensible fluid losses than in the adult. Thus, the infant is prone to develop serious volume deficits in a relatively short period of time. Other groups that are considered at risk for the development of excessive fluid loss include the obese and the elderly. Fat cells contain relatively smaller amounts of water than do other cells, and the percentage of body weight representing fluid is greatly reduced in the obese individual for that reason. A variety of reasons contribute to the problem of fluid balance in the elderly. First, the total percentage of fluid body weight decreases with age. In persons over 65 years of age only 40% to 50% of the body weight may be in fluids. Other problems of the elderly that may complicate fluid balance include reduced nutritional intake, an impaired sense of thirst, chronic illness, and the use of medications that may alter fluid volume and composition.

Possible alterations in the total amount of fluid present in the body include expansion or depletion of the fluid volume. Not only is assessment of the total amount of fluid lost or gained important but also important is the composition of the fluid itself. Changes in the amount and general composition of the body fluid have the potential for ultimately disrupting the osmolality and pH. As stated earlier in the chapter, components of the body fluid include water and various solutes that can be divided into the general categories of electrolytes and nonelectrolytes. Excess and deficit states of water and the various electrolytes will be discussed individually. The results of disruption of the normal isotonic concentrations of water and electrolytes will be discussed in terms of changes in fluid osmolality.

Water loss. The term *dehydration* has been used to describe loss of pure water from the body fluid; however, it has also been used to describe the syndrome accompanying sodium loss. To avoid confusing the different syndromes, use of the term dehydration will be avoided in this discussion of the various deficit states.

Water depletion can result from reduced intake, excessive loss, or hyperosmolarity of the body fluid. Reduced intake occurs when water is unavailable or intake is restricted for long periods of time, as might occur when a patient is undergoing diagnostic testing or prior to surgical procedures. Intake can also be reduced due to the inability to swallow, when the sense of thirst is impaired, or in persons who are unable to obtain fluid for themselves such as an infant or a comatose or paralyzed person.

Excessive loss of water via the kidneys can result from a decrease in the concentrating ability of the kidneys due to either primary renal disease or a lack of ADH. Secretion of ADH may be inhibited or impaired by injury to the hypothalamus or by intake of ethyl alcohol. Conditions in which altered ADH secretion is a major feature are discussed in detail in Chapter 11. Because of the effect of alcohol on ADH secretion, alcoholics tend to lose greater than normal amounts of body water.

Excessive loss of water can also occur through the lungs, skin, and gastrointestinal tract. The presence of a tracheostomy or a pattern of rapid respiration decreases anatomic dead space and results in expiration of a greater than normal amount of water vapor via the lungs. Fever or a hot, dry environment will increase the loss of water through both the lungs and the skin. Mild diarrhea without a propor-

tional electrolyte loss can result in pure water loss, especially in infants and children.

Rapid ingestion or infusion of large amounts of water will cause water loss from diuresis. Water dilutes the extracellular fluid, causing it to become hypo-osmolar in relation to the intracellular fluid. This condition inhibits secretion of ADH, which causes water diuresis. The liver participates in this response as an osmoreceptor. Water is absorbed from the gastrointestinal tract into the splanchic circulation. When the osmolarity of the blood returning to the liver via the portal vein is low, the liver is stimulated to send afferent impulses via the vagus nerve to the hypothalamus, which responds by causing increased excretion of water via the kidneys.

Excretion of excessive amounts of solutes is accompanied by an obligatory water load. These solutes are osmotically active and draw water into the urine to be excreted. Persons with untreated diabetes mellitus excrete large amounts of glucose in the urine. The obligatory water load that is necessary causes the symptom of polyuria and may precipitate a water deficit. This can also be a serious problem in a patient receiving nasogastric tube feedings, which contain large amounts of substances such as dextrose and various amino acids in a concentrated form. During water loss due to solute excess, the patient may gain weight rather than lose and while the water loss is developing will pass large quantities of urine with a low specific gravity. This is different from water loss due to decreased intake, in which the urinary output decreases as the water loss develops, and weight loss is usually quite acute.

Water excess is also referred to as water intoxication or overhydration. This condition rarely occurs as a result of increased intake but may in the case of psychotic persons who develop compulsive water-drinking habits. It has occurred as a result of "water diets," in which people ingest large amounts of plain water to maintain the sensation of fullness and to squelch the desire to eat. Water excess may occur as a result of excessive secretion of ADH and in conditions in which the kidneys do not excrete water normally. Water excess may also develop as a result of iatrogenic causes. For example, dextrose in water solutions may be administered to oliguric patients to increase their urinary output when the oliguria is due to renal insufficiency. Large amounts of water can be absorbed rectally, and children being treated for congenital megacolon with enemas may develop water excess.

The signs and symptoms of water deficit and excess can be found in Table 10-2. Many of these depend on how rapidly the condition developed. With acute water excess, symptoms appear suddenly and dramatically. Violent behavior may alternate with lethargic behavior. Table 10-2 lists the signs and symptoms that occur with a more slowly developing water excess. Pitting edema is not usually seen with pure water excess, and symptoms do not usually become significant until serum sodium levels drop below 125 mEq per liter. It is important to note that *acute* changes in body weight always reflect changes in body fluid balance.

Sodium. To a great extent the quantity of sodium as the principal cation of the extracellular fluid determines the volume of that compartment. Signs and symptoms associated with excess and deficit states of sodium reflect its role in the regulation of extracellular fluid (ECF) volume. Sodium is osmotically active, and water is drawn along with it. Excess sodium may greatly expand ECF volume, leading to circulatory congestion and pulmonary edema. Severe sodium deficit leads to ECF volume depletion, which may be to such a degree that circulatory collapse and shock occur.

The sodium balance is closely regulated and maintained within normal limits despite wide variations in dietary intake. The routes of sodium loss include the skin, kidneys, and the gastrointestinal tract. When intake is reduced, regulatory mechanisms operate to minimize the loss of sodium from the body through these routes.

With an increase in sodium intake, plasma volume also increases, which leads to an increase in the rate of glomerular filtration. This increases the amount of sodium filtered and suppresses the release of renin. Consequently aldosterone secretion is inhibited, leading to an increased urinary loss of Na^+. A third factor, which is probably a hormone, is also thought to be stimulated; it acts to decrease tubular reabsorption of Na^+. When Na^+ intake is decreased, plasma volume also is decreased, causing a drop in the glomerular filtration rate and

Table 10-2. Signs and symptoms of water imbalance

Water deficit	Water excess
Symptoms	
Thirst	Headache (rare)
Change in urinary output: oliguria except in solute excess where polyuria is seen	Drowsiness
	Weakness
Weakness	Disorientation
Disorientation	Apathy and lethargy
Signs	
Flushed skin	Weight gain
Scant body secretions	Skin warm and moist
Tongue appears dry and fissured	Cramps
Mucous membranes feel "sticky"	Hematocrit may be slightly low but usually is unchanged
Weight loss (except with solute excess)	
"Doughy" texture of skin	Serum sodium concentration is low due to dilution
Increased temperature	
Hematocrit may be slightly elevated	
Serum sodium concentration is high	
Personality changes	
Hallucinations, delirium, manic behavior, convulsions, and coma may develop	

renal blood flow, which stimulates the release of renin and consequently aldosterone secretion. Sodium will be reabsorbed by the kidneys as a result.

The Na^+ concentration of fluid entering the colon from the small bowel is similar to that of plasma, and reabsorption of sodium in the colon can reduce the amount of sodium in the feces to very low levels. In the presence of diarrhea, however, this capacity for reabsorption becomes extremely limited, and the concentration of Na^+ in the diarrheal fluid may approximate that of the plasma. Sweating represents a potential source of great Na^+ loss in the presence of reduced intake. Some sodium will continue to be lost in the sweat in spite of a reduced intake. The mechanisms for reducing the amount of sodium lost are least efficient for sweating (see Chapter 11).

A sodium deficit can be the result of reduced intake or excessive loss. Sodium deficit that is symptomatic is not related to the total exchangeable body sodium but only to the Na^+ of the extracellular fluid. Internal shifts of fluid removing Na^+ from the ECF can produce a serious sodium deficit even when there is an excess amount of total exchangeable Na^+ in the body.

A Na^+ deficit is often associated with a deficit of circulating plasma proteins. The reasons for this are not clearly elucidated, although it is thought to be due to a reduction in the lymphatic and venous return of the ECF. Sodium loss from the ECF causes plasma volume to fall because of the drop in the osmotic pressure of the ECF that occurs. Because of the lowered osmotic pressure, water leaves the ECF for the cells. As the volume of the ECF falls, a concurrent reduction in the plasma volume takes place. When the effective circulating volume becomes so reduced that tissue perfusion does not occur, circulatory failure (shock) ensues. This type of shock will not respond to vasopressor drugs but only to replacement solutions of isotonic or hypertonic saline.

As stated earlier, Na^+ is lost through the skin, gastrointestinal tract, and kidneys; excessive loss of Na^+ can occur through any of these routes in the presence of pathologic conditions. Table 10-3 lists the concentrations of electrolytes in the various gastrointestinal secretions and excretions and in the sweat. Sodium may also be lost from the ECF volume due to sequestration in a nonequilibrating compartment in the body. This occurs in burns, in acute venous obstruction, in inflammatory reactions, in peritonitis, and in small bowel obstruction. Fluid can become trapped in these "third spaces," causing a concomitant loss of Na^+.

Sodium loss via the kidneys may occur as a result of primary disease of the kidneys and their regulation or as a result of drugs that increase the excretion of Na^+ ions. Sodium loss via the kidneys may also occur in the presence of diabetic acidosis. The glucose diuresis that occurs causes Na^+ and other electrolytes to be lost in the urine as well.

Sodium deficit may also be the result of severe hemorrhage, loss of bronchial secretions, or as a result of gastric or intestinal drainage and lavage. A sodium deficit is more likely to develop if a person's dietary intake of sodium is limited. Water excess is more likely to develop with a sodium deficit since the osmotic pressure of the ECF is lower than that of the cells, causing water to flow into the cells. The clinical picture of sodium loss depends on how rapidly

Table 10-3. Electrolyte concentration of body excretions and secretions (mEq/liter)

Source	Sodium	Chloride	Potassium	Bicarbonates
Sweat	15-80	15-80	>5	0
Saliva	20-80	20-40	10-20	20-60
Gastric juice	20-100	20-160	5-10	0
Bile	150-250	40-80	5-10	20-40
Pancreatic juices	120-250	10-60	5-10	80-120
Ileum	129 mean	116 mean	11 mean	29 mean
Cecum	80 mean	48 mean	21 mean	22 mean

Table 10-4. Clinical manifestations of excess and deficit states of major electrolytes

	Excess	Deficit
Sodium	*Hypernatremia* Edema, congestive heart failure, hypertension	*Hyponatremia* Weakness, fatigue, anorexia, nausea and vomiting, ↓ mental activity, hypotension, ↓ kidney function, abdominal cramps, diarrhea
Potassium	*Hyperkalemia* Muscle weakness, nausea, colic, diarrhea, paresthesias, muscle irritability, ↑ T waves in ECG, cardiac arrest due to fibrillation (see Fig. 10-6)	*Hypokalemia* Muscle weakness of *all* muscles, paralytic ileus, abdominal distension, glucose not metabolized, lethargy, apprehension, tachycardia, flat or broad T waves, cardiac arrest (see Fig. 10-6)
Calcium	*Hypercalcemia* Formation of calculi, flank pain, deep thigh pain, ↓ muscle tone in smooth and striated muscle, mental confusion, impaired memory, slurred speech, polyuria	*Hypocalcemia* Convulsions, muscle cramps, tingling of fingertips, ears, nose, or toes, tetany
Chloride	*Hyperchloremia* Few clinical problems	*Hypochloremia* Achlorhydria, ↑ respiratory rate, dyspnea

this deficit develops. When a sodium deficit develops rapidly, shock is more likely to develop, and the clinical picture is one of acute circulatory failure. The signs and symptoms of the excess and deficit states of the major electrolytes are included in Table 10-4.

True sodium excess, meaning an increase in the total exchangeable body sodium, is manifested by edema since an excess of Na^+ is always accompanied by a corresponding excess of water. Serum sodium concentrations do not accurately reflect the total amount of Na^+ in the body. The serum sodium concentration becomes elevated when water is lost in excess of solute and decreases when water is present in excess of solute. The serum Na^+ concentration reflects more accurately the relative concentrations of sodium and water rather than the true amount of Na^+ in the body. Edema is discussed later in this chapter as a manifestation of a compartmental fluid shift.

Potassium. It is difficult to determine the total exchangeable body potassium because it is an intracellular ion and serum levels do not accurately reflect the real cellular content. The terms hyperkalemia and hypokalemia refer to the serum concentrations of potassium. *Hyper-* *kalemia,* or *hyperpotassemia,* refers to a greater than normal serum concentration of potassium, while *hypokalemia,* or *hypopotassemia,* refers to a lesser than normal serum concentration of potassium. Potassium balance is maintained through excretion in the urine, sweat, and feces, while the primary source of potassium is the diet. Urinary excretion of potassium will be increased whenever increased Na^+ or anion loads are presented to the distal tubules. There is an inverse relationship between tubular H^+ ion secretion and K^+ excretion. An increase in the output of one will reduce the excretion of the other. This is related also to the renal production of the ammonium ion.

Hyperkalemia does not occur as a result of abnormal retention or accumulation, in contrast to the retention of Na^+, which occurs in a number of pathologic conditions. Hyperkalemia can occur as a result of excessive intake with low urinary output, in the presence of extensive tissue injury as K^+ is liberated from the injured cells, and from administration of a large volume of stored blood. Adrenocortical insufficiency and the presence of respiratory or metabolic acidosis cause the serum K^+ level to rise.

Hyperkalemia in the presence of respiratory and metabolic acidosis is a compensatory mechanism. As the hydrogen ion concentration of the ECF increases, K^+ ions move out of the cells, and H^+ and Na^+ ions move into them.

Hypokalemia may result from dilution after large amounts of K^+-free fluids are ingested or infused. In response to insulin, K^+ moves from the blood into the liver and muscle cells to participate in the conversion of glucose to glycogen. An excessive loss of K^+ may occur via the gastrointestinal tract or the kidneys. Gastric and intestinal secretions contain large amounts of K^+, which is usually reabsorbed into the blood (see Table 10-4), and excessive loss of these secretions can result in a serious K^+ deficit. Urinary loss of potassium will be increased by a high sodium load or excess bicarbonate levels, primary renal disease, and the action of various drugs, specifically diuretics and sodium penicillin G. Diuretics cause excretion of chloride, usually with sodium, potassium, or ammonium ions. Since sodium is not always available for excretion and the kidneys may not be able to form ammonium, potassium is excreted with the chloride. Sodium penicillin G apparently acts as an anion, promoting tubular K^+ excretion. The continued normal urinary excretion of K^+ in persons whose intake is reduced and who are malnourished may result in a K^+ deficit. Secretion of ACTH and adrenal mineralocorticoids will increase K^+ excretion in the urine.

Hypokalemia is related to metabolic alkalosis. Potassium loss will cause a metabolic alkalosis, while a metabolic or respiratory alkalosis will cause hypokalemia. When K^+ moves out of the cells, Na^+ and H^+ ions move from the ECF into the cells to replace K^+ and to maintain electroneutrality. Two Na^+ ions and one H^+ ion replace every 3 K^+ ions lost from the cell. As a result the H^+ ion concentration of the ECF falls, and metabolic alkalosis ensues. Further aggravating this condition is the unavailability of K^+ ions for exchange with H^+ in the renal tubules, which results in a urinary loss of H^+ ions.

Conversely, alkalosis (either respiratory or metabolic) causes hypokalemia. K^+ ions from the ECF move into the cells to allow H^+ ions to move out of the cells into the ECF, thus raising the H^+ ion concentration of the ECF. This is a compensatory mechanism that functions to lower pH to normal levels.

Chronic K^+ deficit causes degenerative changes in the renal tubules, which cause hyposthenuria. Large vacuoles develop in the cytoplasm of the proximal convoluted tubules as a result of disordered electrolyte pumping in the presence of a chronic K^+ deficit. These structural and functional changes are reversible with K^+ replacement therapy. Degenerative changes of the myocardium may also occur. These changes include loss of striation, karyorrhexis, and karyolysis. Leukocytic infiltration of the myocardium and later fibrosis also occur.

The muscles of the body are most grossly affected by changes in the potassium balance due to the role of K^+ in depolarization of the cell membranes of the muscle. Changes in the degree of polarization can prevent the initiation and conduction of the impulse along the muscle. A decreased concentration of K^+ outside the cells (hypokalemia) or an increased concentration of K^+ inside the cells causes *hyperpolarization* so that the degree of depolarization produced by the neurotransmitter is insufficient to initiate an impulse. An increased concentration of K^+ outside the cells (hyperkalemia) or a decreased concentration of K^+ within the cells has an opposite effect, and transmission of the impulse is blocked.

The muscle most seriously affected is the heart. The electrocardiogram (Fig. 10-6) reflects the changes in the state of polarization of the cardiac cells that result from potassium excess and deficit.

Muscle weakness is often the first sign of potassium imbalance. A flaccid muscle paralysis may also occur over a period of days as a result of this imbalance. Paresthesias occur with hyperkalemia, probably as a result of the irritation of nerve endings by the potassium. Mental status usually remains unchanged, although the patient may feel apprehensive.

A disorder that is characterized by hypokalemia is known as *familial periodic paralysis*. These transient attacks of muscular weakness and paralysis occur in response to situations that reduce the K^+ levels in the body, that is, a large

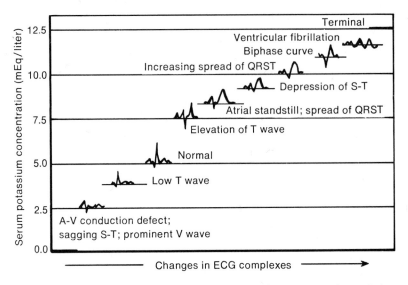

Fig. 10-6. Correlation of increased or decreased serum potassium concentration and electrocardiogram (providing there is no parallel change in Na^+ and Ca^{++}). (From Chatton, M. J., editor: Handbook of medical treatment, ed. 15, Greenbrae, Calif., 1977, Jones Medical Publications.)

carbohydrate meal, or administration of mineralocorticoids, insulin, or dextrose. The attacks occur at normal low K^+ levels. The other signs and symptoms of K^+ excess and deficit are listed in Table 10-4.

Treatment of deficits of both Na^+ and K^+ is by replacement either through increased intake of foods containing these electrolytes, oral supplements (K^+ only) or administration of IV fluids containing isotonic saline or K^+ additives or both. Treatment of K^+ excess is aimed at reducing the potassium concentration as rapidly as possible. This can be done by administering agents that facilitate the movement of K^+ out of the ECF and into the cells. Insulin and glucose are effective transfer agents as is sodium bicarbonate when K^+ excess occurs in the presence of acidosis. Removal of the potassium from the body will also reduce serum potassium levels, and this can be accomplished through dialysis or through the use of a cation-exchange resin, which removes K^+ by exchanging it for Na^+ in the gut. The effects of hyperkalemia (especially the cardiac effects) can be minimized through administration of agents antagonistic to the action of K^+ on the cell membrane, for example, calcium.

Calcium and phosphorus. Calcium exists in the plasma in both bound and ionized forms. The free ionized form is the physiologically active form necessary for blood coagulation, skeletal and cardiac muscle contraction, and nerve function. Regulation of calcium homeostasis is primarily through the function of the parathyroids. Normally the rate of secretion of the parathyroid hormone varies inversely with the ionized calcium level of the plasma via a direct-feedback mechanism. This hormone increases the plasma calcium level by mobilizing calcium from the readily exchangeable reservoir in bone, increasing renal tubular absorption, and increasing absorption of Ca^+ in the intestine, but the latter only in the presence of a metabolite of vitamin D.

Obviously conditions that affect the production of this hormone will have a profound effect on calcium balance. Increased amounts of parathyroid hormone will increase the serum Ca^+ concentration, while decreased amounts of parathyroid hormone will reduce serum Ca^+ concentrations. The parathyroid hormone also increases urinary phosphate excretion, and elevated levels of plasma phosphate can stimulate its secretion. This is not due to a direct effect of phosphate on the glands but is a result of the reciprocal nature of the relationship between calcium and phosphate in the plasma. Elevated plasma phosphate levels lower the cal-

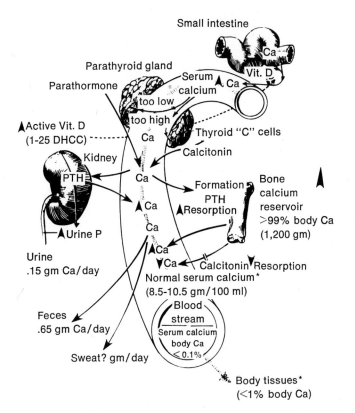

Fig. 10-7. Calcium homeostasis. Control features maintain proper serum calcium that is needed for body tissues. Low serum calcium stimulates absorption of calcium from intestine, retention of calcium by kidney, and release of it from bone. High serum calcium stimulates release of calcitonin, which inhibits calcium resorption from bone. (From Larson, C., and Gould, M.: Orthopedic nursing, ed. 9, St. Louis, 1978, The C. V. Mosby Co.)

cium levels, which in turn stimulates hormone secretion. Compensatory hyperplasia of the parathyroid glands occurs in conditions in which calcium levels are chronically depressed. In renal disease the Ca^+ level is low because the kidneys retain phosphate and are unable to form 1,25-dihydroxycholecalciferol, and a secondary hyperparathyroidism develops. Other hormones that have a major effect on the plasma Ca^+ levels include calcitonin, which decreases plasma Ca^{++} by inhibiting bone resorption, and 1-25-dihydroxycholecalciferol, the active metabolite of vitamin D, which increases intestinal absorption of Ca^+ and mobilizes Ca^+ from the bone to raise plasma Ca^+ levels. Fig. 10-7 schematically illustrates the reciprocal nature of calcium and phosphorus and the interrelationship of parathyroid hormone, vitamin D, and calcitonin in maintain-

ing Ca^+ homeostasis. Other hormones also can affect calcium balance. These include thyroxine, estrogen (if administered for a long time), adrenal steroids, and growth hormone.

Disturbances of calcium metabolism include hypocalcemia and hypercalcemia. A decrease in extracellular calcium generally has an excitatory effect on nerve and muscle cells even though it inhibits transmission at the myoneural junction. The increased activity of the motor nerve fibers results in a symptom complex known as *tetany*. The threshold of peripheral sensory nerve receptors to excitation is also lowered, and sensory changes tend to precede motor changes. Tetany can appear with low normal calcium levels in the presence of increased pH because more plasma protein becomes ionized and binds with the calcium in the alkalotic state.

The neuromuscular irritability of tetany is characterized by paresthesias, carpopedal spasm, Trousseau's sign, Chvostek's sign, and facial muscle spasm. Laryngospasm may be severe enough to cause airway obstruction, and bronchial spasm may simulate an asthmatic attack. Spasm of the abdominal muscles may mimic an "acute abdomen." Convulsions not relieved by anticonvulsant medications and not accompanied by loss of consciousness or aura may also occur. The symptoms of tetany are more pronounced when there is pressure on the motor nerve such as when the legs are crossed. Tetany may be precipitated by exercise or emotional states possibly because of the resultant hyperventilation and respiratory alkalosis and the release of epinephrine.

Changes in mental status, including psychoneuroses and psychoses, may also occur with hypocalcemia. The electrocardiogram is characteristically normal except for prolongation of the QT interval. Other signs and symptoms are listed in Table 10-4.

Hypocalcemia that is a consequence of hypoparathyroidism, parathyroid hormone insensitivity, and lack of vitamin D is discussed in Chapter 14. Hypocalcemia due to hypoproteinemia in which the amount of bound Ca^+ is reduced while the ionized Ca^+ level remains normal is asymptomatic. Hypocalcemia will occur in hyperphosphatemic conditions that result from infusion of phosphate or retention of phosphate such as occurs in renal insufficiency. The administration of large amounts of stored blood may cause hypocalcemia if the excess citrate (added to prevent clotting) binds with calcium. Tetany is more likely to occur if the blood is administered rapidly and if hyperkalemia develops as a result of large amounts of K^+ being released from the stored blood. Certain neoplastic disorders, specifically tumors of the breast, lung, and prostate associated with widespread metastasis, cause increased osteoblastic activity and skeletal uptake of calcium. Tumors that secrete calcitonin also cause hypocalcemia. Hypocalcemia is a well-documented complication of magnesium deficiency secondary to intestinal malabsorption, alcoholism, primary hypomagnesia, and dietary restriction. Hypocalcemia is seen in patients who have increased amounts of fat in the stool (steatorrhea) due to decreased fat absorption because calcium and vitamin D are lost through excretion as calcium salts of fatty acids. This occurs in conditions such as celiac disease, biliary disease, and pancreatic insufficiency (see Chapter 13). A similar mechanism causing hypocalcemia occurs in acute pancreatitis in which large amounts of calcium become fixed by the fatty acids liberated from necrotic mesenteric fat deposits. It has also been postulated that the hypersecretion of glucagon that has been observed in pancreatitis may contribute to hypocalcemia. Hypocalcemia has been reported as a result of glucagon administration.

Tetany is treated by lowering the pH, if alkalosis is present, or by increasing the serum calcium concentration. The cause of the hypocalcemia must be treated, though, in addition to treating the hypocalcemic state itself. Where the cause is increased phosphate retention, phosphate-binding antacids are used to promote intestinal excretion of phosphate. Stored blood should be infused at a rate that does not exceed 1,000 to 1,500 ml per hour. Dietary supplementation with calcium and vitamin D may improve hypocalcemia, but this depends on the cause. Hypocalcemia during pregnancy can be prevented by increasing dietary intake.

A greater than normal serum calcium concentration is termed *hypercalcemia*. The level of elevation of the serum Ca^+ level at which symptoms appear varies among individuals. General symptoms include anorexia, nausea, vomiting, weight loss, easy fatigability, lethargy, headaches, and thirst. Lack of coordination, constipation, and muscle weakness are due to decreased tone in smooth and striated muscle. Polyuria due to impaired renal-concentrating ability is often one of the earliest signs. It has been proposed that an increased calcium ion concentration interferes with active sodium transport across the renal tubule cell membranes by binding with intracellular ATP to form a tight complex calcium–adenosine triphosphate (Ca-ATP). This complex inhibits sodium-potassium-ATPase (Na-K-ATPase), the enzyme necessary for ATP hydrolysis to provide the energy for Na^+ transport. The lesions of metastatic calcification (calcium deposition in various body tissues) tend to first occur in the renal medulla. A characteristic feature of hypercalcemic nephropathy is intrarenal hydronephrosis due to tubular obstruction. Infection, hypertension, and uremia may be long-term complications. Hypercalcinuria favors the development of renal calculi.

Other signs of metastatic calcification appear in the cornea and conjunctiva. *Band keratopathy* is a hazy, grayish opacity seen on the cornea concentric with the limbus. Conjunctival lesions appear as glassy particles and impart a gritty sensation in the eyes. Inflammation often develops as a result of these lesions.

Other manifestations include changes in behavior and emotional state. Apathy, depression, and changes in affect and drive are among these. Acute psychoses are common when serum Ca^+ levels rise above 16 mg/100 ml. Neuromuscular excitability is depressed by hypercalcemia. This is characterized by the decreased muscle tone already mentioned, hyporeflexia (hyperreflexia has occasionally been noted), and increased auditory and visual disturbances.

Acute hypercalcemic crisis may occur when the serum calcium level rises above approximately 16 to 18 mg/100 ml. All the signs and symptoms of hypercalcemia will be present, but the outstanding features will be intractable vomiting with severe volume depletion and electrolyte and acid-base imbalance, fever, altered levels of consciousness including coma or a grossly disturbed mental state, azotemia, and a normal or even above normal serum phosphorus level. Death may occur in this state.

Changes in distribution of body fluid

Disruption of homeostasis can be the result of changes in the distribution of the body fluid. A shift of fluid from the intravascular compartment to the interstitial compartment results in *edema,* the visible swelling of the body tissue. A shift of body fluid from the intravascular compartment to a nonequilibrating *third space* results in depletion of the extracellular volume or hypovolemia. Both conditions may result in reduction of the effective circulating volume of the blood with the effect of reducing tissue perfusion.

Edema. Edema may occur as a result of two interacting mechanisms: the alteration of capillary hemodynamics, favoring filtration out of the intravascular compartment, and the accumulation of sodium and water in the body. The negative interstitial fluid pressure and the interstitial oncotic pressure favor movement of fluid out of the capillary into the interstitium (Fig. 10-4). As fluid begins to accumulate in the interstitium, however, there is an increase in the negative interstitial fluid pressure and a decrease in the interstitial oncotic pressure due to dilution. These pressure changes favor reabsorption into the capillary. Lymphatic flow will also increase in order to remove excess fluid from the interstitium. The pressure changes favoring reabsorption and the increased lymph drainage normally prevent any excessive accumulation of interstitial fluid and account for the fact that there must be a 10 to 15 mm Hg increase in the gradient favoring filtration before edema becomes apparent.

Disruption of the Starling forces in a manner that alters capillary hemodynamics to favor the net filtration of fluid out of the capillary into the interstitium can be the result of increases in capillary hydrostatic pressure, capillary permeability, or interstitial oncotic pressure or of a decrease in plasma oncotic pressure. The capillary hydrostatic pressure remains fairly stable in spite of changes in the arterial pressure because of the resistance provided by the precapillary sphincter. Changes in venous pressure, however, will be reflected by concomitant changes in the capillary hydrostatic pressure since resistance in the venules is not so stringently regulated. Venous pressure can be increased as a result of venous obstruction or an increase in intravascular volume. The edema seen in a limb in which venous thrombosis has occurred is due to the increased capillary hydrostatic pressure in the presence of venous obstruction. The edema seen in renal failure is a result of the increased capillary hydrostatic pressure due to the increased intravascular volume.

Any condition favoring the release and accumulation of protein in the interstitial fluid will cause an increase in the interstitial oncotic pressure. The capillary membrane is normally impermeable to all but very small amounts of protein, restricting its presence to the intravascular compartment. The small amount of protein filtered out of the capillary is normally returned to the circulation via the lymphatics. If the lymph flow is obstructed or reduced, this protein will accumulate and cause an increase in interstitial oncotic pressure. A change in capillary permeability that allows free passage of protein will also increase interstitial oncotic pressure. This mechanism characterizes the formation of edema in burns and allergic reactions. If the protein loss from the intravascular compartment is severe, plasma oncotic pressure may also be reduced. The osmotic pressure generated by the plasma proteins (oncotic pressure) plays an important role in promoting reabsorption of fluid into the capillary from the interstitium. This effect is lost when the plasma oncotic pressure is reduced because of lack of protein, and more fluid will continue to enter and remain in the interstitium. Other factors that decrease the plasma oncotic pressure include an increased loss of protein from the body and a reduction in the synthesis of plasma proteins by the liver.

The presence of edema also indicates an excess amount of the total body sodium, which is accompanied by an obligatory load of water. The sodium excess may serve as either an initiating or a secondary factor in the pathogenesis of edema. Accumulation of an excess amount of sodium in the body is most frequently due to either increased retention or reduced ability to eliminate Na^+ in the presence of normal intake. Most commonly the increased retention of sodium and subsequently water is seen in edematous states as a compensatory mechanism to restore and maintain the circulating volume at near-normal levels while fluid accumulates in the interstitial space. How changes in the circulating volume are sensed and responded to by the kidneys is not completely understood. Sodium retention following a reduction in intravascular volume is thought to be due to both a decrease in the glomerular filtration rate reflecting that reduction and an increase in tubular reabsorption. Increased reabsorption along the entire tubule has been demonstrated in edematous states and is affected by several factors:

aldosterone secretion, increased sympathetic tone, redistribution of renal blood flow away from the outer cortex, increased peritubular oncotic pressure, and absence of a natriuretic (influencing urinary loss of Na^+) hormone. No one of these factors appears to play a primary role in sodium reabsorption, however.

Renal retention of sodium and water as a compensatory mechanism to restore circulating volume is illustrated in conditions such as the nephrotic syndrome, liver disease, and congestive heart failure. With the nephrotic syndrome and liver disease, disruption of capillary hemodynamics is the initiating factor. In both conditions the plasma oncotic pressure is decreased due to the lack of plasma proteins. In liver disease, synthesis of the plasma proteins is depressed, while in the nephrotic syndrome excessive amounts of the plasma proteins are lost in the urine. As the intravascular volume drops, sodium and water retention increases in order to maintain the effective circulating volume. In congestive heart failure, both disruption of capillary hemodynamics and renal retention of sodium and water come into play as primary factors in the pathogenesis of cardiac edema. In the presence of heart failure, venous pressure rises because the heart is unable to pump all of the blood being returned to it. The increased venous pressure will cause an increase in capillary hydrostatic pressure (backward theory). As cardiac output falls in the presence of heart failure, various compensatory mechanisms, among them renal retention of sodium and water, come into play. The resulting increase in circulating volume only serves to intensify the already increased venous and capillary hydrostatic pressures (forward theory). A diagram of the interaction of the disrupted Starling forces and the sodium and water retention that occurs in these conditions is presented in Fig. 10-8.

In contrast to these conditions, increased renal retention of sodium and water plays a primary role in the pathogenesis of cyclic edema seen in menstruating women. The ovarian hormones, estrogen and progesterone, influence the rate of renal sodium reabsorption. When the rate of the secretion of these hormones increases, sodium and water reabsorption will

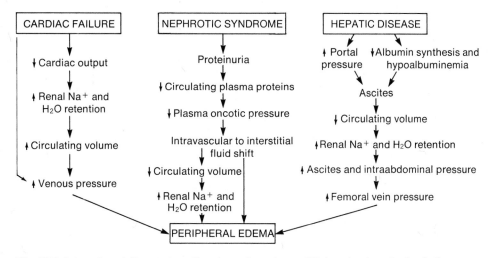

Fig. 10-8. Interaction of disrupted capillary hemodynamics and Na^+ and water retention in three conditions that include edema as a chief manifestation.

Table 10-5. Etiology of edema

Etiologic factors	Associated conditions
Increased capillary permeability	Inflammatory reactions
	Burns
	Trauma
	Allergic reactions
Increased capillary hydrostatic pressure	
Na^+ retention and increased blood volume	Congestive heart failure
	Trauma and stress
	Renal failure
	Refeeding edema
	Adrenocortical hormone secretion
	Drugs: estrogen, phenylbutazone
Venous obstruction	Local obstruction
	Hepatic obstruction
	Pulmonary edema
Decreased plasma oncotic pressure	
Decreased synthesis of plasma proteins	Liver disease
	Malnutrition
Increased loss of plasma proteins	Nephrotic syndrome
	Burns
	Protein-losing enteropathy
Increased interstitial pressure	Lymphatic obstruction
(plasma protein lost to interstitium)	Increased capillary permeability

also increase. As the total amount of sodium and water increases, venous pressure will continue to rise. When venous pressure increases to the point where the capillary hydrostatic pressure is also increased, fluid will move out of the capillary and remain in the interstitial space. This is the basis of the premenstrual edema that many otherwise normal women experience. Birth control pills contain these hormones in varying amounts so that many women taking birth control pills experience edema as an unpleasant side effect. The higher the estrogen content of the pill, the greater the likelihood that edema will develop. Increased levels of these hormones as well as a reduction in plasma oncotic pressure interact to promote edema in the pregnant woman.

The kidneys' inability to excrete sodium while normal ingestion continues will result in the accumulation of an excessive amount of sodium. This occurs when renal function is compromised as a result of disease or direct damage to the nephrons. The edema that accompanies renal failure occurs when the increased levels of sodium and water increase venous pressure to the point where capillary hemodynamics are altered, favoring filtration out of the capillary. Table 10-5 lists the various etiologic factors and the conditions in which these factors play a primary role in the pathogenesis of edema.

When pressure on edematous tissue displaces the edema fluid and leaves an indentation, the edema is described as *pitting edema* (Fig. 10-9). The term *brawny edema* describes a type of edema in which the overlying skin is stretched taut and resembles a pig's skin with pronounced pores. It is hard to the touch, and pressure will not leave an indentation. Brawny edema is the characteristic type of edema that accompanies lymphatic obstruction or occurs following removal of lymph nodes. An example of this type of edema is that seen in the arm of a woman after a mastectomy with removal of the lymph nodes.

The effects of edema are determined by its location and extent. Edema may be generalized or localized, depending on its cause. For example, pulmonary edema is the result of the transudation of fluid into the alveoli that oc-

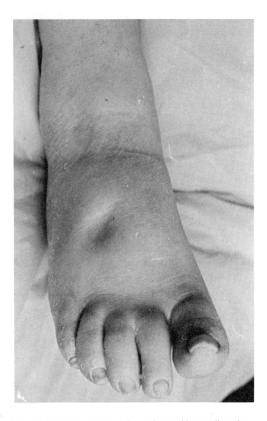

Fig. 10-9. Pitting edema in patient with cardiopulmonary disease. (From Beyers, M., and Dudas, S.: The clinical practice of medical surgical nursing, Boston, 1977, Little, Brown & Co.)

curs when the hydrostatic pressure in the pulmonary capillaries exceeds the plasma oncotic pressure. This occurs when the left side of the heart fails. Pulmonary edema constitutes a life-threatening situation because gas exchange is blocked by the presence of fluid at the alveolocapillary membrane. Laryngeal edema, another form of localized edema, results from increased capillary permeability secondary to allergic reactions or burns of the face and neck with smoke inhalation. With severe laryngeal swelling, airway occlusion may occur. This also is a life-threatening situation since oxygen is prevented from reaching the alveolocapillary membrane. In contrast to these conditions is the localized edema of the feet and ankles that may occur after prolonged periods of sitting or standing. This edema usually causes only minor discomfort and is readily relieved by elevation of the extremities.

Edema in an organ such as the brain, which is enclosed in a limited, nonexpandable space, can have serious consequences. As edema increases and brain tissue swells, filling the cranium, intracranial pressure will increase, and cerebral blood flow will be impaired. Signs of the resulting cerebral dysfunction may include restlessness, changes in the level of consciousness from disorientation and lethargy to stupor and coma, irregular pupillary reaction, papilledema, visual disturbances, headache, vomiting, and weakness or paralysis of parts of the body. Changes in the vital signs will reflect the effects of disruption of the cerebral control centers on vital organ function: increased blood pressure, decreased pulse rate, and depressed respirations often with periods of apnea.

Generalized edema usually first appears in the dependent, gravity-affected parts of the body: in an ambulatory person, the feet and ankles, and in a bedridden person, the sacrum and buttocks. Aside from discomfort, edematous tissue is prone to other problems. The flow of blood to the affected tissue is compromised as a result of the altered capillary hemodynamics. Thus, the delivery of oxygen and nutrients and the removal of wastes is impeded, leading to the development of a state of hypoxia and acidosis that will impair cellular function. As a result the edematous tissue is more prone to breakdown and more susceptible to infection. Pressure sores that develop in edematous tissue are more extensive and more difficult to heal than those in normal tissue. The effects of even a minor amount of pressure on edematous tissue are intensified because of preexisting hypoxic conditions.

The treatment of edema is determined by its effects on the body and its cause. Consideration must be given to the questions of how rapidly the edema fluid can be removed and what the possible consequences of this removal will be to the overall functioning of the body. Obviously the effects of conditions such as pulmonary and cerebral edema are life threatening, and removal of the edema fluid from the lungs and brain must be done in the most expedient way possible. Sometimes removal of edema fluid has serious consequences. Rapid removal of ascitic fluid, for example, can cause a serious depletion of the circulating volume, resulting in hypovolemic shock. It must be remembered that mobilization of the edema fluid through use of diuretic medications is initially at the expense of the plasma volume. Despite this reduction most patients benefit from the use of diuretic medications. However, there are two exceptions: patients with a low effective circulating volume (severe heart failure) and those who have been treated excessively with diuretics. In these two groups of patients the reduction in plasma volume is enough to seriously impair tissue perfusion. It is not enough to treat only the edema; the underlying condition must also be treated. Often treatment of the causative condition is enough to initiate mobilization of the edema fluid, for example, the patient experiencing edema secondary to heart failure. With increased cardiac contractility and output due to digitalis therapy both the backward and forward effects of heart failure that lead to edema formation are minimized. If the underlying condition is not treated the edema will reoccur. Edema due to venous or lymphatic obstruction will not be relieved until the cause of the obstruction is relieved.

"Third space" syndromes. Third space syndromes in which a significant amount of the ECF becomes unavailable to the effective ECF are sometimes referred to as *sequestered edema*. This fluid remains in the body and with appropriate treatment may be mobilized to return to the effective ECF. For all intents and purposes a new fluid compartment is formed in addition to the intracellular and extracellular compartments; hence, the name *third space*.

Conditions that result in large amounts of the ECF becoming trapped outside the extracellular compartment, either in the tissues or in a serous body cavity, include burns, intestinal obstruction, and venous obstruction within a major venous system. Sequestration of fluid around the site of injury is a feature of trauma, either accidental or surgical, accompanied by extensive tissue damage (e.g., crushing injuries, surgery involving massive tissue resection). Bleeding into a body cavity or tissue can also result in a third space syndrome.

A third space syndrome may also result from *peritonitis,* an inflammatory disorder of the peritoneum that can result from damage by a variety of bacterial and chemical agents. The peritoneal membrane functions in the transport of water and electrolytes between the peritoneal cavity and the circulation. As a result of the inflammatory process this function is disrupted, and large amounts of Na^+ and water may be lost into the peritoneal cavity. Additionally, protein may be lost into the peritoneal cavity, thus increasing the osmotic pull of fluid into this third space. Peritonitis is often a complication of untreated intestinal obstruction, in which the increased permeability of the intestinal wall allows bacteria and their toxins and other substances potentially harmful to mucosal tissue (enzymes, etc.) to move out of the bowel into the peritoneum, where they initiate an inflammatory response.

The clinical manifestations of a third space syndrome include those of the pathologic process that originally caused the fluid shift and also the manifestations of depletion of the effective circulating volume. As cardiac output is decreased due to volume depletion, tachycardia and hypotension result. Sympathetic stimulation causes peripheral vasoconstriction, which is manifested by pallor and coldness of the extremities. Oliguria reflects the decreased renal blood flow and the body's attempts to conserve fluid. There will be no weight loss as there is when fluid is lost from the body, however. If the depletion of the effective circulating volume is severe and acute, hypovolemic shock may develop. The rapidity of the fluid accumulation into the third space is an important variable. If the fluid loss from the ECF occurs slowly, the body can compensate by retaining salt and water. If the fluid loss is quite rapid there is not enough time for the compensatory mechanisms to begin to function to restore fluid volume in the ECF, and signs of depletion of the effective circulating volume will become apparent. Fluid therapy must be supportive to maintain tissue perfusion until the sequestered fluid can be mobilized from the third space.

Additional signs and symptoms possibly accompanying the hypovolemic state include those of the electrolyte and acid-base disorders that may accompany fluid depletion. These depend on the composition of the fluid that is lost from the effective circulating volume.

Table 10-6. Alterations in the pH of body fluid

Condition	Other names	Signs and symptoms	Sources	Compensatory mechanisms
Primary base bicarbonate deficit Ketones, chlorides, and/or organic acids replace HCO_3 ions → deficit of base bicarbonate; ratio of 1 part H_2CO_3 to 20 parts HCO_3 is ↓ on HCO_3 side	Metabolic acidosis Primary alkali deficit Uncompensated alkali deficit Nonrespiratory acidosis	Deep, rapid breathing (Kussmaul) SOB on exertion Weakness Stupor Coma Lab findings Plasma pH ↓ 7.35 Urine pH ↓ 6 Plasma HCO_3 ↓ 25 mEq/liter in adults and ↓ 20 mEq/liter in children	Gain of strong acid by extracellular fluid Gain of exogenous acid Metabolic and organic acid overproduction and retention Loss of base from extracellular fluid Renal loss Intestinal loss	Respiratory: ↓ pH stimulates pulmonary ventilation; lungs blow off CO_2, and ↓ CO_2 is available to form H_2CO_3; acid side is decreased Renal: kidneys retain base bicarbonate through preferential excretion of hydrogen ions → acid urine
Primary base bicarbonate excess	Metabolic alkalosis Primary alkali excess	Depressed breathing (rate and depth)	Gain of HCO_3 from extracellular fluid	Respiratory: lungs hold back CO_2 to build up H_2CO_3

Mechanism	Names	Clinical signs / Lab findings	Causes	Compensation
Ratio of 1 part H$_2$CO$_3$ to 20 parts HCO$_3$ is ↑ on HCO$_3$ side, resulting in excess of base bicarbonate	Uncompensated alkali excess / Nonrespiratory alkalosis	Hyperactive reflexes / Muscle hypertonicity / Tetany progressing to convulsions / Lab findings / Plasma pH ↑7.45 / Urine pH ↑7.0 / Plasma HCO$_3$ ↑25 mEq/liter in adults and ↑20 mEq/liter in children / Plasma K ↓4 mEq/liter	Gain of exogenous base / Oxidation of salts of organic acids / Loss of acid from the extracellular fluid / Intestinal loss / Renal loss / Potassium depletion (may be renal or extrarenal)	side; breathing may be shallow and irregular; ↑Pco$_2$ of blood stimulates respiratory center / Renal: kidneys excrete HCO$_3$ ions and retain H ions and nonbicarbonate anions to aid in restoring ratio and pH to normal range → alkaline urine
Carbonic acid deficit of extracellular fluid / Plasma Pco$_2$ ↓ due to hyperactive breathing; ratio of 1 part H$_2$CO$_3$ to 20 parts HCO$_3$ decreased on H$_2$CO$_3$ side	Respiratory alkalosis / Hyperventilation / Primary carbonic acid deficit / Uncompensated carbonic acid deficit / Hypocapnia / Nonmetabolic alkalosis	Convulsions / Tetany / Unconsciousness / Lab findings / pH of plasma ↑7.45 / pH of urine ↑7.0 / Plasma HCO$_3$ ↓25 mEq/liter in adults and ↓20 mEq/liter in children	Anxiety, extreme emotion, hysteria / Intentional overbreathing / Rapid breathing (hyperpnea) / Mechanical overventilation / Oxygen lack / High fever / Encephalitis* / Salicylate poisoning*	Renal: kidneys excrete HCO$_3$ ions and retain H ions and nonbicarbonate anions; urine becomes alkaline; by dropping bicarbonate level proper ratio is nearly restored
Carbonic acid excess of extracellular fluid / Retention of CO$_2$ by the lungs causes an excess of carbonic acid; ratio of 1 part H$_2$CO$_3$ to 20 parts HCO$_3$ increased on H$_2$CO$_3$ side	Respiratory acidosis / Primary CO$_2$ excess / Uncompensated CO$_2$ excess / Nonmetabolic acidosis / Hypoventilation / Hypercapnia	Respiratory embarrassment / Weakness / Coma / Disorientation / Lab findings / Plasma pH ↓7.35 / Urine pH ↓6.0 / Plasma HCO$_3$ ↑29 mEq/liter in adults and ↑25 mEq/liter in children	Any condition that causes retention of carbon dioxide / Asthma / Chronic obstructive lung disease (COLD) / Pneumonia / Occlusion of breathing passages / Barbiturate or morphine poisoning (causes depression of respiratory center)	Renal: kidneys conserve base bicarbonate while excreting hydrogen ions and nonbicarbonate anions → acid urine

*Respiratory center directly affected.

Changes in pH of body fluid

Failure to maintain the hydrogen ion concentration of the body fluid within normal limits so that the pH is maintained at a value between 7.35 and 7.45 results in abnormal conditions known as alkalosis and acidosis. A change in pH indicates a disruption in the normal bicarbonate-carbonic acid ratio of 20:1. Depending on the etiology, clinical conditions in which the hydrogen ion concentration is outside the normal range are classified as either metabolic or respiratory. Disruption of the normal carbonic acid level has a respiratory etiology, while disruption of the normal bicarbonate level has a metabolic etiology. Table 10-6 summarizes the clinical manifestations, causative factors, and compensatory mechanisms that occur in the various states of acid-base imbalance. Table 10-7 presents typical blood gas values obtained in the various disorders before and after compensation occurs as well as in some mixed disorders. Etiologic mechanisms of respiratory acidosis and alkalosis are discussed in Chapter 8, as are the manifestations of acidosis and alkalosis. Fig. 10-10 clearly demonstrates the relationship of the arterial pH and arterial P_{CO_2} and how these are altered in the different conditions.

DISEASE MODELS

Many pathologic conditions are characterized by a severe disruption of chemical equilibrium. Examples of such conditions include congestive heart failure, renal failure, diabetic ketoacidosis, and Cushing's syndrome. These disorders are discussed in detail in other chapters. The effects of stress and thermal injury on

Table 10-7. Acid-base disorders

Terminology	Typical values		
	pH	P_{CO_2}	HCO_3
Respiratory acidosis	7.10	80.0	24.0
Compensated respiratory acidosis	7.40	80.0	48.0
Respiratory alkalosis	7.70	20.0	24.0
Compensated respiratory alkalosis	7.40	20.0	12.0
Metabolic acidosis	7.10	40.0	12.0
Compensated metabolic acidosis	7.40	20.0	12.0
Metabolic alkalosis	7.70	40.0	48.0
Compensated metabolic alkalosis	7.40	80.0	48.0
Mixed respiratory and metabolic acidosis	↓	↑	↓
Mixed respiratory and metabolic alkalosis	↑	↓	↑
Normal	7.40	40.0	24.0

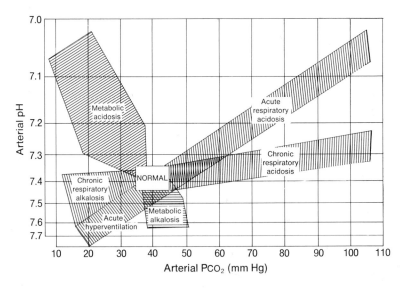

Fig. 10-10. Blood gas interpretation. Acid-base graph that allows diagnosis of acid-base abnormalities from P_{CO_2} and pH.

body fluid homeostasis can also be quite profound.

Effect of surgical stress on fluid homeostasis

Maintenance of fluid homeostasis is precarious in the surgical patient. Potential departures from the normal chemical equilibrium in the surgical patient can occur anywhere on the spectrum between overhydration and dehydration accompanied by a variety of electrolyte and acid-base disorders. Prior to surgery the patient is allowed nothing by mouth, and if he is acutely ill during that time it is highly probable that some disruption of chemical equilibrium has already occurred due to vomiting, diarrhea, or other causes. Fluid loss during surgery can be quite high because of bleeding and evaporation of fluid from the organs while they are exposed to the environment. On the other hand, overhydration can occur as a result of rapid infusion of IV fluid or infusion of excessive amounts due to inaccurate estimation of the fluid loss. Basic to the maintenance of body fluid homeostasis in the surgical patient, however, is the metabolic response that surgical stress evokes.

First, there is tissue damage, which in extensive surgical procedures may be quite severe. In response to this, metabolic processes accelerate to facilitate repair of the tissue. This causes an increase in the utilization of energy, which must be endogenously supplied because the surgical patient is usually fasting. Fluid not only may be lost from the injured area but may be sequestered around the damaged tissue, creating a third space, which further contributes to extracellular fluid volume depletion. Additional fluid may be lost via the skin and lungs in response to the rise in body temperature that

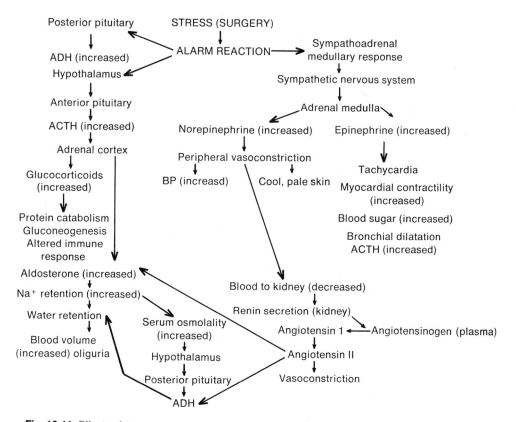

Fig. 10-11. Effects of stress reactions in surgical patient. (Copyright Nov. 1977, the American Journal of Nursing Co. Reproduced with permission from the American Journal of Nursing, vol. 77, no. 11, Nov. 1977).

usually occurs 24 to 48 hours postoperatively as part of the inflammatory response to tissue trauma and the accelerated metabolic processes.

The hormonal and sympathetic responses to surgical trauma (Fig. 10-11) represent protective and restorative mechanisms that allow the body to adapt to the altered physiology and to eventually regain homeostasis. While these particular responses following surgery do not directly affect acid-base balance, the changes in water and electrolyte balance as well as many of the conditions accompanying surgery (gastric suction, shallow breathing, oxygen therapy, etc.) and primary disease condition may have an effect. For example, respiratory acidosis often occurs as a result of the pattern of shallow breathing seen following surgery. The cause of this hypoventilation is multifactorial: a combination of the effects of pain, drugs, anesthetic agents, positioning, and bandages to name a few. The reduction in ventilatory capacity is most severe following thoracic and high abdominal surgery, making these patients more prone to develop respiratory acidosis. Prolonged gastric suction after surgery without adequate fluid and electrolyte replacement may lead to metabolic alkalosis accompanied by severe hypokalemia. Respiratory alkalosis after surgery may be the result of overbreathing due to anxiety or excessive mechanical ventilation either during surgery or after surgery if the patient is placed on a respirator.

Retention of water, which can be attributed to several factors, is most marked following surgery. Stress causes extremely potent direct stimulation of the posterior pituitary, which is responsible for the formation and secretion of ADH. The usual regulation of ADH secretion through osmoreceptor control is overridden by the effect of stress, and dilution due to water retention may cause hyponatremia and decreased serum osmolality. Elevated levels of ADH may persist for 2 to 4 days after uncomplicated surgery. Endogenously formed water that is sodium free also figures in postsurgical water retention. Approximately 1 ml of water is formed with each gram of fat or lean tissue oxidized. Tissue catabolism increases after surgery in order to meet the body's caloric

requirements so this water must be considered in calculating the total amount of water in the body.

Stimulation of the sympathetic nervous system and the adrenal medulla causes increased amounts of epinephrine and norepinephrine to be released. This in turn causes vasoconstriction and decreased blood flow to the kidneys where the juxtaglomerular cells are stimulated to release renin, which activates the renin-angiotensin system to cause aldosterone secretion by the adrenal cortex. Aldosterone causes retention of Na^+ and the subsequent retention of water. Aldosterone secretion is further augmented by any reductions in intravascular volume and to a lesser degree by ACTH secretion.

Adrenocorticotropic hormone (ACTH) is secreted by the anterior pituitary gland in response to the hypothalamic hormone, corticotropin releasing factor (CRF). Stimulation of ACTH secretion consistently occurs as a response to trauma and stress. ACTH stimulates the adrenal cortex to secrete the glucocorticoids and mineralocorticoids, chiefly aldosterone. The glucocorticoids cause increased protein catabolism, which leads to a loss of nitrogen and muscle potassium. Serum K^+ levels will increase initially as the K^+ released from the catabolized cells enters the ECF. Eventually negative potassium and nitrogen balances develop, however. The negative nitrogen balance is due to a combination of factors: direct tissue damage, protein catabolism, and the effects of starvation (the postoperative patient is usually fasting). Serum K^+ levels will eventually fall after the initial slight increase due to the K^+ mobilized from damaged and catabolized cells. Urinary excretion of K^+ increases in the presence of aldosterone as resorption of Na^+ by the distal tubule is accomplished in exchange for K^+. If excessive losses of K^+ due to vomiting, diarrhea, or draining fistulas occurred prior to or since surgery without adequate replacement therapy, the hypokalemia may become quite severe. Increased blood glucose levels and even glycosuria may develop due to glycogenolysis and gluconeogenesis that occur in response to the adrenal hormones. Diuresis usually occurs 3 to 4 days postoperatively, and as Na^+ retention continues, serum osmolality tends to increase. At this time the posterior pituitary responds appropriately to the increased osmolality and secretes ADH to cause water retention and to restore normal serum osmolality.

The duration of the metabolic response to surgery depends on the extent of the injury and the presence of complications. The development of shock, sepsis, or renal failure will further complicate the return to homeostasis and the fluid and electrolyte therapy necessary in the interim.

Effect of burns on fluid homeostasis

Thermal trauma, or burns, represents a massive insult to the normal physiologic functioning of the body and especially to body fluid homeostasis. Burns cause a substantial loss of fluid from the effective ECF and elicit a maximal systemic response to the decreased circulating volume, tissue destruction, anemia, and electrolyte and acid-base imbalances that occur.

The most significant pathophysiologic event that occurs in the immediate postburn period is a fluid shift from the intravascular compartment into a third space around the burn wound. This burn edema, as it is sometimes referred to, is a characteristic feature of a thermal injury and is due to dilation and grossly increased capillary permeability. Formation of the burn edema occurs most rapidly during the first 6 to 8 hours and continues for up to 48 hours after the burn. This 48-hour period is referred to as the stage of *sodium loss and shock*.

The electrolyte composition of this trapped fluid is similar to that of plasma. The plasma protein content of the burn edema is slightly less than that of plasma, but research has documented that the plasma proteins present in the burn edema initially come from the plasma. In severe burns the loss of intravascular oncotic pressure due to the loss of proteins from the plasma results in fluid leaks into the interstitial spaces at sites remote from the burn injury. The formation of burn edema is augmented by the release of bradykinin produced by tissue proteases.

Fluid loss in burns is not only due to the formation and trapping of edema fluid in the third space but also may be due to loss of fluid as exudate (especially in second degree burns) and through vaporization of water from the burn surface. The loss of fluid through vaporization can be very high and is associated with an increased energy expenditure since heat must be generated endogenously to make up for the heat lost from the body surface and to maintain a normal body temperature. The loss of fluid by vaporization peaks between the fifth and tenth days after a burn.

During the first 48 hours after a burn hypovolemic shock may occur and is thought to be related to the Na^+ deficit rather than to the loss of fluid per se. Na^+ is lost from the ECF into the burn edema and moves into the cells to replace K^+. Hyperkalemia is the result of large amounts of K^+ being released into the ECF from damaged cells. The abnormal movement of Na^+ and K^+ may be due to injury-related changes in the function and efficiency of the sodium pump. Hemoconcentration occurs due to the loss of fluid in amounts relatively greater than the solid constituents of the blood. This hemoconcentration is reflected by an increased hematocrit. Urinary output is reduced due to decreased renal blood flow, increased secretion of ADH, and Na^+ and water retention in response to the increased sympathetic, pituitary, and adrenocortical activity caused by stress.

Metabolic acidosis is the result of poor tissue perfusion and release of acidic products of tissue destruction. Blood viscosity is increased as a result of the hemoconcentration, released tissue thromboplastin, and increased platelet adhesion. Widespread thrombosis occurs as a result of damaged vascular endothelium and aggregation of the erythrocytes. Microthrombi develop and block the microcirculation, causing hypoxia of those cells served by that portion of the circulation. Lactic acid will accumulate due to anaerobic metabolism. The combination of lactic acid plus the acidic anions released from traumatized tissue (e.g., PO_4^-) increase the H^+ concentration, and pH falls.

There is a fall in cardiac output after a burn that is related to several factors: decreased plasma volume and hypotension, decreased perfusion to the coronary arteries secondary to hypotension, hypothermia due to evaporative

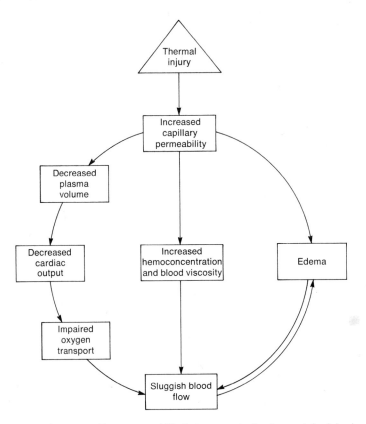

Fig. 10-12. In severe burns, capillary permeability is increased, allowing protein-rich plasma to leak from vascular to intravascular spaces, which causes edema, hemoconcentration, and a decrease in cardiac output.

water loss, and acidosis. Acidosis causes reduced cardiac output and increased total peripheral vascular resistance, which increases cardiac work load. A vicious cycle is established since cardiac function will be further impaired, and reduced tissue perfusion will further contribute to the state of acidosis that already exists. Additionally the release of a myocardial toxin by the burned tissue has been documented by research with extensively burned animals. The release of such a factor in humans has been proposed and may be significant in burns involving 80% of the body surface area. This toxin is thought to directly depress cardiac contractility through a negative inotropic effect. Respiratory alkalosis sometimes occurs after a burn injury as a result of the rapid pattern of respiration elicited by pain and anxiety in the burn victim. Respiratory acidosis may be the result of hypoventilation due to swelling or burn damage of the neck, face, or upper respiratory tract, which occludes the airway (Fig. 10-12).

The second stage occurs after the first 48 hours and is called the stage of *sodium and water reabsorption,* or *fluid remobilization.* As fluid returns to the intravascular compartment from the interstitial space, urinary output increases, and the hematocrit drops. Sodium will be lost with the water during the diuresis that occurs in this stage. As fluid reenters the intravascular compartment, the decrease in the number of red blood cells as a result of thermal destruction becomes apparent. The hemoglobinuria that results from the red blood cell destruction can adversely affect renal function. Hypokalemia occurs during this stage as K^+ begins to move back into the cells from the ECF.

The third stage, *anemia and malnutrition,* or the *convalescent phase,* occurs from the fifth day on. During this stage, signs of a calcium

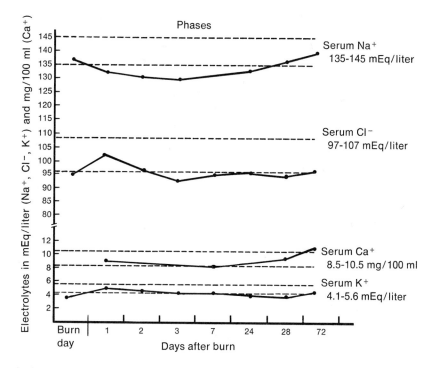

Fig. 10-13. Serum levels of potassium, calcium, chloride, and sodium for 72 days after burn in patient who had second degree (partial thickness) and third degree (full thickness) burns over 40% of his body. (From Beland, S., and Passos, J.: Clinical nursing: pathophysiological and psychosocial approaches, ed. 3, New York, 1975, Macmillan Publishing Co.)

deficit may become manifest, although the causative mechanism is not understood. However, calcium is known to be mobilized to damaged tissue. The major concern during this stage is the negative nitrogen balance that has developed due to a combination of factors: protein destruction at the burn, protein losses in the exudate, inadequate protein intake, increased protein catabolism (due to ACTH secretion), and immobilization. The Na^+ deficit may still be present during this stage also.

Typical changes in serum electrolyte concentrations, fluid intake, body weight, and urinary output that can be expected in a patient who has sustained a thermal injury are presented in Figs. 10-13 and 10-14. Fluid replacement to maintain volume and restore electrolyte levels to normal is critical in the management of the burn patient. Calculation of the amount of fluid lost is based on the surface area and depth of the burn, hence the critical importance of accurate initial assessment of a thermal injury (see also Chapter 6).

Effect of treatment modalities on chemical equilibrium

A variety of treatment measures that are frequently used in the clinical setting have the potential for profoundly disturbing chemical equilibrium. The administration of fluid intravenously is a good example. There are several potential problems that can arise with the use of parenteral therapy. Rapid administration of fluids can cause fluid overload. Electrolyte deficits may occur with the administration of fluid that is hypotonic to the body fluid. Administration of too little fluid can cause a state of fluid deficit in the patient.

The parenteral administration of hypertonic dextrose solutions with amino acids and other supplements (electrolytes, vitamins) is called *parenteral hyperalimentation,* or *total parenteral nutrition.* The amino acids serve as the nitrogen source, and the dextrose serves as the caloric source. This therapy is used to restore and maintain positive nitrogen balance in the patient for whom oral intake is impossible or

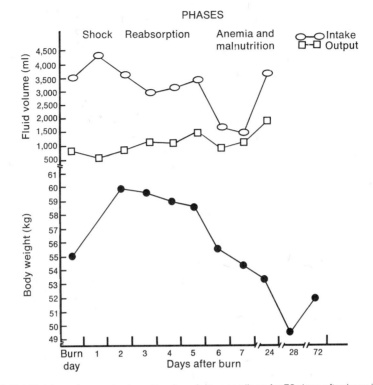

Fig. 10-14. Fluid intake, urinary output, and body weight recordings for 72 days after burn in a patient who had second degree (partial thickness) and third degree (full thickness) burns over 40% of his body. (From Beland, S., and Passos, J.: Clinical nursing: pathophysiological and psychosocial approaches, ed. 3, New York, 1975, Macmillan Publishing Co.)

contraindicated. Fluid and electrolyte disturbances may occur in this form of parenteral therapy just as they do in others. Additionally too rapid an infusion can lead to a hyperosmolar reaction. Vitamin toxicity can cause hypercalciuria.

Patients who are being vigorously treated for ulcer with antacids and frequent milk product ingestion may develop what is referred to as the *milk-alkali syndrome*. This condition is characterized by hypercalcemia and metabolic alkalosis.

Diuretic therapy probably presents the greatest potential hazard to the body's chemical equilibrium. Aside from the side effects of the drugs themselves, the diuresis they produce and the mechanism by which they produce it can lead to severe electrolyte and acid-base disorders, as well as severe volume depletion.

Chemical disequilibrium may also have adverse effects on drug therapy. For example, hypokalemia, or low levels of extracellular potassium, is synergistic with digitalis and thus predisposes the patient to digitalis toxicity.

SUMMARY

This chapter presented an overview to the effects of fluid, electrolyte, and acid-base imbalance on the physiologic functioning of the body. Chemical processes are basic to this functioning, and disruption of the normal equilibrium of these processes can present a serious threat to life. Pathologic conditions that disrupt chemical equilibrium as a result of abnormal intake, elimination, or regulation are discussed in subsequent chapters.

SUGGESTED READINGS

Goldberger, E.: A primer of water, electrolyte and acid base syndromes, ed. 4, Philadelphia, 1970, Lea & Febiger.

Haberich, F. J.: Osmoreception in the portal circulation, Fed. Proc. **27:**1137, 1968.

Manzi, C., et al.: Edema, how to tell if it is a danger signal, Nursing 77 **7**(4):66-77, 1977.

Marcinek, M.: Stress in the surgical patient, Am. J. Nurs. **77**(11):1809-1811, 1977.

Maxwell, M., and Klieman, C.: Clinical disorders of fluid and electrolyte metabolism, ed. 2, New York, 1972, McGraw-Hill Book Co.

Reed, G.: Confused about potassium? Here's a clear concise guide, Nursing 74 **4**(3):21-27, 1974.

Rognes, P., and Maylan, J. M.: Restoring fluid balance in the patient with severe burns, Am. J. Nurs. **76**(12): 1953-1957, 1976.

Rose, D.: Clinical physiology of acid-base and electrolyte disorders, New York, 1977, McGraw-Hill Book Co.

Schrier, R., editor: Renal and electrolyte disorders, Boston, 1976, Little, Brown & Co.

Simmons, D.: Evaluation of acid-base status, Basics R.D., vol. 2, no. 3, Jan. 1974.

CHAPTER 11

Disorders of elimination

AT THE COMPLETION OF THIS CHAPTER THE STUDENT WILL BE ABLE TO:

- Explain the pathophysiologic mechanisms that occur in response to disruption of normal elimination processes.
    Describe the alterations in normal function, dynamics, and regulation that occur in response to disruption of the normal elimination processes.
    Identify compensatory and adaptive mechanisms that occur in response to disruption of the normal elimination processes.
    Describe the clinical manifestations of the altered dynamics and resultant adaptation.
- Cite the etiology of disorders of elimination.
- Cite predisposing factors to the development of disorders of elimination.
- Explain the treatment of disorders of elimination.
    State the goals of treatment.
    Identify the treatment measures.
    Describe the physiologic basis of treatment.
- Describe the physiologic effects of abnormal routes of elimination.

Homeostasis of the body depends on maintenance of chemical equilibrium, which in turn depends on the function of elimination. Through the skin, lungs, and genitourinary and gastrointestinal tracts the body selectively excretes the products of metabolism and any excess substances for which it has no need. Regulation of elimination is the key to the body's retention of those substances vital to its functioning.

This chapter presents an overview of the process and its regulation for each of the major routes of elimination, as well as a discussion of the effects of disruption of the normal processes of elimination on the chemical equilibrium and various organ systems of the body. Additionally, abnormal routes of elimination seen in the clinical situation will be discussed.

The reader is referred to Chapter 8 for a discussion of the elimination of carbon dioxide via the lungs. This chapter deals chiefly with the skin and kidneys as organs of elimination. Altered patterns of elimination via the gastrointestinal tract are only introduced in this chapter; specific disorders causing these disruptions are discussed in Chapter 13.

THE SKIN

The skin serves many important functions in maintaining homeostasis. First and foremost, the skin serves a protective function. It protects the internal organs from the effects of radiation, heat, cold, pressure, chemicals, and microorganisms. Specialized nerve endings in the skin provide cutaneous sensation, which makes an individual aware of potentially harmful conditions. The skin also is important in the retention of body fluids and temperature regulation.

The skin serves as an organ of elimination through perspiration. Under normal conditions, perspiration is more important in terms of body temperature regulation than as a process of elimination per se; however, significant disruption of the body's chemical equilibrium can occur as a result of alterations in the pattern of elimination via the skin.

The excretory function of the skin can be seen when renal failure and uremia occur. The concentration of urea in the perspiration increases. As evaporation takes place and drying occurs, crystals of urea form and appear as a white powder on the skin, usually referred to as *uremic frost*.

Perspiration helps to regulate not only body temperature but also excretion of fluid, sodium, and chloride. Insensible perspiration is mainly composed of water, while sensible perspiration is a hypotonic solution containing primarily sodium and chloride but also lesser amounts of potassium, magnesium, ammonia, and urea. The concentration of the solutes is variable, as is the total amount of perspiration excreted. The rate of excretion depends on environmental temperature and humidity, the amount of clothing worn, the metabolic rate and body temperature, and athletic or physical conditioning to extreme temperature.

Stimulation of the temperature-regulating center of the hypothalamus results in impulse transmission via the sympathetic system to the sweat glands. Upon stimulation the sweat glands secrete a precursor substance from which various substances are reabsorbed as the precursor substance flows through the duct portion of the glands. When sweat production is low, for example, in the basal state, the concentrations of sodium and chloride are also low, probably as a result of the reabsorption of these substances from the precursor secretion before it reaches the surface of the skin. As the rate of sweating increases, the rate of sodium and chloride reabsorption does not increase to a commensurate degree, and consequently the concentrations of sodium and chloride in the sweat increase. This is reflected in the difference between the electrolyte compositions of insensible and sensible perspiration. Reabsorption of sodium in the sweat glands is also under the control of aldosterone, which increases reabsorption of sodium in the ducts of the sweat glands in the same manner as it affects the kidney tubules. Chloride is reabsorbed along with the sodium in order to maintain electroneutrality.

The sodium concentration in perspiration normally is related to dietary intake, but even in the presence of a reduced or nonexistent intake of dietary sodium some sodium will continue to be lost in the sweat. Hence, a great sodium loss can occur as a result of sweating in the normal individual with a reduced intake of sodium. The electrolyte composition of perspiration may also be related to the presence of some underlying disease state. Excess sodium and chloride in the sweat is an important feature of cystic fibrosis. Parents of children with cystic fibrosis have also been found to have greater than normal concentrations of electrolytes in the sweat; however, these differences are of no diagnostic importance since the difference is relatively small. A higher than normal concentration of electrolytes in the sweat, which is nonspecific in nature, may also occur in the presence of chronic pulmonary disease. The normal electrolyte concentration in the sweat is higher in adults than in children. Persons who have become acclimated to a hot environment have a more efficient sweat mechanism; they sweat more, but the concentration of electrolytes in the sweat is less than that of the sweat of a person who has not become acclimated to a hot environment.

Altered elimination patterns

Excessive perspiration. Excessive perspiration can be the result of a variety of conditions, including a hot, dry environment, heavy clothing, vigorous activity or exercise, fever, and fear or anxiety. Sweating occurs in pathologic conditions accompanied by sympathetic stimulation. Sweat is hypotonic, so relatively greater amounts of water than electrolytes will be lost; however, serious depletion of both body water and sodium may occur if the dietary intake of fluid and sodium is restricted or impaired during periods of excessive perspiration. Persons with high electrolyte levels in their sweat are especially susceptible to the development of a sodium deficit. Children with cystic fibrosis must be given supplemental salt during the summer months, and their parents should be advised to watch for signs of sodium depletion. Perhaps the results of excessive perspiration without adequate replacement of water and sodium are best exemplified by the disorders known as heat exhaustion (see Chapter 6). Excessive sweating without water or salt replacement results in hypertonic contraction of the body fluid because water is lost in excess of solute (sodium). Excessive sweating with water replacement but without adequate salt replacement results in hypotonic contraction of the body fluid. The signs and symptoms of these disorders are discussed in Chapter 10.

Cessation of perspiration. Heat stroke is a serious disorder that results from the cessation of sweating following exposure to a hot and usually humid environment. The body is unable to dissipate heat, and the body temperature rises. If heat stroke is not treated, the body temperature will continue to rise, and cell death throughout the body will occur. Central nervous system dysfunction is a feature of this disorder in its prodromal stage; however, most victims are comatose before they receive medical attention (see Chapter 6).

Abnormal elimination due to altered skin integrity

Under normal conditions the skin functions as a barrier to prevent the loss of body fluid to the external environment. When the integrity of the skin is broken, the body may lose significant amounts of body fluid. The fluid lost as a result of open, draining wounds, bedsores, abrasions, or skin lesions such as those seen in exfoliative dermatitis and pemphigus is similar to plasma in terms of electrolyte composition and protein content. A significant disruption of body fluid homeostasis occurs when skin integrity is altered due to a thermal injury (see Chapters 6 and 10). In severe burns, fluid is lost until the burn wound heals or is grafted; therefore emphasis is placed on maintaining adequate fluid and electrolyte replacement, especially in the immediate postburn period.

THE GENITOURINARY TRACT

The organs of the genitourinary system include the kidneys, ureters, bladder, and urethra. The excretory product of this system is

urine, which is formed in the kidneys. The kidneys have excretory, regulatory, metabolic, and endocrine functions and are largely responsible for the control of body fluid homeostasis. The functions of the kidneys include the excretion of metabolic end products, notably the nitrogenous waste products, urea and creatinine. The kidneys can produce glucose under certain conditions. The endocrine functions include the secretion of erythropoietin and renin. Additionally the hydroxylation of 25-hydroxycholecalciferol (25-OH vitamin D_3) to 1,25-dihydroxycholecalciferol ($1,25[OH]_2D_3$), the active metabolite of vitamin D, takes place in the kidney. The presence of this substance is necessary for the parathyroid hormone to have any effect on bone resorption in the maintenance of calcium homeostasis. Maintenance of a constant volume and composition of the body fluids depends greatly on renal response to neural or humoral mediators. For this to occur, renal receptor and effector sites must be intact and functioning.

Kidneys' role

Regulation of body fluid volume, composition, and pH by the kidneys is achieved through selective excretion, which involves the processes of filtration, resorption, and secretion in the functional unit of the kidney, the nephron. The nephron contains the glomerulus in Bowman's capsule, the proximal tubule, Henle's loop, the distal tubule, and the collecting tubule. The nephron is supplied with two capillary beds: the glomerular, which is a high pressure system, and the peritubular, which is a low pressure system that incorporates the vasa recta. Fig. 11-1 illustrates the functional anatomy of the nephron.

Urine formation, composition, and excretion

As blood circulates through the glomerular capillary bed, *filtration,* the first step in urine formation, takes place across the glomerular membrane. Filtration is enhanced and occurs more rapidly here than in other capillary beds because of the high pressure system that exists and the unique construction of the glomerulus and the glomerular membrane (Fig. 11-2). The glomerular filtration rate (GFR) across the

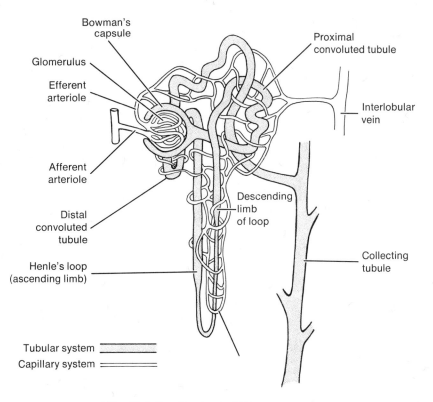

Fig. 11-1. Functional unit of kidney, nephron.

membrane is governed by the Starling forces and therefore is the difference between the sum of the hydrostatic and oncotic forces favoring filtration and the sum of those opposing it in proportion to the relative permeability of the membrane. This relationship is expressed by the following equation:

$$GFR = K_f \,(\textit{favoring forces} - \textit{opposing forces})$$

The favoring forces include the hydrostatic pressure of the glomerular capillary and the oncotic pressure of Bowman's capsule, while the opposing forces include the hydrostatic pressure of Bowman's capsule and the oncotic pressure of the plasma within the capillary. K_f is the filtration coefficient, which normally is a constant, and is a function of the area across which filtration occurs and the permeability of the membrane itself. Both the area and the permeability of the glomerular capillary membrane are greater than that of any other capillary bed within the body.

Changes in the glomerular filtration rate,

then, can be the result of changes in the permeability of the membrane, in the hydrostatic pressure on either side of the membrane, or in the oncotic pressure on either side of the membrane. The potential for alteration of the K_f exists when the glomerular membrane is affected by a pathologic process. The glomerular membrane is highly permeable to water and small solutes but demonstrates a selective permeability to larger solutes such as protein. This relative impermeability to the larger molecules accounts for the normal protein-free composition of the glomerular filtrate, which is similar to plasma in all other respects. This impermeability to protein is important also in maintenance of the plasma volume. The molecular charge of the larger molecules is thought to be responsible for this differential permeability. An example of this concept is the difference between the filtration ratios of albumin and dextran, two molecules of approximately equal size. Albumin normally carries a negative charge, while dextran carries no charge. The fil-

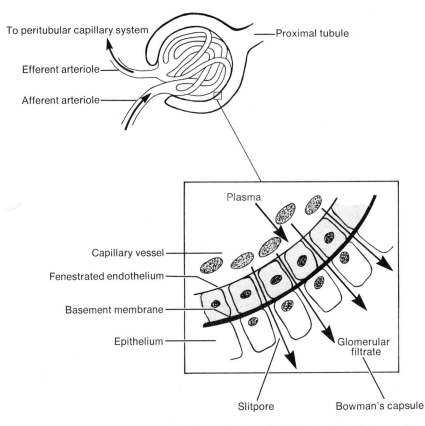

Fig. 11-2. Blood supply of glomerulus and schematic view of cellular structure of glomerular membrane.

tration rate of dextran is much greater than that of albumin under normal conditions. Dextran sulfate, which is the negatively charged form of dextran, is filtered in amounts similar to albumin, however. This effect is thought to be due to the presence of negatively charged proteins in the glomerular capillary wall, which cause electrostatic repulsion of anions in the plasma. Currently under investigation is the possibility that the loss of these negatively charged proteins from the capillary wall is responsible for the change in permeability that allows the increased filtration and urinary loss of protein seen in some renal diseases. A decrease in the surface area of the capillary bed may be the result of diseases in which glomeruli are destroyed or of surgical removal of part of the kidney.

The capillary hydrostatic pressure is determined by the systemic (aortic) pressure and the resistance afforded by the renal arterioles. Aortic pressure is not dissipated as readily in this system as it is in other capillary systems because of the anatomic structure of the renal arterial system. There are few subdivisions between the aorta and the glomerular capillary bed, and the arterial branches that do exist are short with relatively large diameters, allowing pressure to remain high within the system. The glomerular capillary bed, unlike others, is situated between two arterioles, and resistance to blood flow can be increased or decreased at either end, altering the hydrostatic pressure. Arteriolar resistance is intrinsically and sympathetically controlled in addition to being under hormonal control (angiotensin II and prostaglandins). Constriction of the afferent arteriole retards the flow of blood into the glomerular capillary, and both pressure and GFR decrease as a result. Constriction of the efferent arteriole retards blood flow out of the capillary bed, causing an increase in pressure and GFR. Dilation of the respective arterioles has the opposite effect. Intracapsular hydrostatic pressure may be disrupted by obstruction within the urinary tract. The back pressure from the obstruction will increase the hydrostatic pressure within Bowman's capsule, increasing the total of the forces opposing filtration.

As blood moves through the glomerular capillary bed and protein-free fluid is filtered from it, the plasma oncotic pressure rises as the plasma protein concentration increases. At the efferent arteriole, filtration equilibrium is reached, and the filtration gradient equals zero. The filtration gradient is directly related to the plasma oncotic pressure; thus, changes in the concentration of plasma proteins may alter the GFR. Loss of glomerular impermeability to protein will also alter the process of glomerular filtration. The rate of glomerular filtration is an important determinant of solute and water excretion.

The glomerular filtrate, an isotonic solution, is formed at the rate of 130 ml per minute. It is apparent, then, that the kidney tubules reabsorb large quantities of water and solutes. Through the mechanisms of tubular reabsorption and secretion the final composition of the urine is determined. Within the tubules also the kidneys concentrate and dilute urine and in this way maintain the osmolality of the body fluid. Substances are secreted or reabsorbed in the tubules by the process of (1) passive diffusion with electrical and chemical gradients or (2) active transport against such gradients. Segmental functions of the tubules are fairly specific and are summarized in Table 11-1. Most of the active transport processes take place in the proximal tubule, although Na^+ is actively transported out of the tubular fluid of the distal tubule and collecting ducts, and Cl^- is actively pumped out of the ascending limb of Henle's loops. These active transport processes can be inhibited. Pharmacologic treatment of gout is based on the ability of certain drugs to inhibit the mechanism responsible for reabsorption of uric acid.

The concentrating function of the tubules is under the control of ADH, which renders the

Table 11-1. Segmental functions of the renal tubules

Segment	Functions

Proximal tubule	Reabsorption
	  70% filtered H_2O and NaCl
	  Glucose
	  Urea
	  Uric acid
	  Amino acids
	  K^+, Mg^+, Ca^+, HPO^-
	Secretion
	  Organic acids and bases
	  H^+ and NH_3

Henle's loop	Reabsorption via countercurrent multiplier NaCl in excess of H_2O

Distal tubule	Reabsorption
	  Filtered H_2O and NaCl (small fraction only)
	Secretion
	  H^+, NH_3, K^+

Collecting ducts	Reabsorption
	  NaCl
	  H_2O (depends on ADH concentration)
	  Urea
	  K^+ (depends on aldosterone concentration)
	Secretion
	  H^+, NH_3 (pH of urine may be reduced to 4.5-5.0)
	  K^+ (depends on aldosterone concentration)

distal tubule and collecting duct permeable to water. The renal concentrating function also requires that the renal medulla interstitial fluid be hypertonic to plasma. The required medullary hypertonicity is maintained through the countercurrent multiplier and exchanger systems, illustrated in Fig. 11-3, operating within the renal medulla. The anatomic arrangement of the vasa recta allows blood to flow through this hypertonic area without diluting the interstitial fluid. The countercurrent multiplier effect is the result of the active transport of Na^+ without water into the medullary interstitium to increase its osmolality. The countercurrent exchanger arrangement of the blood supply maintains the resulting hypertonicity. The countercurrent mechanism allows a hypotonic urine to

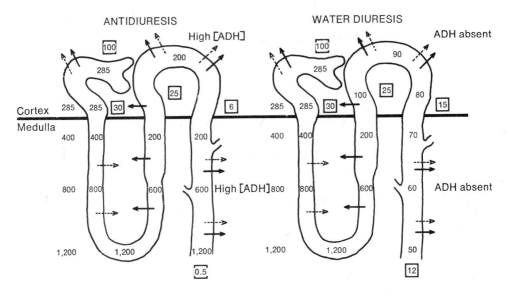

Fig. 11-3. Sodium chloride and water transport in nephron during antidiuresis and water diuresis. Tubular fluid and interstitial concentrations are expressed in mOsmol/kg: large boxed numbers represent percentage of glomerular filtrate remaining in tubule at each site. Note that composition and volume of tubular fluid are essentially the same at end of loop of Henle because excretion of a concentrated or dilute urine is determined primarily in distal tubule and collecting ducts. (From Clinical physiology of acid-base and electrolyte disorders by Rose, D. Copyright 1977 McGraw-Hill Book Co. Used with permission of McGraw-Hill Book Co.)

be delivered to the distal tubule and provides the osmotic gradient that allows the urine to become concentrated in the collecting tubules if ADH is present to increase that duct's permeability to water.

Altered elimination patterns

Disruption of urine formation and excretion will have profound effects on homeostasis. Manifestations of this disruption may include changes in the clearance rates of substances, changes in the amount and composition of the urine and the pattern of its excretion, elevated blood pressure, and the more extreme manifestations of the nephrotic syndrome and renal failure.

Clearance is a technique that allows assessment of renal function through comparison of the excretion rates of urinary substances with the plasma concentrations. Clearance values of substances for which excretion rates remain relatively constant or fixed such as urea and

creatinine provide information on the overall functional capacity of the kidney. Clearance values for substances whose excretion rates vary greatly from day to day, depending on the body's needs, reflect the adequacy of the kidneys' regulatory function.

The principal mechanisms for renal regulation of the composition of the body fluid include reabsorption of Na^+, Cl^-, and bicarbonate and the secretion of the hydrogen ion and K^+. There is a high correlation between the plasma Na^+ concentration and the rate of Na^+ excretion. The rate of Na^+ excretion is altered in the presence of renal disease. In some primary renal disease there is retention of Na^+. Glomerulonephritis is characterized by a reduction in the amount of Na^+ filtered. Retention of Na^+ and water occurs as a compensatory mechanism to restore plasma volume in the patient with the nephrotic syndrome. A salt-losing nephritis may also occur in renal disease where there is selective damage to the

Na$^+$-reabsorbing mechanisms. The kidney is not responsive to mineralocorticoids, and the clinical picture will resemble that of hypovolemia. Where loss of nephron function has occurred, the solute load of remaining nephrons increases, causing an osmotic diuresis.

Osmotic diuresis is the result of an obligatory water load for excretion of substances that are nonreabsorbable (mannitol) or that are present in concentrations that exceed tubular reabsorptive capacity. The diuresis causes an increased loss of sodium chloride and water and is manifested by *polyuria*. In diabetes mellitus, glucose is present in concentrations that exceed tubular reabsorptive capacity so it acts as an osmotic diuretic, causing one of the classic manifestations of that disease, namely, polyuria.

Impairment of the ability to concentrate or dilute the urine may be a manifestation of primary renal disease as well as some other conditions. The inability to concentrate the urine is manifested by polyuria and thirst. If water intake is inadequate, there may also be signs of water loss (see Chapter 10). The inability to dilute the urine may result in water retention if water ingestion is not restricted. Hypo-osmolarity and hyponatremia will develop. If the positive water balance develops rapidly or is great enough, water intoxication will ensue. The concentrating and diluting abilities of the kidney are related to the permeability of the tubules to water, which is controlled by ADH. Syndromes associated with alterations in ADH secretion are discussed later in this chapter. Concentrating ability also depends on medullary hypertonicity, and diluting ability also depends on the delivery of the filtrate to the distal diluting site and sodium transport by the diluting segments.

An increase in blood pressure may also be a manifestation of renal disorders. The secondary hypertension that occurs in renal disease is not completely understood. It is felt that structural damage and changes in the kidney contribute to reduced renal blood flow, which activates compensatory mechanisms that increase blood pressure. The renin-angiotensin system is activated, and both renin and angiotensin II have vasoconstrictive actions. The subsequent sodium and water retention increase blood volume, which contributes to hypertension. Marked activation of the renin-angiotensin system, juxtaglomerular hyperplasia, and excessively high renin levels are the result of renal arterial obstruction. Conversely the kidney may sustain damage as a result of a primary hypertension. Moderate hypertension causes ''benign'' nephrosclerosis, which is characterized by tubular atrophy and glomerular sclerosis (Fig. 9-12). Renal function usually remains fairly intact. Malignant hypertension causes malignant nephrosclerosis. Acute degenerative changes in the arteries and arterioles of the kidney lead to hemorrhagic lesions and basement membrane thickening in the glomerulus. Scarring occurs as the hemorrhagic lesions heal. Obstruction of the vascular bed occurs due to the progressive arterial changes and the scarring. Tubular atrophy and interstitial fibrosis eventually develop (Figs. 11-4 and 11-5). In the more advanced stage, nephrosclerosis impairs renal blood flow and GFR. Hypertension may also stimulate the development of the

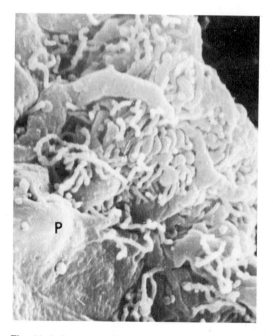

Fig. 11-4. Scanning electron micrograph of glomerulus in severely hypertensive person. Microvilli indicate some injury of podocytes, *P*. (×7,000.) (From Anderson, W. A. D., and Kissane, J. M.: Pathology, ed. 7, St. Louis, 1977, The C. V. Mosby Co.)

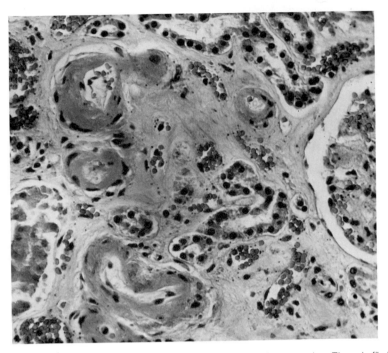

Fig. 11-5. Necrotizing arteriolitis in kidney from case of malignant hypertension. There is fibrinoid necrosis of walls of arterioles, which are swollen and eosinophilic. (Hematoxylin and eosin; ×280.) (From Anderson, W. A. D., and Kissane, J. M.: Pathology, ed. 7, St. Louis, 1977, The C. V. Mosby Co.)

nephrotic syndrome in the pregnant woman, leading to the condition known as *toxemia*.

Renal failure. As stated earlier, the major function of the kidneys is the maintenance of body fluid homeostasis, that is, maintaining the volume, composition, and pH of the body fluid within normal limits. Disruption of all these aspects is demonstrated in the most extreme manifestation of kidney dysfunction, renal failure. The term *renal failure* indicates a loss of renal ability to respond to the ever changing physiologic conditions within the body. The loss of this ability is characterized by impaired volume regulation, electrolyte and acid-base imbalance, and retention of metabolic waste products.

Renal failure may be either acute or chronic. Acute renal failure develops suddenly and is usually reversible. Chronic renal failure develops slowly and is irreversible because of progressive destruction of the renal parenchyma.

The term *renal failure* should be differentiated from the terms azotemia and uremia, which describe clinical conditions that accompany renal failure. *Azotemia* refers to the accumulation of nitrogenous waste products (urea, creatinine, and uric acid) within the body. Azotemia may occur as a result of either circulatory or kidney failure. In circulatory failure these waste products are not delivered to the kidneys, and in kidney failure they are delivered to impaired kidneys which cannot excrete them. The elevated plasma levels of these substances are reflected in the high BUN and serum creatinine values. The retention of nitrogenous waste products is responsible for some of the symptomatology seen in renal failure.

Uremia is the term applied to the clinical syndrome accompanying renal failure when the metabolic and biochemical changes due to renal failure become grossly symptomatic. Impaired volume regulation, electrolyte and acid-base imbalances, and the retention of nitrogenous wastes form the basis of these pathophysiologic changes that affect every organ system in the body.

The degree of the manifestations of uremia may differ depending on whether the renal fail-

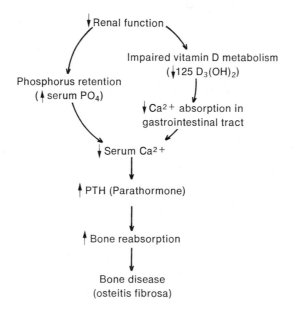

Fig. 11-6. Consequences of disease on nutritional status. Secondary hyperparathyroidism and bone disease occur in acute renal failure when there is retention of phosphorus, decreased absorption of calcium, and impacted vitamin D metabolism. (From Nutrition in clinical care by Howard, R., and Herbold, N. Copyright 1978 McGraw-Hill Book Co. Used with permission of McGraw-Hill Book Co.)

ure is acute or chronic; however, when uremia is severe and progressive, no matter what the cause, death is the ultimate result. The blood urea nitrogen (BUN) and creatinine levels will be high and are often used as an index of the severity of the uremia. The systemic toxicity seen in uremia is thought to be unrelated to the presence of these substances but to be related to the presence of other substances that have a toxic effect on the body and that, through the process of dialysis, can be removed. These toxic substances are believed to be produced through metabolism and normally excreted via the kidneys. They remain unidentified at this time. Some of the signs and symptoms are related to the abnormal volume composition and pH of the body fluid that result when renal control and regulation are impaired.

The clinical manifestations of uremia reveal the widespread effect of the loss of normal renal function on every system of the body. Anemia appears to be related to a decreased red blood cell production and shortened red cell life. Erythropoiesis is depressed as the damaged kidneys cannot produce normal amounts of erythropoietin. Increased red cell destruction may be a direct effect of toxic substances in the blood but may also be due to mechanical factors, as the renal lesions may be traumatic to the red cells as they pass through the renal vascular bed. Defective platelet function is thought to be the cause of the bleeding tendency seen in uremia. Purpuric lesions are often observed on the skin of the uremic patient. Bleeding in the gastrointestinal tract may also occur. Other commonly seen gastrointestinal problems include anorexia, nausea, vomiting, and diarrhea due to a nonspecific gastroenteritis. Pancreatitis may develop due to plugged pancreatic ducts.

Signs of the effect of uremia on the central nervous system are varied and include lethargy, mental depression, tremors and twitching, weakness, and, in more severe or advanced cases, convulsions and coma. These signs and symptoms are probably also related to the electrolyte and acid-base imbalances that are inevitably present. Acidosis, hypocalcemia, increased serum phosphate, hypernatremia, or hyperkalemia may be present. Peripheral neuropathies may also be quite irritating to the patient.

The uremic patient appears to be more susceptible to infection. The immune system is thought to be depressed, which is evidenced by an impaired ability to reject transplanted tissue. Infection in the uremic patient may be overwhelming. Hypervolemia due to Na^+ and H_2O retention may cause pulmonary edema and heart failure. Pulmonary congestion in the uremic patient has been labeled *uremic pneumonitis*. Pericarditis sometimes develops for reasons unknown at this time.

Bone disease is also a fairly common finding and develops via several interacting, complex mechanisms. The damaged kidneys are unable to convert vitamin D to its active form, which results in defective Ca^{++} absorption from the gastrointestinal tract. The serum Ca^{++} concentration may also be depressed as a result of the decrease in GFR, which in turn allows plasma phosphate levels to rise. The hypocalcemia and increased serum phosphate levels serve as a stimulus for increased parathyroid hormone secretion. This causes increased bone resorption (osteomalacia) and hyperplasia of the parathyroid glands (Fig. 11-6).

Acidosis is a major problem in the uremic patient. Acidosis is the result of failure of the kidneys to excrete hydrogen ions and to reabsorb bicarbonate ions. Impaired renal function also allows the accumulation of anions (phosphate and sulfate), which also contributes to the development of acidosis.

Acute renal failure (ARF), the abrupt cessation of renal function, is usually manifested by a urinary output of less than 400 ml per 24-hour period. Complete anuria is seldom seen, and after 10 to 12 days, the oliguric phase of ARF ends, and the diuretic phase begins. Acute renal failure may be the result of a diverse array of diseases and physiologic insults to the body.

A variety of pathologic processes may precipitate acute renal failure, and it is sometimes classified according to prerenal, renal, and postrenal causes. *Prerenal* causes include those conditions in which blood flow to the kidneys is disturbed or in which systemic changes affect kidney function indirectly. *Postrenal* causes include conditions in which the function of the urinary tract is disrupted (obstruction). *Renal* causes are those conditions in which the primary pathologic process occurs within the kidney itself.

The most common cause of acute renal failure is acute tubular necrosis, which may be the result of a variety of disease processes. The mechanisms by which acute tubular necrosis (ATN) occurs include ischemia and direct toxic damage. Sometimes both mechanisms interact in the pathogenesis of ATN. Various drugs and poisons are known to exert a toxic effect on the renal tubules, for example, carbon tetrachloride and ethylene glycol. Mercuric chloride damages tubules directly, but the effects of poisoning on the whole blood cause decreased renal perfusion due to vasomotor collapse, and thus ischemic damage of the tubules is also thought to play a role.

Various theories have been advanced to explain the pathogenesis of acute renal failure after the causative event has occurred. These theories include:

1. The back leak theory: glomerular filtrate leaks into the renal interstitium due to the disrupted integrity of the tubular epithelium and is reabsorbed by the renal capillaries.

2. Tubular obstruction: obstruction occurs as a result of tubular edema or intraluminal debris such as casts and breakdown products of hemoglobin and myoglobin. This theory applies to ARF seen after severe crushing injury in which myoglobin is released in large amounts.

3. Vascular theory: vasoconstriction of the afferent arteriole or vasodilation of the efferent arteriole leads to poor renal perfusion. Decreased permeability of the glomerular membrane must also be considered as a possible factor in this theory.

4. Cell swelling: an ischemic event reduces the amount of metabolic energy available for the active transport process of sodium pumping out of the cell. Because cell membranes are permeable to Na^+, Na^+ would diffuse into the cell, and the resultant rise in cellular osmolarity would cause an osmotic movement of H_2O into the cell. This swelling decreases blood flow and promotes the persistence of ischemia.

5. Renin-angiotensin: according to this theory, tubular dysfunction due to ischemia or toxic injury causes an increased intraluminal Na^+ concentration. Sensed at the macula densa (see Chapter 14), the increased Na^+ concen-

tration stimulates the release of renin, and thus the renin-angiotensin system is activated. Renin and angiotensin II cause constriction of the afferent arteriole.

Chronic renal failure, or renal insufficiency, develops more slowly than acute renal failure. This renal insufficiency is typified by loss of functioning nephrons, which increases the solute load of the remaining functioning nephrons.

Nephrotic syndrome. The presence of protein in the urine is a fairly consistent manifestation of diffuse renal disease. Regardless of the cause of the primary disease process, the symptomatology will ultimately be related to the loss of protein from the body. The pathologic defect basic to proteinuria is usually increased permeability of the glomerular membrane (an exception is the excretion of Bence Jones proteins in multiple myeloma, which is not related to a primary renal defect). The severity of the clinical manifestations is related to the extent of the protein loss. As protein stores are depleted, the resulting aggregate of clinical signs known as the nephrotic syndrome develops: proteinuria, hypoalbuminemia, edema, hyperlipidemia, and lipiduria. The urine appears foamy. Nephrotic crises, which are episodes of severe hypoalbuminemia and anasarca associated with anorexia, nausea, vomiting, and abdominal pain, occur occasionally, but their cause is unknown. A protein loss of 3 g per day or more will precipitate the nephrotic syndrome.

As body protein stores are depleted, hepatic synthesis of albumin is reduced, which reduces the albumin content of the blood. This results in a decreased plasma oncotic pressure, which favors the transudation of fluid into the interstitial spaces. In patients with the nephrotic syndrome there is a generalized, soft, pitting edema with periorbital swelling. Circulating plasma volume is reduced, and sodium retention is stimulated. Lymph flow does increase, and in patients with gross fluid retention, dilated lymphatics can often be identified over the flanks and buttocks.

Because low-molecular-weight plasma proteins (e.g., albumin) are lost preferentially in the urine, high-molecular-weight proteins such as the lipoproteins remain in the plasma. This

contributes to the hyperlipidemia and hypercholesterolemia. The liver also increases its production of cholesterol. The lipiduria is probably the result of increased filtration of some of the smaller lipoprotein molecules and cholesterol esters.

Nephrotic syndrome accompanies those primary renal diseases characterized by glomerular damage, especially membranous and focal glomerulonephritis. The nephrotic syndrome is seen in approximately 5% of patients with systemic lupus erythematosus (SLE) and in 10% to 20% of patients with diabetes mellitus. Diabetic patients with nephrotic syndrome usually exhibit retinal microaneurysms, diastolic hypertension, azotemia due to reduced renal function, and superimposed congestive heart failure.

The causes of nephrotic syndrome can be categorized as follows:

1. Immune complex, autoantibody, or hypersensitivity disease (Figs. 11-7 and 11-8)
2. Hereditary or congenital

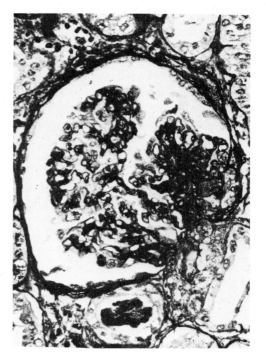

Fig. 11-7. Focal glomerular sclerosis. (From Anderson, W. A. D., and Kissane, J. M.: Pathology, ed. 7, St. Louis, 1977, The C. V. Mosby Co.)

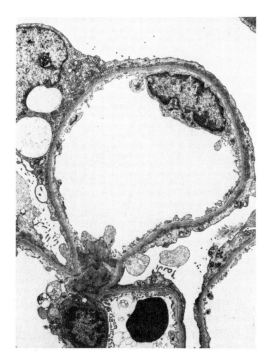

Fig. 11-8. Lipoid nephrosis (minimal change in disease). Note foot flattening. (×4,000.) (From Anderson, W. A. D., and Kissane, J. M.: Pathology, ed. 7, St. Louis, 1977, The C. V. Mosby Co.)

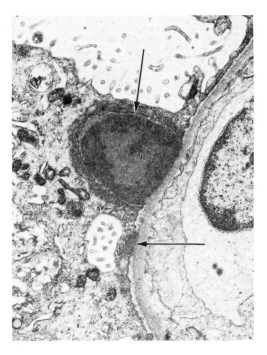

Fig. 11-9. Acute poststreptococcal glomerulonephritis. "Humps" of immune complex outside basement membrane are indicated by arrows. (×60.) (From Anderson, W. A. D., and Kissane, J. M.: Pathology, ed. 7, St. Louis, 1977, The C. V. Mosby Co.)

3. Metabolic disease (sarcoidosis and diabetes mellitus)
4. Pregnancy-induced toxemia
5. Circulatory disease (bilateral renal vein thrombosis)

Treatment of nephrotic syndrome due to primary renal disease is directed toward relief of edema and correction of the hypoproteinemia. Increased dietary protein will provide nitrogen necessary for protein synthesis and build up depleted nitrogen stores (restore positive nitrogen balance). Depending on the cause of nephrotic syndrome, corticosteroid therapy may be successful.

The term *nephrosis* should be differentiated from the nephrotic syndrome. Nephrosis is a term applied to a variety of lesions that are pathologically unrelated. Hence, its meaning, in general, is quite ambiguous and is not always used synonymously with the nephrotic syndrome.

Major causes of altered elimination

The major mechanisms by which primary disruption of genitourinary elimination occurs include inflammation, obstruction, and altered ADH regulation. The mechanisms of disease processes other than primary renal disease that alter genitourinary function are reviewed in terms of the effect they have on renal function. These disease processes are developed in more detail in other chapters of the book.

Inflammation. Inflammation induced by immunologic processes is the basis of the glomerular damage that occurs in a group of diseases classified as *glomerulonephritis*. The primary lesions are glomerular, and other anatomic changes in the kidney occur secondary to them. Glomerular damage has been demonstrated experimentally to be the result of two major immunologic processes: the deposition of antigen-antibody complexes in the glomerular walls and an antibody reaction with antigens

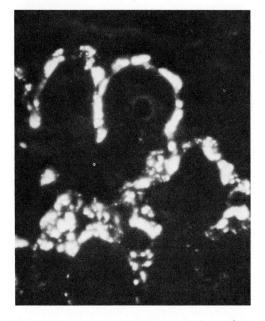

Fig. 11-10. Acute poststreptococcal glomerulonephritis. "Humps" of immune complex stained with fluorescent antihuman complement (C3). (×1,000.) (Courtesy Dr. C. Cornwall, Syracuse, N.Y. From Anderson, W. A. D., and Kissane, J. M.: Pathology, ed. 7, St. Louis, 1977, The C. V. Mosby Co.)

in the glomerular basement membrane (Figs. 11-9 and 11-10).

Acute, diffuse proliferative glomerulonephritis is also referred to as acute poststreptococcal glomerulonephritis; it is the most commonly seen type of glomerulonephritis. The immunologic mechanism in this disorder appears to be the deposition of antigen-antibody complexes within the glomerular walls. This inflammatory disorder occurs at all ages but is frequently seen in children and young adults. It usually follows an acute respiratory or skin infection caused by group A hemolytic streptococci. There is often a latent period between the acute infection and the onset of the glomerulonephritis, which usually develops within 1 to 4 weeks after the onset of the infection. The factors that predispose an individual to the development of streptococcal infection are discussed in Chapter 9.

Glomerular permeability is increased, allowing the escape of protein and red blood cells from the plasma into the urine. There is also a loss of functional glomerular surface area. The

net effect is a reduction in the GFR. The clinical manifestations include a reduction in urinary volume (oliguria) and excretion of a brownish, smoky urine with a high specific gravity, reflecting the proteinuria and hematuria. There is usually a slight to moderate increase in blood pressure, which is thought to result from decreased renal blood flow and the subsequent activation of the renin-angiotensin system. Headache may also be a complaint. Edema occurs and is usually seen as puffiness of the eyelids in the morning that gradually subsides during the day. Edema sometimes becomes severe and generalized. Fluid volume does become expanded as a compensatory mechanism. Treatment is symptomatic, and prevention of complications is of utmost concern. Bed rest is indicated during the acute phase. Sodium and fluid restriction and the use of diuretic and antihypertensive agents may be needed if the edema and hypertension are severe. When edema and hematuria are gone, blood urea nitrogen (BUN) levels return to normal.

Ninety-five percent of the children who develop this disease recover completely. In adults the condition is usually more serious, with only 60% to 70% recovering completely. Death may occur from complications, including acute heart failure or acute renal failure. In others the glomerular lesions persist and progressively worsen, usually causing death from hypertension and renal failure within 2 years. These patients are then classified as having rapidly progressive glomerulonephritis, which also sometimes occurs for no apparent cause.

Proteinuria that persists for several months is consistent with recovery. However, when proteinuria persists for a year or more, it is likely that the glomerular damage is progressing, although there is no clinical manifestation of this. The possibility of progressive glomerular damage is increased if there are also red blood cells and leukocytes in the urine. These patients are most likely to develop chronic glomerulonephritis. There are other types of glomerulonephritis, all of which may eventually reach an end stage in which glomerular function is so depressed that chronic renal failure characterized by uremia and hypertension develops. The rate of progression to this end stage is determined by the type and severity of the preceding glomerulonephritis syndrome. This end stage is referred to as *chronic glomerulonephritis.*

Most patients who develop chronic glomerulonephritis are between 40 and 50 years old. In 70% of the patients there is no clinical history of prior renal disease. In these cases it is often impossible to decide what type of silent glomerulonephritis was present. Pathologic changes in the kidneys in this syndrome include a uniform and equal reduction in size with diffuse thinning of the cortex. The surface may be highly granular, and the renal arteries and branches show arteriosclerotic thickening. If hypertension is present, cortical mottling and hemorrhage may be superimposed on the other pathologic changes.

Severe hypertension accompanying chronic glomerulonephritis will aggravate renal destruction, and renal failure will progress rapidly to death. Where hypertension is less severe, the progress of the renal failure will be much slower, and chronic glomerulonephritis will continue for years.

Pyelonephritis is a bacteria-induced inflammatory disorder involving the renal pelvis,
calices, and parenchyma (Fig. 11-11). It usually occurs secondary to lower urinary tract infection that has ascended. The most common causative organism is *Escherichia coli*. Urinary tract infections occur most frequently in females. Pyelonephritis may occur in acute or chronic forms and may affect one or both kidneys. The acute form causes death only when it occurs bilaterally and is extensive. Particularly when recurrent, the less severe forms may progress to chronic pyelonephritis, which is a leading cause of chronic renal failure.

The most common site of urinary tract infection is the bladder, and it is highly likely that cystitis is a factor in most cases of pyelonephritis. There is evidence that occurrence of the vesicoureteral reflex (reflux of urine from the bladder into the ureters) is enhanced in cystitis. As a result of the inflammatory process, swelling of the ureterovesical valves may cause them to function incompetently. Once the bacteria reach the kidney, they proliferate, and an inflammatory response ensues, often with abscess formation. The irregular and patchy renal lesions seen are characteristic of the random manner in which the bacteria spread from the infected calyces.

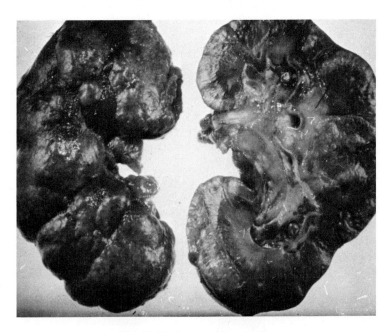

Fig. 11-11. Acute pyelonephritis.

Bacteriuria of over 100,000 organisms per milliliter of urine usually indicates a urinary tract infection. This can reflect infection at any point along the urinary tract. An important determination is whether the renal parenchyma has been involved. A high titer of serum antibody to the infecting bacteria and cellular casts in the urine are fairly accurate indications that the kidneys have been affected. Pyuria can be the result of infection along any portion of the urinary tract. Significant bateriuria in the absence of symptoms of urinary tract infection has been found in the aged and in approximately 1% of healthy schoolgirls and 5% of pregnant women. On reexamination some children have been found to have developed chronic pyelonephritis following symptomless bacteriuria.

Some of the factors that predispose a person to the development of urinary tract infection include urinary tract obstruction, structural abnormalities, certain disease states where resistance to infection is reduced, diabetes mellitus, where there is a general susceptibility to infection, and pregnancy in which uretheric dilatation and stasis of urine occur. Patients with urinary tract obstruction are more likely to develop pyelonephritis for the following reasons: (1) the stagnant urine serves as a culture medium for bacterial growth; (2) obstruction in the absence of structural changes predisposes to intermittent vesicoureteral reflux, and prolonged, partial obstruction causes thickening and dilation of the ureters, which often allows free reflux of urine; (3) obstruction appears to reduce the kidneys' ability to resist infection; and (4) obstruction may lead to renal failure—a condition in which general susceptibility to infection is increased.

The clinical manifestations of acute pyelonephritis include frequency of urination, dysuria, fever, pain and tenderness in the lumbar area, and other systemic signs of an inflammatory process. The clinical manifestations of the chronic form may include a vague history of ill health with a reduced growth rate in children. Urinary constituents may or may not be abnormal, depending on whether the infection is still active. The presenting features are usually hypertension (which occurs in 70% of all patients with chronic pyelonephritis) and the uremia of chronic renal failure.

Obstruction. The major effect of urinary tract obstruction is interference with the flow of urine. An obstruction can occur anywhere along the urinary tract, and the effects depend on whether it is a partial or a complete obstruction. If the obstruction is complete, anuria will be a manifestation, with eventual development of renal failure if the obstruction is unrelieved. Incomplete obstruction results in dilatation of the collecting system. Back pressure from obstruction is eventually transmitted to the kidney. Intracapsular hydrostatic pressure increases, and the GFR decreases. If renal blood flow becomes compromised, ischemic damage to the kidneys can occur with the resultant functional loss of nephrons. This damage may be permanent if the obstruction is of a severe and prolonged nature.

The possible causes of obstruction are many and varied. Obstruction can result from congenital defects in the urinary tract. The position or structure of the organs may be such that urine flow is impeded. Obstruction can result from tumor growth within or outside the urinary tract. Pressure from growth of a tumor of the tissue surrounding the urinary tract may be enough to impair the free drainage of urine. Calculi may form and become lodged in the ureters. Strictures of the ureters or urethra may result from inflammatory damage secondary to infection.

The clinical manifestations of obstruction depend on the cause and extent of the obstruction. Anuria will be present with complete obstruction. With lesser degrees of obstruction, dysuria, hematuria, frequency, dribbling, and nocturia may occur and alter the normal pattern of elimination. If an infectious process is present, the temperature may be elevated. Renal colic is usually intermittent but severe and may radiate from the flank. This pain is thought to be related to the abnormal increase in pressure distal to the obstruction in the renal pelvis. These patients appear pale and anxious, and sometimes they are afraid to move for fear that movement will aggravate the pain. If a renal calculus was the source of the obstruction and it is suddenly relieved, relief from the pain will be immediate.

The more common causes of obstruction are urinary calculi and bladder neck obstruction due to benign prostatic hypertrophy. The appearance of renal calculi is often related to the presence of an excessive amount of calcium in the urine. Hypercalciuria may also occur as a result of hyperparathyroidism, or it may be that idiopathic infection predisposes to stone formation since calcium and phosphate are more soluble at a lower pH, and infection causes urinary pH to rise. The incidence of calculi is increased in patients with hyperuricemia also.

Benign prostatic hypertrophy occurs in men after the age of 50. Hypertrophy may take place in the muscular or glandular structures or both. The reason for the hypertrophy is not completely clear but is thought to be related to changes in the relative amounts of estrogen and androgen due to the aging process. The hypertrophy may impinge on the urethra, the bladder, or both, depending on the portion of the gland that is hypertrophied. The urethra becomes distorted and displaced, and urine flow is impeded. If the bladder wall is also affected such that the normal contour of the bladder is changed, allowing the development of dependent areas within it, complete emptying of the bladder will also be impaired, and urinary stasis will occur in these areas. Stasis predisposes to calculi formation and the development of infection. A complication of prostate hypertrophy is chronic prostatitis, the development of inflammation or infection within the glandular tissues themselves.

Treatment of obstruction is aimed at restoring the normal flow of urine, which sometimes must be done surgically. Another goal of treatment is restoration of normal fluid and electrolyte balance, which may have been disrupted by the obstructive process. If chronic renal damage has occurred, this will be treated through methods already discussed elsewhere.

Altered ADH regulation. Antidiuretic hormone (ADH), or arginine vasopressin, is a hormone synthesized in the supraoptic and paraventricular nuclei in the hypothalamus. The hormone is stored in the posterior lobe of the pituitary. The major stimuli to ADH release are an increase in plasma osmolality and a decrease in the effective circulating volume. Control of plasma osmolality is related to the interaction of ADH release and thirst, which promotes water retention (see Chapter 10). ADH promotes water retention by increasing the permeability of the collecting tubules to water. In the presence of ADH a concentrated urine is excreted. In the absence of ADH a dilute urine is excreted. ADH acts by stimulating collecting-duct adenyl cyclase, which causes the generation of cyclic AMP, which activates a protein kinase responsible for increasing water permeability of the ducts.

Diabetes insipidus is the term applied to a clinical syndrome characterized by diuresis of an extremely dilute urine. The renal concentrating ability is reduced because of a failure of ADH secretion (central diabetes insipidus) or lack of renal response to ADH secretion (nephrogenic diabetes insipidus). An extra 1,200 ml of water will be lost in the urine each day as a result of this. A person with an intact thirst mechanism will maintain normal water balance by increasing his intake. A defect in the thirst mechanism or the inability to ingest water in the presence of this syndrome may result in excessive water loss and an increase in plasma concentration. Patients with central diabetes insipidus will have low levels of circulating ADH, and their polyuria is vasopressin responsive, which constitutes a basis for therapy. This is in contrast to patients with nephrogenic diabetes insipidus, who have normal circulating levels of ADH and vasopressin-resistant polyuria.

Central diabetes insipidus is characterized by loss of renal concentrating ability because of insufficient ADH secretion. The conditions in which the function of the hypothalamus and its tract is disrupted cause central diabetes insipidus. Loss of the posterior pituitary may produce a transient polyuric period. One half the cases of central diabetes insipidus are idiopathic in origin and are thought to reflect cellular degeneration in the hypothalamic nuclei. Other causes include trauma (accidental or surgical, especially hypophysectomy), neoplasms, and hypoxemic encephalopathy.

Symptoms of polyuria and polydipsia begin abruptly in the majority of cases. There is a typical triphasic response following trauma, which is seen clinically after hypophysectomy. During the first 4 to 5 days after the trauma a polyuric state exists that probably represents inhibition of the release of the stored ADH due to hypothalmic dysfunction. This is followed by a 5-day antidiuretic phase, which represents the release of stored ADH from the posterior pituitary. Permanent central diabetes insipidus follows the antidiuretic phase.

Nephrogenic diabetes insipidus may be congenital or acquired, although the congenital form is rare. Acquired nephrogenic diabetes insipidus can be the result of a variety of conditions. The mechanisms through which the lack of renal response to ADH occurs include decreased generation of cyclic AMP, reduced cyclic AMP effect, and interference with the countercurrent function and renal medullary hypertonicity. For example, impaired renal concentrating ability is seen in hypercalcemia and hypokalemia regardless of the cause of the electrolyte imbalance. Research with animals has demonstrated impaired cyclic AMP generation and reduction of medullary hypertonicity. In sickle cell anemia the countercurrent mechanism is impaired due to the sickling of red blood cells in the vasa recta. Hyposthenuria is common since the hypertonicity and low Po_2 of the blood and tortuosity of the vessels in this system favor the sickling process. In renal failure, anatomic changes as well as increased solute excretion per nephron contribute to the loss of renal concentrating ability. Polyuria in patients with renal insufficiency is limited by the loss of functioning nephrons. Various drugs can also impair the ability of the kidneys to respond to ADH. Table 11-2 lists disorders associated with nephrogenic diabetes insipidus and the mechanisms by which they act to limit the renal response to ADH.

In contrast to diabetes insipidus, inappropriate secretion of ADH may also occur in which the ability to maximally dilute the urine is lost. In the *syndrome of inappropriate ADH secretion* (SIADH), water is retained due to enhanced tubular reabsorption, and expansion dilution of the body fluid will occur if normal water intake continues. If the water intake is restricted, water retention will not occur, and the plasma Na^+ concentration will remain normal. Even though plasma sodium concentration is lowered by dilution, the plasma bicarbonate and potassium levels remain unaffected for the most part. Maintenance of HCO_3 concentration appears to be related to the movement of H^+ into the cells and excretion of H^+ in the urine. Intracellular potassium moves out of the cells to maintain plasma K^+ levels and is probably linked to the H^+ movement. A mild hypokalemia may develop.

The mechanisms by which SIADH occurs include increased hypothalamic secretion, ectopic production of ADH, potentiation of the ADH effect, and exogenous administration of ADH. Table 11-3 lists the conditions associated with

Table 11-2. Conditions associated with nephrogenic diabetes insipidus

Mechanism	Conditions
Decreased permeability of collecting ducts through decreased cyclic AMP generation and effect	Hypokalemia Hypercalcemia Congenital (rare) Drugs (lithium, dimethyl chlortetracycline)
Impaired countercurrent function	Renal failure Hypokalemia Hypercalcemia Sickle cell anemia Osmotic diuresis Drugs (Lasix, Edecrin)

Table 11-3. Conditions associated with syndrome of increased ADH secretion

Mechanism	Conditions
Increased production of ADH by hypothalamus	Stress Idiopathic Cerebral neoplasms Disruption of cerebral circulation Infections: pulmonary and cerebral Drugs (Diabinese, Navane, Cytoxan) Miscellaneous: Guillain-Barré syndrome Endocrine disorders
Ectopic production of ADH by nonhypothalamic tissue	Carcinoma: lungs, bronchi, duodenum, pancreas
Potentiation of effect	Drugs (Diabinese)

these mechanisms. The enhanced hypothalamic secretion of ADH seen in certain neural disorders is not completely understood.

Essential hyponatremia has been described in patients with cerebral disorders and certain chronic diseases. It is thought that defective cell metabolism causes a decrease in cell osmolality, which causes the osmoreceptors to signal ADH secretion at a different level of plasma osmolality than normally signals the secretion of ADH. This resetting of the "osmostat" results in a lower plasma Na^+ concentration, which is considered normal for these patients.

THE GASTROINTESTINAL TRACT

The normal function of the gastrointestinal tract in terms of the body's elimination processes involves the formation and excretion of feces. This is accomplished through the mechanisms of ingestion, motility, secretion, digestion, and absorption, which are regulated and integrated by neural and hormonal factors. The membranes of the GI tract are highly specialized and allow an equilibrium to exist between the extracellular fluid and the secretions of the GI tract. Disruption of the normal cycling of body fluid between the extracellular compartment and the GI tract may result in a significant departure from the body's chemical equilibrium. The abnormal loss of GI secretions must be considered in terms of the relative concentration of electrolytes within the fluid in order to predict the ultimate effect of that loss on the body's chemical equilibrium (see Table 10-3 for a listing of the electrolytic composition of various GI secretions). Abnormal elimination through the GI tract may occur via the mechanisms of vomiting, diarrhea, fistulas, and gastric suction. The mechanisms and causes of vomiting and diarrhea are discussed in Chapter 13. The fluid lost is usually isotonic, and the most important deficits involve water and Na^+, with K^+ loss occurring in chronic or more severe diarrhea. Acid-base imbalances may also occur.

Vomiting and gastric suction. Vomiting and gastric suction result in loss of gastric juice, which is the most acid of all the gastrointestinal secretions. Its chief ions are hydrogen, sodium, chloride, and potassium. Loss of gastric juice is most frequently associated with metabolic alkalosis and deficits of sodium, potassium, and occasionally magnesium. If excessive loss occurs, fluid volume deficit may develop, as well as the ketosis of starvation since these patients are usually either unable to eat or are allowed nothing to eat. Ketosis is the result of excessive ketone body production due to metabolism of fat. In the absence of carbohydrate intake a magnesium deficit can also occur. The effects of starvation are discussed in detail in Chapter 12.

Diarrhea, intestinal suction, and ileostomy. Intestinal juice is alkaline and contains a relatively large amount of the potassium ion. Loss of intestinal juice is most often associated with metabolic acidosis and deficits of sodium, potassium, and bicarbonate. Intestinal secretions can be lost as a result of diarrhea, externally applied intestinal suction, or pathologic or surgically created fistulas. The term *diarrhea* is usually applied to a condition characterized by the frequent excretion of loose, runny stools. The basic mechanisms underlying the development of diarrhea are impaired absorption or increased secretion or a combination of these two mechanisms. Normally only 150 ml of water is lost in the stools daily, but this amount will be greatly increased in diarrhea because of its increased fluid content. Severe diarrhea can lead to daily loss of 5 to 10 liters of fluid, and diarrhea in the child can lead to severe fluid and electrolyte imbalances more rapidly than in the adult because of the relatively greater volume of body water in children (see Chapter 13). A fistula is an abnormal passage or opening between the intestines and some body cavity or the external environment. Some disease processes cause fistula formation and are discussed in detail in Chapter 13. An *ileostomy* is a surgically created fistula between the ileum and the abdominal wall, which allows the contents of the small intestine to drain.

SUMMARY

This chapter has presented an overview of the processes of elimination that occur via various routes in the body and the mechanisms by which disruption of the normal elimination processes and patterns may occur. Elimination processes constitute a major means of homeostatic control. It should be apparent to the reader that the loss of this control through disruption of normal elimination processes results in profound chemical disequilibrium, the effects and manifestations of which were discussed in Chapter 10. Restoration of chemical equilibrium is the primary goal of treatment in disorders of elimination; however, correction of the underlying cause of the altered elimination process is necessary to prevent the recurrence of chemical disequilibrium. The reliance on artificial means of maintaining chemical equilibrium becomes necessary in chronic states in which elimination processes are permanently impaired.

SUGGESTED READINGS

Anger, D.: The psychologic stress of chronic renal failure and long term hemodialisis, Nurs. Clin. North Am. **10**(3):449-460, 1975.

Brown, J., et al.: Renal hypertension: role for renin, Postgrad. Med. **53**(suppl. 3):31-34, 1977.

Brundage, D.: Nursing management of renal problems, St. Louis, 1976, The C. V. Mosby Co.

Fearing, M.: Osteodystrophy in patients with chronic renal failure, Nurs. Clin. North Am. **10**(3):461-468, 1975.

Leaf, A., and Cotran, R.: Renal pathophysiology, New York, 1976, Oxford University Press.

Llach, F.: Focusing on the nephrotic syndrome, Drug Ther. Bull. (hospital edition) **3**(2):15-27, 1978.

Michelis, M.: Treatment strategy for the nephrotic syndrome, Drug Ther. Bull., vol. 3, no. 2, 1978.

Schrier, R. W., editor: Renal and electrolyte disorders, Boston, 1976, Little, Brown & Co.

PART FIVE

Pathophysiology of nutritional balance

CHAPTER 12

Mechanisms of nutritional disequilibrium

AT THE COMPLETION OF THIS CHAPTER THE STUDENT WILL BE ABLE TO:

- Explain the interactions of factors that contribute to the metabolic rate and explain how these factors help the organism to maintain the steady state.
- Describe major food sources and explain the regulation of intake of these substances.
- Cite the causes of obesity and describe the abnormalities of adipocytes, blood lipids, and insulin regulation. Discuss ways in which these abnormalities act to disrupt the steady state.
- Describe ways in which starvation may be produced and the metabolic events through which energy is obtained in starving humans.
- Discuss causes of malnutrition and deficiency states and forms that they may take. Relate these states to pathophysiology.
- Describe forms of carbohydrate metabolism disruption and discuss the pathophysiologic mechanisms by which these states disturb normal nutrition.
- Discuss current ideas about the pathophysiology of diabetes mellitus, particularly with reference to the roles of insulin, glucagon, and somatostatin.
- Describe the ways in which juvenile and adult-onset diabetes are alike and how they differ.
- Discuss the diagnosis of diabetes and cite the major signs and symptoms of this disease, relating them to the pathophysiology of diabetes mellitus.
- Compare diabetes to starvation in terms of metabolism, compensatory mechanisms, and symptoms.
- Compare and contrast diabetic ketoacidosis, nonketotic coma, and lactic acidosis.
- Discuss the chronic pathophysiologic mechanisms perpetuated by the diabetic disease process and relate these to the development of specific organ damage.
- Discuss the implications of research into oral hypoglycemic agents and describe other treatment modalities for diabetes mellitus.
- Describe common abnormalities of protein, lipid, purine, and pyrimidine metabolism and ways in which these disorders disturb the steady state.

This chapter and Chapter 13 will focus on pathophysiologic disturbances of nutritional integrity. Nutritonal integrity implies that normal intake, digestion, absorption, metabolism, and elimination of food proceed without interruption or abnormality. Many systems of the body must be functioning well for this to occur. The integrity of the brain and nervous system is required for regulation of food intake in proper amounts when the organism requires caloric energy. The gastrointestinal (GI) tract's patency and normal physiology are required for food to be digested and absorbed. The circulatory system, as the main transport system in movement of nutrients from the GI tract to the liver, adipose tissue, and cells and tissues throughout the body, also plays a critical role in nutritional integrity. The liver and adipose tissue are the major metabolic organs regulating body nutrition and storage of excess calories, and they provide for homeostasis in the open system of food intake, metabolism, and waste disposal. At the cellular level the genetic enzyme complement and endocrine system appear to predominate in the control of food metabolism. Thus, the maintenance of nutrition is a function of all the systems and involves complex mechanisms resulting from the interaction of a great variety of influences.

This chapter will cover various pathophysiologic mechanisms by which nutritional status can be disturbed. These include disorders of food intake and metabolism; some disease models of various nutritional disorders will also be discussed. Specific diseases of the GI tract will be covered in Chapter 13.

METABOLISM

The total processes by which ingested food molecules are utilized either for work by the organism or in the synthesis of new organic compounds is summarized by the term *metabolism*. Man as an open system, constantly seeking the steady state, interacts extensively with the environment and in fact depends on the external environment for his supply of energy, in the form of food calories, and therefore for his very survival. Energy in the molecular bonds of food molecules is converted to work energy, or it may be stored in the organism's glycogen, lipid, and protein. Ultimately all energy that is taken in is returned to the environment, so that the second law of thermodynamics is not violated by living organisms. Energy must be supplied by the ingestion, digestion, absorption, and metabolism of food molecules in order for any physiologic function to proceed. The ultimate source of this energy is, of course, derived from the photons of sunlight, which is converted into food molecules by photosynthesis in green plants. It is therefore the task of metabolism to release in a usable form the energy contained in the carbon-hydrogen bonds of food molecules. The way that the released energy is coupled to function in the cell is determined by the genetic and environmental factors of the particular cell, tissue, or organ. These factors are usually dynamic in nature, as the constantly changing expression of DNA in all cells in response to the external influences will determine the ultimate metabolism of food molecules and the way they are used for energy.

Catabolism and anabolism are the metabolic processes. *Catabolism* is the release of energy in carbon-hydrogen bonds, with some energy being given off as heat and some being coupled to work by the cell. Most functions that require energy for work in the cell, such as movement, cell division, ion transport, and growth, are driven by catabolic reactions. *Anabolic* (synthetic) reactions require energy as well, which is provided by the catabolism of other molecules. Thus, both anabolism and catabolism are inevitably linked, and both require the breakdown of carbon-hydrogen bonds in food molecules.

In order for the energy from food molecules to be used by the cell for work, coupling of this extracted energy to the specific function must take place. The ATP (adenosine triphosphate) molecule is the form in which energy from metabolism is used by the cell. ATP contains high-energy bonds, which when hydrolyzed yield large amounts of free energy. Through oxidative phosphorylation the energy originally present in glucose is transformed into ATP energy. This is accomplished by oxidation of glucose to CO_2 and water through the series of metabolic reactions that comprise the Embden-Meyerhof pathway, the Krebs cycle, and the electron transport chain. The latter two reaction sequences take place in the cytoplasmic mitochondria, organelles whose characteristics have previously been described (see Chapter 7).

The actual coupling of the ATP molecule to cellular work involves intermediate molecules, which are phosphorylated by ATP. The mechanics of such coupling and the identification of intermediate molecules have not been clarified at this date. These reactions are exceedingly complex, as evidenced by the sodium-potassium pump mechanism present in most human cells. It is known that calcium, phospholipid, and ATPase, an enzyme that hydrolyzes ATP, are required for this ion movement, and a number of possible intermediate molecules have been suggested, but the details of sodium pumping are still only known in a rudimentary fashion.

The food molecules ingested by humans normally consist of 40% fats, 45% to 50% carbohydrates, and 12% to 24% proteins. Other molecules that are part of the normal diet (e.g., vitamins, minerals, and nucleotides) are also necessary in order for metabolism to proceed but are not directly hydrolyzed or oxidized by body tissue for extraction of chemical bond energy. The bonds between carbon and hydrogen determine the structure and the energy content of the food molecule; the mechanism by which this energy is extracted is through the biochemical pathways of the cells, which are mediated by enzymes and regulated by the energy needs of the body. The food molecules contain a standard amount of extractable energy, which is measured in *kilocalories*. A kilocalorie is a measure of heat energy. It is the amount of heat needed to raise the temperature of 1 kg of water 1 C.

The oxidation of 1 g of fat releases 9.3 kcal, of 1 g of carbohydrate 4.1 kcal, and of 1 g of protein 4.4 kcal. Determination of the caloric value of different foodstuffs is made by burning appropriate amounts of food and measuring the heat produced in a device known as a *bomb calorimeter*. Another method is determination of oxygen utilization by the oxidation of the food. Animals can be placed in bomb calorimeters to determine the amount of heat liberated by their bodies in the oxidation of their food, or the indirect method may be used, in which case the oxygen utilization and the carbon dioxide release are measured. From these values the *respiratory quotient* can then be calculated:

$$RQ = \frac{\text{Volume of } CO_2 \text{ released}}{\text{Volume of } O_2 \text{ consumed}} \Big/ \text{Unit time}$$

Different food molecules will be metabolized in a living organism with different respiratory quotients. The RQ is in a sense the measure of efficiency of metabolism of the different food molecules. Since the metabolism of glucose requires 6 moles of O_2 and produces 6 moles of CO_2 and 6 moles of water, the ratio in the equation is 1.00. Fat oxidation and protein breakdown are less "efficient" in that the RQ for fats is 0.703 and for proteins is 0.802. RQ is useful, but it should not lead the reader to think that the body oxidizes one com-

pound at a time, even if this compound is presented to the body through ingestion of a meal to the exclusion of other food molecules. The RQ measured in humans is the sum of all the metabolism occurring in a unit of time. There is a metabolic pool of usable interconvertible food molecules in the body, and the liver plays the major role in maintaining the metabolic pool. The RQ does change with disease states, indicating the effect of disease on metabolism. For example, RQ is increased in hyperventilation and alkalosis and decreased in hypoventilation and acidosis. In hyperventilation large amounts of CO_2 are released, thus increasing the numerator of the RQ equation.

Basal metabolic rate (BMR)

When environmental variables such as temperature, nutrition, muscular movement, emotions, and disease states are excluded from the testing conditions, it is possible to measure the basal metabolism of a human being, a value that indicates the minimal energy state of that person in the waking state. It is reported as kilocalories per square meter of body surface per hour. Generally the value for males is higher than for females; the approximate value for a 20-year-old man is 41.4 and for a 20-year-old woman is 36.2. The BMR increases when food is ingested, in fever, during muscular exercise, with sympathetic stimulation, and with hyperactivity of the thyroid gland. It is decreased with sleep, prolonged malnutrition, age, and underactivity of the thyroid gland. In hyperthyroidism the BMR may be increased by 40% to 80% of normal, and with hypothyroidism it may be decreased from 25% to 40% of normal. The metabolism of food molecules in the body constantly supplies heat, which is, of course, required for thermoregulation, and the excess is given off to the environment. (A human can increase his BMR to produce heat [thermogenesis] in a cold environment by shivering but is not able to effectively lower his BMR in a hot environment.) Seventy percent of the energy in food becomes heat energy in the formation and coupling of ATP, and even more is lost when ATP hydrolysis and cellular work occur. Thus, large amounts of the energy in food molecules are returned directly to the

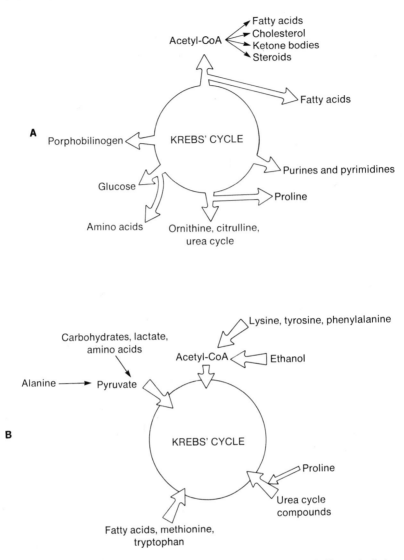

Fig. 12-1. Krebs' cycle plays central role in intermediary metabolism either in **B,** catabolic breakdown of molecules such as glucose, lactate, ethanol, and amino acids for energy, or in **A,** anabolic synthesis of fatty acids, ketone bodies, cholesterol, steroids, glucose, purines, and pyrimidines. Reactions that are favored are determined by needs of body, which in turn influences cellular environment through hormonal and other actions.

environment as heat, emphasizing the open system nature of metabolism.

The metabolism of food molecules is regulated by many control systems in different cells and tissues. The central roles of the liver, the adipose tissue, and the hormones have been known for many years. However, many new and exciting discoveries are being made on the biochemical mechanisms by which carbohydrate, lipid, and protein metabolism proceeds.

Fig. 12-1 summarizes these cellular biochemical pathways. The rates of the separate reaction sequences are regulated by many finely tuned hormonal, enzymatic, and negative-feedback controls. The central role of the Krebs cycle in intermediary metabolism can be seen in Fig. 12-1, which shows the catabolic functions of this mitochondrial reaction series, leading ultimately to the production of high-energy molecules of ATP and formation of water. Glucose

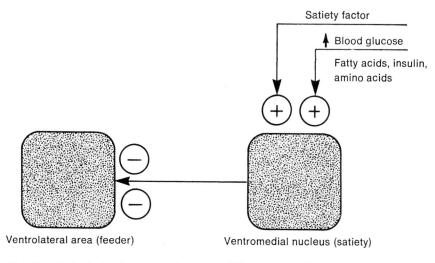

Fig. 12-2. Hypothalamic feeding and satiety center. When ventromedial nucleus is stimulated, it inhibits ventrolateral feeding center. While satiety center is active, organism does not experience hunger or drive to find and consume food.

metabolism is primarily responsible for ATP production, but both proteins and fatty acids can be utilized in intermediary metabolism for energy through conversion into compounds that can enter the Krebs cycle. The Krebs cycle can also be utilized by the cell for anabolic pathways, such as lipogenesis, cholesterol production, porphyrin synthesis, and purine and pyrimidine synthesis. The substrates of the Krebs cycle are, in these situations, used in early steps of the various biochemical, anabolic pathways.

Source of glucose

Before metabolism of glucose can proceed, this monosaccharide must enter the cell through the cell membrane from the bloodstream. Glucose does not appear to enter cells by simple diffusion but must be facilitated by a carrier-mediated process, which delivers the glucose to the interior cytoplasm of the cell. It has been known for years that insulin is required in certain tissues (especially muscle and adipose tissue) for this carrier-mediated diffusion to occur. Recent identification of both insulin and glucagon receptor molecules on many different types of cell membranes is providing a molecular basis for understanding the actions of these hormones. The central role of glucagon in blood sugar regulation is an area of great scientific debate and inquiry, but evidence is accumulating to indicate that it may be as important as insulin. This evidence and its implications will be elaborated on in the section on diabetes.

The glucose that enters the cytoplasm is first metabolized by a series of anaerobic reactions that comprise the Embden-Meyerhof pathway, or anaerobic glycolysis. This pathway converts glucose into pyruvate; depending on the oxygenation requirements of the cells and tissues, pyruvate will either form lactate, which accumulates, or *acetyl-CoA*, which enters the mitochondrial Krebs cycle. The cell must, of course, be endowed with the appropriate enzymes that catalyze the various steps of these metabolic pathways. The enzyme kind and amount is determined by the genetic constitution of the individual cell, and a great variety of genetic enzymatic deficiency diseases has been described. Normal fat and protein metabolism also require enzymatic degradation before these molecules can be utilized in energy production. Again, the enzymes required may be deficient, resulting in a variety of diseases.

Regulation of food intake

The intake of food molecules is regulated in the intact organism, so that the energy needs of the organism are met. The purpose of the GI tract is basically to provide a mechanism by which the organism can take in, process, and absorb food molecules, often in excess of what it needs. Cells take up what they need, with the excess then being stored in the body in the form of fat. The regulation of food supply then is mainly at the level of *food intake,* with the hypothalamus playing an important part in the regulation of feeding and satiety. Certain nuclei in the hypothalamus have been identified as centers of mediation for food intake (Fig. 12-2). The *ventromedial nucleus* has been identified as the *satiety center,* and stimulation of this area results in cessation of appetite; the *ventrolateral area* appears to initiate feeding behavior and has been termed the *feeder center.* The two centers inhibit each other reciprocally, so that when one is stimulated, the other becomes inhibited. Destruction of the ventromedial area of the hypothalamus leads to excessive hyperphagia and obesity in experimental animals, whereas destruction of the ventrolateral area leads to aphagia and wasting. These areas of the hypothalamus are nerve centers, and many nerve pathways pass through the hypothalamus. Thus, it seems probable that many other centers in the brain are responsible for input into the hypothalamic appestat; for example, direct autonomic connections have been demonstrated, implicating a role particularly for catecholamines in feeding and satiety. The actual sensing of the state of nutrition, the gastrointestinal tract status, and the amount of food molecules present and available in the body somehow exerts regulatory effects on the two centers, but the mechanism is poorly understood. *Blood glucose concentration* is thought to be a major regulator of the centers' activities, but fatty acids, amino acids, and insulin have also been implicated. Perhaps some factor is present in the nourished and alimented animal that acts on the satiety center, activating it and thus in turn depressing the firing rate of the feeding center. When food is needed, the satiety factor is no longer present, and the feeder center turns on. The animal feels hunger and will search for food and eat if food is available.

OBESITY

Obesity is defined as that condition in which the body weight is greater than 10% of the ideal weight for the individual's age, sex, and height. Obesity in affluent societies has been estimated to be as high as 49%. It has increased in prevalence in direct relationship to the amount of highly refined, high-sugar food that is readily available to Westerners. The presence of "food cues" as part of the massive advertising campaign exposure that Westerners are unavoidably exposed to also plays a role in the psychologic conditioning to eat sugar-containing, high-calorie foods. Also, in affluent societies, infants are often given high-caloric cereals, sugars, and milk even when they do not particularly want it, creating a condition of infantile obesity that has been shown to be directly related to adult obesity.

The causes of obesity are summarized in Table 12-1. Obesity may develop (1) in patients with hypothalamic tumors as a sequelae to brain trauma or with inflammatory diseases; (2) in patients with a variety of endocrine diseases, such as Cushing's syndrome; (3) in some rare genetic diseases and the more common juvenile-onset diabetics; (4) as the aftermath of drug therapy with phenothiazines or oral hypoglycemic agents; (5) as the result of excessive dietary intake of food; or (6) as the result of inactivity. Animal models for the study of obesity include the *yellow obese mouse* and the *Zucker genetically obese rat, "Fatty."* Human models include lean volunteers who force-feed themselves to the point of gaining 20% to 25% extra body weight. Some studies have also been done on rats with ventromedial hypothalamic

Table 12-1. Causes of obesity

Nature	Causal associations
Essential	Cause unknown
Genetic	In animals, such as the Zucker rat, "Fatty"
Ventromedial hypothalamic injury	Physical: tumors, trauma ?Physiologic: disturbances in regulation
Hyperphagia	Force feeding in lean volunteers
Endocrine disease	Hypothyroidism, diabetes
Psychosocial	Habit, culture, food "cues"

lesions and on humans who have hypothalamic injury caused by trauma or tumors with subsequent hyperphagia and obesity. A number of theories of obesity have been developed from the results of this research. The pathophysiology of obesity is still far from clear, and only certain highlights can be presented here.

Adipocytes

Adipocytes (fat cells) are found predominantly in the subcutaneous tissues and mesentery, although they occur throughout the body in collections called *adipose tissue*. This tissue has been described physiologically as an organ, acting as it does in a fairly uniform way toward stimuli such as hormones, blood concentration of substances, and sympathetic nervous stimulation. The adipose tissue acts as a storage center for excess ingested calories. When the energy needs of the body are less than the calorie intake, then the food molecules are converted to fatty acids, which are carried from the liver as lipoproteins and are taken up by the adipocytes. The absolute amount of adipose tissue can increase in either of two ways. Tissue hypertrophy can occur, with the result that the individual adipocytes enlarge significantly, becoming full of lipid, or the tissue may undergo hyperplasia, in which case the cells divide and increase in total number. There are critical periods in adipose tissue development during which hyperplasia occurs. Not all these periods are well defined, as adipocyte differentiation patterns are not well described, but it is known that

during childhood the adipose tissue may undergo hyperplasia during the period from birth to 2 years of age, from 7 years to 11 years, and during adolescence. It has been shown that the stimulus to hyperplasia is excessive food intake. The cells increase in number and fill with lipid that has formed from excess calories above those required for the body's metabolism and growth needs. In the adult obese individual a childhood history of obesity can often be obtained. It would appear that in these individuals, hyperplasia of the adipose organ has occurred early in life and is irreversible. Furthermore, the hyperplasia conditions these individuals to be obese throughout their lives. A positive correlation has also been found between the underweight state in infants and the same condition in adults.

The hyperplasia that develops in response to overeating during childhood appears to require an intact, functioning pituitary gland. This gland is also required by the embryo in the formation and maturation of the primordial adipoblasts.

In the obese adult the adipose tissue appears to respond to excess calories mainly by hypertrophy of the existing adipocytes. Fig. 12-3 shows the direct correlations between fat cell weight and degree of obesity. Microscopic examination of individual adipocytes shows that these cells bulge with single large droplets of triglycerides surrounded by a cell membrane. The cell can only reach a maximum of lipid content ($\sim$1.0 μg lipid per cell), and this oc-

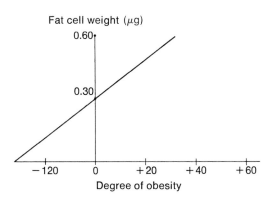

Fig. 12-3. With increasing degree of obesity, adipocytes contain more and more stored lipid.

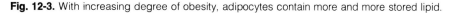

curs in moderately severe obesity. In a sense then if hyperplasia cannot occur, the total degree of obesity is determined by the number of cells available to store fat. Adults with ventromedial hypothalamic damage generally gain up to a maximum of 136 kg (300 lb), while early-onset obesity often results in a much greater weight plateau. However, exceptions do occur, and increased cellularity has been occasionally noted in the remarkably obese, late-onset individual. The ability to respond to excess food intake by adipose tissue hyperplasia may possibly be related to hormonal influences. Possibly pregnancy is a critical period in fat organ development, with hyperplasia occurring during this time in response to hormonal factors. Excess weight gain during pregnancy is notoriously difficult to shed later!

Hyperlipidemia

Increased serum lipids (triglycerides, cholesterol, and fatty acids) are a common finding in obesity. The metabolism of food is directed toward utilization of caloric intake for energy and for storage as fat for later use if excess is ingested. When fatty acids are needed for energy, they are released from the adipose tissue as albumin-bound molecules, which are taken up by the liver, skeletal muscle, and myocardium. These fatty acids are liberated or mobilized from triglyceride molecules in the adipocyte through the action of a hormone-sensitive lipase, which is activated in the cell. Fatty acid mobilization is stimulated by epinephrine, thyroid hormone, glucocorticoids, glucagon, and growth hormone and is inhibited chiefly by insulin. The fatty acids in the blood are taken up mainly by the liver between meals for possible use in energy production, ketone body formation, or triglyceride synthesis there. Chylomicrons, which are similar, lighter, and larger structures formed by the intestinal epithelial cell, carry dietary lipid from the intestinal lymph to the plasma and other tissues, particularly the liver.

The triglyceride molecules formed in the liver are released into the blood attached to protein as structures known as very low-, low-, and high-density lipoproteins. The source of the liver triglyceride, which is carried on lipopro-

teins, is mobilized fatty acids from the adipose tissue and fat ingested in the diet. The lipid is loosely bound to protein in these structures and can be easily cleaved away from the lipoproteins. Lipids are utilized by many other tissues than adipose tissue, liver, and muscle. They are, for example, the backbone of many hormones, and they form the matrix of all biologic cell membranes. Lipid is also important in thermal insulation and as a protective layer around vulnerable internal organs. Cells and tissue that require lipid have ready access to it due to this unique transport system. A blood and tissue enzyme, lipoprotein lipase, facilitates the removal of triglyceride from the lipoproteins. This enzyme is activated by heparin and is concentrated in various parts of the body, particularly adipose tissue, heart, and skeletal muscle. Figs. 12-4 and 12-5 show the liver in fat metabolism and the carriage of lipid.

In obesity the normal regulation of free fatty acid mobilization in response to the needs of the body is greatly disturbed. Two major defects contribute to the elevated free fatty acid and triglyceride concentration in the obese individual. First, total lipid breakdown (lipolysis) in the adipocytes is increased, thus causing excessive mobilization of fatty acids, and second, the regulation of lipolysis and esterification of fatty acids to form triglycerides is abnormal in obesity. Various enzymatic disturbances have also been reported in the adipocytes of obese persons. Normal individuals will experience an elevation of free fatty acids in the blood in response to fasting. This response is minimal or absent in the obese, although the basal level of free fatty acids is increased above normal. The net synthesis of triglycerides from fatty acids in the liver is also increased and poorly regulated in the obese, and insulin regulation of triglyceride formation is disturbed. The obese person appears to make more lipid from ingested carbohydrate than does the normal person, and some reports indicate that the triglyceride that is formed is not removed normally from the plasma by lipoprotein lipase.

The heart of the lipid defects may, however, originate in the insulin resistance and hyperinsulinism that occur in obesity and that result in abnormal fat metabolism.

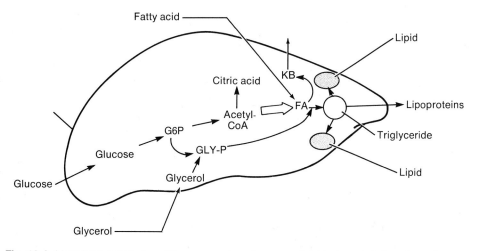

Fig. 12-4. Liver lipid metabolism. When excessive glucose or lipid is ingested, liver forms lipoproteins, which are transported through bloodstream. When food intake is decreased, lipids are delivered to liver from adipose tissue. Lipid infiltration of liver is commonly seen in chronic alcoholism, kwashiorkor, and nutritional marasmus.

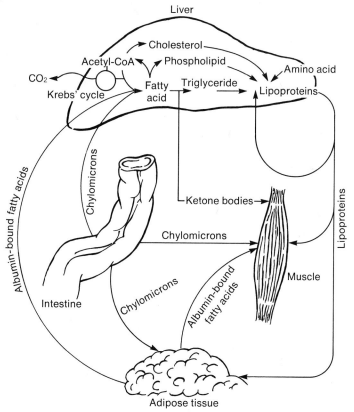

Fig. 12-5. Lipid transport. Lipids are absorbed from intestine as chylomicrons and taken up by liver, adipose tissue, and muscle. In liver, lipids are broken down to fatty acids, which are then either utilized in energy pathways or converted to phospholipids and triglycerides. Triglycerides are transported as lipoproteins from liver to muscle and adipose tissue. Adipose tissue serves as a lipid storage and can release fatty acids either as free molecules or more commonly as albumin-bound molecules when energy needs of body demand it.

Hyperinsulinemia

The finding of increased insulin concentration in the blood in all forms of human obesity is extremely interesting. Some authorities feel that hyperinsulinemia is the primary defect that causes obesity, while others consider it to be a physiologic response to obesity. The elevated insulin concentration is present concurrently with insulin resistance. The pancreas may possibly respond in a compensatory way to primary insulin resistance at the cellular level by increasing its output of insulin. The normal role of insulin in lipid metabolism is to promote lipogenesis and fat storage, so if insulin resistance is present, there may be an increased uptake of free fatty acids by the liver and increased production of triglycerides, which cannot then be taken up normally by the liver, adipose tissue, and muscle. The normal stimulatory effect of insulin on lipoprotein lipase activity is depressed in obesity. Thus, the hyperlipidemia of obesity may actually be caused by the insulin resistance that is commonly found. High-carbohydrate diets aggravate this situation, and physical exercise improves it.

The mechanism of insulin resistance is not known, although abnormal insulin cell membrane receptors have been described. It is possible too that insulin antagonists may exert an effect in obesity. Glucagon and growth hormone are the likely antagonists, but they have both been reported to decrease in obesity in the Zucker rat.

Because of the resistance to insulin some obese individuals have a basal hyperglycemia as well as an abnormal glucose tolerance test, indicating a diabetic predisposition. Cortisol may be important in insulin resistance, and while its plasma concentration is usually normal in obesity, its production and total turnover are increased.

The beta cells of the pancreas are hypertrophied in obesity, and if the beta cells are chemically destroyed by streptozocin in rats with ventromedial nucleus injuries, the expected obesity and hyperphagia are almost completely abolished. Vagotomy also abolishes obesity development in the ventromedial nucleus–injured rat. A causal relationship between the hypothalamus and the hyperinsulinism of obesity is suggested by this experiment. It would appear here at least that excessive deposition of fat requires hyperinsulinism. The development of insulin resistance then would be a secondary response of the tissues to constant exposure to high levels of insulin, so that the tissue becomes more and more tolerant of insulin. Conversely the presence of an increased fat organ in the obese may cause an increased need for insulin for maintenance of the increased adipose tissue mass, thus secondarily creating hyperinsulinemia.

Reversal of the metabolic and hormonal factors (hyperinsulinism, hypertriglyceridemia, hyperglycemia, and glucose intolerance) that are commonly found in obesity can be accomplished by significant weight reduction. Thus, the excessive ingestion of food and the way the body metabolizes this food must be considered the primary cause of most obesity. The reduction of hyperinsulinism in obesity can be accomplished by reduction in the total amount of calories ingested and specifically by a decrease in the ingestion of carbohydrates. Carbohydrates are insulinogenic; in part they also determine or permit the basal response of the pancreatic beta cells to a great variety of other normal stimuli to insulin production. These stimuli include the hormones gastrin, secretin, and cholecystokinin and other gastric peptides, which are all released when food is present in the gastroinestinal tract (Fig. 12-6).

The presence of hyperinsulinemia and insulin resistance in the obese individual clarifies the predisposition of the obese toward the eventual development of diabetes mellitus and thus provides excellent rationale for weight control, particularly in the genetically susceptible adult.

Hyperphagia and thermogenesis

The fatty rat, the animal with ventromedial injury, and obese humans generally are characterized as hyperphagic. They eat voraciously, and their pattern of eating may be altered. The obese person often claims a morning anorexia and may eat fewer meals than the nonobese person. However, the absolute amount of food at a meal is increased, and the intake of sweet-tasting, nonnutritive substances may also be increased. When 3,000 calories are ingested at

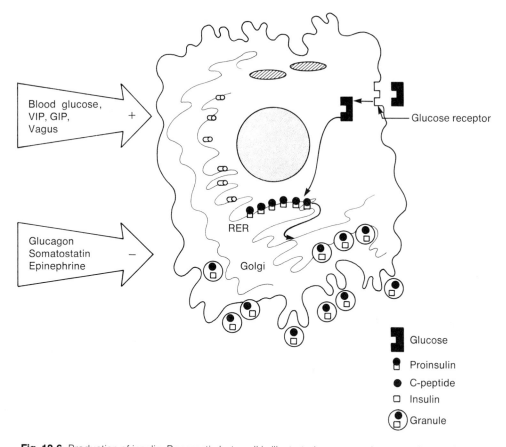

Blood glucose,
VIP, GIP,
Vagus

+

Glucose receptor

Glucagon
Somatostatin
Epinephrine

−

RER

Golgi

Glucose

Proinsulin

C-peptide

Insulin

Granule

Fig. 12-6. Production of insulin. Pancreatic beta cell is illustrated as possessing a membrane glucose receptor site. When glucose is present it attaches first to receptor and then moves into cell. Glucose itself is required in insulin production, which proceeds by protein synthesis along rough endoplasmic reticulum (RER) with formation of proinsulin, which is packaged by Golgi apparatus into granules. Proinsulin is split into insulin and C-peptide. Beta cell is also stimulated by factors other than a rising blood glucose concentration and may be inhibited as well by other factors as shown.

once instead of over the course of the day, an overall elevation of serum lipids occurs. Furthermore, the obese are generally indolent, a factor that contributes not only to the maintenance of their obesity but also to the metabolic and hormonal alterations that perpetuate the obese state.

The hyperphagia of obesity may have many causes. Psychologic conditioning and habit certainly play an important role. Genetic factors may be operative, as evidenced by identical twin studies which show that weight gain over the life span is not markedly different in identical twins. Physiologic abnormalities in the regulation of the feeder and satiety centers of the hypothalamus may be present and yet be al-

most impossible to demonstrate. Parabiotic experiments in mice show that circulating satiety factors are present but are not able to "turn off" the feeder center and "turn on" the satiety center in spontaneous obesity. The hypothalamus is thus unresponsive. There is further evidence that the hypothalamus of the obese person is less sensitive to blood glucose and thus is a defective "glucostat." Obesity is extremely difficult to treat, although recent success has been obtained with behavior modification techniques. Most obese people can be made to lose weight by reduction in caloric intake, but in as much as 80% of this population, the obesity eventually returns.

In volunteers who force-feed themselves to

gain weight in obesity studies, all the metabolic and hormonal patterns of spontaneous obesity in the general population are present, and all parameters return to normal when the excess weight is lost. Weight loss occurs naturally when the diet is self-selected. One interesting factor in these individuals is the requirement that they have to eat a great *excess* of calories to *maintain* obesity once it develops. The fate of these excess calories is not known. It is possible that the excess calories go toward thermogenesis (heat production), which produces a stable body weight even in the face of excess calorie ingestion. Thus, each individual has a "programmed" weight, and excess calories beyond those required to (1) maintain that weight and (2) allow for storage of a certain amount of excess calories in adipose tissue are removed from the body as heat. It is certainly commonplace to find individuals who can eat enormous amounts of food without weight gain, as well as the converse. This has also been shown experimentally in human subjects. Furthermore, in periods of undernutrition, thermogenesis may be decreased so that energy from available calories is directed toward maintenance of nutritional and metabolic status.

Other pathophysiologic effects of obesity

The obese human is at risk for the development of disturbed functioning in many systems of the body, especially diabetes, vascular disease, and cardiac disease.

The effects of obesity upon the physiology of the organism are profound. Probably no system is spared the stress of maintaining this excess tissue.

The respiratory system is compromised, as evidenced by the pickwickian syndrome, which develops in some extremely obese individuals. These people are characterized by high Pco_2, somnolence, massive obesity, and hypoventilation. Studies indicate that a number of mechanisms operate to depress respiration. There is the mechanical effect of obesity upon the ability of the respiratory muscles to function normally —decreased chest cage compliance; there are also biochemical effects on respiratory sensitivity.

The cardiovascular function is affected because of the excess burden on the heart to provide blood supply to additional tissue. Stroke volume and circulating blood volume are both increased. Congestive heart failure, hypertension, stasis ulcerations, and dyspnea are all commonly found in the morbidly obese individual. The hyperlipidemia associated with obesity also appears to predispose these individuals to atherosclerosis, thrombus, and emboli formation, and myocardial infarctions. Hyperlipemic blood is more viscous and coaguable. Obesity also is associated with gallstone development (see Chapter 13). In the genetically susceptible individual, obesity in adult life is related to the onset and severity of diabetes. Degenerative arthritis may develop as a mechanical complication of obesity.

Increased cortisol production and turnover rate may play a role in the predisposition of the obese to a variety of disorders, and therefore in a sense obesity can be considered a stressor, resulting in adrenocortical activation.

The obese individual often has a low self-concept and poor body image, which are reinforced by society. Thus, the obese suffer not only physiologically but also psychologically.

STARVATION

The result of overingestion is accumulation of fat deposits and gain in weight, while undernutrition leads to loss of these energy stores and eventual wasting, or *cachexia*. Undernutrition may result from inadequate or absent intake of food or from inability to absorb or metabolize the calories provided by the food that is eaten. While the juvenile-onset diabetic eats adequate amounts of food (in fact is often voracious), the absolute lack of circulating insulin causes a cellular "starvation," and these children often appear wasted and thin. Cancer, infection, and severe malabsorption can result in a clinical state of starvation. Some infants also respond to emotional and sensory deprivation by the *failure to thrive syndrome* and are in fact starving to death, even though they may eat what are considered adequate amounts of food. *Marasmus* is a clinical term for starvation and cachexia in the infant under 2 years of age; it is seen most often in children who have been totally deprived during their early life. Neglected children of severely disturbed mothers, children growing up in severe poverty, and children suffering from pronounced gastrointestinal tract infections or enzyme deficiencies are all at risk. The child with marasmus often appears to be little more than a skeleton covered with thin flesh and wasted muscles. Generally the dietary deficiency is total, and no one specific nutrient is lacking, as usually occurs in other deficiency diseases.

Starvation may occur in anorexia nervosa, a psychiatric disease in which food is utterly refused. Starvation can occur also, of course, when individuals are isolated without food.

Metabolism

The metabolic processes, as the body adapts to a prolonged fast, are aimed at sparing carbohydrate and protein reserves and utilizing fats. The length of time then that humans can totally abstain from food depends partly on the amount of storage lipid that has been accumulated. Obviously obese people can fast for many weeks longer than their lean counterparts. The average length of time that a human being can go without any food intake is 5 to 6 weeks. During this period most of the energy required for normal metabolism comes from fatty acids and ketone bodies. Certain organs of the body require glucose under normal conditions and are unable to use other sources of energy. Other organs (e.g., muscle) normally utilize fatty acids quite freely in the postabsorptive state after a meal. However, during starvation the glucose-requiring organs can adapt and begin to use ketone bodies and fatty acids. The brain and heart are the most remarkable in this regard. Furthermore, the liver is stimulated by increased glucagon output from the pancreas, which occurs in response to the lowering blood glucose, to produce glucose from available precursors, namely, amino acids. This process is termed *gluconeogenesis*. Fatty acids are removed from the adipose tissue reserves also through the action of glucagon and other stimuli. Thus, almost throughout a starvation fast the liver acts to maintain blood glucose concentration at the normal level, first through glycogenolysis and then through gluconeogenesis. Essentially the same type of response occurs after the ingestion of a very-low-carbohydrate meal, which acts via the intestinal hormones to turn on the production of glucagon, which stimulates gluconeogenesis and also insulin. Insulin stimulates lipogenesis, and some fat eaten in such a diet will be utilized for energy, with the excess being stored by the insulin-stimulated adipose tissue. The insulin produced is not enough to inhibit the production of glucagon in this situation, but if the meal contained sufficient carbohydrates, then a proportionately greater rate of insulin production would ensue. This would depress glucagon production, thus stopping the signal for the liver to split glycogen and produce glucose.

Blood glucose concentration is extremely well regulated, and a variety of sensing mechanisms exist to ensure the maintenance of a fairly constant blood sugar. The liver itself does not require insulin for glucose entry into the cells, so that the blood glucose is more or less equilibrated with liver glucose, which is rapidly phosphorylated upon entering the liver cells. The glucose molecules then may be used for glycogen synthesis or for liver energy metabolism. Glycogen synthesis or breakdown by the liver depends in large part on the insulin: glucagon ratio. Figs. 12-7 and 12-8 diagram the normal liver metabolism when food is constantly being supplied and when fasting is taking place. The metabolic pathways that predominate during prolonged fasting are geared toward the breakdown of glycogen, gluconeogenesis, and ketone body formation, as compared to glycogen synthesis and glucose utilization for energy in the fed state.

Stages

There are metabolic stages in starvation, which are determined by the fuel available for the body to burn for energy. The first 24 hours of a fast are characterized by liver and muscle glycogenolysis, which provides glucose. Free fatty acids are also released from adipose tissue and utilized by muscle as a predominant fuel source. These processes are stimulated by low blood levels of insulin and a high level of glucagon.

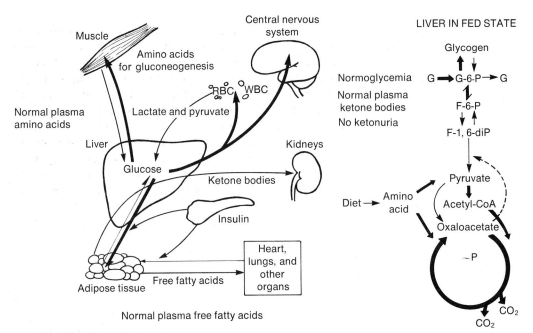

Fig. 12-7. Metabolic interrelationships during fed state. Under normal circumstances, insulin is released when carbohydrate is ingested, promoting glucose utilization and metabolism. Role of Krebs' cycle is indicated to right with glucose entering metabolism through Embden-Meyerhof pathway as pyruvate or being used for glycogenesis. Glycogenolysis and gluconeogenesis are not active at this time. (From Bacchus, H.: Essentials of metabolic disease and endocrinology, Baltimore, 1976, University Park Press.)

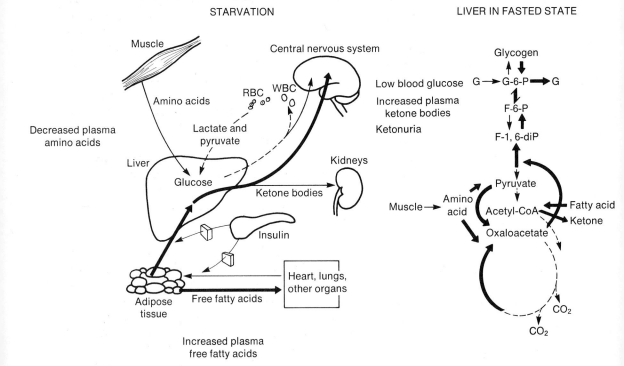

Fig. 12-8. Metabolic interrelationships during fasted state. In starvation due to prolonged fasting, insulin release is inhibited, with fatty acids released from adipose tissue and transported to liver for ketone body formation. Gluconeogenesis and glycogenolysis are both active. (From Bacchus, H.: Essentials of metabolic disease and endocrinology, Baltimore, 1976, University Park Press.)

As the liver and muscle glycogen is removed, the second stage begins, and gluconeogenesis is stimulated. Both amino acids (mainly from muscle protein) and fatty acids are taken up by the liver, and glucose utilization in most tissue of the body progressively decreases. The liver increases the utilization of fatty acids for energy by forming ketone bodies, which are then sent to all the tissues of the body. Ketone body production occurs as the result of a decreased oxaloacetate concentration in the liver cells, which is the result of a decreased anaerobic glycolysis of glucose and increased utilization of oxaloacetate for gluconeogenesis. Thus, the fatty acids that enter the liver from the adipose tissue are dehydrogenated and split into acetyl-CoA fragments; these are then used to form acetoacetate or β-hydroxybutyrate, the ketone bodies. It is thought that fatty acid oxidation in the liver results in high levels of NADH and acetyl-CoA, which cause pyruvate to be carboxylated to oxaloacetate, which then forms phosphoenolpyruvate, thus proceeding toward gluconeogenesis. Amino acids (and thus protein) are spared from utilization for energy production by peripheral tissues. They are utilized for gluconeogenesis by the liver, so that blood glucose is maintained, but the tissues of the body do not take up and use glucose at the normally high rate, having switched to fatty acids and ketone body utilization for their energy needs. Muscle wasting does, of course, occur, as muscle protein must be hydrolyzed to provide amino acids for gluconeogenesis. Muscle protein breakdown appears to be regulated by the insulin:glucagon ratio, being stimulated when the ratio is decreased. The major amino acids released from the muscle are alanine and glutamine, which are then utilized by the liver and also the kidney for gluconeogenesis. The muscle must metabolize its endogenous amino acids to provide these substrates, but the energy needs of the muscle for these mechanisms, as well as its contractility needs, can be met through utilization of fatty acids taken up from the blood. This spares the ketone bodies in the blood, which are the main fuel sources of the brain and myocardium in prolonged starvation.

The development of the terminal phase in starvation is determined by the amount of fat present in the body. The starving individual has a compensated metabolic acidosis because of the keto acids present in the blood. Calcium and phosphorus are depleted, and osteoporosis ensues as the body attempts to maintain these ion stores. Liver failure may occur because of fatty infiltration and is most common in individuals with previous hepatic disease. The basal metabolic rate decreases, and the levels of triiodothyronine decrease, although thyroxine remains at the normal level. There is no significant effect on intellectual function. The hypothalamic satiety center is, however, affected and remains active, and appetite is usually absent during a prolonged fast. (This phenomenon has also been observed in obese individuals on a low-carbohydrate diet and may be due to ketosis.) Emotional stability is also decreased during a prolonged fast.

All these mechanisms may contribute to death, but the primary cause appears to be the loss of all lipid stores and the subsequent massive utilization of protein for energy. The terminal phase of starvation is extremely rapid once it appears. Protein in muscle, cell membranes, and blood is rapidly depleted, causing death within about 24 hours after the lipid reserves are gone. This occurs between 5 and 6 weeks after the start of the starvation fast in a normal lean individual with 15% body fat. People are often reported to suddenly fall down and die during the terminal phase of starvation.

MALNUTRITION STATES
Protein-calorie malnutritions of early childhood

Protein-calorie malnutrition of early childhood is prevalent in economically deprived and underdeveloped areas. *Kwashiorkor* (meaning in Ghandian "the disease that comes after the second child") develops when the total quantity and quality of protein in the diet is deficient. Children who are breast fed are protected from this disease in areas where it is prevalent, but when they are displaced at the breast by a younger sibling and thus forced to eat the common diet, kwashiorkor may result. The diet is characteristically low in protein, with the major source of calories being carbohydrates. Essential amino acids are missing, the protein of-

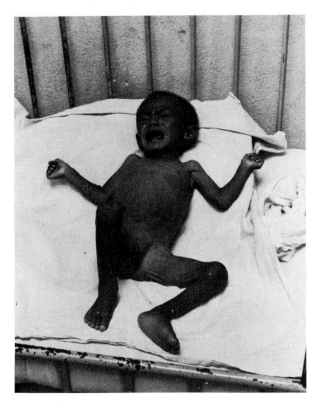

Fig. 12-9. Child in Guatemala suffering from acute malnutrition. There is severe cachexia and no obvious edema. (FAO photograph by Y. Nagata.)

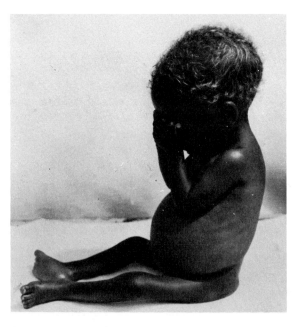

Fig. 12-10. African child suffering from kwashiorkor. Note uncurled, graying hair, edema, and skin lesions. (FAO photograph by M. Autret.)

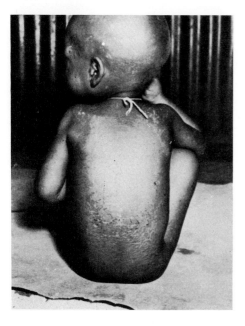

Fig. 12-11. Characteristic "flaky paint" dermatosis of kwashiorkor. (From Williams, S. R.: Nutrition and diet therapy, ed. 3, St. Louis, 1977, The C. V. Mosby Co.)

ten being derived from cornmeal rather than animal protein sources. The symptoms and signs that develop may vary from mild to severe. An important contributing factor to the morbidity is the presence of concurrent parasitic infestation and chronic infections in these children. Kwashiorkor can be contrasted with nutritional marasmus, which also is a common finding in deprived children. In this condition, both protein and calories are deficient, leading to the clinical state of cachexia and starvation previously discussed. Figs. 12-9 and 12-10 show the dramatic contrast between these two deficiency diseases. The child with kwashiorkor is usually characterized by edema, muscle wasting, and growth retardation, and often massive ascites may be present. The infant with marasmus does not have edema and appears wizened and wasted. Other variable findings of kwashiorkor include desquamation (Fig. 12-11), graying of the hair, which may alternate with normal pigmentation along the hair shaft and indicates periods of normal and deficient nutrition, diarrhea, anemia, vitamin deficiencies, and hepatomegaly.

The pathophysiology of protein-calorie deficiency is related to the normal role of proteins. Protein is required for energy, growth, formation of antibodies and enzymes, repair of tissues, and maintenance of blood colloid osmotic pressure and capillary filtration. A certain amount of adaptation and compensation for decreased protein intake will occur. For example, basal metabolic rate, decreased oxygen consumption, decreased nitrogen excretion, and decreased spontaneous activity may all help to maintain the steady state for a certain period. However, over a prolonged period of time, disorders in normal functioning are inevitable. Decreased colloid osmotic pressure accounts for the generalized subcutaneous edema and ascites that are common. Hyponatremia also is common. The edema predisposes these children to slow healing, and ulcers often occur. The edema may actually mask a severe weight retardation, and in fact the moon face and edema are sometimes interpreted as a healthy plumpness. The lack of protein causes protein catabolism with severe muscle wasting. The liver often becomes infiltrated with lipid, but the development of cirrhosis is not common. The pathogenesis of fatty liver in kwashiorkor is not known, but lipoprotein synthesis by the liver may be impaired. The jejunal mucosa also is affected in the disease, becoming flattened and atrophic, and malabsorption and diarrhea occur (see Chapter 13).

The long-term effects of kwashiorkor are growth retardation throughout life and possibly some intellectual impairment, particularly if the child was affected in the first 6 months of life. The other signs and symptoms of kwashiorkor can be eradicated with treatment of the underlying disorder and adequate nutrition.

Variations of marasmus and kwashiorkor with signs and symptoms of both conditions are also common; these are considered "intermediate" forms of the two diseases.

Vitamin deficiencies

Deficiencies in one or more vitamins are common even in Western societies. Vitamin deficiencies also occur secondarily in many disease states. A common role of vitamins in physiologic function is participation as cofac-

Table 12-2. Requirements, functions, and deficiencies of fat-soluble vitamins*

Vitamin	Physiologic functions	Results of deficiency	Requirement	Food sources
A (retinol)	Production of rhodopsin (visual purple)	Xerophthalmia	Adult: male—5,000 IU female—4,000 IU	Liver Cream, butter, whole milk
Provitamin A (carotene)	Formation and maintenance of epithelial tissue Toxic in large amounts	Night blindness Keratinization of epithelium Follicular hyperkeratosis Skin and mucous membrane infections Faulty tooth formation	Pregnancy: 5,000 IU Lactation: 6,000 IU Children: 1,500 to 5,000 IU depending on age	Egg yolk Green and yellow vegetables Yellow fruits Fortified margarine
D (calciferol)	Absorption of calcium and phosphorus Calcification of bones Renal phosphate clearance Toxic in large amounts	Rickets Faulty bone growth Osteomalacia in adults	400 IU (children; pregnant or lactating women)	Fish oils Fortified or irradiated milk
E (tocopherol)	Related to action of selenium Antioxidant with vitamin A and unsaturated fatty acids Hematopoiesis Reproduction (in animals)	Hemolysis of red blood cells; anemia Possible protection of unsaturated fatty acids Sterility (in rats)	Adult: 12 to 15 IU	Vegetable oils
K (menadione)	Blood clotting, necessary for synthesis of prothrombin Possible coenzyme in oxidative phosphorylation Toxic in large amounts	Hemorrhagic disease of the newborn Bleeding tendencies in biliary disease or surgical procedures Deficiency in intestinal malabsorption (sprue, celiac disease, colitis) Prolonged antibiotic therapy Anticoagulant therapy (dicumarol counteracts)	Unknown	Green leafy vegetables Cheese Egg yolk Liver

*From Williams, S. R.: Nutrition and diet therapy, ed. 3, St. Louis, 1977, The C. V. Mosby Co.

Table 12-3. Requirements, functions, and deficiencies of B complex vitamins*

Vitamin	Physiologic functions	Clinical applications	Requirement	Food sources
Thiamine (B₁)	Coenzyme in carbohydrate metabolism TPP—decarboxylation TDP—transketolation	Beriberi (deficiency) GI†: anorexia, gastric atony, indigestion, deficient hydrochloric acid CNS†: fatigue, apathy, neuritis, paralysis CV†: cardiac failure, peripheral vasodilation, edema of extremities	0.5 mg per 1,000 calories	Pork, beef, liver, whole or enriched grains, legumes
Riboflavin (B₂)	Coenzyme in protein of energy metabolism (flavoproteins) FMN (flavin mononucleotide) FAD (flavin adenine dinucleotide)	Wound aggravation Cheilosis (cracks at corners of mouth) Glossitis Eye irritation; photophobia Seborrheic dermatitis	0.6 mg per 1,000 calories	Milk, liver, enriched cereals
Niacin (nicotinic acid) (precursor—tryptophan)	Coenzyme in tissue oxidation to produce energy (ATP) NAD (nicotinamide-adenine dinucleotide) NADP (nicotinamide-adenine dinucleotide phosphate)	Pellagra (deficiency) Weakness, lassitude, anorexia Skin: scaly dermatitis CNS: neuritis, confusion	14-20 mg (niacin equivalent)	Meat, peanuts, enriched grains
Pyridoxine (B₆)	Coenzyme in amino acid metabolism Decarboxylation Deamination Transamination Transsulfuration Niacin formation from tryptophan Heme formation Amino acid absorption	Anemia (hypochromic microcytic) CNS: hyperirritability, convulsions, neuritis Isoniazid is an antagonist for pyridoxine Pregnancy: anemia	2 mg	Wheat, corn, meat, liver
Pantothenic acid	Coenzyme in formation of active acetate (CoA)—acetylation	Contributes to: Lipogenesis Amino acid activation Formation of cholesterol Formation of steroid hormones Formation of heme Excretion of drugs		Liver, egg, skimmed milk
Lipoic acid (sulfur-containing fatty acid)	Coenzyme (with thiamine) in carbohydrate metabolism to reduce pyruvate to active acetate Oxidative decarboxylation	Undetermined (see Thiamine)		Liver, yeast

*From Williams, S. R.: Nutrition and diet therapy, ed. 3, St. Louis, 1977, The C. V. Mosby Co.
†GI = gastrointestinal; CNS = central nervous system; CV = cardiovascular.

Continued.

Table 12-3. Requirements, functions, and deficiencies of B complex vitamins—cont'd

Vitamin	Physiologic functions	Clinical applications	Requirement	Food sources
Biotin	Coenzyme in decarboxylation (synthesis of fatty acids, amino acids, purines); deamination	Undetermined		Egg yolk, liver
Folic acid	Coenzyme for single carbon transfer—purines, thymine, hemoglobin Transmethylation	Blood cell regeneration in pernicious anemia but not control of its neurologic problems Megaloblastic anemia Macrocytic anemia of pregnancy Sprue treatment Aminopterin is folic acid antagonist	400 μg Pregnancy: 800 μg Lactation: 600 μg	Liver, green leafy vegetables, asparagus
PABA (part of folic acid)		Treatment of rickettsial diseases Anemias (see Folic acid)		Same as folic acid
Cobalamin (B$_{12}$)	Coenzyme in protein synthesis Formation of nucleic acid and cell proteins—red blood cells Transmethylation	Extrinsic factor in pernicious anemia—combines with intrinsic factor of gastric secretions for absorption; forms red blood cells (with folic acid) Sprue treatment (with folic acid)	3 μg	Liver, meat, milk, egg, cheese
Inositol	Lipotropic agent (?)	Undetermined		Citrus fruit, grains, meat, milk
Choline	Lipotropic agent Forms nerve mediator—acetylcholine	Fatty liver—hepatitis, cirrhosis (undetermined in human nutrition)		Meat, cereals, egg yolk

tors in enzymatic reactions. Enzyme-mediated reactions are of many different types and are involved in all the metabolic activities of the organism. Therefore, the signs and symptoms of the various vitamin deficiencies (Tables 12-2 and 12-3) are often extremely variable, depending on which functions are most compromised.

Other nutritional deficiencies

In addition to deficiencies in the intake of calories (as proteins, carbohydrates, and lipids) and vitamins, a great variety of other nutritional deficiencies is possible. The minerals in the diet are essential for normal function in many cases, and if they are deficient, disease may result. Again the body will compensate for as long as possible by a variety of adaptive mechanisms. However, prolonged mineral deficiencies can cause serious disease (e.g., anemias).

Iron. Hypochromic anemia, or iron deficiency, is the most common anemia, particularly among women and during pregnancy. Iron is normally required in hemoglobin manufacture, forming the heme portion of this molecule. When the hemoglobin concentration in the blood decreases to less than 10 g/100 ml, anemia is present. The organism adapts to the anemia, which threatens oxygenation of the cells and tissues, by manufacturing more erythrocytes and by decreasing metabolism and activity. Pallor and fatigue, dyspnea upon exertion, tachycardia, and neurologic manifestations are all signs of anemia.

Vitamin deficiencies may also produce megaloblastic anemia in folic acid or vitamin B_{12} deficiencies. Failure to absorb vitamin B_{12} in the ileum when gastric intrinsic factor is lacking results in pernicious anemia. The red blood cells are large, and many reticulocytes are present as well. Vitamin B_{12} and folic acid are required in the normal maturation of the erythrocyte in the bone marrow.

Hemolytic anemia of the premature infant may be due to inadequate vitamin E intake in formulas, which is reversible when these infants are treated with vitamin E preparations.

Calcium. Calcium is an essential mineral required for muscle contraction, bone formation, and many enzyme-mediated reactions. Its absorption requires vitamin D and parathyroid hormone, and its absence either through dietary deficiency or by disordered absorption (e.g., vitamin D deficiency) causes rickets, osteomalacia, and tetany.

Magnesium. A deficiency in magnesium may be brought about by decreased intake, increased output (diuretics), or impaired absorption. It is fairly common in poorly nourished alcoholics, as are most of the other deficiencies. Magnesium activates numerous enzyme reactions and deficiency is associated with neuromuscular abnormalities. It has been suggested that hypomagnesemia in combination with alkalosis is the cause of the delirium tremors of alcohol withdrawal, although the mechanism is not as yet clearly defined.

Zinc. Zinc is an essential mineral, which functions in combination with enzymes, such as carbonic anhydrase. It is required for protein synthesis by certain tissues and for wound healing; it may function in vitamin A metabolism. Zinc deficiency may develop when intake is decreased, such as in the alcoholic, or when malabsorption occurs (e.g., cystic fibrosis). Zinc may be removed from the blood by the action of certain medications (penicillamine), which act as chelating agents. Oral contraceptives also have been reported to lower zinc levels. The symptoms of deficiency are extremely variable, from impairment of growth to abnormalities in the sensation of taste.

Other minerals. Numerous other minerals may be ingested in the diet in decreased or excessive amounts. When excessive amounts of such minerals as lead, copper, or iron are present either in the blood or stored in tissue, numerous pathophysiologic disturbances may occur. Some of the effects of environmental chemical agents are discussed in Chapter 6.

GENETIC AND METABOLIC DISTURBANCES
Carbohydrates

Carbohydrates are essential components of the human diet, being utilized for energy production in every cell of the body in the form of glucose. Indeed, if intake is inadequate, the body's metabolism gears toward the production of glucose from other dietary constituents. Defective absorption in the GI tract, inadequate intake, or abnormal metabolism of glucose all will lead to pathophysiology of nutritional integrity. The problems involved in inadequate intake, such as occurs in starvation or prolonged fasting, have already been discussed. Inadequate absorption may occur in gastrointestinal diseases, such as malabsorption or diarrhea. Certain gastrointestinal enzymes may be deficient, causing poor polysaccharide or disaccharide breakdown in the gut, which then leads to decreased absorption. Lactase deficiency will result in inefficient hydrolysis of lactose to glucose and galactose, and therefore uptake of this disaccharide cannot occur.

Enzymatic deficiencies. The most common disturbances in carbohydrate metabolism are related to the cellular metabolism of these compounds. Cellular enzymatic deficiencies, which are most commonly genetic in nature, are well described in erythrocytes. Hemolytic disease results in anemia with hepatomegaly, splenomegaly, hematuria, and jaundice. The two major enzyme deficiencies that have been described in erythrocytes are of pyruvate kinase and glucose-6-phosphate dehydrogenase (G6PD). Both conditions are quite rare, but a mild form of the latter has recently been described in 35% of the American black population. This type is essentially asymptomatic except when the erythrocytes are severely stressed by administration of certain oxidant-like drugs (primaquine and sulfa drugs) or by infection. Then hemolytic anemia will develop. The worldwide distribution of G6PD deficiency parallels the distribution of falciparum malaria, as do sickle cell anemia and thalassemia, and thus is thought to provide a selective advantage to those who carry the mutated gene. The malarial protozoa requires certain metabolic and protein characteristics, which are decreased in the G6PD-deficient erythrocyte.

Other enzymatic deficiencies that interfere with carbohydrate metabolism are the glycogen storage diseases, resulting from defective breakdown of glycogen into glucose subunits. Glycogen therefore accumulates in various organs of the body, particularly liver, kidney, and muscle. There are a number of forms, all genetic in nature, with a variety of symptoms and prognosis. Muscle weakness and growth retardation are major symptoms in most forms.

Another condition of disturbed carbohydrate metabolism is *galactosemia,* which is caused by the accumulation of large amounts of the sugar galactose or its products of metabolism, in particular galactitol, within the blood and tissues. The congenital form has been associated with mental retardation, kidney damage, and lens cataracts. All described forms of this disease are due to deficiencies in the enzymes normally involved in galactose metabolism.

Hypoglycemia. Hypoglycemia is an abnormally low blood glucose concentration that can be symptomatic of many disorders. The symptoms of acute hypoglycemia reflect the effects of widespread sympathetic nervous system activation, which is stimulated by low blood glucose concentration and which activates glycogenolysis. When the blood glucose falls to less than 40 mg/100 ml (normal is 80 to 110 mg/100 ml), the individual experiences palpitations, weakness, sweating, dizziness, and hunger. Prolonged hypoglycemia may result in serious central nervous system dysfunction, leading to convulsions and coma. Fig. 12-12 diagrams the normal regulation of blood glucose.

The etiology of spontaneous hypoglycemia is generally an abnormal regulation of insulin production in response to stimuli. It is a common finding in prediabetics in the postprandial state and is due to an overproduction of excess insulin in response to the meal. This causes the

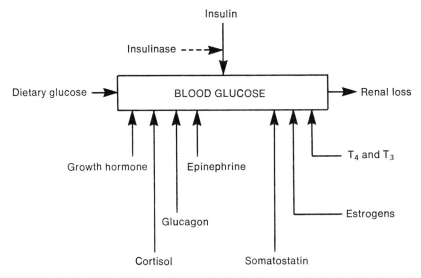

Fig. 12-12. Regulation of blood glucose. Ingested carbohydrate supplies body with glucose for fuel energy under normal circumstances. Regulation of blood glucose is controlled by many factors indicated. Growth hormone opposes action of insulin on hexokinase reaction and promotes release of fatty acids and ketone bodies, which are also anti-insulin. Cortisol stimulates gluconeogenesis. Epinephrine and glucagon both promote glycogenolysis. Somatostatin inhibits both insulin and glucagon. Estrogens are anti-insulin, and thyroid hormone increases carbohydrate absorption from gut.

blood glucose levels to drop markedly after the meal has been absorbed and the products of digestion and absorption have been distributed to the blood and tissues. This response occurs typically 3 hours after a meal, particularly one high in carbohydrates, if no other nourishment has been taken since the meal. The development of hypoglycemia can be averted in these patients by providing a low-carbohydrate, high-protein meal with a snack just before the third hour after the meal.

Hypoglycemia may occur in conditions in which the output of insulin in the unstimulated as well as stimulated state is extremely high. This might occur in patients with insulinomas, or insulin-producing tumors. The treatment is surgical extirpation when possible. Insulin reactions in the diabetic are also a common cause of hypoglycemia, and immediate ingestion of carbohydrates alleviates the condition.

Hypoglycemia of a postprandial nature also occurs in many postgastroenterostomy patients. The cause of this disorder is believed to be rapid absorption of nutrients in a meal due to rapid gastric emptying into the duodenum through an impaired or absent pylorus. The excessive absorption stimulates the pancreas to produce large amounts of insulin, which results in a lowered blood sugar. This form of hypoglycemia may also be treated by a low-carbohydrate, high-protein diet.

Hypoglycemia may develop from certain genetic enzyme deficiencies that interfere with the metabolism of glucose by the liver. It is also a symptom of hypopituitarism and Addison's disease, in which there is hypofunction of the pituitary and adrenal cortex and reduced corticosteroid production. Corticosteroids are normally antagonistic to the actions of insulin.

Proteins

Abnormalities in the absorption and metabolism of proteins are less common than the disorders of carbohydrates just discussed. Amino acid absorption can be impaired in malabsorption syndromes, and metabolism of amino acids is also affected by certain genetic enzymatic deficiencies. It will be recalled that dietary protein is broken down into small peptides and amino acids in the digestive tract by peptidases and removed from the GI tract through the mucosal cells and into the portal vein. Amino acids are then carried to the liver and other tissues for utilization. Fig. 12-1 illustrated the entrance of amino acids into anabolic and catabolic reactions via the Krebs cycle. The amino group is removed from the amino acid by transamination or deamination, reactions that are enzymatically mediated. The nitrogen is metabolized as ammonia, which may then enter the urea cycle or may be taken up by glutamine, which is acted upon by glutaminase in the kidney, releasing the ammonia into the urine. Certain amino acids are considered essential since they cannot be synthesized in the body. These are isoleucine, leucine, lysine, methionine, phenylalanine, threonine, tryptophan, and valine.

A deficiency of protein intake whether as the result of malabsorption, inadequate intake, or excessive loss (burns, excessive catabolism, neoplasms) leads to clinical states associated with negative nitrogen balance. Inadequate intake, exemplified by kwashiorkor, has been previously described. Protein deficiency is associated with decreased resistance to infection, stressors, and traumatic agents. Protein may be lost from the gut in protein-losing enteropathies such as are seen in cancer, ulcers, colitis, and tuberculosis, or it may be lost through the action of catabolic hormones such as cortisol, thyroid hormone, and estrogens and in cachectic wasting associated with malignant tumors. Defective enzymes may result from genetic disease, or alteration in the amount and nature of proteins may be observed. Abnormalities in plasma proteins are associated with a great variety of diseases, including multiple myeloma, cirrhosis, kidney disease, muscular dystrophy, protein-calorie deficiency, and hereditary disorders.

Abnormalities in the metabolic pathways in which the various amino acids are involved can lead to a great variety of clinical manifestations.

The diverse nature of these diseases is due to the multiple roles of protein in cellular metabolism, division, growth, movement, ion transport, buffering, and indeed almost any function. Protein serves structural, enzymatic, and immune functions, and both the nature and the amount of available protein is determined by the availability of amino acids and by genetic regulation of the metabolic pathways.

Lipids

Disorders of intestine-to-liver lipid transport. Fat is required in the diet and is essential for energy production, hormone and bile salt synthesis, and cell membrane integrity. The absorption of fat and the role of lipid in energy maintenance have already been described. Certain clinical disorders exist in which intestinal lipid metabolism is disturbed. Pancreatic diseases in which decreased pancreatic lipases are released into the bowel will result in malabsorption of lipid. This is seen in cystic fibrosis, in which the pancreatic ducts become blocked with thick mucus, and pancreatic degeneration and fibrosis thus ensue. Release of adequate lipase, which is then inactivated by excessive acid, also may occur (e.g., in Zollinger-Ellison syndrome). Micelle formation in the intestinal lumen may also be interrupted in various disorders of bile salt metabolism. These include bile duct obstruction, bowel surgery such that the enterohepatic circulation of bile salts is interrupted, and ingestion of the drug cholestyramine.

Inefficient absorption of lipid micelles also may occur in various disease processes, including celiac disease (see Chapter 14). Celiac disease is associated with fat malabsorption, steatorrhea, diarrhea, and protein-losing enteropathy, to such a degree that sometimes the blood albumin levels are decreased. Other processes that affect this aspect of lipid absorption include bowel ischemia due to mesenteric artery occlusion, hookworm, and the drug neomycin.

The synthesis of triglycerides inside the intestinal mucosal cell may be disrupted if the activity of the required cellular enzymes is impaired. This phenomenon occurs in Addison's disease. The formation of chylomicrons, which transport the lipid formed inside the intestinal cell to the liver and other tissues, may also be disturbed. This is observed in congenital abetalipoproteinemia, in which the formation of globulin, which is required in the formation of chylomicrons and lipoproteins, is disturbed.

Hypobetalipoproteinemia may be seen in conjunction with some malabsorption syndromes and in severe debilitation.

Whipple's disease interferes with the transport of lipid from the intestinal cell. The disease process involves infiltration of the lamina propria of the small intestine and distortion of the intestinal villi. This represents a barrier through which nutrients cannot easily pass, thus causing malabsorption.

Obstruction of the intestinal lymphatic drainage may occur in a great variety of diseases and may be severe enough to impede the absorption of chylomicrons into the intestinal lacteals. Lymphatic flow can be impaired by such factors as tumors, tuberculosis, Whipple's disease, trauma, and infection.

Disorders of lipid transport in serum. The normal pathways of lipid transport have previously been discussed (see Fig. 12-4). Triglycerides and cholesterol are mainly carried from the liver to the peripheral tissues as lipoproteins. Fatty acids are also transported in the plasma from the adipose tissue to the liver and other tissues as albumin-bound molecules.

Disorders of lipid transport include hyperlipoproteinemias and hypolipoproteinemias. The hyperlipoproteinemias may be either inherited or acquired. The inherited forms include diseases in which lipoprotein lipase is deficient, in which hyperbetalipoproteinemia with normal triglycerides occurs, or in which hyperprebetalipoproteinemia is present, to name a few. Acquired hyperlipoproteinemias may also be found in pregnancy, diabetes, pancreatitis, hypothyroidism, nephrosis, liver disease, and multiple myeloma. The symptoms that may be associated with hyperlipoproteinemia depend on which lipoproteins are involved. Abdominal pain, premature atherosclerosis, xanthomas, and pancreatitis are sometimes found.

The hypolipoproteinemias are mainly inherited disorders such as congenital β-lipoprotein deficiency, hypobetalipoproteinemia, and familial high-density lipoprotein deficiency (Tangier's disease). The signs and symptoms of these disorders include malabsorption, retinitis, neuropathy, abnormally shaped erythrocytes (acanthocytes) in abetalipoproteinemia, and acanthocytes and orange discoloration of the tonsils in Tangier disease. The abetalipoproteinemias are remarkably asymptomatic.

Purines and pyrimidines

This chapter would not be complete without some mention of the various conditions that can disturb the metabolism of purines and pyrimidines, the nitrogenous bases that are the backbone of DNA and RNA. These bases are derived both from dietary intake and from cellular synthetic pathways. The most common disorder of purine synthesis is gouty arthritis, in which excessive uric acid accumulates in the blood and tissues (see Chapter 4). Excess uric acid develops either as the result of increased synthesis or decreased excretion of purine compounds. Approximately 0.3% of the population have this abnormality, which is thought to have a hereditary background. Pyrimidine metabolism involves the formation of orotic acid, and a hereditary orotic aciduria has been described. This condition is associated with megaloblastic anemia, growth and developmental retardation, and renal disease. Treatment is aimed at administration of uridine, which is deficient in this disease.

DISEASE MODEL: DIABETES MELLITUS

Diabetes mellitus is a common inherited disorder of carbohydrate metabolism caused by either an absolute lack of circulating insulin or an inability to use available endogenous insulin, leading to hyperglycemia, and a variety of other metabolic tissue and cardiovascular effects. Inheritance is thought to be multifactorial, rather than simply recessive, and the influence of environmental factors (i.e., obesity) upon the development of the adult-onset type is critical in the *penetrance* of the genes that determine the expression of diabetes. The degree and nature of diabetes is extremely variable, and while it is possible to identify prediabetics in the population, it is very difficult to predict the possibility of diabetes among populations of genetically "susceptible" individuals.

Insulin production

Fig. 12-6 shows the functional morphology of the insulin-secreting beta cell of islands of Langerhans in the pancreas. Insulin is produced by these cells in response to the stimuli indicated. Probably the major stimulus is increased blood glucose concentration, but the effects of the vagus nerve, gastrointestinal peptides, glucagon, and somatostatin are all considered important in regulation of the response. The release of insulin by the beta cell requires calcium, zinc, and glucose itself. The packaging and extrusion of insulin-containing granules by the beta cell is termed *emiocytosis*.

The beta cell is thought to possess glucose receptors on its membrane, which allow glu-

Table 12-4. Effects of insulin on tissues (summary of the three major target organs of insulin)

Liver	Adipose tissue	Muscle
Increased glycogen synthesis	Increased glucose transport	Increased glucose transport
Decreased gluconeogenesis	Increased formation of α glycerophosphate and triglyceride synthesis	Increased oxidative metabolism of glucose
Increased triglyceride synthesis	Increased fatty acid transport into adipocytes by activation of lipoprotein lipase on adipocyte membrane	Increased glycogen synthesis
Increased very-low-density lipoproteins		Increased amino acid transport and protein synthesis
Decreased glycogenolysis	Decreased cyclic AMP, decreased activity of hormone-sensitive lipase in adipocyte, and decreased triglyceride mobilization	Decreased amino acid release from muscle cell

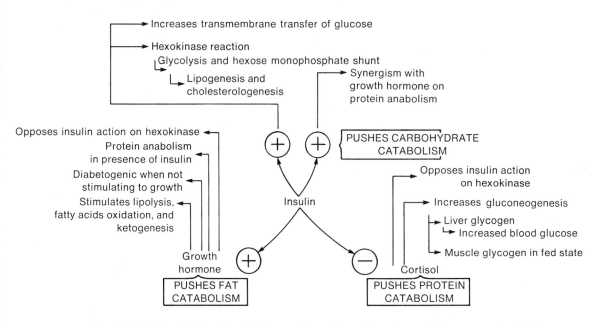

Fig. 12-13. Role of insulin on metabolism and opposing actions of growth hormone and cortisol.

cose to initially attach to the cell and then move through the membrane and become metabolized. This initiates the formation by the endoplasmic reticulum of *proinsulin*. The Golgi complex is thought to then somehow cleave away a section of proinsulin, known as the C-peptide, leaving insulin. Both molecules are then released by emiocytosis in beta granules. The insulin becomes active in the bloodstream and is free to act on muscle, adipose tissue, and other insulin-dependent sites, facilitating the entry of blood glucose into these cells, and to act on liver glucose metabolism.

The mechanism by which insulin facilitates glucose entry into cells is not completely understood. The entry appears to be facilitated by diffusion, which requires a membrane-bound carrier mechanism. Insulin receptors have been identified in many cells and appear to be membrane glycoproteins. Binding of insulin to these receptors may in some way activate the glucose-carrier system, perhaps by dramatically altering the mosaic structure of the lipoprotein membrane. Not all cells require insulin for glucose entry, although some of them nevertheless appear to have receptor sites. The liver, blood cells, and brain do not need insulin in order for rapid glucose entry to occur.

Glucose utilization by the body is much more complex than simple dependence on glucose entry into cells. Insulin is known to have both profound and subtle effects (Table 12-4) on metabolism generally, most of which contribute in some way to the maintenance of normoglycemia. The whole direction of insulin function appears to be toward glucose utilization, fat storage, and protein anabolism (Fig. 12-13).

The diabetic individual may have a pancreatic defect such that the production and release of insulin through the above mechanisms is depressed. However, in only 10% of diabetics does a true insulin lack occur, most often it is associated with juvenile diabetes, which commonly results in weight loss, growth retardation, and volatile ketoacidosis. The other form of diabetes is maturity- or late-onset diabetes; it is characterized by a decreased and abnormally regulated insulin release in response to increased blood glucose, rather than an absolute insulin deficiency. It has therefore been suggested that the primary cause of this type of diabetes rests with the pancreatic beta cell glucoreceptor. Occasionally normal insulin release or hyperinsulinism is reported in this form of diabetes.

The hyperinsulinism may, however, be only relative, in that if total body obesity is taken into consideration, the insulin levels may actually be lower than normal. A common finding in maturity-onset diabetes is insulin resistance, even if hyperinsulinism is found, causing a relative insulin deficiency in terms of cellular transport and metabolism. This is, of course, reminiscent of obesity, in which the same phenomenon occurs. Indeed, the development of diabetes in the genetically susceptible obese may occur in response to the tremendous secretory demands of excess tissue upon the pancreas, resulting eventually in inability of the beta cells to respond to stimuli. The high level of circulating insulin in obesity can perhaps by itself "insulinize" cells, thus making them resistant and thereby further increasing the demand for insulin from the already compromised pancreas. Eventually a state is reached in which clinically apparent diabetes, characterized by hyperglycemia, abnormal glucose tolerance, and possibly ketoacidosis, occurs. At this point the pancreas is unable to regulate the blood glucose concentration in a normal manner, and changes in diet and life-style and perhaps exogenously administered oral hypoglycemic agents or insulin are required. It has been possible to show an inverse correlation between level of circulating insulin and the number of binding sites in cells, thus lending credence to the idea that increased blood insulin causes cellular insulin resistance. The number of insulin receptors and the concentration of insulin can be controlled by dieting, and oral hypoglycemic agents appear to increase both the number of receptors and amount of insulin binding to cells.

The current controversy over the importance of glucagon in the pathogenesis and pathophysiology of diabetes was prompted by the discovery of the hypothalamus hormone *somatostatin*, which is a growth hormone–release suppressor and which has the property also of inhibiting the pancreatic release of both insulin and glucagon. Somatostatin has been shown to ameliorate both experimental and human diabetes and thus has implicated glucagon in diabetes. Glucagon is a hormone released by the pancreatic alpha cells and has also recently been shown to be released by the gastrointestinal tract. It is stimulated normally by low blood glucose and insulin and suppressed by high blood glucose and insulin. Thus, after a meal, an expected rise in insulin and drop in glucagon occurs. Glucagon's main known action is on liver glycogenolysis and involves activation by glucagon of the liver cell membrane adenyl cyclase system, which produces a cascade of events leading to the eventual enzymatic degradation of glycogen to glucose. Glucagon then is normally responsible for maintenance of the blood glucose concentration between meals, as glucose in the presence of insulin is removed from the blood to the insulin-dependent tissues.

It has been suggested by Unger and associates (1976) that diabetes is a *bihormonal* disease and that the pancreatic hormone glucagon is perhaps more important in blood sugar regulation than is insulin. This represents a great challenge to traditional thinking on the role of insulin, which has been considered the major regulator of blood glucose. Unger has shown that insulin is decreased and glucagon increased in human diabetes and that the normal effect of glucose on glucagon release is lost in the diabetic. Therefore, the glucagon level following a meal is extremely high, and the hyperglycemia of diabetes may actually be partly caused by glucagon-stimulated glycogenolysis. Treatment of the diabetic with somatostatin results in decreased blood glucagon and decreased blood glucose concentration, even in the presence of hypoinsulinism. The insulin that most diabetics must take may act by suppressing glucagon release, and somatostatin is considered a possible future drug of choice for diabetes. This hormone has recently been synthesized in the laboratory by *Escherichia coli* plasmids, an experiment that may prove to be a prototype for hormone synthesis of all types in the future.

On the other hand, Felig and associates (1976) have presented data that implicates insulin as the major regulator of blood glucose and its deficiency, either absolute or relative, as the main cause of diabetes. He suggests that the effect of somatostatin in diabetes is due to an inhibition of carbohydrate absorption in the gastrointestinal tract. Further support for the primacy of insulin in the pathophysiology of diabetes comes from experiments in which glucagon is infused. The effect on glycogenolysis is observed to be extremely transient in both normal and diabetic individuals. Furthermore, during prolonged 2- to 4-day infusions of glucagon in diabetics who receive their usual doses of insulin, no change in blood sugar is observed. When insulin is not administered to juvenile, insulin-dependent diabetics, a fivefold to fifteenfold increase in blood glucose concentration occurs as glucagon is administered. Thus, only when insulin was absolutely deficient did glucagon produce a diabetic hyperglycemia. These experiments demonstrate a major role for insulin in the pathogenesis of diabetes.

The role of glucagon is perhaps best related to its transient action on liver glycogenolysis. Glucagon may act by preventing the hypoglycemia that would probably develop following a low-carbohydrate, high-protein meal. Insulin increases markedly after a high-protein meal, and this should therefore cause a decrease in hepatic glucose output (see Table 12-3), resulting in possible hypoglycemia. However, glucagon is also stimulated by protein, and a transient effect of glucagon on the liver, which may be enough, nevertheless, to increase liver output of glucose to three times normal, acts to raise blood glucose in the presence of insulin, thus providing for maintenance of the steady state.

The diabetic patient produces more glucagon than normal in response to a high-protein meal, and liver glycogenolysis is therefore higher than normal. This response lasts for 2 hours, and by that time liver glucose output returns to normal levels even though glucagon production continues. However, hyperglycemia is still manifested by the diabetic, indicating an inability of the blood glucose to be transported into the cells, due to the relative insulin lack in the diabetic.

Diagnosis

The signs and symptoms of diabetes mellitus may develop insidiously. The major symptoms are polydipsia, polyphagia, and polyuria. The individual may complain of headaches and weakness and have other vague feelings of malaise. There is often a family history of diabetes, and obesity may be present, particularly in females. Women often have a history of repeated miscarriages and report having extremely large infants, often in excess of 4,500 g (10 lb) in birth weight. Patients may also report postprandial hypoglycemia. Occasionally cataracts and xanthomas may be present, and some patients may show early signs of vascular disease, particularly in the feet. Intermittent claudication is frequently present, and the feet are cold and hairless, all signs that indicate atherosclerotic changes in leg vessels. Ophthalmoscopic examination may show vascular changes in eyegrounds, and neurologic examination may show neuropathy. Signs of infection or a history of susceptibility to infection may be present as well.

Diagnosis is done on the basis of a glucose tolerance test, as the blood glucose may not be particularly elevated at the time of blood sampling, and the urinary glucose and ketones are absent in most cases. The normal and diabetic glucose tolerance tests are diagramed in Fig. 12-14. The diabetic blood glucose concentration remains over 160 mg/100 ml at 1 hour following the glucose meal and is over 120 mg/100 ml at 2 hours after the glucose meal. If the test is continued, hypoglycemia may develop in certain individuals. The deficiency in the diabetic appears to be a delayed peak insulin secretion in response to elevated blood glucose, occurring about 2 hours after a meal in the diabetic and much earlier, usually within 30 minutes after a meal, in the normal individual. Thus, the diabetic remains hyperglycemic after a meal for a much longer period than normal.

The effects of excess glucose in the blood are still being investigated in many laboratories, but the idea that the glucose molecule in excess does not have a toxic effect on cells is gradually being discarded. Glucose, for example, has been shown to have an effect on the polyol pathway (in which glucose is metabolized to sorbitol and then to fructose) in the walls of vessels and in the lens of the eye. These effects may contribute to atherosclerosis and cataracts, both of which are serious complications of diabetes.

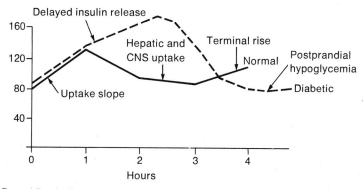

Fig. 12-14. Dotted line indicates a diabetic glucose tolerance test (GTT), and unbroken line shows normal response to glucose "meal." Due to delay in insulin release following glucose ingestion, prediabetic and diabetic experience prolonged period of postprandial hyperglycemia.

Pathophysiologic manifestations

Diuresis. Glucose causes osmotic diuresis when the blood glucose is elevated to levels that exceed the capacity of the kidney to reabsorb it. Glucose remains in the tubular filtrate and is excreted in the urine. Due to the establishment of hyperosmolarity by excess glucose molecules, water will osmose from the interstitium and through the tubular cells in order to reach an isosmotic concentration. Electrolytes as well are present and retained in the tubular filtrate. The increased water drawn to the tubular filtrate will dilute Na^+ ions and cause the reabsorption of Na^+ to be diminished. The loss of water and electrolytes results in increased extracellular osmolarity and cellular dehydration. Therefore, these patients will have an extreme thirst (polydipsia) in order to replace the fluid that has been lost through the polyuria of osmotic diuresis.

Metabolism. Figs. 12-7, 12-8, and 12-15 show the patterns of metabolism in the fed state, the fasted state, and the diabetic state. Diabetes resembles starvation in that fatty acids by necessity become the major source of energy when glucose cannot be taken up the insulin-dependent cells. Thus, ketone bodies are formed in the liver and carried via the bloodstream to the heart, lungs, and other organs for utilization. This produces a state of ketonemia, along with the hyperglycemia and metabolic acidosis, since the ketone bodies are acidic in nature. The development of ketoacidosis may be precipitated by a number of factors in the diabetic, including infection, stress, surgery,

emotional disturbance, and pregnancy; in fact, the prediabetic may show overt diabetes at these times, and thus the penetrance of the disease is precipitated by such factors. The most common cause of diabetic ketoacidosis is, however, omission of insulin in the diabetic patient.

Diabetic ketoacidosis. The signs and symptoms of ketoacidosis include ketonuria, dehydration following polyuria, dry skin, acetone odor on the breath, tachycardia, hypotension, central nervous system depression, and Kussmaul breathing, which is a pattern of respiration in which heavy, labored hyperpnea occurs. Other more variable signs include abdominal pain, anorexia, nausea, and vomiting. The appearance of diabetic ketoacidosis constitutes a medical emergency requiring immediate treatment. Ketosis without acidosis can usually be treated outside the hospital and can be differentiated from metabolic acidosis by a blood pH of over 7.3 and a HCO_3^- of over 15 mEq/liter. Since the dehydration that develops in this state contributes markedly to the pathophysiology of increasing ketoacid concentration and cardiovascular effects of hypovolemia, an immediate measure is hydration to correct the hypovolemia and hypotension. Other goals of therapy are to block lipolysis and promote lipogenesis. Therefore, insulin is administered promptly, usually intravenously in the crystalline zinc form. The acidosis will be corrected by the rehydration and insulin administration if renal function is not impaired, but alkali is often given during the acute stage in the

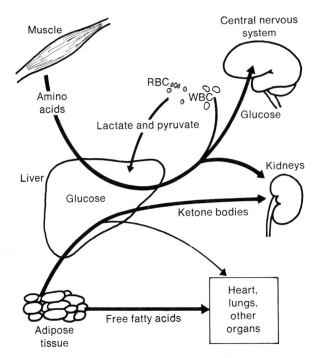

Fig. 12-15. Diabetic ketoacidosis. In diabetic, absence of insulin or presence of cellular refractoriness to insulin results in utilization of fatty acids for ketone body formation and amino acids for gluconeogenesis. Central nervous system requires glucose for energy and is supplied with glucose at expense of muscle protein. Insulin is not required for glucose transport in brain. Other tissues can utilize fatty acids and ketone bodies, but increased concentration of these substances in plasma leads to metabolic acidosis. (From Bacchus, H.: Essentials of metabolic disease and endocrinology, Baltimore, 1976, University Park Press.)

form of sodium bicarbonate when the pH is 7.0 or below. Electrolytes are also replaced as soon as the patient is rehydrated and kidney function is normal. Potassium chloride (20 to 30 mEq per hour) is usually added to the intravenous infusion. The patient in diabetic coma should become stabilized about 8 hours after therapy is instituted. If untreated, the diabetic in ketoacidosis will eventually drop into a deeply stuporous and then comatose state, and respiratory and cardiac failure will cause death.

Other forms of diabetic coma. It has become apparent that ketoacidosis is not the only possible cause of central nervous system depression and coma production in the diabetic. Two other major etiologies have been identified: *hyperosmolar nonketotic coma* and *lactic acidosis.*

Hyperosmolar nonketotic coma (Fig. 12-16) develops most frequently in diabetics with sufficient insulin production to depress excessive lipolysis but not enough to permit glucose utilization and transport across cell membranes. Thus, hyperglycemia is present and induces osmotic diuresis, leading to thirst and subsequent ingestion of fluid, most of which often contains large amounts of sugar. The plasma osmolarity is often in excess of 350 mosmol/kg, and the blood glucose is often greater than 600 mg/100 ml. These abnormalities produce a major change in the sensorium and lead often to a condition of increased fluid intake, thus aggravating the hyperosmolarity and hyperglycemia. The blood and urine tests for ketones are negative or show a slight increase in concentration. The osmotic diuresis, which dilutes the sodium and other ions present in the tubular filtrate of the kidney, will increase the concentration gradient against which sodium is reabsorbed, so that absolute hyponatremia develops. However, in terms of the extracellular fluid, hyperosmolarity is present, as water is

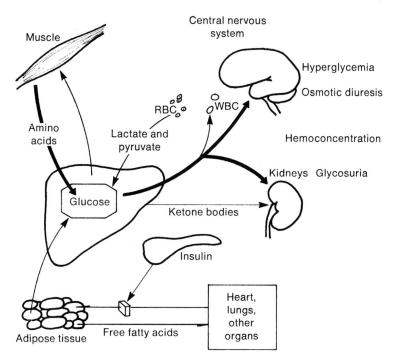

Fig. 12-16. Hyperosmolar nonketotic coma. There is enough insulin for lipogenesis but not enough to permit glucose transport across cell membranes. Thus, hyperglycemia occurs without ketosis. Dehydration can lead to hypovolemic shock. (From Bacchus, H.: Essentials of metabolic disease and endocrinology, Baltimore, 1976, University Park Press.)

being lost in excess of solute through the kidney. The glomerular filtration rate will decrease drastically as the hyperosmolarity develops, and both azotemia and further increases in blood glucose result. This condition may develop quite slowly, in contrast to ketoacidosis, and may be precipitated by renal disease, cerebrovascular accidents, cardiovascular disease, infections, sepsis, and stress. The mortality rate approaches 40%. The treatment is rehydration, administration of small, spaced doses of insulin, and replacement of potassium, as hypokalemia is a serious problem in these individuals and is exacerbated by the restoration of glucose metabolism.

Lactic acidosis in diabetics can cause a comatose state that carries with it a high mortality rate. The blood sugar may be normal, while blood keto acids are often increased. There is often dehydration, hypotension, and hyperventilation. Lactic acid is produced normally in amounts of 1,500 mmol per day in adults but is equally utilized to form pyruvate.

Generation of excess lactic acid is an effect of cellular hypoxia, which results in increased anaerobic glycolysis, a high NADH:NAD ratio, and defective oxidative metabolism. Cellular hypoxia is, of course, a condition found in a number of disease states, as well as being a normal occurrence following muscular exercise. Diabetics often have chronic disease conditions that predispose them to cellular hypoxia. These include cerebrovascular and cardiovascular disease, which may produce tissue ischemia. Another important precipitating factor is the drug phenformin-HCl, an oral hypoglycemic agent commonly used in diabetes, which acts by depressing gluconeogenesis. This would favor lactate accumulation by depressing the Cori cycle. Phenformin also is reported to stimulate anaerobic glycolysis by altering the NADH:NAD ratio. Thus, the action of this drug in combination with other factors in susceptible diabetics can cause lactic acidosis. The treatment of lactic acidosis is aimed at alleviating the acidosis and treating the underlying cause of the excessive lactic acid production, which, of course, may be multifactorial and complex.

It should be mentioned that a coma may also occur in severe hypoglycemia, which may be induced in the diabetic by insulin overdose. Therefore, the differential diagnosis of coma in the diabetic must also include the possibility of insulin reaction. The treatment is infusion of a bolus of glucose, which has a dramatic and immediate arousing effect.

Chronic complications in diabetes. While most diabetics can be maintained by diet and oral hypoglycemic agents or insulin, the development of long-term chronic pathologic changes in many tissues and organs is frequently a concomitant of the disease. In general, the juvenile-onset diabetic with an absolute loss of insulin production capability is most susceptible to complications, but all diabetics may exhibit complications to some degree. These major complications are retinopathy, neuropathy, peripheral vascular disease, atherosclerotic heart disease, and nephropathy. To a large degree all these conditions can be in part or fully explained by characteristic changes that occur in small and larger blood vessels, namely, diabetic microangiopathy and macroangiopathy. The pathogenesis of these vascular conditions is a matter of much debate at the present time, and the basic etiology is unknown. Nevertheless, these vascular changes account for most of the mortality directly caused by diabetes.

The primary lesion in microangiopathy is thought by some to be capillary basement-membrane thickening and biochemical changes in the glucoprotein composition of this structure. These changes appear to occur slowly over the life span of the diabetic, leading eventually to interruption in the patency of the vessels involved and thus to hypoxia and ischemia of the area supplied by these vessels. It is possible that the cells that produce the basement membrane are at fault in the diabetic and that some abnormal metabolic functioning is responsible for basement membrane alterations. The hyperglycemia present in diabetes may cause these cellular alterations, as might the insulin resistance. Another possibility is the increased growth hormone and irregular fluctuations in its concentration that often are observed in diabetes. Hypophysectomy delays the development of diabetic microangiopathy when patients are provided with all the pituitary hormones except growth hormone.

Diabetic *macroangiopathy* also occurs, but it is not well characterized. Medial calcification, which is correlated with the degree of glucose intolerance, has been observed, and roughening of the contours of the vessels occurs. These specific changes are to be differentiated from atherosclerosis, which arises in the intima and is also common in the diabetic; atherosclerosis is most likely related to hyperlipidemia. All of the vascular changes will, however, act together to cause a deficient oxygenation of tissues and specific changes related to hypoxia and ischemia of various organs.

Nephropathy. A specific and distinctive lesion occurs in the kidney of the diabetic and may develop even before the diabetes is overtly manifested. It is a round hyaline mass in the glomerulus, the Kimmelstiel-Wilson nodule. Other nonspecific changes in the vessels of the kidney also occur and are the results of thickening of the basement membrane of the capillaries. Ischemia of the glomeruli result from this microangiopathy, and the disease process is termed *diffuse intercapillary glomerulosclerosis*. The kidney is often hypertrophied, and both kidneys are usually involved. The incidence of renal involvement in diabetes appears to be extremely high, but overt kidney disease such as nephrosis and renal failure may not result. The manifestation of renal involvement usually begins with proteinuria. Edema may also develop, and hypertension may be aggravated. Frank nephrosis is not common but can develop. The eventual outcome of progressive renal nephropathy is azotemia, uremia, and eventually death in kidney failure. The treatment of diabetic nephropathy usually is symptomatic and often involves reduction in insulin. This is apparently due to a decreased degradation of circulating insulin by the damaged kidney. Renal hemodialysis and transplantation are also possible treatments.

Retinopathy. Diabetic retinopathy develops with time, and 80% of those diabetics known to have the disease for 20 years have some degree of retinopathy. Occasionally in the juvenile diabetic retinopathy develops rapidly, causing blindness by late adolescence. There is a positive correlation between the severity of retinopathy and the degree of vascular disease in general. There are a number of types of retinopathy, the two most common being caused by progressive accumulation of hard, lipidlike exudates or by obstruction of the retinal circulation. Diabetic retinopathy causes more blindness in the United States than does any other condition.

Neuropathy. Diabetic neuropathies are of three major types: (1) symmetric sensory disturbances, (2) asymmetric sensory and motor disturbances, and (3) autonomic neuropathies. Neuropathy of one sort or another is common in all diabetics. The signs and symptoms can be extremely variable and the differential diagnosis quite complicated. Many times peripheral polyneuropathy of a predominantly sensory nature occurs, and the diabetic may have peculiar sensations in both the upper and lower extremities. Eventually motor impairment may also result, causing weakness. Usually these processes are bilateral, but asymmetric neuropathy may also occur. Autonomic neuropathy often is found in conjunction with peripheral neuropathy and is most frequently exhibited by postural hypotension. Other possible effects of autonomic neuropathy include impotence, gastrointestinal disturbances, paralytic bladder, and extraocular muscle paralysis. The pathophysiologic basis of neuropathy was traditionally based on ischemic changes in the nerves due to angiopathy of the vessels that supply them. Recent work on glucose metabolism with accumulation of sorbitol implicates this substance in the pathogenesis of neuropathy. Sorbitol retention may lead to injury and decreased nerve conduction velocity and may also interfere with the metabolism of Schwann cells, which produce myelin. Segmental demyelination of the nerves is a common finding in diabetic neuropathy.

Atherosclerotic coronary artery disease. The development of atherosclerosis and the pathophysiologic manifestations of this process were discussed in Chapter 9. The diabetic is more at risk, at least in Western societies,

to develop coronary artery disease, and the same factors that predispose the normal individual to atherosclerosis also operate in the diabetic. Coronary artery disease and myocardial infarctions occur with high incidence among diabetics, irrespective of sex, and at an earlier age than in the normal population. The pathophysiology of atherosclerosis is no clearer in the diabetic than in the nondiabetic. Multiple factors appear to be involved, including hyperglycemia, hyperlipidemia with hypertriglyceridemia, high cholesterol level, hypertension, obesity, physical inactivity, behavior pattern type A, and smoking.

The evolution of acute atherosclerotic plaques is not inevitable and is dependent on many factors, including genetic predisposition, physical and emotional stressors, obesity, diabetes, hypertension, physical indolence, and cigarette smoking. There is no question that the development of atherosclerosis and the associated coronary artery disease, cerebrovascular disease, and peripheral vascular disease are accelerated markedly in the diabetic. Furthermore, evidence is accumulating to suggest that reduction of hyperglycemia and a diet low in carbohydrates and saturated fats with weight reduction and exercise can all contribute to an amelioration of atherosclerotic disease.

The signs and symptoms of atherosclerosis are related to the degree of plaque deposition and the anatomic location of the involved vessels. The incidence of myocardial infarction and cerebrovascular accidents is high, and atherosclerosis contributes to the peripheral vascular disease.

Peripheral vascular disease. The diabetic patient often suffers greatly from impaired circulation, particularly of the extremities. Such individuals often show evidence of ulceration, infection, and eventually gangrene, phenomena that develop most commonly in the feet. Signs of peripheral vascular disease of the lower extremity include pallor on elevation of the foot and rubor or hyperemia upon dependence of the limb. Venous filling time is a good test of the adequacy of tissue perfusion in the leg. When major arterial occlusion occurs in an extremity, the patient is extremely susceptible to infection, and ulceration may eventually progress to abscess and cellulitis and ultimately to necrosis and gangrene. Amputation of the part is the only recourse at that time. Surgical revascularization is done when the tissue ischemic process is in a fairly early stage. A significant percentage of the diabetic patients with venous stasis and ulceration do not have peripheral vascular disease per se. They often have a history of minor trauma to the part, which rapidly develops into the progressive ulcerative process just described. It is not understood exactly what mechanisms are operative in this situation, but neuropathy and angiopathy may both play roles. These patients obviously cannot benefit from revascularization surgery, and treatment is aimed at alleviation of discomfort, avoidance of further trauma, and maintenance of factors that aid in wound healing.

Diabetics also often have an associated dermopathy, which may be related to peripheral vascular disease, to insulin, or to the diabetic disease process itself. Furthermore, the diabetic is more susceptible to infections of the skin and all other tissues as well, and a constant vigilance must be maintained so that early treatment can be instituted. Prevention of infection is a major factor in those who care for diabetics in the hospital and the home.

Physiology of treatment

There are two major forms of diabetes, juvenile and adult-onset, and the treatment of these two conditions differs greatly. The juvenile diabetic and some lean, adult-onset diabetics have a total or nearly total lack of insulin even at basal levels. The obese, maturity-onset form is characterized by adequate or increased insulin, but the cells are insulin resistant, and fasting hyperglycemia and an abnormality in insulin regulation are present. Thus, the juvenile diabetic requires insulin throughout life, while the maturity-onset diabetic may be able to be regulated by diet, weight control, exercise, and drugs. The question of administration of the oral hypoglycemic agents or insulin to these diabetics is a matter of serious consideration since the findings of the University Group Diabetes Program (UGDP) have been made available. This study of the long-range problems of diabetics on insulin or oral

hypoglycemic agents showed that treatment of hyperglycemic, obese adults with either insulin or oral hypoglycemic agents did not reduce the mortality or affect the incidence of microangiopathy. In fact, the UGDP studies indicated that cardiovascular disease–related mortality was higher in patients receiving tolbutamide and phenformin than in patients receiving placebos or insulin. This occurred despite the fact that the fasting blood glucose concentration in these individuals was on the average 112 mg/100 ml. Therefore, it would seem that drug treatment of adult-onset diabetics might not be warranted and that diet alone could be used to maintain these individuals. The diabetic diet has traditionally been low in carbohydrates and high in fat. The observation that diabetics in Asia and Latin America have a much lower incidence of cardiovascular disease than do North American diabetics implicates exogenous factors, most probably dietary. The diet that now appears most protective of cardiovascular disease is *high in starch, low in refined sugars, and low in saturated animal fats*. This diet derives 25% to 35% of its calories from fat, one third of which is polyunsaturated. Between 40% and 55% of the calories are derived from carbohydrates, which are mainly starch, with the rest of the sugars being derived from fruits, vegetables, and milk. This limits the total cholesterol intake to 300 to 400 mg per day. The aim of this diet is not only to control refined sugar and saturated fats but also to control calories. Apparently when the calories are controlled, a diet high in starch does not produce uncontrolled hyperglycemia or hyperlipidemia.

Utilization of insulin is also under scrutiny for adult-onset diabetics and presents a problem when the adult diabetic with fasting hyperglycemia does not lose weight. These patients often require insulin to control hyperglycemia, since they do not limit their calories, control their weight, and follow prescribed diets.

Normally 30 to 50 units of insulin is released daily into the portal vein from the pancreas and thus is immediately removed in large part by the liver, providing for hepatic control mechanisms on blood insulin concentration. This is not the case when insulin is injected parenterally and therefore is absorbed irrespective of need. It is recommended that the diabetic be administered the least possible amount of insulin to control his fasting hyperglycemia. Certain situations may arise that will increase the need for insulin. These include surgery, pregnancy, infections, and glucocorticoid administration. Exercise may decrease the need for insulin, as will significant weight loss in the obese individual.

SUMMARY

This chapter has described the patterns of abnormal nutrition that may develop under diverse conditions of pathophysiology. These ranged from absolute lack of nutrients causing starvation to abnormalities in the metabolism of required nutrients, leading to absolute or relative excess or deficit. The possibilities of abnormalities in these thousands of processes by which the body maintains its homeostasis are overwhelming. There has been no attempt to provide a comprehensive catalogue of these conditions. Rather, it is hoped that the mechanisms through which possible abnormalities may occur have been clarified, so that the student will be able to conceptualize and transfer this knowledge.

The following chapter describes abnormalities of the GI tract and accessory organs. It is recognized that normal nutrition is impossible without structural and functional integrity of the GI tract, and disorders there are extremely common, representing pathology that all practitioners of health sciences will meet on an almost daily basis.

SUGGESTED READINGS

Albrink, M., editor: Clinics in endocrinology and metabolism: obesity, vol. 5, Philadelphia, 1976, W. B. Saunders Co.

Bacchus, H.: Essentials of metabolic diseases and endocrinology, Baltimore, 1976, University Park Press.

Charney, E., et al.: Childhood antecedents of adult obesity, N. Engl. J. Med. 295:6-9, 1976.

Eaton, R., Convay, M., and Schade, D.: Endogenous glucagon regulation in genetically hyperlipemic rats, Am. J. Physiol. 230:1336-1341, 1976.

Felig, P., Wahren, J., Sherwin, R., and Hendler, R.: Insulin, glucagon, and somatostatin in normal physiology and diabetes mellitus, Diabetes 25:1091-1099, 1976.

Fiser, R., and Fisher, D.: Current understanding of the pathogenesis of obesity, South. Med. J. 68:931-933, 1975.

Fried, P., et al.: Effects of ketosis on respiratory sensitivity to carbon dioxide in obesity, N. Engl. J. Med. 294: 1081-1086, 1976.

Kryston, L., and Shaw, R., editors: Endocrinology and diabetes, New York, 1975, Grune & Stratton.

Levine, R., and Luft, R., editors: Advances in metabolic disorders, vol. 7, New York, 1974, Academic Press.

Levine, R., and Pfeiffer, E., editors: Lipid metabolism, obesity, and diabetes: impact upon atherosclerosis, Stuttgart, 1974, Georg Thieme Verlag KG.

Maugh, T., II: Diabetes (III): new hormones promise more effective therapy, Science 188:921-923, 1975.

Maugh, T., II: Hormone receptors: new clues to the cause of diabetes, Science 193:250-252, 1976.

Maxwell, M., and Kleeman, C., editors: Clinical disorders of fluid and electrolyte metabolism, ed. 2, New York, 1972, McGraw-Hill Book Co.

Mountcastle, V., editor: Medical physiology, ed. 13, St. Louis, 1974, The C. V. Mosby Co.

Powley, T., and Morton, S.: Hypophysectomy and regulation of body weight in the genetically obese Zucker rat, Am. J. Physiol. 230:982-987, 1976.

Unger, R. H., and Orci, L.: Physiology and pathophysiology of glucagon, Physiol. Rev. 56(4):778-826, 1976.

CHAPTER 13

Disorders of digestion, absorption, excretion, and metabolism

AT THE COMPLETION OF THIS CHAPTER THE STUDENT WILL BE ABLE TO:

- Relate general principles of nutritional balance to the various disorders discussed.
- Cite the major disorders of motility of the gastrointestinal tract and describe the pathophysiologic mechanisms that may result from disruptions in normal motility.
- Describe the normal secretory functions of the gastrointestinal tract and relate how various disorders of secretion disrupt the steady state.
- Discuss pathophysiologic mechanisms that are perpetuated in cholera and describe the possible commonalities of these mechanisms with other disorders of the gastrointestinal tract.
- Cite the normal absorptive properties of the gut and describe disease mechanisms by which alterations may occur.
- Compare the normal pattern of inflammation and immune responsiveness with the various inflammatory and infectious disorders of the gastrointestinal tract described in this chapter.
- Describe how inflammatory or infectious disorders of the gastrointestinal tract can disturb the steady state and perpetuate further pathophysiology.
- Describe the pathogenesis, pathophysiology, signs and symptoms, and treatment of gallbladder and pancreatic disease and relate these disturbances to normal intestinal function.
- Compare and contrast hepatitis with cirrhosis of the liver in terms of pathogenesis, pathophysiology, signs and symptoms, and natural history of the disease.
- Show how the development of cirrhosis interferes with normal metabolism of the liver, affects other organ systems, and is treated.

GASTROINTESTINAL DISORDERS

Gastrointestinal (GI) disorders will be considered here as abnormalities of motility, absorption, and secretion and as inflammatory disorders. It should be recognized at the outset that many conditions actually fall into more than one of these categories. For example, many inflammatory conditions have a profound effect on GI motility and secretion but are not considered as primary disorders of motility or secretion.

Disorders of motility

The motility of the GI tract is regulated through many nervous and hormonal mechanisms, which act in response to such variables

as distension, food content and amount, pH, activity, metabolism, and blood supply. It should be recalled that the function of a motile GI tract is to grind and mix the food with digestive secretions, disperse it into an absorbable state, and move it caudally through the digestive tract.

Esophagus. Obstruction, either physical or physiologic, and inflammation are two important causes of impaired esophageal motility. The upper esophagus consists of striated and skeletal muscle, while the lower esophagus is smooth muscle. Peristaltic waves move through the esophageal wall, propelling the bolus of food mixed with secretions from the upper esophageal sphincter to the stomach in about 5 seconds. When *dysphagia,* or difficulty in swallowing, develops as a sign of disease, the individual cannot propel the bolus at the normal rate and complains that the food "sticks in his throat"; he may gag in the attempt to swallow the food. Dysphagia is the most common symptom of esophageal disease, but is also seen in other conditions such as goiter, hiatal hernia, and certain neuromuscular conditions. It is also found in psychiatric patients and is termed *globus hystericus*. The most common cause of dysphagia in infants is obstruction caused by congenital malformations of the esophagus, including atresia and tracheoesophageal fistula.

When dysphagia develops, it is often associated with obstruction of the esophagus, such as might occur with esophageal carcinoma, hiatal hernia, or goiter. A physiologic obstruction is one in which the cause is a functional disruption rather than a purely physical barrier, for example, *achalasia,* a disorder in which the esophagus becomes dilated and hypertrophied. Achalasia is due to degeneration of the ganglionic nerve supply of the esophagus. Patients who have suffered brain damage to the swallowing center in the medulla may also have a physiologic obstruction. Other neuromuscular conditions that interrupt swallowing include poliomyelitis, polymyositis, and scleroderma.

Inflammation of the esophageal lining can occur whenever irritation is present, such as would be caused by reflux of gastric acid into the esophagus, or as the sequelae to ingestion of toxic or highly irritating substances such as lye. As with inflammation elsewhere in the body, fibrosis can eventually result, causing strictures in the lumen. The esophagus also reacts to irritation by spasm, thus creating an obstruction to the passage of the bolus. Reflux of acid from the stomach can occur when the cardiac sphincter muscle tone is poor and in *hiatal hernia,* which is a herniation of a portion of the stomach through the opening in the diaphragm through which the esophagus passes. It is very common but asymptomatic in the majority of those individuals discovered to have one. In others the predominant symptoms appear to be related to pressure and acid reflux.

Stomach. The musculature and nervous supply of the stomach provides resting muscle tone for the fundus and corpus of the stomach.

The pyloric antrum also has muscle tone and can contract actively, as can the rest of the stomach when a peristaltic wave passes over it. Peristalsis at a rate of three per minute allows for emptying of food from the stomach into the duodenum. The innervation of the stomach is of two types: *extrinsic,* through both vagal and sympathetic fibers, and *intrinsic,* through ganglionic plexuses, which can be stimulated by the vagus nerve or can become inherently active, much like a primitive, independent nervous net. Furthermore, the smooth muscle of the stomach, and indeed of the entire GI tract, is capable of rhythmic automaticity and is controlled by pacemaker cells that can initiate peristaltic waves, which are conducted through the gut in a one-way direction by the smooth muscle. The intestine appears to have an irreversible cephalocaudad polarity, so that peristalsis can only be conducted in one direction even when a segment of intestine is removed, reversed, and then inserted back into the GI tract.

Distension of the stomach activates receptors in the wall, activating vagal afferent fibers, which transmit the signal to the brain and then to efferent vagal fibers, which when fired will cause muscle contraction in the muscularis layer of the stomach. The major slowing down of the contraction wave is at the duodenum. Hormonal mechanisms such as the enterogastric reflex or enterogastrone release also inhibit gastric emptying.

Important disorders of stomach motility are vomiting, hypermotility, and disorders of gastric emptying.

Vomiting. Vomiting and the often associated sensation of nausea are the most commonly experienced phenomena related to gastric motility. These are symptoms of a great many disorders, ranging from overindulgence in rich and abundant food, to labyrinthine disease, to mental illness. The mechanism by which vomiting occurs is forcible contraction of abdominal muscles, expiration against a closed glottis, and a reverse peristaltic wave, which originates in the pyloric antrum. Increased heart rate, pallor, salivation, sweating, faintness, and other signs of generalized autonomic nervous system arousal are often associated with a vomiting episode. The pathway by which vomiting

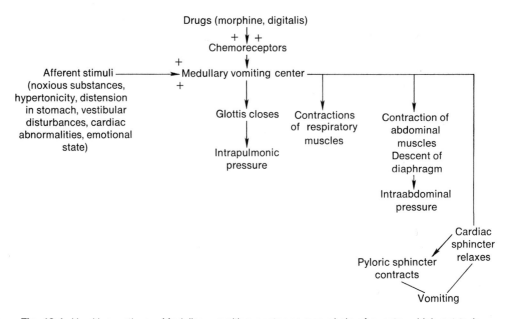

Fig. 13-1. Vomiting pathway. Medullary vomiting center causes chain of events, which act to increase intra-abdominal pressure, increase intrapulmonic pressure (thus compressing esophagus), and relax cardiac sphincter while pylorus contracts. Thus, chyme moves in antiperistaltic direction.

is effected is illustrated in Fig. 13-1. Initiation of the vomiting pathway can be either through stimulation of afferent fibers by irritating substances, which are conveyed to the vomiting center of the brain, or through stimulation of the vomiting center by pathways of nerve fibers from other areas of the brain, such as the hypothalamus or cerebral cortex.

Hypermotility. Gastric hypermotility is often associated with emotional states of anxiety and fear; this is also true for the rest of the GI tract. Hypermotility of this type is caused by excessive parasympathetic firing. Irritation of the stomach lining may also cause hypermotility.

Disorders of gastric emptying. Normally the emptying of chyme into the duodenum is regulated by waves of peristalsis, which occur at a rate of three per minute and which sweep across the pyloric antrum, the pylorus, and the duodenum, causing the expulsion of fluid chyme in spurts from the stomach into the duodenum. Obstruction to the flow of chyme can occur, resulting in an increase of gastric pressure and eventually vomiting. The enterogastric reflex and the release of the hormone enterogastrone inhibit gastric emptying and may be stimulated by irritation of the duodenum.

A major disorder of gastric emptying in infants is *congenital pyloric stenosis*. In this condition the pyloric sphincter is hypertrophied and may actually be cartilaginous in consistency, causing a narrowing of the lumen of the pylorus and dilation of the stomach. The pylorus may be enlarged enough to be palpated; it feels like an olive and is located midway between the umbilicus and the costal margin. The muscle of the pylorus may go into spasm, contributing to the most dramatic sign of this condition: projectile vomiting after feeding, which in some cases may be extremely forceful. The disorder is usually manifested by the third week of life and is more common in males. The polygenic inheritance of pyloric stenosis was discussed in Chapter 2. The treatment may be surgical, but the condition resolves itself in many cases. However, dehydration, electrolyte imbalances, and malnutrition may develop and be severe enough to demand surgical intervention (pylorotomy).

The *dumping syndrome* is another disorder of gastric emptying; it is seen in individuals after pyloric surgery or vagotomy. There appears to be either an anatomic or a physiologic loss of antral control over gastric emptying. The

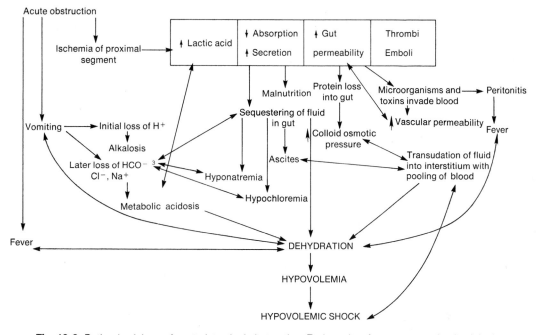

Fig. 13-2. Pathophysiology of acute intestinal obstruction. End results of numerous pathophysiologic mechanisms that are perpetuated by acute intestinal obstruction are vascular dehydration, hypovolemia, and shock.

rate of gastric emptying is markedly increased, with the signs and symptoms, such as sudden weakness, nausea, diarrhea, and hypermotility of the GI tract, appearing after meals.

Any condition that obstructs the stomach outlet, such as tumors, ulcers, edema, or fibrosis resulting in stenosis, will inhibit the rate and degree of gastric emptying. However, the development of symptoms may be quite slow, as the stomach is able to compensate for obstruction to outflow as long as the antral musculature remains intact and functional.

Intestine. The normal motility of the GI tract is characterized by peristalsis and rhythmic segmentation in the small intestine and mass movements, haustral churning, and pendular movements in the large intestine, as well as defecation, which is primarily a function of the distal colon, rectum, and anus.

Decreased motility. *Obstruction,* either acute or chronic, is the major cause of abnormally decreased motility of the intestines. The causes of intestinal obstruction are many, including tumors, foreign bodies, inflammatory conditions, strangulated hernias, and congenital defects.

Acute intestinal obstruction can be so severe as to compromise life in as short a period as 24 hours. Weakness, prostration, and finally irreversible shock ensue. The pathophysiology of intestinal obstruction is illustrated in Fig. 13-2. The prominent symptoms are pain, which is due to stretching of the gut (the gut can stand cutting and tearing without pain), nausea and vomiting, constipation, distension, and absence of motility. The location of the obstruction is important in predicting the pattern of electrolyte changes that will be observed. A low obstruction can cause an initial period of vomiting, which depletes the body of water, H^+, and Cl^-, causing a metabolic alkalosis. However, the usual outcome is a metabolic acidosis, as the obstruction will eventually cause vomiting of fecal material, which is highly alkaline. Obstruction is often mechanical in nature, such as might occur when a loop of bowel is strangulated, which not only causes a mechanical impediment to the flow of fecal material but also results in ischemia of the strangulated loop of bowel due to impairment of the local blood supply. The small intestine becomes ischemic more quickly than the large intestine but is also able to recover and repair more rapidly. Generally, gastrointestinal ischemia that lasts longer than 2 hours will cause irreversible damage. This will result in the rapid development of septic shock, as the ischemic bowel permeability is drastically increased. An obstruction of the intestines results in distension of the intestine above the obstruction, and large amounts of gas accumulate. The normal absorptive functions of that segment are greatly impaired within 6 to 12 hours, with the secretion of Na^+ and water into the ischemic segment increasing until up to 50% of the plasma volume may be sequestered in the proximal segment of intestine. The major effect of such a net increase in secretion over absorption is that hypovolemic shock, hyponatremia, hypochloremia, and acidosis develop. The mucosa that suffers occlusion of its blood supply allows plasma proteins to leak into the gut lumen, and toxins and bacteria of the normal flora pass from the gut into the bloodstream. Septic shock ensues and aggravates the severe cardiovascular effects of the hypovolemia. The pressure in the proximal segment of the obstructed bowel may increase to the point that perforation results, and peritonitis is inevitable. Furthermore, the ischemic gut, besides being a prime site for infection, may also become thrombosed, and emboli may be thrown off to other organs. Fig. 13-2 also shows how one effect of acute intestinal obstruction will aggravate and perpetuate another effect: examples of pathologic positive-feedback loops that act in a concerted manner to destroy the steady state. For example, the dehydration that is a common sign of intestinal obstruction is the result of a number of mechanisms such as fever, sequestration of fluid in the ischemic gut, vomiting, and pooling of blood. As dehydration continues, the development of hypovolemic shock is also perpetuated, and the shock state itself, with its profound decrease in cardiac output and blood pressure, only aggravates the gut ischemia further, thus promulgating continuing dehydration.

Fifty percent of all acute small intestine obstructions in adults are caused by *strangulated hernias*. A loop of bowel becomes caught as it protrudes through a weak area in the abdominal wall, such as an inguinal ring and rapidly becomes hypoxic and then ischemic, resulting in obstruction to the passage of material through the tract.

Other important causes of acute obstruction, particularly in the large intestine, are volvulus, diverticulosis, and paralytic ileus in adults and intussusception in children. *Volvulus* is a condition in which the intestine becomes twisted on itself. Infarction of the bowel is a common side effect. *Diverticulosis* is characterized by the presence of hypertrophic rings, which then alternate with herniations of the mucosa and submucosa through sacs in the muscularis, usually in the colon. This condition may be either congenital or acquired, and it is believed that a low residue diet of the type found in most industrialized and civilized societies is etiologic. *Meckel's diverticulum* is a special congenital case in which a single outpuching of the small intestine results from the vestigial remnant of an embryonic duct. Diverticula in general are prone to inflammation, impaction with fecal material or foreign bodies, fibrosis, and fistula development. Spastic, colicky pain is common, and acute obstruction occasionally develops.

Paralytic ileus is a common cause of intestinal obstruction following abdominal surgery. It is also seen in hypokalemia. The small intestine becomes atonic, and peristalsis is absent. Distension, pain, and absence of bowel sounds are important symptoms, and if it does not resolve itself, not only is the flow of gastrointestinal contents interrupted but the vascular supply can become compromised by the increasing distension. Any handling or manipulation of the peritoneum, the abdominal organs, and the gut itself may set up this reflex response. In some patients it can be avoided or relieved in part by diet and exercise.

Intussusception is a condition found most commonly in children under 2 years of age and is caused by the telescoping of a segment of the small intestine upon itself, usually near the ileocecal valve. The symptoms are quite characteristic, and the condition usually appears suddenly in an otherwise healthy child. The major symptoms are paroxysms of acute abdominal pain, which are then followed by periods of normal activity. Gradually, however, vomiting begins and may proceed until fecal material is vomited, blood is passed rectally, and the child becomes more and more lethargic. Intussusception often will suddenly reduce itself spontaneously or following an enema, and surgery is thus avoided.

Motility of the gut may also be compromised by more chronic obstructive conditions, such as might be caused by slowly growing tumors or interruptions in the myenteric plexuses, which are involved in normal peristalsis, or in the vagal or sympathetic extrinsic controls over normal motility. *Hirschsprung's disease* is an excellent example of neuromuscular obstruction. It is a congenital condition, also called congenital megacolon, in which the ganglia of Auerbach's and Meissner's plexuses are absent from birth in the distal colon. This results in enormous distension of the proximal segment of the colon with fecal material, as the muscle cells of the affected segment are unable to contract normally to permit defecation because mass-movement peristaltic waves are inhibited.

An extremely common disorder of motility is constipation. Constipation may be caused by destruction of any of the nervous elements in the normal defecation reflex, which over a long period of time produces atony of the rectum and colon and thus a progressively weaker defecation reflex. This phenomenon is observed in individuals who rely on laxatives and stool softeners for regular bowel movements, some of which are known to destroy nervous elements in the gut and in individuals who continually supress the urge to defecate. Constipation may also be a primary abnormality of the motility of the sigmoid and descending colon, such that the gastrocolic and duodenocolic reflexes cannot operate. These disorders of defecation do not often result in acute intestinal obstruction, as described above. Low obstruction of this nature does not result in proximal ischemia, and absorption and secretion are not impaired. Individuals have been known to have been constipated for over a year without apparent adverse effects on their general health. Up to 100 pounds of accumulated feces may burden such individuals, but no toxic effects on their physiology have been observed.

Increased motility. Certain susceptible individuals will respond to a variety of stimuli by intestinal hypermotility. Emotional stress may cause irritability of the colon, and *diarrhea* characterized by frequent, watery, mucus-filled stools occurs.

Diarrhea is not always accompanied by hypermotility of the gastrointestinal tract, however. Most common causes of diarrhea, such as infection, toxic foods, and emotional anxiety, actually are accompanied by a decreased colonic luminal pressure and depressed motility, such that any small increase in colonic pressure will set up a mass movement of feces in the caudal direction. When the diarrhea is caused by hypermotility and cramping, the condition is known as a *spastic irritable colon*.

Disorders of secretion

Different parts of the gastrointestinal tract have different secretory and absorptive functions (Table 13-1). Pathophysiology of any one of these functions can occur, and in many cases, disruption of one function can have a profound effect on another.

Gastric secretion

Peptic ulcers. The major disorder of secretion of the gastrointestinal tract is peptic ulceration

Table 13-1. Secretory and absorptive functions of gastrointestinal tract

	pH	Secretion	Digestion	Absorption
Mouth		Saliva	Carbohydrates	
Esophagus		Mucus		
Stomach	2-4	HCl; pepsin; intrinsic factor; mucus	Begins protein digestion	Alcohol
Small intestine	Duodenum, 6; ileum, 8	Pancreatic enzymes; HCO_3^-; bile; Na^+; water; K^+	Most digestion of proteins, carbohydrates, lipids	Minerals; amino acids; Na^+; glucose; lipids; vitamins; water
Large intestine	8	HCO_3^-; Na^+; Cl^-; K^+; water		Water; Na^+; K^+; HCO_3^-; Cl^-

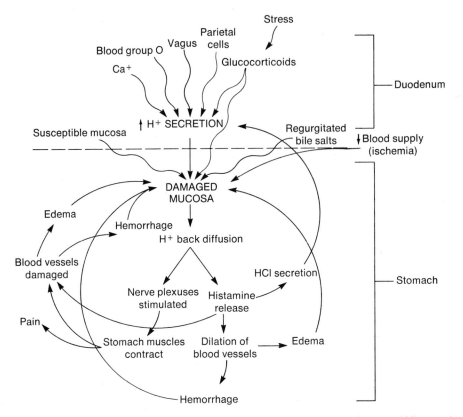

Fig. 13-3. Duodenal and gastric ulcer pathophysiology. In duodenal ulcer, an increased H$^+$ secretion is implicated; in gastric ulcer, a normal H$^+$ secretion in presence of a damaged mucosal barrier is etiologic. Either mechanism results in ulceration, a process that sets up positive-feedback situations such that ulceration is further perpetuated.

of the stomach or more commonly the duodenum (Figs. 13-3 and 13-4). This is a common condition of the twentieth century (affecting 10% of all Americans) with an increased incidence in men, particularly under the age of 50. It has been associated with increased levels of stress and anxiety in many cases. Estrogen may protect against peptic ulceration. There is some evidence of a hereditary predisposition, with the duodenal type occurring more commonly in individuals with blood group O and the gastric type in individuals with blood group A. The gastric peptic ulcer appears to be associated with a breakdown in the normal stomach mucosal defenses to the highly acid stomach secretions, while duodenal peptic ulcer pathogenesis implicates a primary increased acid secretion. Increased HCl secretion causes a breakdown in the mucosa, which then ulcerates.

STOMACH. The acidity of stomach gastric juice is very high, the pH becoming as low as 2.0 when acid is being actively secreted. This acid is certainly capable of totally digesting and destroying the epithelial lining of the stomach. The fact that it does not is remarkable. The protective mechanism whereby autodigestion is prevented is through (1) the secretion of a slightly alkaline layer of mucus that coats the surface of the gastric epithelium, (2) dilution of the acid by food and secretions, (3) prevention of diffusion of the HCl from the lumen back into the cells, and (4) regulation of gastric pH by negative-feedback mechanisms that act mainly on the gastrin-releasing antral cells. It should be recalled that a marked diffusion gradient for HCl exists between the gastric lumen and the epithelial cells. Diffusion of HCl down this gradient is prevented in part by the presence of nonpermeable tight junctions between adjacent epithelial cells. The gradient for diffusion

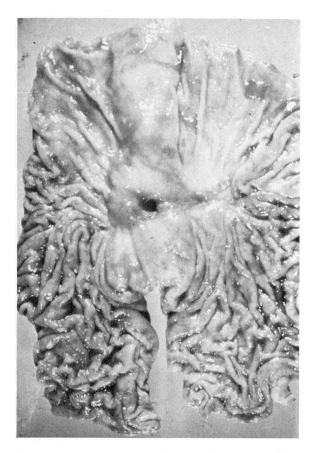

Fig. 13-4. Very well circumscribed peptic ulcer. (Courtesy Department of Pathology, University of Tennessee, Memphis.)

across the epithelial cell membrane will also increase as HC1 concentration in the lumen is increased. If the barriers to diffusion are broken down in any way, there is a tendency, governed by purely physical laws, for the HC1 to back diffuse down its gradient into the epithelial cells. It has been speculated that a *gastric peptic ulcer,* which is very often associated with a lower than normal basal HC1 concentration, is caused by such a breakdown in the epithelium, rather than by a hypersecretion of HC1. The diffusion barrier may be interrupted by aspirin, alcohol, inflammation, and perhaps regurgitated bile salts. The detergentlike properties of bile salts, which may be regurgitated into the stomach from the duodenum, may cause the barrier to break down. These substances strip away the surface mucus and can solubilize the membrane lipids, thus increasing the permeability of these cells, allowing mas-

sive back diffusion to take place. The pathophysiologic mechanism by which the ulcerative process is perpetuated is illustrated in Fig. 13-5. The refluxed bile salts cause damage and H^+ back diffusion, which further aggravates the mucosal damage, resulting in ulceration. The primary disorder may then be a delay in gastric emptying and motility of the stomach, a process that is in large part mediated by duodenal receptors, which may be CO_2 sensors and which respond to acid stimuli by decreasing the rate of emptying. The actual mechanism by which bile is refluxed forward into the antrum is not well understood, however.

Davenport has described a possible mechanism by which aspirin can damage the mucosal barrier. Chronic aspirin users are subject to the development of gastritis, bleeding, and peptic ulceration of the stomach. Aspirin is known to damage the mucosa, causing slight bleeding

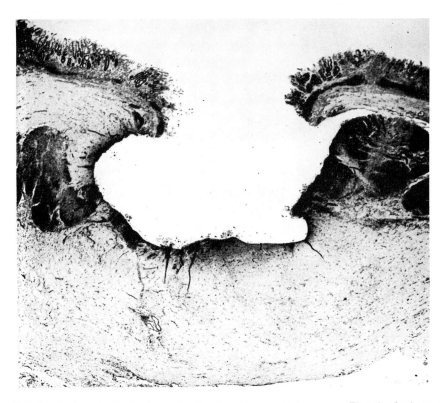

Fig. 13-5. Peptic ulcer. A chronic ulcer extending through muscularis mucosa. Fibrosis of submucosa and base of ulcer provides evidence of continuing process. (×8.) (From Anderson, W. A. D., and Kissane, J. M.: Pathology, ed. 7, St. Louis, 1977, The C. V. Mosby Co.)

(around 2 ml) in almost all people and massive hemorrhage in those who are for some reason susceptible. Damage to the mucosa occurs when the aspirin is unbuffered and thus present in the un-ionized state, for it is most soluble in membrane lipids then and can rapidly diffuse through the cell membrane into the mucosal epithelial cells. There it ionizes at the neutral pH of the interior of the cell, so that the un-ionized form is quickly removed almost as soon as it enters the cells. This sets up a steep downhill diffusion gradient for the un-ionized form from the lumen into the cells. The ionized form of aspirin can damage the mucosa, and once this occurs HCl can back diffuse, and hemorrhage may eventually result from the damage. Alcohol is another substance that can be absorbed by the stomach mucosal cells, due to its great lipid solubility, and it is known to enhance the damaging effect of aspirin.

It is believed that minor damage to the stomach mucosa may actually occur in normal individuals with every meal, but the continuous renewal of the gastric epithelium counteracts this process, so that the effect is minor.

DUODENUM. While breakdown in the normal mucosa appears to be the major cause of a stomach peptic ulcer, hypersecretion of acid appears most important in the etiology of *duodenal peptic ulcer*. Evidence for this theory comes from the observation that vagal activity is increased, especially during fasting and at night in ulcer patients. The vagus, it will be recalled, acts to increase the release of HCl by stimulating pyloric antrum cells, which produce the hormone gastrin; *gastrin* acts via the bloodstream of the parietal cells of the stomach, causing them to respond by secreting HCl. The vagus is normally stimulated by distension, the presence of food in the stomach, higher centers of the brain such as the cortex, and the feeding- and satiety-regulating centers of the hypothalamus. Its basal rate of firing appears to be increased in ulcer patients even when these normal stimulating factors are absent (Fig. 13-4). Experimentally, peptic ulcer can be produced by the administration of excess acid or excessive gastrin release. The Zollinger-Ellison syndrome, which is characterized by the presence of peptic ulceration in patients with a gastrin-secreting pancreatic tumor, also points to the importance of acid hypersecretion. Individuals with blood group O are often found to have an increased secretion of HCl, and further evidence is found in the association of peptic ulcer with an increased parietal cell mass.

The most common symptom of peptic duodenal ulcer is intermittent epigastric pain, which is usually most pronounced when the stomach is empty. The pain is thought to be due to increased irritation of the damaged and hyperemic mucosa by HCl, leading to stimulation of the nerve plexuses in the stomach, which results in local muscular contraction. The pain is relieved by eating. The pain that typifies gastric ulceration is often present after a meal, but this is a variable finding. The major complication of peptic ulceration of either the stomach or duodenum is hemorrhage, which may be sudden and life threatening. Ulcers may also become chronic inflammatory sites, which can fibrose and cause obstruction. The ulcer may become so excavated that perforation through the gut or stomach wall occurs, leading to massive hemorrhage, peritonitis, and shock. Ulcer symptoms are characteristically episodic, and long periods of time may occur between them. Anticholinergic drugs, bland, high-fat diet, complete alcohol abstinence, and frequent small meals are generally recommended for the treatment of ulcer. There is, however, no good evidence that a bland diet can alleviate this disease.

Surgical treatment is subtotal distal gastric resection and occasionally vagotomy for duodenal ulcers with removal of a large part of the gastrin-secreting pyloric antrum and the parietal cell mass. The surgical treatment for gastric ulcers is the same, but the parietal cell mass is usually preserved.

Stress ulcers. The pathophysiology of stress ulcers has never been clearly described. The occurrence of an acute gastritis and the almost immediate appearance of multiple, well-circumscribed gastric ulcers following head injury, surgery, trauma, burns, and sepsis have led to numerous postulates for their occurrence. Circulating peptides, corticosteroids, and acid hypersecretion have all been suggested. Recent research, however, has led to the suggestion that three factors must exist for this phenomenon to occur. These are the presence of acid, the presence of bile salts or other agents that will increase H^+ permeability through the mucosal cells, and the occurrence of a period of decreased mucosal blood flow, such as might occur during a bout of profound hypotension associated with a shock state. Menguy has shown that hemorrhagic shock in rats is associated with diffuse foci of mucosal necrosis within 15 minutes and with gross ulceration leading to gastric hemorrhage within 45 to 60 minutes. He suggests that a sudden cellular energy deficit causing cellular necrosis, such as is observed in hypovolemic shock induced by hemorrhage, results in damage to the mucosa, leading to stress ulcer formation. Furthermore, it is apparent that the lesions formed during the initial period of gastric hypoxia will be aggravated by the HCl, which continues to form when gastric function is returned to basal levels. Thus, the gastric permeability to H^+ must be considered not as a static barrier but rather as a dynamic and changing tolerance of the mucosa that depends on the maintenance of a variety of factors at steady state values.

Achlorhydria. Achlorhydria is depression or total absence of HCl and pepsinogen secretion by the stomach caused by atrophy of the gastric mucosa. The stomach pH that results is usually between 7.0 and 8.0. The absence of an acidic stomach environment is not an insurmountable impairment to normal digestion, but the absence of intrinsic factor production in achlorhydria does result in major pathology. *Intrinsic factor* is produced by the stomach mucosa; it is a proteinaceous substance required by the ileum to absorb vitamin B_{12}. The intrinsic factor is thought to bind the highly charged vitamin complex as the first step in its subsequent pinocytosis by intestinal epithelial cells. It is of interest that both intrinsic factor and vitamin B_{12} are rather large molecules, and when bound together they form an unusually massive complex for the cell membrane to transport. It is the opposite for most other digestive and absorptive processes, where larger molecules are broken down into smaller fragments to facilitate their absorption by the mucosa. When vitamin B_{12} absorption is inhibited in the absence of intrinsic factor, red blood cell maturation is delayed and deficient, so that anemia results. This is termed *pernicious anemia* and is treated by injections of the needed vitamin B_{12}, which delivers the vitamin directly into the bloodstream, thus bypassing the gut entirely.

Achlorhydria is associated with atrophic gastritis in less than 20% of the cases. Atrophic gastritis is present in about half of the individuals with gastric peptic ulcers and is also associated with an increased incidence of gastric carcinoma.

Intestinal secretion. The major function of the small intestine is to disperse and digest the larger molecules of food substances into readily absorbable form, which mainly occurs in the duodenum, and to then absorb these molecules through the intestinal lining cells and into the capillary blood or lymphatic fluid of the intestinal lacteals. This process is a major function of the jejunum. The small and large intestines participate in both the secretion and later reabsorption of tremendous amounts of fluids and electrolytes, which aid the digestive and absorptive processes. In a sense there is a circulation of about 9,000 ml of isotonic fluid from the blood, through the intestinal lining cells, into the lumen of the gut, back out through the cells, and eventually a return of this fluid to the blood. Only 1,500 ml of fluid is taken in through the diet, and only 150 ml is normally excreted in the feces.

Disorders of secretion can originate at many levels of the gut and can involve fluid or mucous secretion. For example, disordered gastric emptying, such as might occur with the dumping syndrome, results in the sudden influx of a large amount of highly acid and often hypertonic fluid from the stomach into the duodenum. This will result in osmosis of water into the duodenum, and this rush of chyme may overwhelm the limited capacity of the colon to absorb water and electrolytes, so that fluid diar-

rhea may result. Thus, excessive secretion has occurred in response to the loss of regulation of gastric emptying that occurs in the dumping syndrome. A low, unbuffered gastrointestinal tract pH can by itself inhibit the absorption of water and Na^+ as well, thus further contributing to the net secretion.

Another condition that can result in abnormal fluid secretion has been described in individuals with secretin-releasing pancreatic tumors. Large amounts of secretin are released and cause excessive secretion of large amounts of highly alkaline fluid from the pancreas, which is poured into the duodenum. Net secretion and Na^+ and water reabsorption impairment result.

Increased mucous secretion in the lower bowel is a common response both to a variety of bowel inflammations and in certain tumors.

Cholera. The best-described disorder of intestinal fluid secretion is the infectious disease *cholera,* which is caused by the organism *Vibrio cholerae.* Individuals with cholera may lose up to 16 liters of diarrhea fluid per day from their gastrointestinal tract as massive secretion of fluid from mainly the jejunum and ileum into the lumen occurs. The mechanism of action for cholera toxin is currently under investigation, but considerable evidence has accumulated to implicate the adenyl cyclase system of the mucosal cells as the site of action for cholera toxin. It has been suggested that adenyl cyclase, which converts ATP to cyclic AMP, may be required in the control of Na^+ secretion into the bowel lumen. Prostaglandins may be mediators of this process. There is conflicting evidence for an actual secretion of Na^+ into the gut, however. The increased concentration of sodium in the gut may be the result of depressed Na^+ absorption rather than an actual secretion of Na^+. Considerable evidence does exist for stimulation of HCO_3^- and Cl^- active transport into the lumen by cholera toxin, which has an extremely protracted action. The result of such activations is a reversal of the normal direction of fluid and electrolyte movement in the intestine. The colon is presented with large amounts of fluid containing Na^+, Cl^-, and HCO_3^- and is unable to absorb these ions and fluids efficiently. Thus, cholera stool composition is approximately the same as ileal fluid. Glucose and amino acid absorption, which are Na^+ dependent, are normal in cholera, even in the presence of large fluid secretion into the gut lumen. Oral fluid replacement in cholera therefore is often high in amino acids and glucose, as their transport mechanisms may actually increase absorption of Na^+, water, and other electrolytes.

It would appear that the many forms of infectious gastroenteritis that afflict humans may actually mimic the interferences of normal water and electrolyte movement observed in cholera. A number of other organisms elaborate enterotoxins that appear able to act on intestinal secretion. The most noteworthy among these are *Escherichia coli* and *Staphylococcus aureus,* which are known to be common agents for diarrheal diseases.

Disorders of absorption

Of all the gastrointestinal functions, the function of the jejunum is the most compromised by the various clinical malabsorption syndromes common in humans, as most foods are absorbed in this segment of the small intestine. When protein and carbohydrate digestive products are not absorbed in the jejunum, due to some disease process, the osmotic pressure of the jejunum increases, and Na^+ and water reabsorption are impaired, resulting in an increased flow and load of liquid material into the ileum and colon.

Malabsorption may be due to disease of organs such as the liver, gallbladder, or pancreas, such that digestive enzymes or bile is deficient, or it may be caused by primary disorders of the intestinal tract itself.

A primary malabsorption syndrome is *lactose intolerance,* which is caused by a genetically determined lack of lactase, an enzyme required to break down lactose in milk into a form that can be readily absorbed by the gut mucosa. It also acts to cause an osmotic diarrhea (Fig. 13-6). It can be seen that the absence of the enzyme required to break down the ingested food molecules results in a large concentration

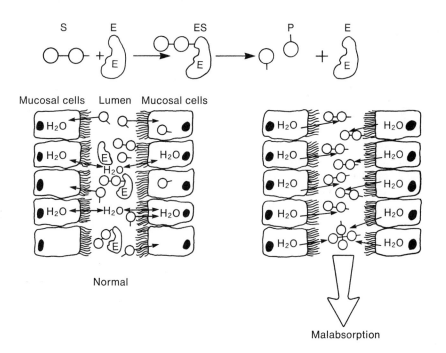

Fig. 13-6. Osmotic diarrhea in malabsorption. When a normally absorbable substance that is broken down by an intestinal enzyme into smaller units so as to be able to pass through mucosal cells remains in lumen due to a deficiency of enzyme, an osmotic gradient is created. Substance accumulates and creates a hypertonic luminal fluid, with water moving into lumen, causing a fluid diarrhea. *S* = substance; *E* = enzyme; *ES* = enzyme substance complex; *P* = products.

of these molecules in the lumen of the intestinal tract, which acts to osmotically pull water from the luminal cells into the gut, thus causing a large volume of fluid to move through the tract and be expelled as diarrhea. Lactase deficiency may develop in the aged as well and may be treated by addition of the enzyme to milk.

Other malabsorption syndromes may act differently to cause the characteristic diarrhea, malnutrition and weight loss, and other signs of starvation that are common to all malabsorption disorders. *Celiac disease,* for example, may result in the formation of toxic products, which then act directly on the gut mucosa to damage it and diminish its normal regulatory capacity for secretion and absorption. Celiac disease in children and *nontropical sprue** in adults appear to be the same disease process. There is evidence that a genetic predisposition to these conditions is present. The most outstanding finding in these disorders is an inability to digest gluten and gliadin, proteins found mainly in wheat. Toxic peptides may be produced when these large molecules are not broken down completely, and these peptides may then act on the small intestinal mucosa to cause characteristic damage. There are generally hypertrophic changes associated with inflammation in this condition. Flattening of the jejunal villi is also common, and the ability of the intestinal cells to secrete intestinal hormones, such as cholecystokinin and secretin, is affected. This results in impaired fat absorption, causing a common sign of malabsorption: *steatorrhea,* or fat in the stools. Many abnormal enzyme activities of the intestinal cells have been reported as well. Fermentation of undigested food by large intestine bacteria gives rise to large amounts of flatus and frothy, offensive stools. These histologic and physiologic changes revert to normal when a gluten-free diet is administered. This disorder may have an immune hypersensitivity etiology,

or it may be accompanied by an increased gut permeability to antigens normally sequestered in the gastrointestinal tract. The major signs and symptoms of celiac disease and nontropical sprue are diarrhea, steatorrhea, malnutrition, weight loss in the presence of an increased appetite, abdominal distension and bloating, hypocalcemia, anemia, and edema.

Many other malabsorption conditions cause morphologic changes in the intestinal structure. Kwashiorkor, caused by a protein-calorie deficiency, is usually accompanied by a chronic diarrhea. Atrophic changes in the jejunal mucosa, with resultant malabsorption of glucose and disaccharides, and diarrhea result, further debilitating an already severely malnourished child.

Malabsorption of Na^+ and water has also been described in association with scleroderma, Crohn's disease, and ulcerative colitis. Increased secretion of K^+ into the lumen may also occur in these conditions. The extensive use of laxatives may result in Na^+ and water depletion, which may become chronic and debilitating. Certain laxatives (senna and cascara) also can cause atonia of the colon by irreversible damage to the myenteric nerve plexuses.

Defects of intestinal amino acid transport such as in cystinuria and tryptophan malabsorption can occur, and protein malabsorption is often observed in pancreatic disease, stasis of the small intestine, gastrectomy, celiac disease, and Crohn's disease.

Fat malabsorption resulting in steatorrhea is common in many gastrointestinal conditions; it is particularly common in cystic fibrosis, celiac disease, ileal resection (such that the overall absorptive surface is decreased), and in any condition that results in the loss of bile salts (cholelithiasis, hepatic disease). When large amounts of fat are retained, hypocalcemia may develop, with signs of tetany, since the fatty acids form insoluble calcium soaps, resulting in GI calcium loss. Vitamin and mineral deficiencies are common in most malabsorption syndromes, and specific vitamin malabsorption also may occur (pernicious anemia). Endocrine disease, diet, drugs, surgery, intestinal factors, and systemic influences may all interfere with absorption of vitamins, minerals, and other food molecules.

---

*Tropical sprue, another disorder of absorption, may be due to bacterial overgrowth secondary to mucosal injury. It is acquired in the tropics but may actually appear 20 years after an individual has migrated from the tropics. It is characterized by sugar, fat, and vitamin B_{12} malabsorption and steatorrhea. It should be differentiated from nontropical sprue, as its etiology and pathogenesis are entirely different.

Inflammatory and infectious disorders

Inflammation and infection of the gut have been alluded to previously as being responsible for disorders of secretion, motility, and absorption. There are a number of disease models that illustrate the pathophysiology of gastrointestinal inflammation.

Stomach

Acute gastritis. Acute gastritis is so common among the human population that the signs and symptoms need hardly be mentioned. It can occur in response to ingestion of highly irritating or toxic substances, such as aspirin or alcohol, or it can be the result of infection of the stomach by *Staphylococcus* or *Clostridium botulinum*. Stress, burns, and head injuries also provoke a gastritislike response that may lead to the development of numerous gastric ulcers (Curling's and Cushing's ulcers; see Stress Ulcers). The stomach mucosa responds to all the above agents by increasing the rate of cell turnover of the epithelial lining, and thus the disease process may be self-limiting, with the renewal of the epithelium providing an adequate surface, and the damaged, necrotic cells produced by the gastritis being sloughed away. If the exposure is particularly intense or long, the mucosa may respond with an acute inflammatory response characterized by hyperemia, edema, infiltration, and occasionally by hemorrhage.

The symptoms of acute gastritis are nausea, vomiting, and often diarrhea if the intestine is involved. A severe but fairly common response is hematemesis, which may lead to a significant loss of blood. Acute gastritis may predispose the individual to the further development of ulceration of the gastric mucosa.

Chronic gastritis. Chronic gastritis is associated with atrophy of the gastric mucosa and the possible development of pernicious anemia. The etiology of this disorder is not well understood at this time, but the incidence does increase with age. An autoimmune background has been suggested, as chronic thyroiditis, an autoimmune disease of the thyroid gland, is often found in individuals with pernicious anemia.

Intestine

Acute gastroenteritis. This infectious or inflammatory response of the gastrointestinal tract is common to all who have traveled in foreign countries or have eaten contaminated food. It is also seen frequently among infants, in whom it can be extremely virulent. For the most part the condition is mild and self-resolving, causing diarrhea, nausea, vomiting, and often systemic symptoms such as malaise and fever. Acute gastroenteritis can be caused either by the direct infection of the GI tract lining by a pathogenic organism such as *Salmonella* or *Shigella,* or indirectly by the ingestion of bacteria that produce toxins, such as the neurotoxin of *Clostridium botulinum*. The latter is the cause of the most severe form of food poisoning. Gastroenteritis may also be caused by imbalance in the normal bacterial flora of the gut. Most travelers' diarrhea probably occurs through the latter mechanism. Local strains of normal gut flora, such as *Escherichia coli,* may be acquired by the traveler, and a temporary upset in the normal flora may occur, causing the signs and symptoms of acute gastroenteritis.

Generally pathogens invading the GI tract tend to localize in a particular segment of the gut and accumulate there in amounts of 10^7 to 10^8/g of tissue. This phenomenon may be peculiar to the specific pathogen or may be related to the anatomy and physiology of the gut.

Many pathogenic organisms cause gastroenteritis by actual binding with the mucosal cells of the GI tract, causing an effect similar to cholera, which results in increased secretion of salt and water into the gut lumen. Other organisms may act by causing a rush of chyme from the small intestine, which contains large amounts of undigested foods that can act osmotically to increase water secretion into the gut and that can also result in fermentation by large intestinal flora. Large amounts of gas and foul-smelling liquid stool result. The organism responsible for botulism acts by elaborating a neurotoxin that affects motor nerve synapses and causes abnormal GI tract motility in this manner. The *Clostridium botulinum* neurotoxin causes an early severe diarrhea, but this is later followed by a prolonged constipation. Viruses have been implicated as causative agents of acute infantile gastroenteritis, and identification of these reoviruses was first made in 1973.

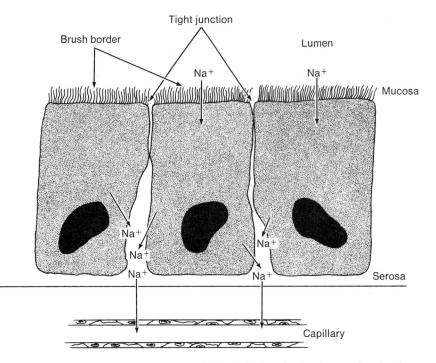

Fig. 13-7. Pathway of molecules through intestinal wall. Na^+ and other ions and molecules move through intestinal epithelial cells at brush border and then are actively transported at lateral cell surfaces. Na^+, glucose, and amino acid transport are all believed to be linked.

The pathophysiology of fluid diarrhea is given in the box at right. The normal physiology of water and solute balance requires that the 7,500 ml of water, 1,000 mEq Na^+, 40 mEq K^+, and 750 mEq Cl^- secreted into the gut each day be reabsorbed by the intestinal epithelium, so that the final outputs of these substances will be small. This reabsorption mainly occurs in the jejunum, ileum, and colon. If it is not complete, either because the mechanisms for reabsorption are impaired, interfered with, or overcome, or because the transit time to this fluid in the gut is shortened, fluid diarrhea may result. Sodium reabsorption appears to involve active transport at the lateral cell membranes of the mucosal cells. Movement of Na^+ into the mucosal cells from the lumen is passive but appears to be coupled to glucose and amino acid absorption. Therefore, any defect that interferes significantly with Na^+ reabsorption may also deplete the body of energy-producing food molecules and water.

Whenever the load in the intestine is increased over the ability of the intestine to reab-

CAUSES OF DIARRHEA*
Normal gut mucosa
Increased gastric emptying
Abnormal upper GI secretions
Hypertonic load
Increased motility
Abnormal gut mucosa
Disorders of absorption
Celiac disease
Acute gastroenteritis
Sugar malabsorption
Laxatives (?)
Inflammatory diseases
Disorders of secretion
Celiac disease
Mucus-secreting tumors
Unabsorbed bile acids
Cholera

*Modified from McColl, I., and Sladen, G.: Intestinal absorption in man, London, 1975, Academic Press.

sorb, malabsorption and diarrhea are possible. Osmotic diarrhea occurs when the number of osmotically active particles increases, such as might be seen in malabsorption of specific nutrients, which are therefore left behind in the gut. This causes hypertonicity of the luminal contents, driving excess water into the lumen. The gut may also be defective in absorption of food, fluid, and electrolytes. When either of these processes occurs, the colon is overwhelmed by fluid and electrolytes that it cannot absorb, and fluid diarrhea results. Diarrhea may result from increased motility of the small intestine, which causes an osmotic rush of fluid fecal material through the large intestine; this rush of fecal material may be aided by the accumulation of the products of fermentation of undigested food by the large intestine bacteria. Some invading organisms that cause gastroenteritis may destroy the colonic mucosa, and decreased water reabsorption may result, contributing to the development of diarrhea. Volume overload of this type may not be accompanied by increased gut motility.

Superinfection. The normal intestinal flora itself may become imbalanced by antibiotics, such as ampicillin, which are broad spectrum in nature. These drugs may act on components of the normal flora, destroying an innocuous species and thus removing a source of competition for food molecules in the gut. Populations of pathogens that are normally very small or absent then begin to grow and may invade the mucosa, causing *mucous enterocolitis*. A common causative organism that may invade and cause ulceration and necrosis of the colon wall is *Staphylococcus aureus*. The enteritis that occurs in this case is prolonged rather than acute. It has been recently suggested that consumption of sour milk products, high in lactobacilli, may counteract this effect of the broad-spectrum antibiotics. The problem of superinfection also may occur in the oral cavity and the vagina.

Ulcerative colitis. Ulcerative colitis is classified along with Crohn's disease as an inflammatory bowel disease. However, there are some important differences between them in terms of location and characteristic lesions (Table 13-2).

Ulcerative colitis is more common under the age of 30 and is occasionally associated with certain behavior patterns and stress states. There is a familial nature to the disease also. Individuals with ulcerative colitis sometimes

Table 13-2. Differences between ulcerative colitis and Crohn's disease

Signs and symptoms	Ulcerative colitis	Crohn's disease
Ulcerations	Usually superficial, involving only mucosa	Deep; may invade many layers
Strictures and fistulas	Rare	Common
Involvement of small intestine	Rare	Extensive
Granulomas	Rare	40%-80%
Continuity	Contiguous	Often skips areas
Thickening of bowel wall	Occasionally slightly increased	Thickened
Anal and perianal lesions	Rare	Common
Cancer incidence	Increased risk	Normal risk

have attitudes of hopelessness and hidden hostility. They are usually overachievers and will attempt impossible tasks. The disorder is characterized by chronic hemorrhagic ulceration of the colon and usually the rectum, which is commonly associated with diarrhea, melena, pain, and fever. Occasionally systemic manifestations appear, including arthritis, liver disease, uveitis, and skin lesions. The cause of ulcerative colitis is unknown, but increasingly the theory that an immunologic abnormality is etiologic is being accepted. Diet has also been implicated as a factor. One theory of pathogenesis suggests that *cross-reactivity* of normal gut antigens with bacterial floral antigens results in the destruction and erosion of the normal mucosa. The bacteria present in the gut may invade a damaged mucosa more easily, thus perpetuating the disease process. Evidence for an immunologic component is also given by the fact that T cell function is disturbed in patients with ulcerative colitis.

The disease typically arises in the left colon, and the earliest sign is tiny abscesses in the crypts of Lieberkühn, which cause the mucosal cells to slough away from the surface, leaving behind ulcerations that eventually coalesce and occasionally invade deep into the muscular coatings of the intestine. Intense hyperemia may be present as an accompaniment to ulcerative changes. The inflammation that is part of this process often takes on the characteristics of a chronic process. However, fibrosis is rare in this condition. Chronic loss of blood and fluids through bloody diarrhea often results in anemia and debilitation. Defects in fluid and electrolyte absorption may be present. Morphologic abnormalities of the mucosa include the development of pseudopolyps and fistulas. The course of ulcerative colitis is characterized by periods of remission and exacerbation. Treatment includes management of diarrhea, bleeding, and anemia, prevention and treatment of secondary infection through drug therapy, and surgical colostomy or ileostomy (depending on the degree of involvement of the colon and rectum). It has been previously noted that long-standing chronic ulcerative colitis is associated with an increased incidence of colon carcinoma. A further complication may be the development of *toxic megacolon,* which is due to the destruction of the myenteric nerve plexus. Massive dilation and obstruction of the colon may occur and require emergency intervention.

Crohn's disease. This condition should be mentioned in contrast to ulcerative colitis. It is much less common than ulcerative colitis, and the etiology, the area of bowel involved, and the pathologic changes are different, but the two conditions are often confused, particularly if Crohn's disease is present in the left colon. Crohn's disease can affect both the small and large intestine, and it is characterized by a chronic hyperemic granulomatous response of the mucosa of unknown etiology. The acute condition is usually a regional ileitis that is self-resolving in the majority of cases. The chronic regional enteritis is characterized by intermittent diarrhea, anorexia, abdominal pain, and weight loss. The lesions that develop in the gastrointestinal tract are likely to become suppurative and transmural, and fistulas frequently form communicating channels from one section of the intestine to another. There are often intermittent patches of enteritis so that areas of affected bowel are followed by disease-free areas. The disease is also one in which remissions and exacerbations occur over the course of many years, and most of the treatment during acute stages is symptomatic. Antibiotics and corticosteroids are the major drugs used in the treatment of Crohn's disease, and surgical intervention is often necessary to excise diseased segments of bowel.

Acute appendicitis. A discussion of inflammatory conditions of the intestine would not be complete without inclusion of acute appendicitis, which is the most common cause for emergency surgery to the abdomen but which has been steadily declining in incidence in recent years. Acute appendicitis is the result of obstruction and inflammation leading to ischemia of the vermiform appendix, which may result in necrosis and perforation of the appendix and subsequent abscess formation or peritonitis. The earliest and most significant symptom of appendicitis is pain, which is caused by distension of the serosa due to inflammatory edema. Obstruction of the appendix (e.g., by a foreign body or fecalith or even by lymphatic hypertrophy due to systemic infection) will result in edema, which can compromise the vascular supply to the appendix. This will increase the permeability of this segment of the intestines, and bacterial invasion of the wall of the appendix by organisms of the normal flora then results in infection and inflammation. The appendix may rupture, causing either a local or generalized peritonitis.

The symptoms of acute appendicitis are pain and rebound tenderness, which usually eventually localize over McBurney's point, nausea and vomiting, anorexia, diarrhea, and systemic signs of inflammation such as leukocytosis and fever. If perforation of the appendix occurs, the pain becomes generalized, and the patient will lie very still and rigid. Many conditions simulate the symptoms of appendicitis, making this condition surprisingly difficult to diagnose.

Other conditions that will cause an "acute abdomen" include ruptured gallbladder, perforated duodenal ulcer, pancreatitis, a ruptured tubal pregnancy, sickle cell crisis, and gastrointestinal conditions such as diverticulitis.

DISORDERS OF THE GALLBLADDER

The gallbladder's function is to store and concentrate the bile produced in the liver and then to release it into the duodenum through a physiologic "sphincter," the sphincter of Oddi, when it is required for fat digestion. The major stimulus to release of bile from the gallbladder is mediated through the intestinal hormone cholecystokinin, which is a product of endocrine cells in the duodenum that are activated by fats, proteins, and hypertonic solutions. Cholecystokinin has a stronger effect on gallbladder contraction than does stimulation by the vagus nerve, but both mechanisms act to contract the gallbladder and relax the sphincter of Oddi, allowing bile to squirt into the duodenum at the ampulla of Vater. The gallbladder can store as much as 500 ml of bile between meals, which the organ concentrates by reabsorbing fluid and salt through its mucosal lining. Many organisms do not have a gallbladder, and humans are quite easily able to adapt to the accidental or surgical loss of the gallbladder. In this case the bile ducts themselves dilate and can actually compensate for the absence of the gallbladder by concentrating the bile.

Bile is required in the absorption of lipids that have been taken in and digested in the small intestine. Bile contains salts, acids, and pigments that serve to provide a medium for emulsification of dispersed fatty acids, mixtures of glycerides, and cholesterol. This is necessary for the preliminary absorption of these molecules by the intestinal epithelial cells. When the gallbladder's release of bile is obstructed by gallstones or stenosis of the ducts, the gallbladder often enlarges and may become inflamed and eventually fibrotic. The formation of gallstones with or without overt disease occurs in about 10% of the population. Stones may vary in size from a gravelly mixture to those large enough to totally fill the lumen of the gallbladder. Stones may form when the blood cholesterol is significantly increased, such as might occur in diabetes or during pregnancy; when hemolytic anemia occurs and results in hyperbilirubinemia; when biliary stasis occurs; or when the gallbladder is inflamed or infected. Gallstones are generally of a mixed nature, containing cholesterol, bilirubin, and calcium, and are multifaceted and brown. When bile acids are somehow decreased in the bile, the constituents can precipitate and coalesce, thus forming a stone.

Cholelithiasis

Cholelithiasis is the clinical term for gallstones (Fig. 13-8), accretions that form in the gallbladder. The signs and symptoms of gallstones vary. Whenever gallstones do form, they

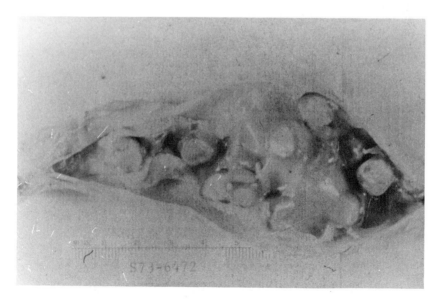

Fig. 13-8. Gallstones. Entire gallbladder is filled with stones and purulent material. (Courtesy Department of Pathology, University of Tennessee, Memphis.)

are often free to move into the cystic duct, the common bile duct, and even into the liver via the hepatic ducts. Pancreatitis may also result from obstruction of the pancreatic duct. The most common symptom of gallstones is a colicky pain, believed to be caused by spasm of the sphincter of Oddi, which is a reflex response to gallbladder epithelium irritation or obstruction of the cystic or common bile duct by a gallstone. Obstruction of the common bile duct, if not relieved, will lead to jaundice, a yellowish discoloration of the skin due to the accumulation of bile pigments in the liver, which then "spill over" into the blood. Before it is apparent, there may be a pruritus. Jaundice is also associated with acholic stools and dark, frothy urine. Jaundice is often first observed in the sclera of the eye but may eventually be evident on all skin surfaces. Obstruction of the bile duct also leads to swelling of the gallbladder with accumulated mucous secretions and eventually inflammation and infection, which often is purulent. The gallbladder may become gangrenous even when symptoms are absent, and the presence of gallstones will usually result in acute or chronic cholecystitis. While most cholecystitis is caused by cholelithiasis, a primary infection or inflammation of the gallbladder can itself result in stone formation. Common infective organisms include *Staphylococcus, Streptococcus,* and enteric organisms, which may reach the gallbladder through the blood or lymph or by contact with infected neighboring organs. *Salmonella* may be carried in a chronically inflamed gallbladder and excreted in the feces, serving as a source of contagion.

Abnormal bile constituents may themselves be found in the bile and then may injure the gallbladder mucosa, resulting in inflammation and occasionally secondary infection.

Cholecystitis

Inflammation of the gallbladder may be either acute or chronic. An acute inflammation begins in the mucosal layer of the organ; it may develop as a primary infection, although more commonly it is superimposed on a preexisting chronic cholecystitis that was initially caused by gallstones. The gallbladder becomes dilated and filled with bile, blood, and pus. Infarction of the organ may result from vascular occlusion. The major symptoms are intense pain, malaise, nausea and vomiting, and if perforation has occurred, signs of local or diffuse peritonitis. Chronic cholecystitis may be the sequela of an acute attack of cholecystitis and is almost always associated with the presence of gallstones of either the pure or mulberry type. The major symptoms are vague pain in the upper right quadrant of the abdomen and fat intolerance. The gallbladder may be large enough to palpate, and if the stones contain sufficient calcium salts, they may be visualized by roentgenography. If obstruction is present, jaundice may be another important sign.

The usual treatment for cholecystitis is removal of the gallbladder, particularly if gallstones are present, after the acute inflammation has been relieved by medical intervention.

Cancer

While gallbladder cancer is not common, when it is present it may be overlooked by the patient as causing signs and symptoms of gallstones. The great majority of these tumors are columnar cell carcinomas, and they cause symptoms of inflammation and obstruction.

Congenital anomalies

Surgeons have often observed that the common bile duct, hepatic ducts, cystic duct, and pancreatic duct show great anatomic variety. Occasionally the gallbladder is absent or is found encapsulated by hepatic tissue. The ducts may be abnormally joined to each other or present in a duplicated form. The presence of stenosis or atresia of the common bile duct in the newborn represents the most serious of these anomalies.

DISORDERS OF THE PANCREAS

The pancreas has both exocrine and endocrine functions, but its role in gastrointestinal physiology is basically as an exocrine gland, providing a volume of bicarbonate-containing fluid and a separately regulated juice containing a high concentration of digestive enzymes. The innervation of the pancreas is through the vagus nerve and sympathetic fibers, and the hormonal regulation, which is most important, is via cholecystokinin and secretin release by duodenal endocrine cells. The pancreas provides its secretion to the duodenum via the pancreatic duct, and the patency of this duct is an absolute requirement for the functional integrity of the pancreas and also for normal digestion to take place. The function of the gland may also be compromised by inflammation or carcinoma.

Pancreatic insufficiency

Cystic fibrosis. This hereditary recessive homozygous condition is a disorder of most if not all exocrine glands. However, its primary manifestations are related to respiratory and digestive tract dysfunction. The mucus secreted in these tracts is more viscous than normal, and 80% of affected children have pancreatic insufficiency. The cause of pancreatic dysfunction is related to obstruction of the pancreatic ductules and ducts, causing the lobules of the pancreas to atrophy, with eventual development of fatty infiltration and loss of function. The pancreatic secretions in cystic fibrosis have a greatly lowered enzyme concentration, HCO_3^- level, and fluid composition. Twenty percent of the affected newborns develop *meconium ileus,* caused by the accumulation of viscous meconium in the small intestine, which leads to obstruction. Surgical correction is usually required, but the general development of the infant will continue to be impaired. Malabsorption results from the pancreatic insufficiency, and steatorrhea is common. These children also appear undernourished and usually have symptoms of chronic obstructive lung disease, which may lead to cor pulmonale and heart failure. Most of the signs and symptoms of cystic fibrosis can be directly attributed to obstruction of the pancreas, intestines, respiratory tract, liver, and reproductive tract by highly viscous, abnormally composed mucus. The treatment is then symptomatic, and pancreatic enzymes are usually administered to aid digestion. Vigorous treatment from infancy onward has led to the survival of some patients into adulthood.

Other causes of pancreatic insufficiency. A number of diseases have been described that are directly caused by a specific pancreatic enzyme deficiency. These conditions are rare and seem to be associated with genetic defects. Included in this category are pancreatic lipase deficiency, amylase deficiency, and trypsinogen deficiency. All these conditions are associated with maldigestion and often steatorrhea.

Inflammation

Acute pancreatitis. Acute pancreatitis has a mortality rate higher than 20%; it is found in conjunction with biliary tract disease in more than 50% of the patients and in conjunction with alcoholism in at least 4% of the patients. The actual etiology of acute pancreatitis is not clear, although whatever the cause, the primary lesion is a chemical inflammation caused by pancreatic enzymes and secretions, which leads to necrosis of the cells of the gland. The presence of gallstones in the pancreatic duct, reflux of bile into the glands, toxins, and direct infecting organisms have all been suggested. Acute pancreatitis thus appears to be associated with either duct obstruction or increased pancreatic secretions. It is often hemorrhagic and typically has an acute onset characterized by nausea and vomiting, severe left-sided radiating pain, and a rigid, tender abdomen. These symptoms often follow the ingestion of large amounts of food or alcohol. The white blood cell count may be elevated, and pancreatic enzymes such as amylase may appear in high concentration in the blood.

The pathophysiology of acute pancreatitis is associated with the possibility of irreversible shock in the early stages of the disease process and with the possibility of autodigestion of the gland in later stages. The pancreas responds to the chemical inflammation initially by edema, and as much as 30% of the plasma volume may become entrapped in the gland, leading to hypovolemia. The possibility of shock is even greater if hemorrhage, ischemia, and cellular necrosis develop, as the tissue sloughs off the organ, and infection, abscess, and gangrene are probable. Furthermore, the glandular cell membranes become autodigested by the pancreatic enzymes, which have escaped into the interstitium and perpetuated the inflammatory response, causing more enzymes to be released into the interstitium, a pathophysiologic positive-feedback situation. These enzymes can then act on other organs and tissue around the pancreas, and grayish discoloration around the loin or umbilical area is a late and serious sign of tissue autodigestion by pancreatic enzymes. The enzymes released into the bloodstream from the pancreas may themselves promote a systemic vasodilation through the kallikrein-kallidin-bradykinin system (see Chapter 4). This activation contributes to the development of shock, which then may rapidly become irreversible. Shock has been prevented in experimental animals by the administration of a kallikrien inhibitor, aprotinin. A major diagnostic test for acute pancreatitis is elevation of serum amylase over 1,000 Somogyi units. This enzyme does not appear to have any dangerous side effects when it is present in the blood. Other conditions such as mumps and renal failure can result in an elevated serum amylase, however. Elevated lipase does present problems, a major one being fat necrosis of the pancreas. Furthermore, the liberation of large amounts of free fatty acids by pancreatic lipase will result in hypocalcemia, as Ca^{++} is taken up by the free fatty acids, which then form calcium soaps. Trypsin may increase in the blood and interfere with the coagulation cascade, leading to a prolonged prothrombin time. The gland apparently "shuts down" almost completely during an attack of acute pancreatitis so that although anticholinergics are commonly administered, the need for them is questionable. Other treatment is aimed at fluid and electrolyte replacement, antibiotic therapy, and pain relief. The course of acute pancreatitis is generally short, unless a chronic inflammation of the gland develops.

Chronic pancreatitis. Chronic pancreatitis is caused by residual damage from the acute disease. Dull persistent pain is characteristic, and acute attacks may recur. Pancreatic secretion is minimal, and malabsorption and steatorrhea are common. Jaundice, due to stricture of the common bile duct, and diabetes mellitus are also often found. The chronically inflamed pancreas may become fibrotic and calcified, and calculi may form in the gland. Why some individuals experience chronic or relapsing pancreatitis is obscure, but alcoholism appears to be an important contributing factor, being present in at least a third of the patients. Relapse may be prevented in some patients by complete alcohol avoidance.

Cancer

Cancer of the pancreas (see also Chapter 3) is increasing in incidence, being the fourth most common cause of cancer mortality in men. The tumor may be present as a primary cancer or may be the result of metastases from cancers of the lung, breast, thyroid, kidney, or skin melanoma. Primary pancreatic tumors are generally adenocarcinomas and are extremely malignant, metastatic, and invasive. The signs and symptoms are associated with obstruction of the lobules, ductules, and pancreatic duct, which is often obstructed early in the growth of the tumor, as most pancreatic cancer arises in the head of the gland. The symptoms (epigastric pain, flatulence, nausea, malaise) may be so vague in the early stages of the disease, however, that a diagnosis is not made until extensive invasion and metastases have occurred. The treatment therefore is usually only palliative.

DISORDERS OF THE LIVER

The liver organ is essential for life and functions as a regulator in many homeostatic systems (Fig. 13-9). It also is able to withstand and repair damage in a remarkable way. The liver is subject to viral infection, to metastases, and to toxic stimuli.

Viral hepatitis

Three viruses are known to be associated with viral hepatitis: hepatitis A virus, hepatitis B virus, and possibly a non-A, non-B (NAB) virus. The A virus is known to cause the short-incubation, low-mortality infectious hepatitis; the B virus has been associated with what was formerly termed *serum hepatitis;* and the non-A, non-B virus is associated with a small percentage of hepatitis that seems clearly not due to infection with the other more common viruses. The short-incubation (1 month) form of viral hepatitis has been associated with outbreaks in institutions where a large number of people and unsanitary conditions coexist.

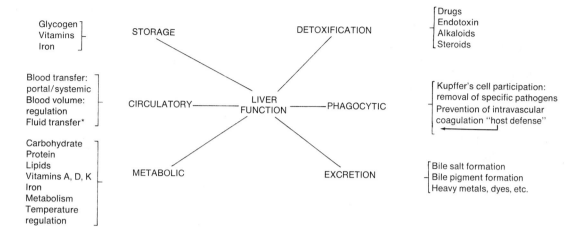

Fig. 13-9. Physiologic functions of liver can be divided into metabolic, excretory, phagocytic, detoxification, storage, and circulatory categories.

Serum hepatitis was so named because it was thought that it was solely transmitted through the infected serum, a fact that has been shown to be untrue. The incubation of this form of hepatitis is usually about 3 months, and the mortality associated with it is much higher.

Both hepatitis A and hepatitis B usually have an associated *icterus,* or jaundice, a staining of the skin, mucous membranes, and body fluids with bile pigments, particularly bilirubin. It is often first observed in the sclera of the eye, and even before that it can be detected by examination of the tympanic membrane.

Bilirubin is formed from hemoglobin breakdown in reticuloendothelial cells. It is conjugated to plasma protein in a form that cannot be excreted in the urine. In the liver the complex is bound to glucuronic acid and forms water-soluble complexes, which are excreted through the bile. The complexes are degraded by intestinal bacteria into stercobilinogen (urobilinogen). Most of this is excreted, some is recirculated, and urobilinogen can be filtered and excreted by the kidneys.

The appearance of a dark and frothy urine also may precede the clinical appearance of jaundice, and the stools may be acholic if the primary cause of the jaundice is obstruction of the flow of bile into the small intestine. In 29%

to 40% of patients with hepatitis, stools may be gray during the first week of jaundice. Jaundice can be produced by hemolytic processes, by obstruction to the flow and release of bile, and by primary hepatocellular disease (Table 13-3).

Hepatitis A. Infection with hepatitis A is indicated by virus particles in the feces and other body secretions, even before a clinical infection is apparent. The infection is usually transmitted through the fecal-oral route, although, if eaten raw, mollusks in polluted water, have been reported to be fomites and have caused several epidemics. The signs and symptoms appear at the end of a prodromal period, with fatigue, weakness, and mild gastrointestinal disturbances being common. A striking aversion to cigarettes also occurs, and patients may complain of pruritus even before jaundice is present; some may have systemic signs such as joint pain, which may reflect the presence of circulating immune complexes. There may be fever, lymphadenopathy, hepatomegaly, and jaundice (which reflects liver cell disruption in bile production). The fundamental lesion in both common types of hepatitis is cellular necrosis. The liver is capable of remarkable regeneration, a process that occurs by budding of remaining liver lobules, and complete regeneration may take place when even

Table 13-3. Mechanisms of jaundice production (normal blood bilirubin is 0.5 mg/100 ml)

Mechanism	Signs	Urine	Feces	van den Bergh test*
Increased breakdown of erythrocytes	Anemia, reticulocytosis, abnormal erythrocytes in blood	Normal (acholuric)	Fecal urobilinogen increased	Indirect positive
Infection or toxic damage to liver cells	Decreased hepatic function	Contains bile salts and bilirubin	Fecal urobilinogen decreased	Direct positive
Bile duct obstruction	Digestive disturbances, high fecal fat	Contains bile salts and bilirubin	Fecal urobilinogen often absent	Direct positive

*The direct van den Bergh test is for conjugated bilirubin, whereas the indirect one tests for bilirubin or bilirubin-protein complexes.

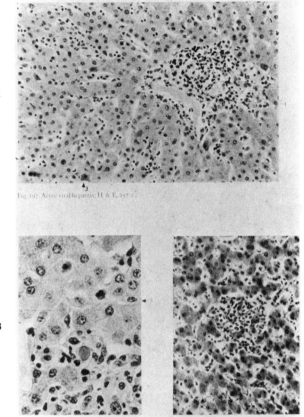

Fig. 13-10. Hepatitis. **A,** Inflammation of acute viral hepatitis. **B,** Inflammatory cells and necrosis of infected parenchymal cells at higher magnification. **C,** Chronic hepatitis in which chronic inflammatory cellular infiltrate and fibrotic scarring are present. (Courtesy Department of Pathology, University of Tennessee, Memphis.)

as much as 70% of the liver is destroyed. Recovery from hepatitis is then dependent on a balance between cell loss and cell regenerative capability and also upon loss of hepatic function. When all the cells become necrotic, death is inevitable. Hepatitis A is associated with a high recovery rate, and usually has a 6-week course.

Hepatitis B. The incidence of this form of viral hepatitis increases in populations of individuals who have received blood transfusions and in drug addicts who may commonly use and share infected needles and syringes. A large number of asymptomatic hepatitis B carriers exist, particularly in the tropics, and the virus may be found in the blood, as well as in saliva, tears, nasal secretions, and menstrual fluid and in blood-sucking insects who have picked up the virus from infected individuals.

The B virus has been difficult to isolate and characterize and appears in the blood as a virion, called the *Dane particle,* which contains the hepatitis B surface antigen on its outer shell. This viral antigen is also termed the *Australian antigen,* since it was originally described in the blood of an Australian aborigine. The central core of the Dane particle contains viral RNA and a DNA polymerase, which is required for the particle to be infective. The surface antigen is also present in the free form in the blood in spherical and tubular shapes. It has been suggested that the Australian antigen may actually be a serum protein produced by the host. These particles do, however, appear to be synthesized in hepatic cells. Blood from infected carriers has been shown to contain this antigen, and its presence in very small concentration still renders the blood potently infective. The presence of surface antigen in the blood is a diagnostic test for hepatitis B.

Hepatitis B generally presents as a more virulent liver disease than hepatitis A and is sometimes associated with the development of chronic hepatitis in those who recover. The prodromal period is characterized by general malaise, joint swelling, rash, pruritus, gastrointestinal symptoms, and hepatomegaly. The appearance of jaundice is accompanied by more marked nausea and vomiting, but occasional cases are anicteric, and the diagnosis may be quite difficult.

Pathologic damage. Hepatocellular necrosis is associated with abnormal elevation of liver enzymes in the serum as well as impaired liver function in regard to storage and excretion (Fig. 13-10). The degree of liver parenchymal cell damage may be evaluated by the degree of elevation of serum aminotransferase activity (SGOT [serum glutamic-oxaloacetic transaminase] and SGPT [serum glutamic-pyruvic transaminase]). Necrosis of only 1% of the liver cells will result in a doubling of the normal serum enzyme activity. Activation of these enzymes is achieved by the liver cell membrane as the enzymes are released. The ratio of SGOT to SGPT is an important indicator of viral hepatitis; this ratio is decreased in early liver damage, although both enzymes increase in absolute amount and activity. The SGPT is normally found in liver cell cytoplasm only, while the SGOT is present in both cytoplasm and mitochondria and is not released at the same rate as SGPT. Other enzymes do increase in concentration and activity in the plasma, indicating liver cell damage, but their measurement is not widely used in diagnosis of liver disease.

Necrosis of the parenchymal liver cells is not the only pathologic feature of hepatitis. Inflammation and leukocyte infiltration are certainly prominent signs, occurring in the portal tracts, periportal space and in the lobules of the liver (Fig. 13-10).

The bile canaliculi and ductules can become dilated and filled with bile-containing material, which may be related to microvilli damage in the canaliculi or to a disorder of the bile-secreting hepatocyte.

Both forms of hepatitis may result in a cirrhotic process of liver destruction, leading eventually to liver failure. Cirrhosis is due to massive necrosis, which leads to fibrosis (Fig. 13-11).

Cirrhosis

In cirrhosis the normal liver parenchyma becomes replaced with fibrous, collagenous tissue, eventually resulting in loss of hepatic function (Fig. 13-11). The major types of cirrhosis include cardiac cirrhosis, which is caused by backward congestive heart failure; postnecrotic cirrhosis; biliary cirrhosis, which is caused by bile tract obstruction leading to hepatocellular damage; and portal or Laennec's cirrhosis, which is usually associated with chronic alcoholism.

Cirrhosis is often but not always preceded by fatty infiltration of the liver (steatosis). Fatty liver and somteimes cirrhosis can be caused by the following:

1. Nutritional disorders resulting from, for example, starvation, kwashiorkor, obesity, or surgical jejunoileal bypass

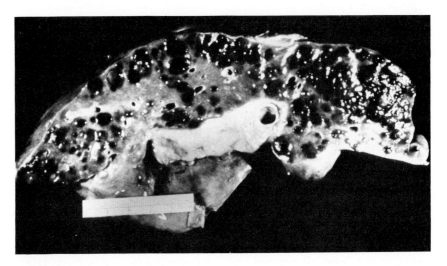

Fig. 13-11. Postnecrotic cirrhosis. Hemorrhagic damaged liver results from acute liver infection. (Courtesy Department of Pathology, University of Tennessee, Memphis.)

2. Obstruction in the biliary system
3. An apparently autoimmune disorder that causes infiltration of the biliary system with immune complexes
4. Sequelae to infections and poisons (e.g., carbon tetrachloride)
5. Iron storage disorders (e.g., hemochromatosis) that lead to tremendously elevated iron concentrations; copper storage disease (Wilson' disease)
6. Ethanol ingestion

While cirrhosis caused by agents other than alcohol may differ somewhat from Laennec's cirrhosis, all these conditions share many common features. Laennec's cirrhosis, being by far the most prevalent form, will be discussed in detail in this chapter.

Laennec's (portal) cirrhosis. There are 6.5 million alcoholics in the United States alone, and in nearly one third of these individuals the possibility of liver cirrhosis is very real. It may take between 5 and 20 years of chronic alcohol ingestion for Laennec's cirrhosis to become evident. It is usually preceded by a theoretically reversible fatty infiltration of the liver cells, which is possibly caused by a fundamental defect in lipid metabolism or secretion and storage. The lipid may represent as much as 40% of the liver weight, as compared to a normal value of 3%. The composition of the lipid is mainly triglycerides and free fatty acids. Triglycerides are normally found in liver cells in small amounts and appear to be present in two "compartments." One compartment is in free exchange with the plasma, while the other compartment seems to hold the lipid and turn it over to the plasma at a very slow rate. It is possible that in fatty liver this second compartment enlarges and sequesters much of the liver cell lipid, thus causing an increased cellular concentration of lipid. The liver appears yellow and greasy and enlarges significantly.

Fatty liver (steatosis). Serum triglycerides are normally taken up by the liver cells and hydrolyzed there into glycerol and free fatty acids. Triglycerides, which are synthesized in the liver, and which may accumulate in huge amounts in steatosis, may be derived from lipid in the diet or in the body fat reserves. (The intestinal digestion, absorption, and ultimate delivery of fats to the liver cell was described in Chapter 12.) The liver may utilize the free fatty acids formed from triglyceride hydrolysis for energy or may convert them to phospholipids, cholesterol esters, or triglycerides once again. The lipids formed in the liver cells are packaged into lipoproteins, which circulate in the blood, delivering the lipids to cells throughout the body, including adipose tissue. Fatty acids may be mobilized from adi-

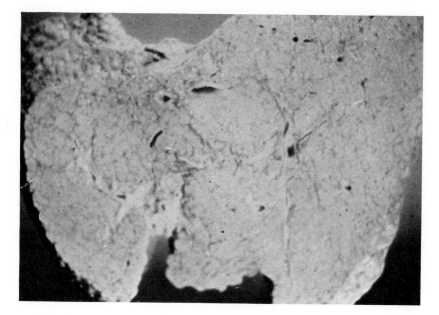

Fig. 13-12. Fatty liver. Extensive fatty infiltration is first event in sequelae leading to Laennec's cirrhosis. (Courtesy Department of Pathology, University of Tennessee, Memphis.)

pose tissue into the blood in a variety of circumstances. The fatty acids become bound to albumin in the blood, and about one third of these fatty acids are taken up by the liver and handled as previously described. Fatty acid mobilization from the adipose tissue is increased by lowered blood glucose concentration, glucagon stimulation, corticosteroids, somatotropin, thyroid hormone, sympathetic nervous system stimulation, or epinephrine and norepinephrine. A decrease in blood glucose, which stimulates release of fatty acids from the adipose tissue, may be important in the etiology of fatty liver that is associated with starvation or malnutrition states. A decrease in fat mobilization may be accomplished by agents that block the stimulators and by insulin. Possible mechanisms whereby fatty liver may be produced are (1) increased fatty acid concentration in the blood and thus increased delivery to the liver, (2) increased triglyceride formation, and (3) decreased synthesis or release of lipoproteins. In alcoholics the development of fatty liver precedes the necrotic and fibrotic secondary changes of cirrhosis. It was long held that the cause of fatty liver in alcoholics was primarily due to the severe nutritional impairment commonly found

in the chronic alcoholic. The discovery that alcohol was a direct hepatotoxin established the idea that both malnutrition and hepatotoxic effects synergistically acted together to produce fatty liver. It was, however, believed that fatty liver and cirrhosis due to the chronic ingestion of alcohol could be prevented by the ingestion of a nutritionally adequate diet. However, it has been shown that the administration of ethanol in a total liquid diet that was nutritionally adequate produced fatty liver but not cirrhosis. Recently the baboon has been studied by Lieber and De Carli, who showed that it will develop not only fatty liver but also cirrhosis when fed an adequate diet with large amounts of alcohol over time. The development of cirrhosis occurred in less than a year in some animals. This species is genetically close to humans and lives much longer than most laboratory animals. The development of cirrhosis in baboons indicates that malnutrition is not the primary cause of cirrhosis in alcoholics.

The actual mechanism by which alcohol induces increased liver triglyceride is, however, not well understood. Nonalcoholic volunteers who ingest large amounts of alcohol over a period of a day or two are noted to have increased liver triglycerides as an almost immediate effect of the imbibition. Ethanol may act primarily by stimulating the sympathetic nervous system to activate lipid mobilization from the adipose tissue. Ethanol may also act at the level of the liver cell, inducing enzymatic reactions, some of which act to detoxify alcohol and to perhaps interrupt other enzymatic reactions, leading to eventual triglyceride accumulation in the liver. Alcohol may inhibit reactions that lead to fatty acid oxidation or may interfere with the incorporation of fatty acids into phospholipids and cholesterol, thus leading to an increased yield of triglycerides. These possible mechanisms are currently being analyzed in laboratories.

Fatty liver itself may cause severe signs and symptoms, such as hepatomegaly, abdominal pain, indigestion, and anorexia. Necrosis of the cells may develop in an acute manner in this clinical entity, leading to *acute alcoholic hepatitis,* a precirrhotic lesion. The development of fatty liver prefaces the eventual development of cirrhosis if the individual continues to imbibe alcohol. If alcohol ingestion is stopped, the fatty liver can revert to normal, and cirrhosis can be avoided. The progression of fatty liver to cirrhosis appears to require that significant cell necrosis occur. The types of fatty liver that are due to causes other than alcohol and that do not develop into cirrhosis are associated with very little or no necrosis. Therefore, it has been suggested that the underlying pathologic process that leads to fatty liver in the alcoholic may also result in cirrhosis, since fat accumulation in liver cells is not in itself the cause of necrosis (Fig. 13-12).

Pathophysiologic effects. The liver in portal cirrhosis is generally golden yellow, and the surface is often stippled and nodular, resembling the surface of a football, which is caused by destruction of parenchyma and later repair. The absolute amount of connective tissue is increased, and fibrosis is diffuse. Alcohol causes a net increase in serum proline and hydroxyproline, amino acids required for the biosynthesis of collagen by fibroblasts. This may either reflect a primary effect of ethanol on proline metabolism and collagen synthesis or may be the result of increased collagen synthesis and deposition in the diseased liver. The fibrosis is also directly related to the necrosis and represents repair of the liver by connective tissue replacement. Infiltration and deposition of hemosiderin in the parenchymal cells are other features.

The major signs and symptoms of cirrhosis are related to the pathophysiologic processes perpetuated by a fibrotic, necrotic, functionally impaired liver. The normal function of the intact healthy liver was depicted in Fig. 13-9, and the essential nature of these functions is quite apparent. Failure of the liver to adequately perform these functions can result in a great variety of signs and symptoms. The cirrhotic patient will suffer general ill health, as evidenced by easy fatigability, frequent infections, weight loss, and general malaise. While muscle wasting is an important development, weight loss is not always apparent, if ascites is present. Aside from generally poor health, specific symptoms are usually present from which a diagnosis of cirrhosis can be made.

JAUNDICE. Jaundice is not invariably present in cirrhosis but is relatively common, particularly in the later stages of the disease. Many conditions cause jaundice (see Table 13-3). In cirrhosis, hepatic parenchymal cells fail to metabolize bilirubin, and the increased serum bilirubin stains the elastic tissue, causing jaundice. Localized edema may give rise to pigmented areas, particularly if the edema fluid contains protein, since bilirubin is normally albumin bound.

PORTAL HYPERTENSION. Portal hypertension is the most significant complication contributing to mortality from liver cirrhosis. The liver in cirrhosis is usually enlarged, but in advanced disease associated with severe portal hypertension the liver may be shrunken and hardened. The absolute amount of fibrous tissue, however, is invariably increased. The nodules of regenerative tissue and the increased fibrous nature of the liver both act to compress blood vessels, and general narrowing of portal venules occurs. This results in increased back pressure in the portal vein. Increased hepatic artery flow and mass, which causes abnormal communications to form between the hepatic artery and the portal vein, may also occur, and both factors contribute to the development of portal hyper-

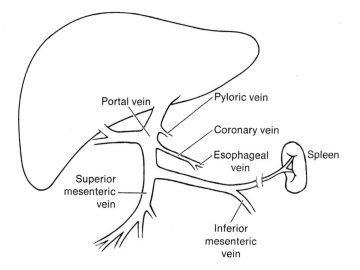

Fig. 13-13. The splanchnic veins. Venous drainage of splanchnic organs. When portal hypertension develops, other vessels can become engorged, leading to stasis and hypoxia of respective organs.

tension, as the absolute amount of blood will increase in the portal vein, and there will be increased resistance to blood flow from the portal vein into the portal venules and sinusoids of the liver. Increased back pressure in the portal system will contribute to elevated hydrostatic pressure not only in the portal vein but also in the vessels that feed into this vein, namely, the coronary vein, pyloric vein, superior and inferior mesenteric veins, and splenic vein. These veins all receive multiple tributaries before emptying into the portal vein (Fig. 13-13). The liver, it will be recalled, is a relatively anoxic organ, receiving arterial blood via the hepatic artery, and venous blood from the gastrointestinal tract and many abdominal organs. The liver microcirculation is so arranged that low-pressure portal blood and high-pressure arterial blood mix in the liver sinusoids, which are drained by hepatic venules. The parenchymal cells that make up the bulk of the liver cell mass form lobules from which a central vein emerges. The sinusoids themselves are lined with phagocytic reticuloendothelial cells such as Kupffer's cells. The blood flow through the liver is regulated by respiration (increasing upon inspiration) and by sympathetic innervation of the vessels. The flow through the liver in different areas is highly variable, and generally the splanchnic bed circulation will be profound-

ly decreased during stress, exercise, shock states, and any other phenomenon that will propagate sympathetic nervous system firing. The general adequacy of splanchnic circulation is ultimately dependent on the ability of the liver circulation to handle the portal venous blood. If acute obstruction occurs in the portal vein, due to a thrombus or injury, death follows almost immediately. This effect was shown by a Russian surgeon, Nicolai Eck, who devised the now famous Eck fistula, a portalcaval shunt. When portal blood flow is suddenly occluded, rapid hypovolemic shock due to an enormous increase in filtration forces causes massive extravasation of fluid into the abdominal cavity and throughout the splanchnic bed. More slowly developing portal occlusion is compatible with life, due to the ability of the cardiovascular system to form collateral vessels, which are able to shunt the high-pressure portal blood into lower pressure veins, "decompressing" the portal circulation.

Canalization of collateral vessels is particularly prominent (1) in the esophagus, where fragile collateral vessels shunt blood from the coronary vein into the azygos vein, which drains into the superior vena cava; (2) in the rectum, where collateral vessels connect the middle and superior hemorrhoidal veins to the inferior hemorrhoidal vein, which drains into

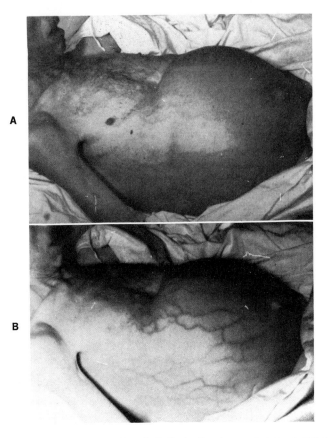

Fig. 13-14. Collateral circulation and ascites. **A,** Patient with advanced cirrhosis of liver shows marked ascites. **B,** Infrared photography is used to demonstrate multiple collateral vessels that are present. (From Schiff, L.: Diseases of the liver, Philadelphia, 1975, J. B. Lippincott Co.)

the inferior vena cava; (3) in the splenic vein, which forms anastomoses into the left renal vein; and (4) in the portal vein itself, which forms connections into the epigastric veins. The cirrhotic patient often will demonstrate the presence of multiple, large collateral abdominal veins, which are grossly visible on the abdomen (Fig. 13-14). A consequence of this sometimes massive collateralization is dilation of the walls of the collateral vessels, which are themselves not particularly strong, and also of the veins, which were not designed to carry the extra volume of blood and higher pressures that are imposed by the cirrhotic liver disease. These vessels then out-pouch, forming local areas of dilation called *varices* as illustrated in Fig. 13-15. Pressure in these varices is increased even above that in the vein of which they are a part due to the modified Laplace equation, which

states that the tension, T, in a tube is proportional to the pressure, P, times the radius, R, divided by the wall thickness, h; $T = PR/h$. Thus, factors that cause a decrease in vessel elasticity or increase in radius result in decreased distensibility of the vessel and therefore a rise in pressure. While veins are much more distensible than arteries, the degree of stretching that takes place when varices are formed is probably significant enough to account for the tendency of varices to rupture. When esophageal or more commonly gastric varices rupture, blood under great pressure, due to the concomitant portal hypertension, is poured out, and a life-threatening hemorrhagic emergency is present. Furthermore, clotting factors produced by the liver may be deficient, and prothrombin time is often increased, contributing to the hemorrhage. The treatment of such hemorrhage

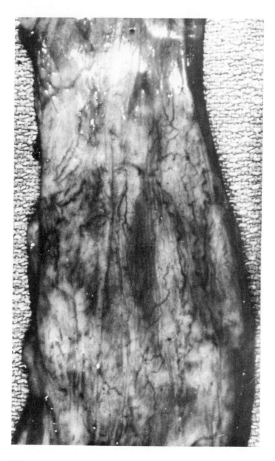

Fig. 13-15. Esophageal varices. Swollen varices and extensive collateral circulation are evident in this segment of esophagus from patient with Laennec's cirrhosis. (Courtesy Department of Pathology, University of Tennessee, Memphis.)

is aimed at attempts to stop the bleeding either directly by insertion of ballooning tubes, which can be pulled so as to exert pressure on the bleeding gastric varices and laterally on the esophageal walls if bleeding is occurring from esophageal varices, or physiologically by administration of vasopressin. The first hemorrhage from bleeding varices has, however, a high associated mortality. There is some evidence that massive upper gastrointestinal bleeding in cirrhosis can also occur from gastric erosion and ulceration.

Surgical decompression shunts are performed to alleviate the portal hypertension that is commonly associated with cirrhosis and that results in varices. The portacaval shunt has been the most common surgical procedure, although other techniques are presently being used. The portal vein is dissected away from the liver and inserted into the inferior vena cava, an operation that will prolong life in many cirrhotics, although the death rate associated with hepatic failure in these individuals is still very high.

ASCITES. The common finding of ascites in Laennec's cirrhosis, which is usually found in conjunction with portal hypertension, suggests that the two processes are related, a conjecture that has much experimental backing. It is thought that hepatic lymph formation occurs in excess of that which the hepatic lymphatics can remove, due to sinusoidal hypertension. The same phenomenon probably occurs in mesenteric and intestinal capillaries. Another possible factor contributing to ascites formation in cirrhosis is abnormal albumin metabolism, acting to cause hypoalbuminemia and resultant decrease in colloid osmotic pressure. Loss of protein into the ascites fluid accounts at least partially for hypoalbuminemia. Ascitic pressure forces on renal perfusion may also initiate renin release with subsequent aldosterone-produced Na^+ and water retention. Hyperaldosteronism can occur through impaired degradation of the hormone by the diseased liver, and plasma volume may actually be expanded in cirrhosis, further accounting for the hypoalbuminism. These positive-feedback mechanisms are diagramed in Fig. 13-16. Treatment of ascites is aimed at removal of the excess fluid by paracentesis, dietary restriction of Na^+ and sometimes fluid, and a high-calorie diet that contains a moderate restriction of protein (no greater than 50 g per day). The diseased liver is not able to metabolize proteins well, and excess protein can precipitate the development of hepatic coma. Diuretics may be administered as well if the ascites fails to respond to medical management. In general the development of ascites indicates that serious pathophysiologic processes are being perpetuated, and the prognosis is poor, with about 25% of cirrhotic patients with ascites dying within a year. Most do not die from fluid loss due to ascites but from hepatic coma or gastrointestinal bleeding, complications associated with the liver pathology.

OTHER SIGNS AND SYMPTOMS. The individual

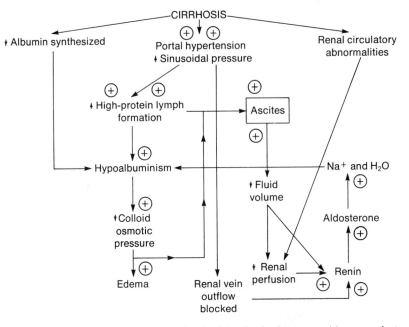

Fig. 13-16. Pathophysiology of ascites formation in cirrhosis. Ascites caused by many factors that are present in advanced cirrhosis. Edema is also perpetuated by interaction of these factors.

suffering from Laennec's cirrhosis may have a great variety of symptoms, which are related to the multisystemic effects of liver disease. Fever, neuropathy, cardiovascular disturbances, renal failure, and endocrine imbalance have all been reported in this disease.

Physiology of treatment. The most obvious therapy for alcoholic liver disease is complete abstinence of alcohol, which can result in complete reversal of fatty liver and, if enough parenchymal cells are present, reversal of cirrhosis by regeneration of these cells. The architecture of the liver will change with regeneration of new parenchyma, but functional capacity is preserved. The mechanisms by which budding of new regenerative parenchyma occurs are not known, but a blood-borne factor may be involved. However, abstinence is generally not observed by cirrhotic patients, and so the true potential for recovery from this disease is not known.

The complications of cirrhosis must be treated vigorously as patients with this disease are susceptible to many problems that can interact and produce rapid deterioration. These complications include hypokalemia caused by

the presence of hyperaldosteronism, hypoxia, renal disease (the hepatorenal syndrome), infection, and encephalopathy, as well as jaundice, portal hypertension, gastrointestinal hemorrhage, and ascites, the hallmarks of the disease. In general the course of cirrhosis is marked by many crises, which require emergency management. The patient's diet may be an important part of his daily management; it is generally high in carbohydrates, moderate or restricted in protein, low in sodium, and supplemented by vitamins. Attention to fluid and electrolyte status is important, particularly since many cirrhotic patients are placed on diuretics. Corticosteroids have been used in the care of the cirrhotic patient. The physiology of corticosteroid action in Laennec's cirrhosis may be based on interference with fibrosis in the diseased liver. Corticosteroids decrease the activity of protocollagen proline hydroxylase and induce the enzyme collagenase in fibroblasts, increase the collagenolytic activity of hepatic cell lysosomes, and decrease the absolute amount of endoplasmic reticulum in fibroblasts. All these actions may inhibit the deposition of collagen fibers in the liver, thus slowing down the development of hepatic fibrosis. The long-term treatment of cirrhotics by corticosteroids is, however, limited due to their side effects, which may aggravate other pathophysiologic mechanisms operating in the disease.

Hepatic coma

The terminal stage of most liver disease is the development of hepatic coma due to liver failure. Hepatic coma can also develop as an acute phase in an otherwise reversible liver disease. Encephalopathy is observed in advanced cirrhosis and can be considered an early stage of hepatic coma. Thirty-six percent of individuals with cirrhosis die in hepatic coma. The onset is insidious, with major symptoms related to encephalopathy causing a diminished level of consciousness, which is often indicated by drowsiness and confusion, irritability, and a characteristic flapping tremor (asterixis). A comatose state follows, from which most patients do not recover. Anatomic changes in the morphology and amount of nerve cells have been reported.

The pathogenesis of encephalopathy and hepatic coma traditionally has been thought to be due to ammonia intoxication. Ammonia ingested in the diet or that arises from the action of gut bacteria normally is removed from the portal blood by the liver and is used in the formation of urea. Urea is then released into the bloodstream and excreted by the kidney. Blood ammonia is elevated in hepatic coma, but the degree of elevation cannot be correlated with the degree of encephalopathy. Ammonia has been shown experimentally to have a direct toxic action on brain cells and possibly may act by inhibiting acetylcholine synthesis or by causing the accumulation of GABA (gamma-aminobutyric acid), an inhibitory brain neurotransmitter. Ammonia may also inhibit cerebral energy metabolism. Common precipitating factors in the development of hepatic coma include increased dietary protein, which would give rise to increased ammonia, and gastrointestinal bleeding, which results in deposition of large amounts of blood in the gut. This blood is high in aromatic amino acids and would also give rise then to increased ammonia due to bacterial breakdown. Other precipitating factors include azotemia, sedatives, tranquilizers, and analgesics.

There are, however, several features of hepatic coma that cannot be explained by ammonia intoxication. These include the increase in brain serotonin and tryptophan found experimentally in hepatic coma. It is possible that "false neurotransmitters" are formed in coma, leading to the development of encephalopathy. L-dopa has been occasionally reported to wake people from hepatic coma in a dramatic manner. Another possible culprit in the pathogenesis of hepatic coma is *alpha-ketoglutaramate,* which is elevated in the cerebrospinal fluid during coma, and also short-chain fatty acids, which are increased and which may act synergistically with ammonia. The pathogenesis of hepatic coma is therefore an area of continuing research.

Treatment. Treatment of the patient in hepatic coma is complicated by the impairment of drug metabolism and detoxification that commonly occurs in liver damage. Thus, administration of hypnotics, analgesics, and sedatives must be carefully considered. Morphine, which is conjugated by the liver, can precipitate hepatic coma, while meperidine hydrochloride (Demerol) can be administered without serious side effects (in terms of liver function), since it is not handled by the liver. Long-acting short-chain barbiturates are normally excreted by the kidney and can be given to patients with liver disease, while the short-acting long-chain barbiturates are metabolized by the liver. Therefore, phenobarbital can be administered to patients with liver disease, albeit with caution. Paraldehyde is an extremely potent sedative, which is also metabolized by the liver, and its odor can be present on the breath of a cirrhotic patient for several days after its administration. Anesthesia may provoke serious effects in the cirrhotic patient. Chloroform in particular is extremely toxic to an already damaged liver.

Antibiotics may be administered to the patient in hepatic coma, particularly neomycin, 4 g per day, to sterilize the lower GI tract. This is an attempt to remove a major source of ammonia. Dietary protein is restricted for the same reason. If upper-GI-tract bleeding has occurred, the stomach may be aspirated to remove blood, which can serve as a source of amino acids and therefore ammonia. Corticosteroids are also administered frequently.

Attempts at removing ammonia from the circulation have been attempted both pharmacologically and physically with exchange transfusions and hemodialysis. These have met with limited success. More radical procedures have included colonic surgery for intractable cases.

Prognosis. The nature of the coma varies from patient to patient. Individuals may go in and out of deep stuporous states, and treatment may result in complete awakening and loss of all signs of encephalopathy. Occasionally death will occur as the result of bronchopneumonia, sepsis, or gastrointestinal hemorrhage, or death may occur naturally in the deep comatose state. The longer and deeper the coma, the less likely it is that the patient will recover.

SUMMARY

This chapter has presented various disease states as models of pathophysiologic alterations in normal digestion, absorption, excretion, and metabolism. These conditions are best understood and appreciated against the background of nutritional derangements presented in Chapter 13. Maintenance of the steady state of nutritional balance is a requirement of all physiologic functions in every organ system.

Special disruptive effects of the diseases discussed in this chapter must not be underestimated, however. These effects can cause severe pathophysiology by themselves or can contribute in more general ways to nutritional disequilibrium.

SUGGESTED READINGS

Anderson, W. A. D., and Kissane, J. M.: Pathology, ed. 7, St. Louis, 1977, The C. V. Mosby Co.

Davenport, H. W.: Physiology of the digestive tract, ed. 3, Chicago, 1971, Year Book Medical Publishers.

Dowling, R. H., and Riecken, E. O.: Intestinal adaptation, New York, 1974, F. K. Schattauer Verlag.

Drasar, B. W., and Hill, M. J.: Human intestinal flora, London, 1974, Academic Press.

Hawk, W. A.: Primary inflammatory bowel disease, facts and fancy, Ostomy Quart. **11:**3-4, Fall 1974.

Hunt, J., and Knox, M.: Slowing of gastric emptying by acids, J. Physiol. **222:**187-207, 1972.

Johnson, L. R., editor: Gastrointestinal physiology, St. Louis, 1977, The C. V. Mosby Co.

Lieber, C. S., and De Carli, L. M.: Alcoholic liver injury: experimental models in rats and baboons, Adv. Exp. Med. Biol. **59:**379-393, 1975.

McColl, I., and Sladen, G.: Intestinal Absorption in Man, London, 1975, Academic Press.

Mendeloff, A., and Dunn, J. P.: Digestive diseases, Cambridge, Mass., 1971, Harvard University Press.

Menguy, R., Desbaillets, L., and Masters, Y.: Mechanism of stress ulcer: influence of hypovolemic shock on energy metabolism in the gastric mucosa, Gastroenterology **66:** 46-55, 1974.

Popper, H., and Schaffner, F., editors: Progress in liver diseases, vol. 5, New York, 1976, Grune & Stratton.

Rhodes, J., and Calcraft, B.: Aetiology of gastric ulcer, Clin. Gastroenterol. vol. 22, 1973.

Robbins, S., and Angell, M.: Basic pathology, Philadelphia, 1976, W. B. Saunders Co.

Schaffner, F., Sherlock, S., and Leevy, C.: The liver and its diseases, New York, 1974, Intercontinental Medical Book Corp.

Schiff, L., editor: Diseases of the liver, Philadelphia, 1975, J. B. Lippincott Co.

Wakim, K.: Basic and clinical physiology of the liver, J. Int. Anesth. Res. Soc. vol. 44, no. 5, Sept.-Oct. (suppl.) 1965.

Watson, D. W.: The problem of chronic inflammatory bowel disease, Calif. Med. **117:**25, 1972.

PART SIX

Pathophysiology of reproductive and endocrine integrity

CHAPTER 14

Endocrine system: disorders and mechanisms

AT THE COMPLETION OF THIS CHAPTER THE STUDENT WILL BE ABLE TO:

- Describe the pathophysiologic conditions characterized by endocrine dysfunction.
  Explain the mechanisms through which endocrine dysfunction is precipitated.
  Describe the alteration in normal function that occurs.
  Identify the effects of endocrine dysfunction on energy production, chemical equilibrium,
    growth, and development.
  Describe the clinical manifestations of endocrine dysfunction.
- Cite the etiology and predisposing factors of endocrine dysfunction.
- Describe the physiologic basis of treatment.

Adaptation of the physiologic processes to the ever changing conditions of the external and internal environment is the result of a finely tuned process of neuroendocrine regulation. The nervous system detects changes in the environment and transmits this information via afferent impulses to the brain, where efferent impulses directing motor and autonomic activity are generated. Afferent impulses are also relayed to the hypothalamus, which activates the endocrine system and integrates its activity with that of the nervous system. While nervous system responses tend to be immediate, hormonal effects occur more slowly and over a longer period of time. Through this control system the functions of the various organ systems are regulated and coordinated with one another to meet the body's needs for energy production, chemical equilibrium, development, growth, and reproduction. The physiologic response to stress is probably the most dramatic example of the role of neuroendocrine mediation in promoting adaptation. Disruption of either component of this control system will result in a departure from the normal adaptive processes. This chapter will deal with disruption

of the endocrine regulatory mechanisms, the effects of these disruptions on the physiologic processes and homeostasis, and the etiologic factors involved in these disruptions.

The endocrine system is comprised of seven glands, which secrete biologically active chemical substances called hormones into the bloodstream. These glands include the pituitary, thyroid, parathyroid, adrenal glands, pancreas, ovaries and testes. In addition to these glands, many organs also secrete hormones into the bloodstream: secretin and glucagon are produced by the intestine, gastrin by the stomach, and renin and erythropoietin by the kidney to name a few. This chapter will discuss dysfunction of the components of the endocrine system specifically, with the exception of the ovaries and testes, which are discussed in Chapter 15, and the pancreas, which is discussed in Chapters 12 and 13.

HORMONAL ACTION AND SECRETION

Hormones regulate existing cellular function; they do not initiate new biochemical activities but regulate already existing enzymatic and

379

chemical reactions. This catalytic action is limited to those target tissues specifically responsive to a particular hormone, although some hormones may have important effects on their tissues of origin as well. An example of this is the necessity of cortisol in the blood from the adrenal cortex for the synthesis of epinephrine in the adrenal medulla. Target tissue specificity is guaranteed through the necessity of interaction between the hormone and a specific target tissue receptor, which responds only to that particular hormone. The hormone-receptor interaction also serves as the first step in the process of hormonal action.

At the present time two main mechanisms of hormonal action have been identified. Enzymatic regulation may occur as a result of activation or deactivation of enzymes present within the target tissue or through induction of enzyme synthesis. The first mechanism, *activation or deactivation of existing enzymes,* is mediated through the adenyl cyclase–cyclic adenosine monophosphate (cAMP) system. The enzyme adenyl cyclase is located within the cell membrane; it becomes activated when the hormone binds at its receptor site. Adenyl cyclase converts ATP to cAMP. Prostaglandins are thought to regulate the activity of adenyl cyclase and thus regulate the cellular response to a hormone. The extent and nature of the regulatory function of the prostaglandins remains to be elucidated through research. Within the target cell, cAMP activates protein kinases, which in turn convert inactive enzymes to active enzymes, probably through phosphorylation reactions.

Hormones that act through this "second messenger" mechanism produce their effects fairly rapidly, for example, catecholamines, glucagon, vasopressin (ADH), parathyroid hormone, gastrin, adrenocorticotropin, luteinizing hormone, thyroid-stimulating hormone, thyrotropin-releasing hormone, and follicle-stimulating hormone. cAMP is deactivated by the enzyme phosphodiesterase, which can be inhibited by xanthines such as caffeine and theophylline. These compounds then will prolong the action of cAMP and augment the hormonal effects that it mediates.

The second mechanism of hormonal action, *enzyme synthesis,* is typical of the action of the steroid hormones and involves entry of the hormone into the cell. The hormone binds with a specific binding protein in the cytoplasm of the cell. This hormone-protein complex is then transported into the nucleus of the cell, where it combines with specific sites on the chromatin. The subsequent derepression of DNA allows that segment to be transcribed and form messenger RNA to direct protein synthesis. These two mechanisms just described do not represent the complete picture of hormonal action but only two mechanisms that research has documented to date. Other mechanisms are required to explain the extremely rapid and possibly direct action of the steroids on vascular walls to affect blood pressure. Insulin-mediated transport of glucose into the cell occurs without an increase in cAMP and therefore must be explained by some other mechanism.

Hormonal secretion is regulated through feedback control. In other words, the presence of the hormonal substance itself or a substance produced by the target tissue in response to the hormone will affect further secretion of that hormone. An example of negative-feedback control is the relationship between parathyroid hormone and the serum calcium level. When the serum calcium concentration is low, parathyroid hormone secretion increases. As the serum calcium concentration rises, the parathyroid hormone secretion is reduced. Two hormones may be involved in a system regulated by both positive- and negative-feedback controls. An example of this is the regulation of thyroid hormone secretion. The thyroid hormones are released in response to pituitary thyroid-stimulating hormone (TSH). When the level of the thyroid hormones is increased, TSH release is inhibited, a negative-feedback mechanism. TSH release is enhanced by hypothalamic thyrotropin-releasing hormone (TRH), secretion of which is stimulated by low levels of thyroid hormone, a positive-feedback mechanism. When thyroid hormone concentration is low, TRH secretion is stimulated, which in turn stimulates TSH secretion and subsequently thyroid hormone secretion. (See Fig. 1-2.)

It has already been stated that the hypothalamus provides neurohormonal integration in the

Table 14-1. Hypothalamic regulatory hormones (factors)

Hormone	Action
Releasing hormones	
CRH (corticotropin-releasing hormone)	Stimulates secretion of ACTH (adrenocorticotropin)
TRH (thyrotropin-releasing hormone)	Stimulates secretion of TSH (thyroid-stimulating hormone)
GHRH (growth hormone–releasing hormone)	Stimulations secretion of GH (growth hormone)
PRH (prolactin-releasing hormone)	Stimulates secretion of prolactin (also called lactogenic hormone)
LHRH/FSHRH (releasing hormone for luteinizing hormone and follicle-stimulating hormone)	Stimulates secretion of LH (luteinizing hormone) and FSH (follicle-stimulating hormone)
MRH (melanocyte-stimulating hormone–releasing hormone)	Stimulates secretion of β-MSH (beta melanocyte-stimulating hormone)
Inhibitory hormones*	
GHRIH (growth hormone release–inhibiting hormone [also called somatostatin])	Inhibits secretion of GH (growth hormone)
PRIH (prolactin release–inhibiting hormone)	Inhibits secretion of prolactin
MRIH (melanocyte-stimulating hormone release–inhibiting hormone)	Inhibits secretion of β-MSH (beta melanocyte-stimulating hormone)

*Inhibitory hormones are not necessary for the other four hormones of the anterior lobe of the pituitary gland since they are tropic hormones, which promote hormone release in the target tissues. The blood levels of these target tissue hormones serve to inhibit further secretion of the pituitary hormones through a negative-feedback mechanism.

maintenance of homeostasis. The hypothalamus activates the endocrine system through its effect on the anterior lobe of the pituitary gland; it controls the release of the tropic hormones from the pituitary. This action is accomplished through the release of hypothalamic releasing hormones or hypothalamic release-inhibiting hormones. Table 14-1 lists the various hypothalamic regulatory hormones and their actions. Through the tropic hormones, which are stimulated by the hypothalamic hormones, the anterior lobe of the pituitary gland regulates the function of many of the endocrine glands. Thus, internal regulation of endocrine function is achieved via the hypothalamic-pituitary axis. Because of the interrelatedness and antagonistic effects of many of the endocrine hormones, this internal regulation provided by the pituitary is also necessary for the maintenance of the steady state.

ENDOCRINE DYSFUNCTION

Endocrine disease is characterized by disruption of normal hormone production and activity. An alteration in hormonal synthesis, release, target tissue interaction, or degradation may serve as the basis for endocrine dysfunction. The primary mechanism involved in most conditions characterized by endocrine dysfunction is an abnormal amount of the hormone substance within the body. Greater than normal amounts of hormone may be the result of hyperfunction of the gland or a tumor of the gland. Tumors that occur in endocrine glands are not subject to the usual feedback controls, and therefore hormone levels may be grossly elevated or reduced. The syndromes caused by multiple tumors of the endocrine glands, or *multiple endocrine adenomatosis* (MEA), do not occur often. The clinical picture is one of multiple, complex endocrine dysfunction.

An increasing number of hormone-producing neoplasms arising from nonendocrine tissue have been identified. This process is referred to as ectopic hormone production, and the resulting syndrome of endocrine dysfunction superimposed on the neoplastic process is referred to as an *ectopic hormone syndrome*. The most frequently seen syndrome of this type is excessive ACTH and parathyroid hormone secretion associated with neoplasms of the lungs. Excessive ectopic production of vasopressin is most frequently associated with bronchogenic carcinoma and results in the syndrome of inappropriate antidiuretic hormone secretion (SIADH), which is discussed in more detail in Chapter 11.

Inadequate hormone production may be the result of a loss or a reduction in glandular function. Causes include congenital hypoplasia, surgical removal of the gland, destruction due

example

to radiation, inflammation, or pressure from surrounding tissue, or atrophy of unknown cause. The congenital absence of a necessary enzyme may inhibit hormone production. This usually causes hyperplasia of the gland as the body attempts to compensate.

Another mechanism of endocrine dysfunction may be an abnormal response of the target tissue to the hormonal substance. A lack of response may be due to lack of a hormone receptor or of the "second messenger" substance. The effect of the latter is seen in pseudohypoparathyroidism, in which a lack of cAMP due to defective renal and bone synthesis causes a lack of response to parathyroid hormone. Prostaglandins have been found to be related to endocrine activity and changes in cAMP. One theory is that the prostaglandins serve as a connecting link between polypeptide–hormone receptor interaction and the activation of adenyl cyclase, the enzyme necessary for cAMP formation. The synthesis and release of prostaglandins by tumor cells has been demonstrated in syndromes of endocrine dysfunction accompanying certain tumors. The physiologic role of prostaglandins continues to be an area of research and holds some promise for broad applications to clinical medicine in the future.

Metabolic degradation of hormonal substances takes place in the blood, liver, kidney, and possibly in the target tissues. If an organ's ability to degrade a hormone is reduced, a properly functioning control system will reduce the secretory rate of the hormone to maintain normal plasma levels. Obviously if the control system is also impaired, an excess of the hormonal substance may develop. An alteration in the normal chemical process of the degradation of testosterone, making its degradation similar to that of other steroids, will increase or perpetuate androgenic potency. Another mechanism through which endocrine dysfunction can occur is the conversion of biologically inactive hormone precursors into active hormones in nonendocrine tissue.

Variation in the internal rhythmicity of hormonal secretion may also precipitate endocrine dysfunction. Hormone secretion for the most part is episodic, occurring in response to an intrinsic rhythm based on diurnal sleep-wake patterns. Normally, the secretion of growth hormone peaks shortly after sleep has begun, while ACTH and cortisol secretion peak at the end of the sleep period and beginning of the activity period. Because the systemic effects of growth hormone are inhibited by cortisol, this pattern allows growth hormone to exert a maximal effect. If this pattern were disrupted in a manner that allowed hormonal peaks to coincide, the systemic effects of growth hormone would be minimized.

General manifestations

The manifestations of endocrine dysfunction reflect the aberrant hormonal regulation. Weakness and easy fatigability reflect alterations in energy metabolism. Abnormalities of growth and development (especially sexual development) are more obvious manifestations of disrupted endocrine regulation of the growth and reproductive processes. Weight gain must always be carefully evaluated for a possible endocrine-related cause. The most serious endocrine dysfunctions characterized by weight gain are diabetes mellitus and insulinoma. Moderate weight gain accompanies hypopituitarism and hypothyroidism. Cushing's syndrome is characterized by the loss of adipose tissue in the extremities with an increase in the abdominal fat pad and development of a fat pad on the back, which is referred to as *buffalo hump*. This is due to appetite stimulation by cortisol and the increased availability of glucose for fat synthesis. It is not known why the fat localizes in the specific way it does, however.

Hypertension can be a sign of volume expansion due to sodium retention or accelerated cardiac activity with increased cardiac output in response to hormonal changes. Changes in respiratory rate and depth (especially increases) and changes in appetite may signal changes in the metabolic rate due to altered hormonal regulation. Other signs of a possible endocrine problem include changes in the appearance and texture of the skin and pattern of hair growth, arthropathies, tetany or convulsions, edema, extreme thirst (polydipsia), and frequent urination (polyuria). Any of these signs must be evaluated carefully for possible endocrine etiology. Manifestations of the specific endocrinopathies are discussed in more detail.

GLANDULAR DYSFUNCTION AND HORMONAL IMBALANCE STATES
Pituitary gland

Dysfunction of the pituitary usually takes the form of either anterior or posterior lobe dysfunction, although both lobes may be affected simultaneously. Abnormal secretion of ADH by the posterior pituitary is discussed in Chapter 11. Table 14-2 summarizes the effects of the pituitary hormones. The anterior lobe of the pituitary, as already mentioned, exerts much control over developmental, energy-producing, and reproductive processes. The pituitary exerts this control through both direct action on the tissues and through regulation of other glandular secretions via tropic hormones.

Hypopituitarism. Complete absence of all the anterior lobe pituitary hormones is rare. More commonly seen is a decrease in the amount of all of the anterior lobe hormones.

CLINICAL MANIFESTATIONS OF HYPOPITUITARISM

1. Inhibited growth and development (in children) due to lack of growth hormone
2. Manifestations of adrenocortical (except aldosterone) and thyroid hormone deficiencies due to lack of tropic hormones (see Table 14-3); aldosterone secretion continues due to its regulation by factors other than ACTH
3. Hypogonadism: loss of secondary sex characteristics, oligomenorrhea or amenorrhea, and decreased spermatogenesis due to deficiency of tropic hormones, which affect reproductive functions
4. Paleness due to lack of MSH and subsequent reduction in pigmentation
5. Central diabetes insipidus due to vasopressin deficiency; polyuria and decreased specific gravity of the urine are manifestations

---

Table 14-2. Pituitary hormones: target tissues and actions

Hormone	Target tissue	Action
Anterior lobe		
ACTH (adrenocorticotropic hormone; also called corticotropin)	Adrenal cortex	Stimulates synthesis and release of corticosteroids and adrenocortical growth
TSH (thyroid-stimulating hormone; also called thyrotropin)	Thyroid gland	Stimulates synthesis and release of thyroxine and triiodothyronine (thyroid hormone)
GH (growth hormone)	Nonspecific (has a generalized effect)	Promotes growth through protein anabolism, insulin antagonism, and lipolysis
Prolactin (also called lactogenic hormone)	Mammary glands	Stimulates production of breast milk
LH (luteinizing hormone; also called interstitital cell–stimulating hormone [ICSH])	Follicle (female)	Stimulates ovulation, progesterone secretion, and luteinization of ovarian follicle
	Testes (male)	Stimulates secretion of testosterone
FSH (follicle-stimulating hormone)	Follicle (female)	Stimulates maturation of follicle and secretion of estrogen
	Testes (male)	Stimulates spermatogenesis
Intermediate lobe		
α-MSH and β-MSH (α and β melanocyte-stimulating hormones)	Melanocytes	Promote pigmentation (secretion increased in pregnancy and may have a retarding effect on normal cycle)
Posterior lobe*		
Vasopressin (ADH or antidiuretic hormone)	Collecting ducts of kidney	Promotes water retention by increasing permeability of collecting ducts to water
Oxytocin (release is stimulated by infant's suckling of breast)	Mammary glands; uterus	Ejection of breast milk; stimulates uterine contraction (exogenous oxytocin used to induce labor in full-term pregnancy)

*Synthesized in hypothalamus and stored in posterior pituitary; transported between hypothalamus and posterior pituitary bound to neurophysines.

Isolated deficiency of a single pituitary tropic hormone is more likely to be the result of hypothalamic dysfunction rather than primary pituitary dysfunction. The manifestations of hypopituitarism differ somewhat between adults and children. In the adult the primary manifestations are related to the decrease in the tropic hormones, although thyroid and adrenal function will not be as severely depressed as is usually seen in primary disorders of those glands. Hypogonadism is most frequently seen. When hypopituitarism occurs while growth and development are still progressing, the outstanding features are stunted growth and delayed maturation with depressed sexual development. This latter condition is referred to as *pituitary dwarfism*.

Pituitary dwarfs may be a normal size at birth, and growth may proceed normally in the first few years of life. Eventually, however, growth will be retarded, and other signs and symptoms of hypopituitarism will become apparent. The manner in which growth is stunted may be the result of the following mechanisms: growth hormone deficiency, inadequate growth hormone secretion (possibly due to hypothalamic dysfunction), failure of growth hormone to generate *somatomedin,* or an end-organ defect in which the tissues fail to respond to growth hormone and somatomedin. This latter mechanism is thought to be responsible for the short stature of Pygmies.

Postpubertal hypopituitarism, or Simmonds' disease, is characterized by an insidious onset with vague, nonspecific symptoms. The initial manifestation of this condition may be severe adrenal insufficiency, which occurs as a result of stress. A variant of this disease process is Sheehan's syndrome, or hypopituitarism resulting from infarction of the pituitary due to hypotension secondary to hemorrhage during labor and delivery. A characteristic of this syndrome is the inability to secrete breast milk due to lack of prolactin after delivery. Other predisposing factors to Sheehan's syndrome include enlargement of the pituitary, which occurs during pregnancy, and a low-pressure vascular supply. Other causes of hypopituitarism in general include pituitary tumors, congenital abnormalities, infections, and vascular abnormalities.

Most pathology of the anterior lobe of the pituitary is secondary to tumors that may be hormonally active or inactive. Pituitary tumors that are active hormonally and that cause increased secretion of the tropic hormones are discussed later in the chapter as is increased growth hormone secretion.

Other signs and symptoms of hypopituitarism are listed in the box on p. 383. The characteristic paleness seen in patients with hypopituitarism is due to the lack of melanocyte-stimulating hormone (MSH) as a result of dysfunction of the surrounding pituitary tissue. This can be an important point in differentiating between primary and secondary adrenal hypofunction. The excessive secretion of ACTH and MSH seen in patients with primary adrenal hypofunction causes them to appear hyperpigmented. Where pituitary dysfunction results in secondary adrenal hypofunction, pigmentation is reduced due to the lack of MSH.

Treatment of hypopituitarism consists of appropriate hormonal replacement, nutritious diet, and surgery or irradiation for removal of a tumor. Growth hormone is not administered as part of the hormonal replacement regime in postpubertal hypopituitarism.

Hyperpituitarism. Growth hormone affects most of the body tissues rather than a specific target organ. Growth hormone promotes growth through its protein anabolic effect, with the result of positive nitrogen and phosphorus balances, and through its ketogenic and diabetogenic actions, which increase fat utilization and decrease carbohydrate utilization for energy. Amino acid transport into the cell and mitosis are increased, which promote increased cell size and proliferation. Excessive and prolonged secretion of growth hormone is usually the result of a pituitary tumor and causes *acromegaly* in the adult and *giantism* in the child.

Giantism is characterized by proportional growth that occurs before epiphyseal closure. This results in vertical overgrowth, with these patients reaching heights of 244 cm (8 ft.) or greater. Once epiphyseal fusion has occurred, the effects of acromegaly will become superimposed. Acromegaly is characterized by disproportionate growth and thickening of the long

---

CLINICAL MANIFESTATIONS OF ACROMEGALY

Increased tissue growth due to excessive growth hormone secretion
1. Bones (especially flat bones) become disproportionately widened, which results in enlargement of the hands and feet, lengthening of the lower jaw, causing it to protrude (prognathism), and widening of the bridge of the nose; teeth separate, and malocclusion occurs secondary to the growth of the jaw
2. Arthropathy occurs due to bone overgrowth around the joints and predisposes to osteoarthritis
3. Skin thickened with deep creases and folds and oversecretion of glands
4. Palpable enlargement of visceral organs, especially liver and kidneys
5. Enlargement of tongue, vocal cords, laryngeal cartilage, and lips causes speech to become disarticulate and voice to deepen

Endocrine interactions
1. Descreased carbohydrate tolerance due to antagonistic effect of growth hormone on insulin
2. Hypermetabolism without hyperthyroidism, although thyroid may be enlarged and hyperthyroidism may occur in 20% of the patients
3. Hyperadrenocortical effects
4. Hyperlibido and hypertrophy of genitalia; hyperfunction is characteristic of early stages of acromegaly; this changes to hypofunction with all the signs and symptoms of hypopituitarism later in the course of the disease
5. Secretion of prolactin causing gynecomastia in the male and galactorrhea in the female

Psychologic effects
1. Emotional lability
2. Psychologic disturbances

---

bones since the bones cannot elongate after closure of the epiphyses. The extremities, the face, and especially the nose appear enlarged. The lower jaw is lengthened so that the teeth project beyond the upper jaw. Approximately 50% of acromegalic patients have visual disturbances due to upward displacement of the tumor into the optic nerves. Arthropathy, carpal tunnel syndrome (tingling of the thumb and middle three fingers), hypertrophy and hyperplasia of cardiac muscle with eventual cardiac decompensation, and myopathy may become apparent before overt anatomic changes occur. Diabetes mellitus is found in 25% to 50% of the patients with acromegaly and can be of two types: (1) endogenous insulin production continues but cannot overcome the inhibitory effects of the growth hormone; and (2) exhaustion of the pancreatic islet cells occurs, and insulin deficiency develops. Other signs and symptoms of acromegaly are given in the box above. Acromegaly may follow a prolonged course, while the average life expectancy for the giant is 21 years of age. Death may occur from cardiac failure, diabetic acidosis, respiratory insufficiency, or as a result of tumor-related complications.

Thyroid gland

The thyroid gland secretes three hormones. Calcitonin is secreted in response to high serum calcium concentrations in the plasma; it lowers the serum Ca^+ level by increasing bone deposition. Thyroxine (T_4) and triiodothyronine (T_3) are iodinated amino acids that play a key role in the regulation of the metabolic rate and are necessary for growth and for maturation and development of the central nervous and skeletal systems. These two hormones are referred to collectively as *thyroid hormone*. Secretion of thyroid hormone occurs in response to the hypothalamic secretion of thyrotropin-releasing hormone (TRH), which in turn stimulates pituitary secretion of thyroid-stimulating hormone (TSH). Adequate levels of thyroid hormone in the blood inhibit secretion of TSH and probably TRH via a negative-feedback loop. Glandular concentrations of thyroid hormone are maintained via autoregulation through iodine uptake and release in an as yet unexplained manner.

Production of thyroid hormone requires adequate dietary intake of iodine. Uptake of iodide by the gland occurs via an energy-dependent, trapping mechanism. Uptake of iodide by the gland is increased in hyperthyroid states and decreased in hypothyroid states. Changes in glomerular filtration also affect iodide uptake. A decrease in glomerular filtration rate will result in increased uptake of iodide because of the resultant decrease in renal clearance.

Enlargement of the thyroid gland is termed *goiter* and is the result of prolonged secretion of TSH. The term *euthyroid goiter* is applied to various noninflammatory conditions that result in enlargement of the thyroid gland without hyperthyroidism. This type of goiter is probably preceded by and for a time accompanied by inadequate amounts of thyroid hormone due to depressed synthesis. The reduction in synthesis may be due to either a dietary lack of iodine or impaired enzyme activity secondary to genetic defects or goitrogenic substances. Under these conditions, excessive TSH secretion and the resulting hyperplasia of the gland are compensatory changes that may increase thyroid hormone production enough to prevent hypothyroidism.

Hypothyroidism. The state of deficient thyroid hormone production is called hypothyroidism. It results in *myxedema* in adults and *cretinism* in children. The clinical manifestations of myxedema are related to the degree of hypothyroidism present and reflect a slowing of the metabolic processes. Vague complaints of dry skin, forgetfulness, and intolerance for cold characterize mild forms. In more severe forms, the metabolic and vital functions will be noticeably reduced. A decrease in heat production reflects the reduced metabolic rate, and as a result of reduced endogenous heat production, cold intolerance develops. There is a noticeable weight gain, and motor function and reflexes are slowed. Mentation is slow, and the voice becomes characteristically husky and slow.

Depression of hepatic function leads to carotenemia, a yellowish discoloration of the skin due to reduced conversion of carotene to vitamin A, and increased plasma cholesterol levels. This latter effect may lead to accelerated atherosclerotic processes in the hypothyroid patient.

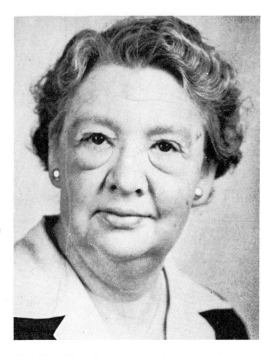

Fig. 14-1. Mxyedema, a condition caused by hyposecretion of thyroid gland during adulthood. (Courtesy Dr. Edmund E. Beard, Cleveland, Ohio. From Anthony, C. P., and Thibodeau, G. A.: Textbook of anatomy and physiology, ed. 10, St. Louis, 1979, The C. V. Mosby Co.)

Cardiac function is also depressed, and cardiac muscle may become weak and flabby. Protein and electrolytes accumulate in the interstitial spaces, resulting in edema. The patient has a characteristic puffy, drowsy appearance (Fig. 14-1). Other signs and symptoms are listed in Table 14-3.

Myxedema coma is a serious medical complication of myxedema. It may be precipitated by any type of stress. All the manifestations of hypothyroidism in their most extreme form are present. This state is characterized by loss of consciousness, hypotension, and bradycardia that may precipitate vasomotor collapse, hypoventilation, and seizure activity. Thyroid preparations must be immediately administered, and glucose may be administered for the hypoglycemia.

Cretinism is characterized by severe permanent stunting of both mental and physical development. Before the use of iodized salt became widespread, the most common cause of

Table 14-3. Clinical manifestations of hypothyroidism (myxedema)

Causative mechanisms	Signs and symptoms
↓ Energy production due to decreased metabolic reactions	Weakness; lassitude and easy fatigability, lethargy
↓ Heat production	Cold intolerance ↓ Body temperature ↓ Cardiac output and rate
↓ Oxygen requirements	↓ Blood pressure ↓ Respiratory effort Dyspnea on exertion
↑ Blood lipids up ↑ Cholesterol due to depressed liver function	High incidence of atherosclerosis and coronary artery disease
↓ Tissue synthesis	Capillary fragility with bruising; dry, flaky skin; dry, brittle nails; dry, sparse hair; anemia (↓ bone marrow metabolism)
↓ Reproductive function	↓ Libido and fertility
Fluid shift due to accumulation of protein and electrolytes in intestinal space	Puffy appearance of face; edema
Mental status	Apathy; speech slow
↓ Gastrointestinal activity	Weight gain; constipation; decreased appetite

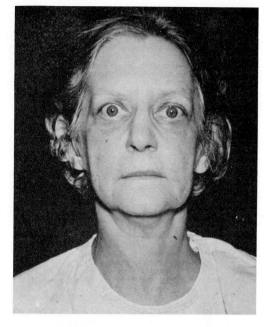

Fig. 14-2. Graves' disease caused by hypersecretion of thyroid gland. (Courtesy Dr. William M. Jefferies, Cleveland, Ohio. From Anthony, C. P., and Thibodeau, G. A.: Textbook of anatomy and physiology, ed. 10, St. Louis, 1979, The C. V. Mosby Co.)

cretinism was maternal iodine deficiency. Congenital anomalies, autoimmune disease, maternal ingestion of iodine, and medications to depress thyroid function may result in cretinism. Characteristically the face has a short forehead, wide, puffy eyes, and large nose. The child appears short and fat with short, broad hands. Umbilical hernias are common as a result of the hypotonic abdominal musculature. In addition to the lack of normal development, the manifestations are those of hypothyroidism (see Table 14-3). Once the typical clinical picture has developed, it is too late to prevent permanent mental retardation.

The causes of primary hypothyroidism include a lack of or destruction of thyroid tissue or inability to synthesize thyroid hormone. Chronic lymphocytic thyroiditis (Hashimoto's disease) is an inflammatory state that results in glandular enlargement, usually without accompanying hormonal imbalance; however, hypothyroidism may occur. It is believed to have an autoimmune etiology. Causes of secondary hypothyroidism include hypothalamic and pituitary disorders in which thyroid hormone secretion is absent due to lack of tropic hormone stimulation of the thyroid gland.

Treatment of hypothyroidism involves administration of supplemental thyroid preparations with the goal of increasing the metabolic rate. Dosage must be gradually increased to acclimate the systems (especially the cardiovascular) to the demands of increased metabolism. Dosage requirements are not static but increase with stress and decrease with age. Abrupt withdrawal of the drug may precipitate myxedema coma. The manifestations of drug toxicity are those of hyperthyroidism. A pulse rate of 100 is usually an indication to withhold the medication.

Hyperthyroidism. Hyperthyroidism or thyrotoxicosis is the result of excessive secretion of thyroid hormones. *Graves' disease* is the

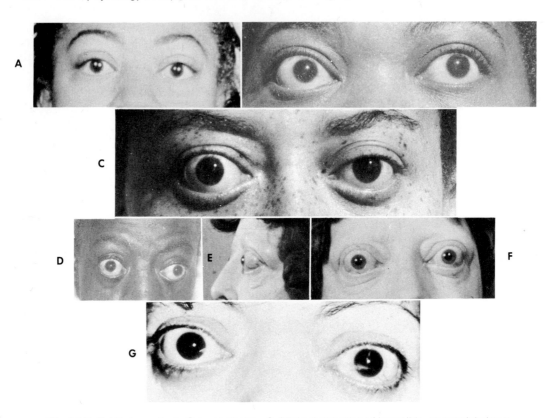

Fig. 14-3. Ophthalmopathy in Graves' disease. **A,** Minimal retraction of lower lids, no exophthalmos. **B,** Lid retraction with mild exophthalmos. **C,** Asymmetric exophthalmos. **D,** Ophthalmoplegia. **E** and **F,** Infiltrative ophthalmopathy with severe exophthalmos. **G,** Residual corneal scar in left eye after unilateral malignant exophthalmos. (From Schneeburg, N. G.: Essentials of clinical endocrinology, St. Louis, 1970, The C. V. Mosby Co.)

most common form of hyperthyroidism; it is accompanied by thyroid gland enlargement and exophthalmos, or protrusion of the eyeballs, which imparts a characteristic staring appearance (Figs. 14-2 and 14-3). Because of these features it is also referred to as *exophthalmic goiter*.

This disease has been demonstrated to be due to an autoantibody that reacts with the thyroid cell surface receptor for TSH. Plasma TSH levels are below normal due to the pituitary suppression of TSH by the high levels of thyroid hormone in the blood. This antibody is called long-acting thyroid stimulator (LATS), and its effects on the thyroid are much longer in duration than those of TSH.

The clinical manifestations of hyperthyroidism are the opposite of those seen in hypothyroidism (Table 14-4). The cardiovascular system is most severely affected. In some patients cardiovascular manifestations may be the only ones. High-output heart failure may be the result of the heart's inability to increase cardiac output to the degree required to maintain adequate tissue perfusion and to meet the increased metabolic demands. Cutaneous vasodilation causes a drop in peripheral resistance, which must be compensated for in order to maintain tissue perfusion. Treatment of hyperthyroidism depends on the severity of the manifestations and the age and ability of the patient to comply with the treatment regimens. Treatment may include surgery, antithyroid drugs, iodine treatment, and use of radioactive iodine.

Thyrotoxic crisis, or thyroid storm, is manifested by the extremes of the clinical manifestations of hyperthyroidism. Hyperthermia, heart failure, and severe nervous system dysfunction are all manifestations of the hypermetabolic state that exists. This condition can be precipi-

Table 14-4. Clinical manifestations of hyperthyroidism

Causative mechanisms	Signs and symptoms
↑ Catabolism and heat production	Muscle wasting (negative nitrogen balance); weight loss; increased appetite; fatigue (at first ↑ physical stamina); heat intolerance
↑ Sensitivity to catecholamines	Sweating; heat intolerance; tachycardia and palpitations; warm hands and feet; ↑ nervousness and irritability; tremors and ↑ Achilles reflex time; increased susceptibility to infection
↑ Cardiovascular activity	Tachycardia and palpitations; ↑ cardiac output and ↑ blood pressure; congestive heart failure (high output)
↑ Gastrointestinal activity with ↑ motility	Diarrhea; weight loss; nausea and vomiting
Speech	Rapid speech; hoarseness
Mental status	Emotional instability
Reproductive activity	Oligomenorrhea or amenorrhea

tated by stress such as trauma or severe infection. It is usually fatal but has become relatively rare with the use of antithyroid drugs.

Calcium homeostasis

Calcitonin is secreted by the C cells of the thyroid gland, and its major effect is to lower serum calcium levels through a reduction of bone resorption activity. The role of calcitonin is closely related to that of parathyroid hormone and vitamin D in the maintenance of calcium, phosphate, and bone metabolism. This interrelationship is briefly discussed in Chapter 10 in terms of calcium homeostasis. The active metabolite of vitamin D that participates in the maintenance of calcium homeostasis is considered to be a hormone because it is produced in the body and transported in the blood to a distant site to produce its effects. The functions of calcitonin, parathyroid hormone, and vitamin D will be discussed as a whole due to the interdependent roles they play in maintaining calcium homeostasis, which in turn largely determines

skeletal homeostasis. Alterations in calcium and skeletal homeostasis can be either manifestations or causes of disruption of the normal action and secretion of these hormonal substances. Disruption of normal parathyroid function sometimes occurs as a secondary, compensatory response to pathology occurring in another part of the body that affects calcium metabolism.

Parathyroid glands

The parathyroid glands secrete parathyroid hormone (PTH) in response to a fall in the serum ionized calcium level. Control of the secretion of parathyroid hormone is via a negative-feedback mechanism; a low serum calcium level stimulates parathyroid activity, while high serum calcium levels suppress it. A rise in serum phosphate levels will also stimulate parathyroid activity, but this effect is not a result of the increased phosphate per se but rather a result of the decreased serum calcium concentration that occurs due to the reciprocal nature of these two ions. Magnesium activates an intermediary in the calcium-mobilizing effects of PTH, and changes in the serum magnesium may affect PTH effectiveness. This may be the basis of the hypocalcemic state that accompanies low serum magnesium.

The bones and kidneys are the primary target organs of PTH. In the bone tissue, PTH exerts both short- and long-term effects that increase bone resorption and serum calcium levels. First, it stimulates osteocytic osteolysis, which rapidly increases serum calcium. PTH also stimulates bone tissue to form osteoclasts and retards the transformation of osteoclasts into osteoblasts. In the kidneys, PTH enhances renal tubular reabsorption of calcium and increases urinary excretion of phosphorus, sodium, potassium, amino acids, and bicarbonate. The mild acidosis that results from excretion of bicarbonate also enhances bone resorption. PTH also stimulates the renal conversion of 25-hydroxycholecalciferol to 1,25-dihydroxycholecalciferol, the active metabolite of vitamin D necessary for PTH to have its full effect on bone, and exerts direct effects on calcium metabolism as well. This hydroxylation is inhibited by calcitonin and high serum phosphate levels, while low serum phosphate levels stimulate it.

In the bone, 1,25-dihydroxycholecalciferol stimulates the formation of osteoclasts and prolongs their life span, effects similar to those of PTH. Both hormones must be present for either to be completely effective in bone tissue. 1,25-Dihydroxycholecalciferol also increases calcium reabsorption in the gut and calcium and phosphorus reabsorption in the renal tubules (see Fig. 10-7).

The target organs of calcitonin, which is secreted in response to high serum calcium levels, are similar to those of PTH. The bone effects and the inhibition of the hydroxylation of 25-hydroxycholecalciferol are antagonistic to those of PTH. Calcitonin does increase urinary calcium excretion, but it also has a phosphaturic effect similar to PTH. Calcitonin is currently being utilized as a therapeutic agent in certain hypercalcemic states and in Paget's disease of the bones, in which excessive and abnormal bone resorption and formation take place in a random, uncontrolled manner. Medullary cancer of the thyroid causes hypersecretion of calcitonin; however, serum Ca^+ levels usually remain within normal limits.

Hypoparathyroidism. Hypoparathyroidism is characterized clinically by hypocalcemia and hyperphosphatemia with decreased bone resorption and increased bone density due to the consequent reduction in calcium mobilization from the bones. The clinical manifestations include those of hypocalcemia (see Chapter 10). These patients frequently suffer ectodermal problems, which include dry skin, brittle nails, and thin hair. Frequent monilial infections of the nails, pharynx, and vagina may occur in patients with idiopathic hypoparathyroidism. Dental abnormalities include softening, late eruption, poor development, and defects in the enamel. Eye problems that may develop are irreversible and include cataracts, conjunctivitis, and photophobia. In chronic hypoparathyroidism, personality changes sometimes occur, including psychoses and mental retardation. Calcification in the basal ganglia, frontal regions, dentate nucleus, and cerebellum of the brain sometimes occurs but is not always related to the signs of parkinsonism that are seen in some hypoparathyroid patients.

The most frequent cause of hypoparathyroidism is surgical removal of or damage to the parathyroid glands. This may occur inadvertently during thyroid surgery or as a result of interruption of the blood supply to the glands. The hypoparathyroidism that follows is temporary in approximately one third to one half of these patients. A type of latent hypoparathyroidism may also follow thyroid surgery, in which the serum calcium level remains normal, but the return to a normal serum calcium level following a hypocalcemic episode will be extremely slow.

Hypoparathyroidism occurs physiologically in the neonate and is thought to be related to the development of tetany in infants who are fed high-phosphate cow's milk. Hypoparathyroidism during the neonatal period may also occur as a result of maternal hypercalcemia. There is a 25% chance of fetal death and a 50% chance of tetany developing during the first 3 weeks of life in the presence of maternal hyperparathyroidism.

There are two types of idiopathic hypoparathyroidism: early onset and late onset. The early-onset type appears to be an inherited condition that affects males and usually is manifest during the first year of life. It is generally very mild. This condition is different from hypoparathyroidism due to congenital absence of the parathyroid and thymus glands (DiGeorge's syndrome), which occurs sporadically in both males and females. The characteristics of this condition include failure to thrive, diarrhea, hypocalcemic tetany, and lymphopenia with increased susceptibility to infection. These infants tend to die early. The other type of idiopathic hypoparathyroidism, which has its onset later in life, occurs more frequently than the early-onset type. This type does not appear to be hereditary in nature, and there is some evidence of an autoimmune etiology. Addison's disease and pernicious anemia have been associated with this condition.

Treatment of hypoparathyroidism involves administration of calcium and vitamin D to correct the hypocalcemia. Hormone replacement therapy is impractical at this time, since it involves frequent intramuscular injection of parathyroid hormone. The hormone extract is ineffective when given orally because it is destroyed by digestive enzymes. Serum calcium levels are usually maintained in the low-normal range. Symptoms are usually absent at this level, and the hypercalciuria that is a common sequela to exogenous calcium administration is kept at a minimum. Formation of renal calculi is sometimes a complication of this form of therapy as is hypervitaminosis D, which causes hypercalcemia to develop. Even with treated hypoparathyroidism in which the serum calcium level is normal, serum phosphate levels remain elevated. Treatment of the hyperphosphatemia by dietary restriction or administration of either aluminum hydroxide gels, which limit intestinal absorption, or probenecid, which increases urinary phosphate excretion, is not usually necessary.

The condition of pseudohypoparathyroidism also bears mentioning. It is a rare, hereditary disorder in which there is no pathologic involvement of the parathyroid glands. The parathyroid hormone level is usually normal but sometimes elevated. The defect is in the target tissue (bone and kidney), which fails to respond to the hormone. A lack of cAMP seems to be the most plausible theory at this time to explain this failure of the target tissue to respond to PTH.

Hyperparathyroidism. Hyperparathyroidism is characterized by hypercalcemia and the sequelae to the chronic hypercalcemic condition: renal calculi and skeletal disease due to increased bone resorption. Renal calculi occur in approximately 75% of all patients with hyperparathyroidism, and in many of these patients, renal calculi are the only clinical manifestation of the hyperparathyroid state. In hyperparathyroidism there is an increase in the urinary excretion of calcium and phosphate, and renal calculi form as a result of these substances precipitating out into the urine. Pathologic changes in the kidney (hypercalcemic nephropathy) may progressively worsen.

Skeletal involvement occurs in approximately one third of the patients with hyperparathyroidism. This bone disease is referred to as *osteitis fibrosa cystica generalisata* and is characterized by increased bone resorption, replacement of normal bone tissue with a highly cellular fibrous tissue, and formation of cysts and tumors. The manifestations of this skeletal disorder include

pain and pathologic fractures. The pain may be local or diffuse and may become quite severe. The bones may be tender to palpation and the muscles weak and atrophied also.

The other signs and symptoms of hypercalcemia occur in approximately one third of the patients with hyperparathyroidism. The clinical manifestations of hypercalcemia are discussed in Chapter 10. Duodenal ulcer and pancreatitis also may be present in the hyperparathyroid state. The incidence of duodenal ulcer is close to 30% in hyperthyroid patients. Research has not documented a direct causal relationship, but there does seem to be a direct relationship between the plasma calcium level and the serum gastrin level and gastric secretory rate. The etiology of the increased incidence of pancreatitis in hyperparathyroidism is thought to be related to the calcium-dependent conversion of trypsinogen to trypsin. The theory is that the increased calcium content accelerates the conversion reaction, increasing the amount of trypsin, which causes inflammatory changes in the pancreas. Other possible etiologic mechanisms that continue to be examined include direct injury to pancreatic cells by the PTH, obstruction of the pancreatic duct by calculi, and thrombotic or embolic vascular damage associated with the excess PTH or hypercalcemia.

The causes of hyperparathyroidism may be classified as primary, secondary, or tertiary. *Primary hyperparathyroidism* applies to conditions in which the pathologic process affects the parathyroid glands directly and the feedback control of PTH secretion is lost so that hypercalcemia develops. Primary hyperparathyroidism may be the result of adenoma, hyperplasia, and carcinoma. Treatment of primary hyperparathyroidism is by surgical removal of the hyperfunctioning tissue.

Secondary hyperparathyroidism refers to conditions in which excessive secretion of PTH and parathyroid gland hyperplasia occur as compensatory mechanisms in response to chronic hypocalcemia. Serum calcium levels remain within normal limits since the feedback mechanism continues to operate effectively. Chronic hypocalcemia is a feature of vitamin D deficiency and calcium deprivation states. It accompanies steatorrhea since calcium and

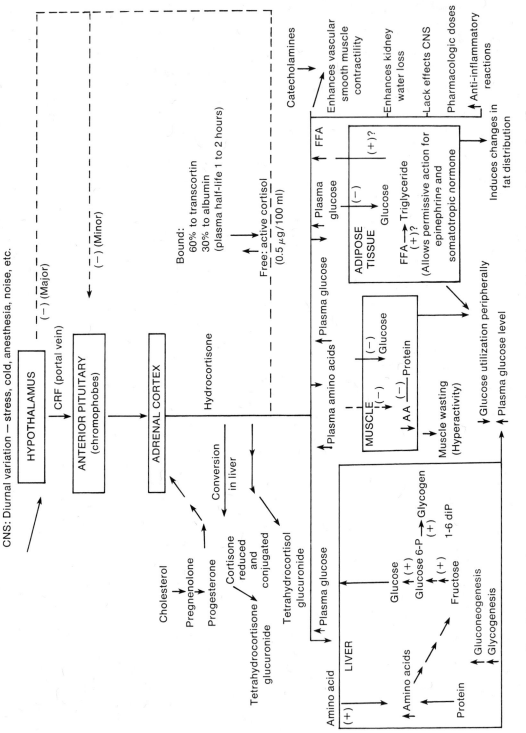

Fig. 14-4. Actions of hormones of adrenal glands. **A,** Actions of glucocorticoids. Adrenal cortex: hydrocortisone.

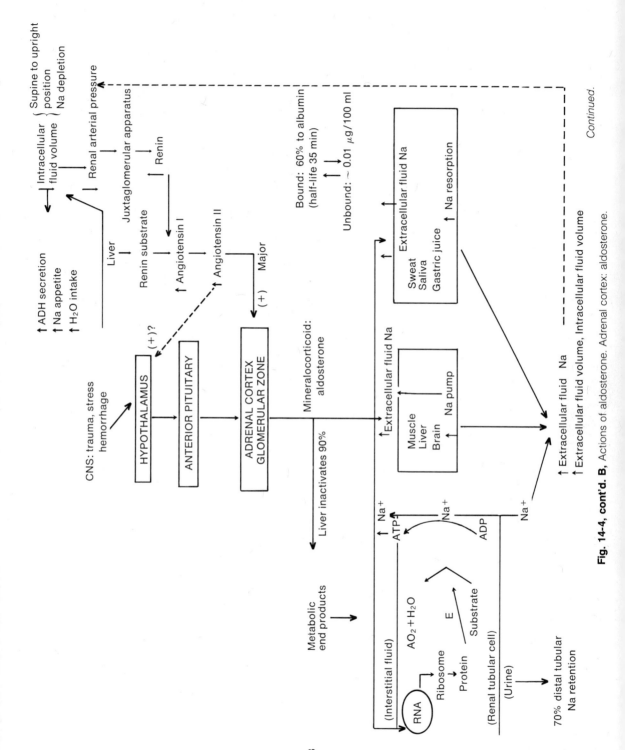

Fig. 14-4, cont'd. B, Actions of aldosterone. Adrenal cortex: aldosterone.

Continued.

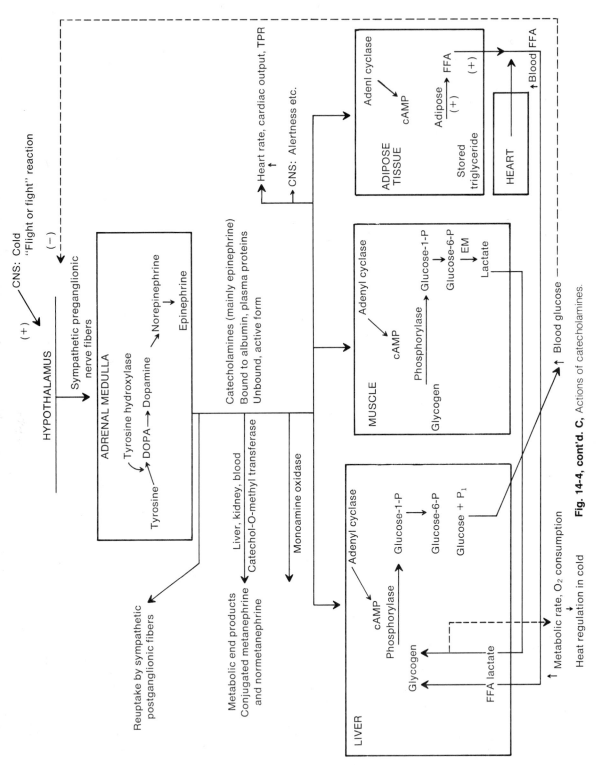

Fig. 14-4, cont'd. C, Actions of catecholamines.

vitamin D are lost through excretion bound to fatty acids. In chronic renal disease, chronic hypocalcemia is the result of the hyperphosphatemia that occurs and its reciprocal effect on the serum calcium. Hypercalcemia may develop if the normal feedback control is lost; this is referred to as *tertiary hyperparathyroidism*. It can be the result of adenoma formation in the hyperplastic tissue. Tertiary hyperparathyroidism sometimes occurs in patients with chronic renal disease who have been successfully treated with renal transplantation. Parathyroidectomy sometimes becomes necessary in these patients.

Adrenal glands

The adrenal glands are comprised of an inner portion, the medulla, and an outer portion, the cortex. The hormones secreted from each area serve diverse physiologic functions (Fig. 14-4), although they all play a major role in the physiologic adaptation to stress (see Chapter 6). The adrenal medulla secretes the catecholamines epinephrine and norepinephrine and can be considered a specialized type of sympathetic ganglion. The function of the adrenal medulla is not essential to life since the sympathetic nervous system also secretes catecholamines. The adrenal cortex secretes three classes of hormones: the glucocorticoids, the mineralocorticoids, and the sex hormones. The function of the adrenal cortex is essential to life. Death follows removal or loss of the adrenal glands without adequate glucocorticoid and mineralocorticoid replacement therapy. Disruption of the normal hormonal secretion of the adrenal cortex and medulla will be discussed separately.

Adrenocortical disruption. The hormones of the adrenal cortex are collectively termed *steroid hormones* and are derived from cholesterol via similar pathways. Progesterone serves as an intermediary in the conversion of pregnenolone to the various steroid hormones. The synthetic pathways of the glucocorticoids and adrenal androgens differ from that of the mineralocorticoid aldosterone in terms of the control mechanisms governing the synthesis and release of those hormones from the various histologic areas at the adrenal cortex. The synthesis and secretion of the glucocortoids and

adrenal androgens by the two inner layers of the cortex, the fascicular zone and the reticular zone, are under the control of adrenocorticotropin (ACTH). Control of the synthesis and secretion of aldosterone by the outermost layer of the adrenal cortex, the zona glomerulosa, is multifactorial, with the renin-angiotensin system probably exerting the greatest influence and ACTH exerting a minimal influence.

ACTH controls the synthesis of the glucocorticoids and adrenal androgens by increasing the amount of free cholesterol that enters the mitochondria to be converted to pregnenolone through activation of the adenyl cyclase–cAMP mechanism. It also stimulates cortical growth. Pituitary secretion of ACTH is primarily regulated by a negative-feedback mechanism involving a hypothalamic regulatory hormone and circulating levels of cortisol, the major glucocorticoid, and cortisollike steroids. In response to decreased blood levels of cortisol the hypothalamus is stimulated to secrete corticotropin-releasing hormone (CRH), which in turn stimulates pituitary secretion of ACTH. Increased blood levels of cortisol inhibit pituitary secretion of ACTH and to a lesser degree hypothalamic secretion of CRH.

ACTH secretion is also subject to diurnal variation and the effects of stress. ACTH and cortisol secretion usually peak in the morning hours shortly after a person normally rises and are most depressed at night. Reversal of sleep-wake patterns will reverse this diurnal variation. Loss of this episodic diurnal pattern of secretion may be an early sign of adrenocortical hyperfunction, or Cushing's syndrome.

The ACTH response to stress is mediated through the hypothalamic release of CRH. The response to stress can occur at any time during the day and if sufficiently strong can override negative-feedback inhibition.

Secretion of aldosterone is controlled by the renin-angiotensin system, the potassium concentration of the extracellular fluid, and ACTH. The juxtaglomerular cells of the afferent arteriole of the glomerulus secrete renin in response to renal hypoperfusion. Specialized renal reception cells participate in the regulation of renin secretion. These include stretch receptors in the afferent arteriole, which respond to lack of

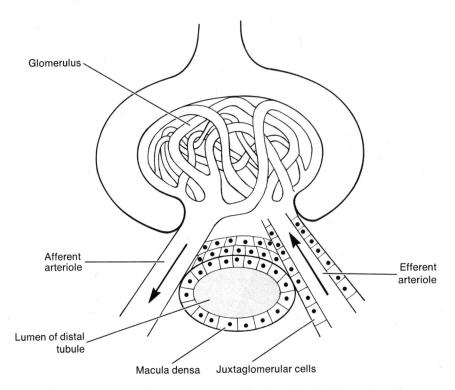

Glomerulus

Afferent arteriole

Efferent arteriole

Lumen of distal tubule

Macula densa   Juxtaglomerular cells

Fig. 14-5. Juxtaglomerular apparatus: specialized renal cells that secrete renin.

stretch, and the cells of the macula densa, which are thought to respond to changes in the sodium chloride load. Stimulation of renin secretion is also mediated by the catecholamines and sympathetic innervation of the kidney. When an individual is in a hypotensive state, less blood is delivered to the kidney, thus stimulating the stretch receptors of the afferent arteriole. Due to the decreased glomerular filtration rate less sodium chloride is delivered to the macula densa, thus stimulating these cells, and sympathetic activity increases due to stimulation of the arterial baroreceptors. Fig. 14-5 illustrates the anatomic arrangement of the juxtaglomerular apparatus.

Renin is converted into angiotensin II, which stimulates the release of aldosterone from the adrenal cortex. Control of further secretion of renin is provided via a negative-feedback mechanism in which both angiotensin II and aldosterone participate. Systemic pressure is increased due to the vasoconstrictor properties of angiotensin II and the restoration of effective circulating volume by aldosterone. The increase in systemic pressure augments renal perfusion

and glomerular filtration rate (with an increased glomerular filtration rate, tubular sodium chloride delivery is enhanced), and further secretion of renin is thus inhibited.

There is also a direct relationship between aldosterone secretion and plasma potassium concentration. Elevated plasma K^+ levels will stimulate aldosterone secretion via a direct effect on the zona glomerulosa. This mechanism is also controlled by feedback inhibition. The feedback regulation of aldosterone secretion via the renin-angiotensin system and plasma K^+ concentration is summarized in Fig. 14-6. Angiotensin II and potassium appear to act by stimulating the conversion of cholesterol to pregnenolone in the zona glomerulosa. ACTH appears to play a minor role in aldosterone secretion. The permissive nature of this role is demonstrated by the fact that aldosterone secretion in response to volume depletion in hypophysectomized animals is extremely low. Aldosterone exerts its renal effects through the hormonal mechanism of activating protein synthesis.

Adrenocortical disease can be the result of

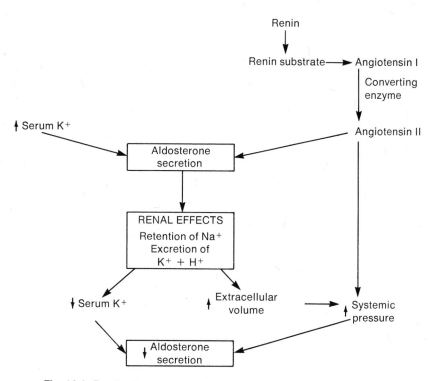

Fig. 14-6. Feedback regulation of aldosterone via two distinct mechanisms.

hyperfunction or hypofunction and is manifested by an excess or deficit of glucocorticoid or mineralocorticoid or an excess of the adrenal sex hormones.

Cushing's syndrome. Cushing's syndrome is the result of excessive cortisol and to a lesser extent adrenal androgen production and secretion in the body. The clinical manifestations are an exaggeration of the normal effects of cortisol on the body. Disordered fat metabolism results in truncal obesity and a round plethoric face referred to as *moon face* (Fig. 14-7). There is a peculiar localization of fat with an increase in the abdominal fat pad, a buffalo hump on the back, and a loss of fat in the extremities. Hypercholesterolemia leads to accelerated atherosclerotic processes. Protein wasting is the result of the catabolic actions of cortisol. Muscle wasting and thin, easily bruised skin due to loss of the perivascular supporting tissue are manifestations of protein wasting. Weakness and easy fatigability result from loss of muscle tissue and K^+ depletion. Loss of K^+ and hypertension are secondary to the mineralocorticoid effects of cortisol. Glucose intolerance, which

is manifested by hyperglycemia and glycosuria, develops in 90% of the patients, while frank diabetes mellitus develops in only 20%. This is due to the antagonistic effect that cortisol has on insulin action. Androgen excess presents with acne, hirsutism, and oligomenorrhea or amenorrhea in women.

Loss of the diurnal variation of cortisol secretion is one of the earliest signs of Cushing's syndrome. The release of growth hormone and its effectiveness are inhibited by cortisol, and thus the protein catabolic effects are enhanced and growth processes retarded. Melanocyte-stimulating hormone is usually secreted in excess with ACTH so that hyperpigmentation is a feature of Cushing's syndrome.

Loss of the protein matrix and demineralization of the bones lead to osteoporosis. Cortisol is antagonistic to 1,25-dihydroxycholecalciferol, which leads to reduced intestinal absorption of calcium and inhibits activation of bone cells. Secondary hyperparathyroidism develops with the result of increased loss of calcium from the bones. Pathologic fractures frequently complicate untreated cases with collapse of the

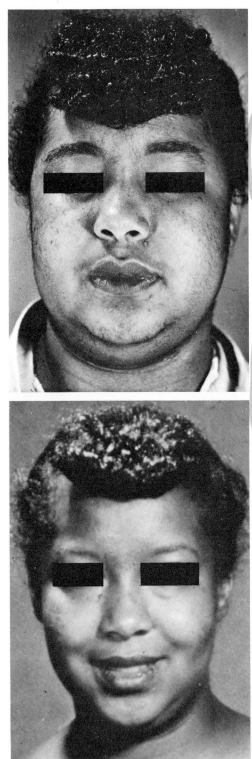

vertebrae constituting a most serious complication.

Extreme emotional lability is demonstrated by these patients. The range of emotional disorders may extend from euphoria to irritability and depression, with frank psychosis occasionally occurring.

The excessive cortisol secretion that causes Cushing's syndrome occurs as a result of hyperfunction of the adrenal gland. This hyperfunction may be the result of either excessive stimulation of the gland or a defect in the gland itself. Cushing's syndrome may also be iatrogenically caused (see Iatrogenic Endocrinopathies). Approximately 75% of the patients with endogenous Cushing's syndrome have bilateral adrenal hyperplasia secondary to excessive ACTH stimulation of the adrenals. In approximately 70% of all cases of Cushing's syndrome the excessive ACTH production is of pituitary origin, while in the rest the excessive ACTH production is the result of tumors in tissues that normally have no endocrine function and that produce an ACTH-like substance. Pituitary oversecretion of ACTH may be due to a pituitary adenoma; however, in the majority of cases the cause is obscure, and disturbances of the neurohypothalamic control of corticotropin releasing factor (CRF) have been proposed as a possible etiology.

Possible disturbances in neurohypothalamic function that may increase ACTH secretion include abnormal release of neurotransmitters and a decreased inhibitory effect by the limbic system on CRF release. Support for this theory of a neurohypothalamic etiology of Cushing's syndrome lies in the observation that tumors of the hypothalamus and hydrocephalus are sometimes associated with it. Additional evidence obtained by administration of antiserotonin and anticholinergic agents to dogs has demonstrated a reduced response to stimuli that normally affect

Fig. 14-7. Cushing's syndrome, result of chronic excess glucocorticoids. **A,** Preoperatively. **B,** Six months postoperatively. (Courtesy Dr. William M. Jefferies, Cleveland, Ohio. From Anthony, C. P., and Thibodeau, G. A.: Textbook of anatomy and physiology, ed. 10, St. Louis, 1979, The C. V. Mosby Co.)

the hypothalamus (pyrogens and hypoglycemia) and altered ACTH and cortisol secretion in response to these agents.

Approximately 25% of patients with Cushing's syndrome have tumors of the adrenal glands. The tumor may be an adenoma that becomes encapsulated in the adrenal tissue or a carcinoma that tends to invade the adrenal vasculature and thus metastasize.

The treatment of Cushing's syndrome depends on the etiology. Adrenalectomy may be necessitated by the presence of an adrenal tumor. If both adrenals are removed, the patient must be placed on replacement steroid therapy. Surgery and irradiation therapy are used for pituitary tumors. The neurotransmitter antagonists are being investigated for their possible application in Cushing's syndrome. Other pharmacologic agents that have been used for years are those that suppress adrenal function by inhibiting biosynthesis of steroids and destroy adrenocortical cells.

Aldosteronism. Aldosteronism may be primary or secondary. Primary aldosteronism (Conn's syndrome) is due to pathology arising within the adrenal glands, while secondary aldosteronism is due to pathologic conditions that occur outside the endocrine system and that cause the excessive stimulation of aldosterone secretion. In primary aldosteronism the secretion of aldosterone is no longer under normal feedback control in that it is not maintained by the appropriate stimuli nor is it inhibited by the factors that normally suppress it.

The causes of primary aldosteronism include adrenal hyperplasia in the zona glomerulosa and adrenal adenoma and carcinoma. Secondary aldosteronism occurs with conditions that decrease renal perfusion and that are sensed by the kidney as a reduction in circulatory volume. Bartter's syndrome is a condition in which excessive renin secretion due to hyperplasia of the renal juxtaglomerular apparatus causes secondary aldosteronism.

The clinical manifestations of aldosteronism are exaggerations of the normal effects of aldosterone, which are summarized in Fig. 14-8. There is an increased retention of Na^+ and increased urinary excretion of K^+. Metabolic alkalosis is the result of this shift of hydrogen ions into the cells to replace K^+ and maintain electroneutrality. Hypertension develops as a result of the increased blood volume and renal changes that occur. Hypertension will not be

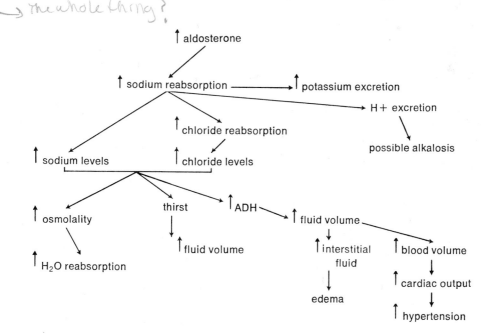

Fig. 14-8. Effects of increased aldosterone. (From Krueger, J. A., and Ray, J. C.: Endocrine problems in nursing, St. Louis, 1976, The C. V. Mosby Co.)

seen with secondary aldosteronism occurring in response to depletion of the effective circulatory volume. The other manifestations of aldosteronism reflect the electrolyte imbalance that occurs. Muscular weakness, paralysis, paresthesias, and tetany occur in response to hypokalemia and alkalosis.

Renal changes, which cause a loss of renal concentrating ability, occur in response to K^+ depletion (see Chapter 10). Polyuria and nocturia are symptoms that reflect this loss. The K^+-depleted kidney appears to be susceptible to infection, and signs of pyelonephritis develop.

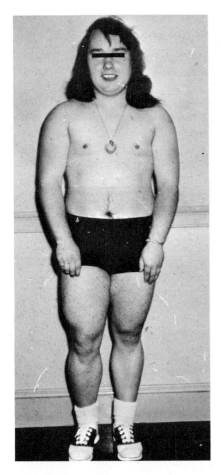

Fig. 14-9. Virilizing tumor of adrenal cortex of young girl. Tumor secretes excess androgens, thereby producing masculinizing adrenogenital syndrome. (Courtesy Dr. William M. Jefferies, Cleveland, Ohio. From Anthony, C. P., and Thibodeau, G. A.: Textbook of anatomy and physiology, ed. 10, St. Louis, 1979, The C. V. Mosby Co.)

Headache is commonly seen in this disorder and is often accompanied by vomiting and visual disturbances.

Adrenogenital syndrome. The adrenogenital syndrome constitutes a group of disorders that are caused by excessive adrenal secretion of the sex hormones. These syndromes occur most frequently when cortisol synthesis is impaired and the normal feedback inhibition to ACTH secretion is lost. Excessive ACTH secretion causes adrenal hyperplasia and excessive secretion of the sex hormones, since their synthesis is not inhibited. Causes of loss of cortisol-synthesizing ability include congenital defects and tumors.

Virilization and development of masculine secondary sex characteristics are the results of excessive androgen secretion in the female and immature male. The effects of androgen excess on a young girl are shown in Fig. 14-9. Masculinization in the mature female is manifested by deepening of the voice, beard growth, hypertrophy of the clitoris, irregular menses, and infertility. Feminization of the male due to adrenocortical tumors is rare.

Adrenocortical insufficiency. Adrenocortical insufficiency can occur in either acute or chronic forms. The chronic form is called *Addison's disease*. The causes of adrenocortical hypofunction may be primary, due to a disorder within the adrenal glands, or they may be secondary, due to pituitary dysfunction or administration of synthetic steroids for therapeutic purposes without appropriate withdrawal. Adrenocortical insufficiency secondary to lack of ACTH is usually not as severe as the primary form because of the patency and control of the zona glomerulosa. Primary adrenocortical insufficiency is usually idiopathic and is thought to have an autoimmune etiology, but it may also have a chronic infectious cause. In fact, the commonest cause of Addison's disease in Europe was tuberculosis, which caused destruction of the adrenals. Acute adrenocortical insufficiency may occur with septicemia or acute (meningococcal) infection. This is called the Waterhouse-Friderichsen syndrome; prompt treatment is necessary to prevent death.

The clinical manifestations of adrenocortical insufficiency are those of decreased mineralocorticoid and glucocorticoid secretion. The early stages are characterized by lassitude, anorexia, nausea, and vomiting. As the disease process advances, hypotension and hypoglycemia occur. The skin is highly pigmented and may be surrounded by areas of vitiligo, or patchy depigmented areas. In addition to the chronic manifestations, acute exacerbations called *crises* can be induced by physiologic or psychologic stress. These crises are characterized by severe vomiting, hypotension, weakness, diarrhea, and hypoglycemia. Without treatment coma and death will ensue. Treatment of Addison's disease is through hormonal replacement.

Disruption of the adrenal medulla. Because catecholamines are secreted by the sympathetic nervous system, hypofunction of the adrenal medulla does not produce pathologic manifestations. Medullary tumors appear to be the only distinct cause of adrenal medullary hypersecretion. The most common pathologic condition associated with hypersecretion of the adrenal medulla is *pheochromocytoma,* a benign, encapsulated tumor that causes hypertension, hypermetabolism, and hyperglycemia. The increased secretion of the catecholamines is intermittent; hypertension may at first be paroxysmal, later becoming continuous. Headache, palpitations, visual disturbances, sweating, nervousness, tremors, loss of appetite and weight, attacks of blanching or flushing, and heat intolerance are all symptoms that reflect the hypertension and hypermetabolism. The most extreme manifestations of hypertension may occur, namely, arrhythmias and congestive heart failure. Treatment is usually through surgical excision of the tumor.

IATROGENIC ENDOCRINOPATHIES

Prolonged administration of high doses of steroid medications may produce the features of Cushing's syndrome. Exogenous steroid therapy suppresses ACTH secretion, which leads to atrophy of the zona fasciculata and the zona reticularis of the adrenal cortex and thus to suppression of the secretion of those hormones. Patients being treated with synthetic steroids, in fact, have a form of iatrogenically induced Cushing's syndrome and are susceptible to many of the same problems: osteoporosis, gastric ulcer, increased susceptibility to infection, masking of an underlying infectious process, and extreme emotional lability.

Abrupt termination of the exogenous hormone will cause a state of adrenocortical insufficiency to develop. To withdraw a patient from exogenous steroid therapy, dosage should be tapered and the drug withdrawn slowly so that glandular function can return.

SUMMARY

This chapter presented an overview of the major mechanisms by which endocrine dysfunction can occur. Specific endocrinopathies were discussed in terms of the mechanism of the basic dysfunction and the manifestations of that dysfunction. The interrelatedness of the component glands of the endocrine system cannot be stressed enough. The role of the hypothalamus in providing neuroendocrine integration ensures that endocrine function remain a finely regulated process in tune with the specific needs of the body at any given time.

SUGGESTED READINGS

Brown, J., et al.: Thyroid physiology in health and disease, Ann. Intern. Med. **81**:68-81, 1974.

Hallal, J.: Thyroid disorders, Am. J. Nurs. **77**(3):418-432, 1977.

Hershman, J., and Pittman, J. A.: Control of thyrotropin secretionin man, N. Engl. J. Med. **285**:997-1006, 1971.

Mackin, J. F., et al.: Thyroid storm and its management, N. Engl. J. Med. **291**:396-1398, 1974.

Montgomery, R., Dryer, R. L., Conway, T. W., and Spector, A. A.: Biochemistry: a case oriented approach, ed. 2, St. Louis, 1977, The C. V. Mosby Co.

Newton, D., Nichols, A., and Newton, M.: Corticosteroids, Nursing 77, **7**(6):26-33, 1977.

Said, S.: The lung in relation to hormones, Basics R.D., vol. 1, no. 3, Feb. 1973.

Schteingart, D.: Cushing's disease, an update, Drug Therapy **3**(2):53-63, 1978.

Sutherland, E. W.: Studies on the mechanism of hormone action, Science **177**:401, 1972.

Thorn, G., et al.: Harrison's principles of internal medicine, ed. 8, New York, 1977, McGraw-Hill Book Co.

Williams, R. H.: Textbook of endocrinology, ed. 5, Philadelphia, 1974, W. B. Saunders Co.

CHAPTER 15

Reproductive system: disorders and mechanisms

AT THE COMPLETION OF THIS CHAPTER THE STUDENT WILL BE ABLE TO:

- Differentiate between normal and abnormal patterns in the reproductive cycle.
- Explain pathophysiologic mechanisms underlying reproductive dysfunction.
- Describe the various manifestations of reproductive dysfunction in terms of the disruption of normal reproductive functions and resultant compensatory mechanisms that occur.
- Identify etiologic and predisposing factors in disorders of reproductive function.
- Explain the physiologic basis of treatment of various disorders of the reproductive system.

The major physiologic function of the reproductive system is the procreation of new life and the perpetuation of the species. In the human species the creation of new life through reproduction is also viewed as a visible expression of love between two individuals. Based on this view, the human reproductive capacity and function take on profound psychologic and even spiritual significance. The impact of reproductive dysfunction is usually felt by more than one individual. The acceptance of such a dysfunction and the ability and willingness to deal with it effectively are greatly determined by the value systems of the individuals involved. The effects of psychosocial factors on the progression of any pathophysiologic process must always be considered. This is especially true for diseases of the reproductive system.

The reproductive process involves fertilization of the ovum, maternal adaptation to pregnancy, fetal growth and development, fetal separation, and adaptation to extrauterine life. This reproductive ability is primarily under endocrine control, although it is also influenced by various neural and metabolic factors. This chapter discusses the effects of reproductive dysfunction in terms of the manifestations and mechanisms of this dysfunction. Disorders of sexual differentiation are discussed in Chapter 2.

The female ovary and the male testis serve both exocrine and endocrine functions. The exocrine function is gametogenesis, or the production of ova and sperm. The endocrine function is secretion of the sex hormones, which control sexual development and function. The hormones of the female serve the additional function of preparing the body for and maintaining pregnancy. Gonadal function is under the control of the pituitary-stimulating hormones, the release of which is mediated by the hypothalamus. Feedback inhibition is provided by the sex hormones. Activation of testicular and ovarian function occurs at puberty in response to increased levels of the pituitary stimulating hormones.

The functions of the testis include secretion of the male sex hormones (androgens), the major one being testosterone, and spermatogenesis. Control of these functions is provided by two pituitary trophic hormones: follicle-stimulating hormone (FSH), which regulates sper-

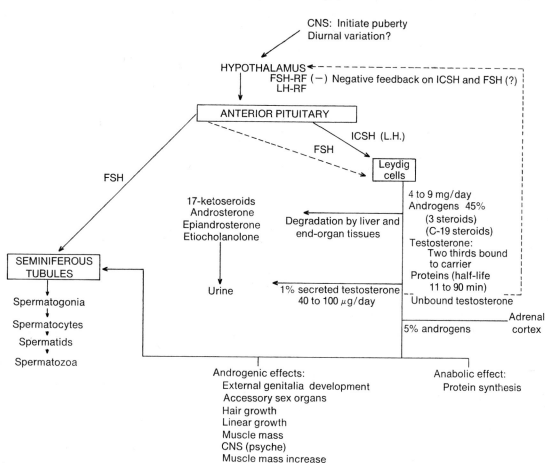

Fig. 15-1. Testes: control and function, including testosterone secretion and actions.

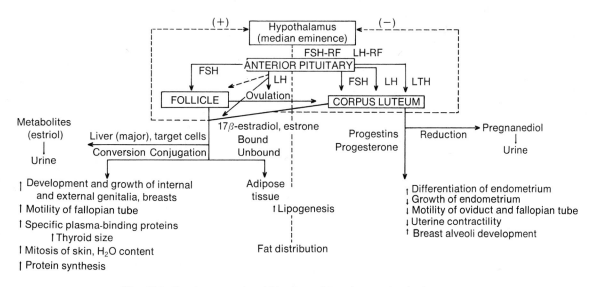

Fig. 15-2. Ovaries: control and functions of female reproductive hormones.

matogenesis, and luteinizing hormone (LH), or interstitial cell–stimulating hormone (ICSH) as it is sometimes called, which regulates testosterone production by the Leydig cells of the testis. Fig. 15-1 illustrates the functions of the testis under pituitary and hypothalamic control. Estrogen is also produced by the testis in very small amounts.

At puberty, testosterone is necessary for the development of the secondary sex characteristics in the male. Another function of testosterone is development of normal male sex organs and sex characteristics during fetal life. During the last 3 months of fetal development, testosterone is required for the normal descent of the testes into the scrotum. Testosterone secretion in the fetus, however, is under the control of the hormone chorionic gonadotropin, which is secreted by the placenta.

Reproductive ability in the female begins at puberty and ends at menopause (climacteric) when estrogen secretion diminishes. The ovaries secrete the female sex hormones, estrogen and progesterone (Fig. 15-2). In contrast to gonadal function in the male, which is continuous, gonadal function in the female is cyclic. The menstrual cycle can be characterized by two phases: preovulatory and postovulatory. During the preovulatory, or follicular, phase, growth and maturation of the ovarian follicle and a gradual thickening of the endometrium occur. The growth, development, and involu-

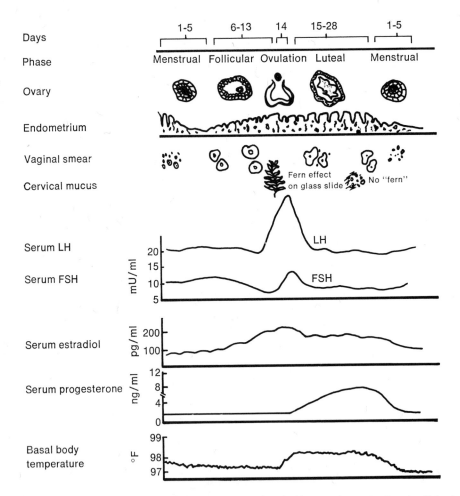

Fig. 15-3. Humoral, secretory, and cellular events associated with normal menstrual cycle. (Adapted from Ryan, W. G.: Endocrine disorders: a pathophysiological approach, Chicago, 1975, Year Book Medical Publishers.)

tion of the corpus luteum occur during the postovulatory, or luteal, phase. The whole purpose of these cyclic events is maturation and release of the ovum and preparation of the uterus to receive the fertilized ovum. This cycle normally occurs over a 28-day period, although individual cycles may vary between 21 and 35 days. It may be interrupted by fertilization and implantation of the ovum. Control of the cycle, which is hormonal, is summarized below.

FSH stimulates several follicles to begin to develop in the ovary; however, only one will continue to mature, while the others involute. The maturing follicle produces estrogen, and the increased estrogen level is thought to stimulate the rise in both LH and FSH just before ovulation. LH is thought to stimulate progesterone secretion, which in turn induces produc-

tion of an enzyme that attacks collagen in the follicular wall. The follicle ruptures, releasing the ovum, which enters the fallopian tube. The ruptured follicle fills with yellow, lipid-containing luteal cells (the corpus luteum), which produce progesterone under the influence of LH. The high concentrations of estrogen and progesterone inhibit the release of FSH, preventing the development of any new follicles. During this period the blood supply to the endometrium increases and glycogen deposition occurs in preparation for implantation of a fertilized ovum. If fertilization does not occur, the levels of estrogen and progesterone drop as the corpus luteum degenerates, and endometrial bleeding and shedding (menstruation) occur. FSH will again be stimulated by the decreased concentrations of these hormones, and follicular develop-

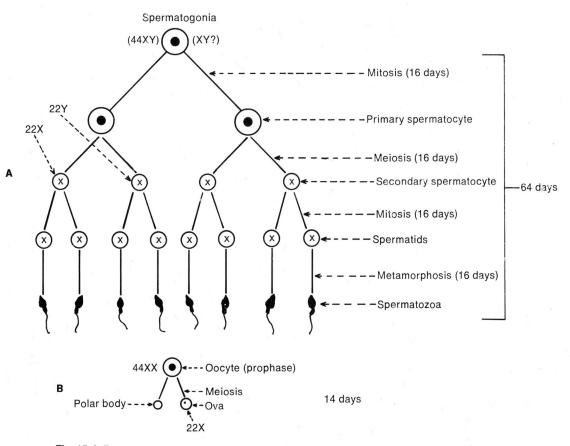

Fig. 15-4. Events associated with spermatogenesis, **A,** and oogenesis, **B.** (Adapted from Ryan, W. G.: Endocrine disorders: a pathophysiological approach, Chicago, 1975, Year Book Medical Publishers.)

ment will begin again. The hormonal and cellular events of the menstrual cycle are summarized in Fig. 15-3, which includes the histologic changes that occur in the cervix and vagina. Fig. 15-4 diagrams the processes of oogenesis and spermatogenesis.

If fertilization and implantation occur the corpus luteum continues to provide estrogen and progesterone until approximately the third month of gestation. The placenta produces chorionic gonadotropin (CG), which serves as the stimulus for the function of the corpus luteum at this time. Later in the pregnancy the placenta takes over production of these hormones and the secretion of CG diminishes. During pregnancy, estrogen stimulates growth of the uterine muscle mass. Progesterone exerts an inhibitory effect on uterine smooth muscle, preventing muscular contraction and hence expulsion of the fetus, and also stimulates formation of glandular tissue in the breast. The concentrations of estrogen and progesterone decrease prior to the onset of labor, or parturition. The decrease in progesterone allows the rhythmic uterine contractions that characterize labor to occur and removes the inhibitory effect that it exerts on prolactin release, allowing lactation to begin.

MANIFESTATIONS OF DISORDERS OF THE REPRODUCTIVE SYSTEM

Disorders of the reproductive system may become apparent through a variety of clinical manifestations. The three classic symptoms that typify the normal menstrual cycle include pain, bleeding, and discharge. Alterations in the normal state of any of these symptoms may indicate pathology. The general character of these symptoms is important, but the characteristics of their occurrence within the menstrual and reproductive cycles are just as important if not more so. Bleeding after the onset of menopause or between menstrual periods is an example of this; what is considered normal in one part of the reproductive cycle may represent dysfunction in another part of the cycle. Polymenorrhea is considered normal in the pubertal adolescent, but in the mature female this symptom may indicate underlying pathology such as endometrial cancer. Infertility, abnormal discharge from

the breast, vagina, or penis, abnormalities of lactation, and gynecomastia are other potential manifestations of disorders of the reproductive system. Many of these manifestations apply chiefly to disorders of the female reproductive system.

Pain

Dysmenorrhea is the term applied to the lower abdominal and pelvic pain that occurs with normal menstruation. *Primary dysmenorrhea* is usually considered a benign condition that occurs principally in young adults and adolescents. It tends to decrease with maturity and particularly after the first pregnancy. *Secondary dysmenorrhea* is seen in women in their late 20s and early 30s and is indicative of coexisting organic disease, which may include inflammatory and infectious processes, cervical stenosis, pelvic congestion, endometriosis, and adenomyosis. The pathogenesis of primary dysmenorrhea is unclear, and probably a number of interrelated factors are responsible. Factors postulated to play a role in its development include mechanical obstruction of the menstrual flow by a small cervical outlet, anxiety, uterine hypercontractility, and vascular spasm.

Dysmenorrhea is characterized by pain in the lower abdomen, which may be sharp and crampy or dull and constant. It begins approximately 12 to 14 hours before flow begins and lasts for 24 to 48 hours. It is sometimes associated with headache, fatigue, irritability, nausea, vomiting, and diarrhea. The pain may radiate to the thighs, upper legs, and back.

The syndrome of premenstrual tension and edema often accompanies dysmenorrhea. This syndrome is characterized by malaise and fatigue often beginning up to 1 week before the menstrual flow begins. The fluid retention may cause marked edema. Headaches with a tendency toward migraine are the most characteristic complaint of this syndrome and probably reflect a certain degree of cerebral edema.

Bleeding

Vaginal bleeding or the lack of it must first be assessed in terms of whether it is occurring in the pregnant or nonpregnant state.

Amenorrhea is the absence of menstruation;

it is considered normal before menarche, after menopause, and during pregnancy and lactation. *Primary amenorrhea* is the failure of menstruation to begin. It may be present if a girl reaches 18 years of age without having menstruated. *Secondary amenorrhea* is the cessation of menstruation following the initiation of menstruation at the menarche. Primary amenorrhea is usually the result of ovarian dysfunction or hypothalamic-pituitary disorders. Secondary amenorrhea may be due to endocrine dysfunction but is also frequently a feature in a number of general illnesses. An example of this is the patient with chronic renal failure who has ceased to menstruate with the onset of renal failure but who had previously experienced normal menstrual cycles. Secondary amenorrhea can be the result of psychologic stress and anxiety, the effects of which are probably mediated via the hypothalamus.

Dysfunctional bleeding in the adolescent is related to immaturity of the pituitary-ovarian axis and the presence of anovulatory menstrual cycles. Progesterone secretion is insufficient, and therefore complete shedding of the endometrium does not occur. The consequence of this is irregular periods of bleeding. Dysfunctional uterine bleeding in the menopausal or postmenopausal woman may indicate a pelvic malignancy. Cervical erosion and polyps, both benign lesions, are frequent causes of intermenstrual bleeding or excessive menstrual flow. Bleeding usually occurs with no discomfort. Uterine fibroids are another form of benign tumor that causes abnormal bleeding, pain, and pressure. These most commonly occur in women of child-bearing age. Surgical removal of the tumors and often hysterectomy are necessitated by this condition.

Bleeding during pregnancy. Bleeding during pregnancy is often indicative of a serious complication. Potential causes of bleeding during early pregnancy include abortion, ectopic pregnancy, and hydatidiform mole. Bleeding after the 28th week of gestation is considered antepartal hemorrhage due to abnormal placental separation.

The term *abortion* implies the termination of pregnancy prior to the time the fetus has sufficiently developed to survive. The term *mis-carriage* is applied when abortion occurs spontaneously. Spontaneous abortion in the early months of pregnancy is usually preceded by the death of the fetus. Early fetal death may be the result of an abnormality in the developing embryo or reproductive tissue or systemic disease of the mother. Abnormalities of development appear to be the most common cause of early fetal death. The mechanisms by which these malformations develop are discussed in Chapter 2.

Clinically, spontaneous abortion can be grouped according to the following classifications: threatened, inevitable, incomplete, missed, or habitual. One half or less of the women who bleed during early pregnancy actually abort. A *threatened* abortion is characterized by vaginal bleeding or bloody, vaginal drainage during the first half of pregnancy. This may or may not be accompanied by low back pain and mild abdominal cramping. Slight bleeding at the time the normal menstrual cycle would have occurred is considered physiologic.

Inevitable abortion is characterized by rupture of the membranes and cervical dilation. Prior to the tenth week of pregnancy the fetus and placenta are likely to be expelled together. After the tenth week the placenta is likely to be retained either completely or in part. This causes bleeding, which is the main sign of *incomplete abortion*. Signs of a threatened abortion may appear upon death of the fetus. After this the uterus will no longer enlarge, and mammary changes revert. Most *missed abortions* terminate spontaneously after a period of time with no ill effects to the mother. Occasionally, coagulation defects develop, which are probably mediated by the thromboplastin from the dead fetus. The incidence of missed abortion is increasing with the use of potent progestational compounds to treat threatened abortion. *Habitual abortion* refers to three or more consecutive abortions.

Ectopic pregnancy is the result of implantation of the fertilized ovum outside the uterine endometrium. The most common site of ectopic implantation is the fallopian tubes. Two general mechanisms have been implicated in ectopic pregnancy: (1) an increase in the receptivity of ectopic tissues (especially tubal tissue) to the fertilized ovum and (2) conditions that prevent or retard the passage of the fertilized ovum into the uterine cavity. This pregnancy normally cannot go to term, although some cases of ovarian pregnancies going to term have been reported. Ectopic pregnancy usually terminates through rupturing, which constitutes an emergency situation.

A *hydatidiform mole* is a benign tumor of the placenta in which some or all of the chorionic villi are converted into a mass of clear vesicles. The incidence of this disorder appears to be quite high in some parts of the world (mainly Asia and Mexico), and it usually affects women in the end of their child-bearing years. Persistent bleeding, which can be either ''spotty'' or hemorrhagic, and rapid uterine enlargement are characteristic. Additionally, the manifestations of hypertension, absence of fetal activity and heart sounds, and increased thyroxine secretion without hyperthyroidism are seen. Treatment involves the immediate termination of the mole and later follow-up for possible malignant changes since it is the most common lesion preceding choriocarcinoma.

Bleeding that occurs during the later part of pregnancy is usually due to abnormal separation of the placenta from the uterine site of implantation. There are two conditions in which this mechanism is operative: abruptio placentae and placenta previa. *Abruptio placentae* is a condition in which a normally situated placenta becomes separated. Bleeding occurs between the placenta and uterine wall and results in formation of a decidual hematoma (concealed hemorrhage). External bleeding may or may not occur. The extreme form, in which at least one half the placenta is separated, presents with pain, uterine rigidity, absent fetal heart tones, and hypovolemic shock. In less severe forms, fetal heart sounds may be audible although abnormal. Acute renal failure and consumptive coagulopathy (DIC; see Chapter 5) are complications of this disorder. Abruptio placentae is considered a hemorrhagic emergency. Possible causes include trauma, a short umbilical cord, sudden uterine decompression, hypertension, and compression or obstruction of the vena cava, which increases venous hydrostatic pressure distal to the site of compression or obstruction.

In *placenta previa* the placenta is abnormally attached to the lower uterine segment over or near to the cervical internal os. Multiparity and advancing age seem to predispose women to the development of this disorder, which is characterized by painless hemorrhage in the latter part of pregnancy. Many abortions in early pregnancy may be the result of misplaced placental tissue. In the latter part of pregnancy the lower segment of the uterus stretches and thins out, which results in tearing of the placental attachments. The stretched myometrium is unable to compress the bleeding vessels, and hemorrhage occurs. This hemorrhage occurs without warning in a woman who has previously been in good health. It may occur during sleep, so that she wakes up to find herself in a pool of blood. The development of placenta previa necessitates emergency delivery by cesarean section.

Discharge

Discharge from any body orifice must be assessed in terms of amount, color, consistency, and accompanying odor. The various infectious processes that affect the male and female reproductive systems can often be identified through the discharges they produce. Abnormal changes in the character of the vaginal discharge during the menstrual cycle may be indicative of underlying pathology. Discharge from the male or female breast (other than during lactation) may indicate an underlying pathologic process.

Leukorrhea is the term applied to any vaginal discharge other than blood. The mucous glands of the cervix are the chief source of leukorrheal discharge, which normally is a clear, viscid, alkaline mucus. The amount of this discharge increases and its consistency changes at the time of ovulation. A change from the normal secretion to a thin, watery, profuse secretion in the menopausal and postmenopausal woman is usually indicative of cell breakdown, which suggests a metastatic process. Vulval irritation and contact dermatitis also may alter the amount and character of the vaginal secretion as can forgotten tampons and other foreign bodies inserted into the vagina.

Infertility

Failure to conceive may be the result of infertility in either of the partners, the incidence

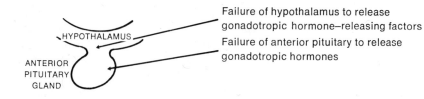

Failure of hypothalamus to release
gonadotropic hormone–releasing factors

Failure of anterior pituitary to release
gonadotropic hormones

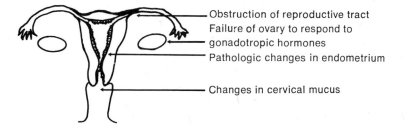

Obstruction of reproductive tract

Failure of ovary to respond to
gonadotropic hormones

Pathologic changes in endometrium

Changes in cervical mucus

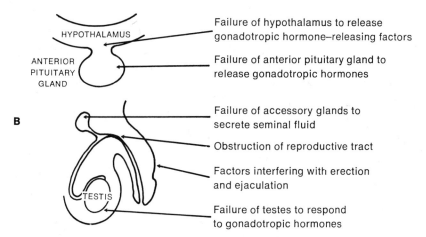

Failure of hypothalamus to release
gonadotropic hormone–releasing factors

Failure of anterior pituitary gland to
release gonadotropic hormones

Failure of accessory glands to
secrete seminal fluid

Obstruction of reproductive tract

Factors interfering with erection
and ejaculation

Failure of testes to respond
to gonadotropic hormones

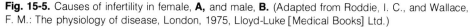

Fig. 15-5. Causes of infertility in female, **A,** and male, **B.** (Adapted from Roddie, I. C., and Wallace, F. M.: The physiology of disease, London, 1975, Lloyd-Luke [Medical Books] Ltd.)

of infertility being equally common in both sexes. For conception to occur it is necessary for the ovary to produce an ova and for viable, motile sperm to be deposited near the cervix. The reproductive tract of the female must permit free passage of the sperm and ova. For further development to occur, implantation of the fertilized ova must take place in a suitable uterine endometrium. The deposition of sperm depends on adequate production of sperm and seminal fluid and a patent delivery system. Failure in meeting any of these conditions or failure of the pituitary to secrete gonadotropic hormones or of the gonads to respond to the pituitary stimulus can cause infertility. Fig. 15-5 graphically illustrates the points at which normal fertility in the male and female can be impaired.

Mechanical obstruction within the female reproductive tract is the most common cause of female infertility. Obstruction may be due to inflammatory changes following infection within the reproductive system. It is this mechanism that is responsible for female infertility after an untreated gonorrheal infection. The development of scar tissue and adhesions in the peritoneal cavity as a result of surgical procedures, or a peritoneal inflammatory reaction may also cause obstruction of the female reproductive tract. This mechanism accounts for the infertility that often accompanies endometriosis. Alterations in the cervical mucus may prevent penetration by the sperm. Pathologic changes in the endometrium may prevent implantation. Infertility may also be the result of an immunologic reaction to sperm. Approximately 15% of all cases of female infertility are the result of hormonal failure: failure of the pituitary to release gonadotropic hormones or failure of the ovary to respond to them.

Spermatogenesis will be impaired by lack of gonadotropic hormones or failure of the testes to descend into the scrotum, since the increased abdominal temperature inhibits sperm production. Damage to the prostate gland and seminiferous vesicles may reduce the volume and alter the composition of seminal fluid. Changes in the seminal fluid will impair the motility of the sperm. Inflammatory damage to the seminiferous tubules or ducts will cause obstruction, which prevents the release of sperm. Inflammatory damage to the seminiferous tubules may occur as a complication of mumps. Failure to attain an erection and ejaculate is an obvious cause of male infertility. Control of these functions is provided by psychologic and neurologic factors.

Treatment for infertility depends on the cause. Obstruction may be relieved by various surgical procedures. Ovulation may be induced by hormonal therapy. Hormonal therapy to stimulate spermatogenesis has been tried but has not proven to be very successful.

Disorders of lactation

Female breast development at puberty is due to the action of estrogen, which stimulates development of the ducts, and progesterone, which stimulates alveolar growth. Prolactin influences the secretion of these hormones and thus promotes breast development. Galactorrhea, or milk production, normally occurs in the female following pregnancy. During pregnancy the breasts enlarge and develop in response to placental hormones. Milk production is enhanced by suckling, which produces neural stimuli that promote prolactin secretion. The absence of lactation after pregnancy is characteristic of Sheehan's syndrome (see Chapter 14), or pituitary necrosis caused by delivery. Galactorrhea in nonparturitional females and in males is abnormal and is inevitably accompanied by increased prolactin secretion. Galactorrhea is frequently associated with a pituitary tumor, although it may accompany administration of certain drugs (L-dopa, rauwolfia, alkaloids, tranquilizers, antidepressants) and endocrine disorders.

Gynecomastia

Gynecomastia, or enlargement of the male breast, is a normal and transitory finding in approximately one half of all normal males at puberty. Gynecomastia in the male adolescent must be evaluated in terms of whether development of secondary sex characteristics is also occurring, since puberty is a time when gonadal dysfunction and disorders of sexual differentiation become apparent. Klinefelter's syndrome is a disorder of sexual differentiation in which gynecomastia may occur; the gynecomastia that accompanies this syndrome is usually more severe than that seen in normal males. There is a high correlation between the occurrence of male breast cancer and Klinefelter's syndrome.

Gynecomastia may also occur secondary to testicular tumors. It often accompanies liver disease and is thought to be due to the inactivation of estrogen, which occurs as a result of liver dysfunction. Gynecomastia may be a manifestation of an endocrine disorder or may occur as a side effect to therapy with certain drugs. These drugs include digitalis, steroids, androgens, psychotropic drugs, spironolactone, phenothiazine, and marijuana. Gynecomastia may also occur as an idiopathic disorder.

DISEASE MODEL: ENDOMETRIOSIS

Endometriosis demonstrates many of the manifestations just described. Its incidence has increased markedly in the developing nations over the last 20 years, and it may possibly come to be thought of as a disease induced by societal conditions in much the same way as respiratory disease or cancer is induced by environmental conditions. Endometriosis is seen most commonly in women from the upper socioeconomic level who are between the age of 30 and 40, although it may appear before the age of 30, and some cases of teenage endometriosis have also been reported. Frequent pregnancy beginning at a young age appears to impart some "immunity" to this disease. Many women who develop endometriosis delayed getting pregnant until they were older, a fairly popular recent trend in modern society. Endometriosis also occurs more commonly in women who have had repeated surgeries for dilation and curettage of the uterus, possibly a reflection of a more affluent and liberal modern society. The "typical" patient has been described as a perfectionist who is intelligent, overanxious, and underweight. It is interesting to note that this personality type is more frequently found in fast paced, goal-oriented, "advanced" societies.

Endometriosis is a condition in which tissue resembling that of the uterine endometrium is found in extrauterine locations but mainly in the pelvic cavity. The most common sites include the ovaries, uterine ligaments, rectovaginal system, pelvic peritoneum, covering the organs of the pelvis, umbilicus, laparatomy scars, hernial sacs, appendix, vulva, vagina, cervix, tubal stumps, and lymph glands. It has also occasionally been found in sites such as the pleural and pericardial cavities, the arm, and the thigh.

This displaced endometrial tissue is not a tumor per se but does represent a type of abnormal cellular proliferation. If the endometrial tissue is functional, it undergoes maturation and sloughing in the same manner as uterine tissue. Endometriosis with ovarian involvement is most commonly seen and is usually the functioning type, capable of response to hormonal stimulation. Cysts form within the endometrial tissue and fill with blood. These cysts may undergo atrophy and become fibrotic, or they may rupture, releasing blood into the peritoneal cavity. This blood plus the blood from the functioning tissue causes an inflammatory reaction in the peritoneal cavity. As a result of this inflammation, scar tissue forms, and adhesions develop. These adhesions cause obstruction of the tubes, which will prevent ovulation and implantation. Rupture of the endometrial cyst, which causes major abdominal bleeding, constitutes an emergency situation.

There are several theories as to the pathogenesis of endometriosis. Many persons believe there is more than one possible mode of origin for this disorder and that no one theory explains all cases. The "classic" theory is labeled the *retrograde menstruation theory,* in which viable endometrial tissue is believed to be deposited in the peritoneum due to transtubal regurgitation of menstrual blood. These endometrial particles are then believed to implant and grow on the surfaces where they were deposited. Another theory is based on the fact that the endometrium and peritoneum are derived from the same embryologic tissues. This theory, the *coelomic metaplasia doctrine,* asserts that the peritoneal mesothelium undergoes metaplasia and that the aberrant tissue develops as a result of abnormal cellular differentiation. The *hematogenous spread* of endometrial tissue is a viable theory for explaining the rare cases that sometimes develop in sites distant from the uterus. Endometrial tissue has been found in the pelvic lymph glands during menstruation, leading to a theory that implicates the lymph glands in the spread of endometrial tissue.

Endometriosis is characterized clinically by pain, abnormal bleeding, and infertility. The severity of the signs and symptoms is not related to the extent of the pathology. Approximately 25% of the women so affected exhibit no signs and symptoms. Infertility is commonly seen and is a result of the obstruction of the fallopian tubes by adhesions. Ovarian involvement and dysfunction cause *metrorrhagia,* or irregular intermenstrual bleeding. Excessive bleeding may occur during the menstrual period. Dysmenorrhea is frequently associated with endometriosis. With ureterosacral involvement the dysmenorrhea is sometimes referred to the lower sacral and coccygeal regions. The dysmenorrhea and dyspareunia are thought to be related to increased tension in the tissues due to premenstrual and menstrual swelling and thickening of the endometrium. Dyspareunia and constipation or pain on defecation are also more commonly seen with ureterosacral involvement.

Abdominal pain may be the result of an endometrial cyst leaking blood. This pain can be quite severe; it can mimic the pain of pelvic inflammatory disease or of a ruptured ectopic pregnancy or appendix. The signs of "acute abdomen" will be present (see Chapter 13).

The above signs and symptoms may also be seen in various benign and malignant neoplastic conditions of the female reproductive system. On rare occasions, endometriosis can mimic a large bowel cancer with rectal bleeding and palpable masses. The relationship of the rectal bleeding to menstrual flow should be explored to determine the nature of the pathology.

Treatment of endometriosis varies, depending on the severity of the symptoms. Pregnancy can cause atrophy of the lesions. Hormonal therapy may be used for relief of symptoms. Surgical treatment may involve simple cauterization or excision of the aberrant tissue, removal of the ovaries (since ovarian function stimulates its proliferation), or hysterectomy. Obviously the last two measures are extreme and are usually avoided for as long as possible in young women who still desire children.

MECHANISMS OF REPRODUCTIVE DYSFUNCTION

Reproductive dysfunction can cause a lack of maternal adaptation to pregnancy, disruption of normal fetal growth and maturation, difficult parturition, and inability of the neonate to adapt to extrauterine life. Many pathologic processes may develop during the reproductive period that will evoke these conditions. Those processes most commonly encountered in the clinical situation and the role of pre-existing maternal disease states in evoking these conditions are discussed in this chapter.

Lack of maternal adaptation to pregnancy

Normally during pregnancy the mother's body adapts to the growing fetus in order to meet its needs as well as her own. This adaptation involves complex physiologic changes in nearly every system of her body. Occasionally a pathophysiologic process develops that prevents complete adaptation of the mother to the new physiologic state of pregnancy. The course of the pregnancy or the life of the mother may be seriously jeopardized, or the symptoms may evoke only minor discomfort. Pathophysiologic conditions that impair maternal adaptation to pregnancy include hyperemesis gravidarum, toxemia, and polyhydramnios.

Hyperemesis gravidarum is characterized by excessive nausea or vomiting that may cause severe fluid and electrolyte abnormalities in the pregnant woman. A moderate degree of nausea and vomiting is often experienced by otherwise normal women during the first trimester of pregnancy. The etiology of the nausea and vomiting of pregnancy is unclear but may be related to the presence of chorionic gonadotropin, since the incidence of nausea and vomiting is higher (1) during the periods of pregnancy when the secretion of this hormone normally peaks and (2) in cases of hydatidiform mole in which levels of this hormone remain high.

Preeclampsia is a condition in which hypertension (diastolic pressure of at least 90 mm Hg or systolic pressure of 140 mm Hg), induced by pregnancy, appears after the twentieth week of gestation. This hypertension may be associated with proteinuria or edema or both. Edema of the face or arms or an acute weight gain, exceeding 1 kg (2 lb.) per week, immediately suggests preeclampsia. *Eclampsia* refers to the occurrence of convulsions in a preeclamptic woman in whom no neurologic disease coexists. Hypertension is one of the factors responsible for a significant number of maternal and perinatal deaths. Preeclampsia and eclampsia occur most often in a first pregnancy. They may occur in subsequent pregnancies but usually only if a predisposing factor such as chronic vascular disease or diabetes mellitus is present. Multiple fetuses, diabetes mellitus, placental disorders, and dietary deficiencies are predisposing factors to the development of preeclampsia and also eclampsia. Other signs and symptoms depend on the severity. There may be headache and visual disturbances ranging from blurring of vision to blindness in severe cases. Epigastric pain and vomiting may occur.

Vasospasm due to increased vascular reactivity appears to be the basic pathophysiologic event in eclampsia. A pressor response that can be induced in the pregnant woman by assumption of the supine position after lying in the lateral recumbent position has been demonstrated and can be used to identify women in whom pregnancy-induced hypertension is most likely to develop. The etiology of this increased vascular reactivity is not known. Vascular spasm and cerebral edema are responsible for the cerebral and visual problems that occur.

Theories of uterine ischemia, hypovolemic compensation, and protein-poor diets have been proposed to explain the pathogenesis of eclampsia. The uterine ischemia theory proposes that the uteroplacental circulation is impaired secondary to uterine distension and that the hypoxia causes release of metabolic substances, which stimulate Na^+ and water retention. A more recent theory is that of vasospasm occurring as a compensatory measure in response to the normal salt loss of pregnancy, which causes hypovolemia and activates Na^+-retaining mechanisms.

Glomerular function is also adversely affected: glomerular filtration rate (GFR) is reduced, and degenerative changes in the glomerulus (Fig. 15-6) allow the loss of protein (albumin) in the urine. Na^+ and water retention occurs due to many factors: the decreased GFR and increased secretion of ADH, aldosterone, and corticosteroids.

The objectives of treatment of eclampsia include prevention of convulsions, safe delivery of a healthy child, and prevention of residual

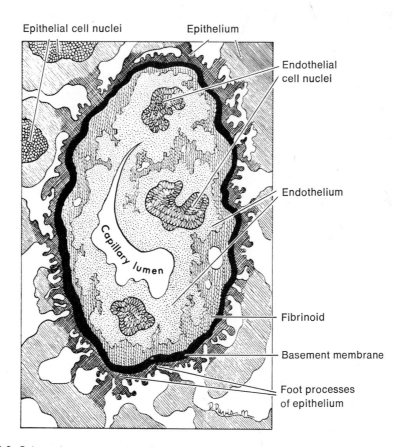

Fig. 15-6. Schematic representation of electron micrograph showing renal glomerular capillary in woman with preeclampsia. Note swelling of endothelial cells and greatly narrowed lumen but normal basement membrane. (From Sandberg, E.: Synopsis of obstetrics, ed. 10, St. Louis, 1978, The C. V. Mosby Co.)

hypertension. Treatment involves bed rest, a high-protein diet, and magnesium sulfate to prevent and control convulsions. Presently there are questions regarding the value of Na⁺ restriction and the use of diuretic medications in the treatment regimen. According to the pathogenic theory that implicates Na⁺ loss, sodium should not be restricted but rather increased.

Hydramnios, or *polyhydramnios,* refers to an excessive quantity of amniotic fluid. Hydramnios presents a serious threat to the viability of the fetus, as the incidence of prematurity in cases of hydramnios is twice the overall rate. Fetal malformation accompanies 20% of all cases of hydramnios. Hydramnios is present in nearly all cases of esophageal atresia and in approximately one half the cases of anencephalus.

The effects of hydramnios on the mother range from discomfort and difficult breathing due to the extreme size of the abdomen to such serious complications as abruptio placentae, postpartum hemorrhage, and uterine dysfunction. Compression of the major veins by the grossly expanded uterus can cause edema of the lower extremities and vulva. The mother usually tolerates hydramnios better if it develops slowly. Rapidly developing hydramnios can cause severe pain and intense dyspnea.

Tenseness of the uterine wall can make palpation of the fetus difficult if not impossible. Difficulty in eliciting fetal heart tones due to the excess fluid and obvious uterine enlargement are other characteristic signs. When hydramnios is diagnosed, further examinations by roentgenograms and ultrasound should be made to determine the presence of multiple fetuses or fetal abnormalities.

The mechanisms that cause this condition may be associated with the fetus's ability to swallow and inspire amniotic fluid and to urinate. Observations regarding the occurrence of abnormal amounts of amniotic fluid with certain types of fetal malformations tend to support this idea. Fetal malformations in which the ability to swallow is impaired are almost always accompanied by hydramnios, while fetal malformations that cause anuria are almost always accompanied by *oligohydramnios,* in which the amount of amniotic fluid is decreased.

Disruption of normal fetal growth and maturation

The duration of pregnancy is normally 40 weeks from the first day of the last menstrual period, which allows enough time for full development of all the fetal tissues and organs. A shorter than normal gestational period causes incomplete structural and functional development of fetal organs and tissues. A longer than normal gestational period may also result in problems for the fetus.

A low birth weight in an infant may be the result of a normal rate of fetal growth for an abnormally short gestation period, an impaired rate of fetal growth in a normal gestational period, or both a shortened gestational period and an impaired rate of growth. A low birth weight is generally considered to be below 2,500 g. Birth is considered premature when the gestational period is less than 38 weeks from the first day of the last menstrual period. Birth is considered postmature when the gestational period is 42 weeks or more. The actual birth weight must be considered in light of the norms that have been obtained for the various gestational ages to determine if fetal growth retardation has occurred. Infants are usually classified as small for gestational age when their actual birth weight falls below the tenth percentile of the norms for that gestational age.

A variety of mechanisms may be responsible for fetal growth retardation. The influence of maternal factors on fetal growth and development is discussed in Chapter 2. Other factors that influence fetal growth are classified as either fetal or placental in origin. Included among the fetal factors are the presence of multiple fetuses, chromosome disorders, and chronic infection. A placental villitis of unknown etiology has been found in the placentas of fetuses in whom growth retardation was marked. Other placental factors include a small placenta or one in which the blood supply is interrupted.

A problem with fetal growth should be suspected if during the latter half of pregnancy the mother fails to gain weight or the uterus is smaller than expected for the gestational age of the fetus. Death of the growth-retarded infant is most likely to occur during the last 2 or 3 weeks of pregnancy. The growth-retarded infant may tolerate labor and delivery very poorly, and preterm delivery is often indicated. In the absence of intrinsic disease the prognosis for these infants is generally good with rapid and steady weight gain following delivery.

Prematurity is characterized by lack of development of the organ systems. This lack of development accounts for many of the problems seen in the premature neonate. The development of idiopathic respiratory distress syndrome is thought to be related to the lack of alveolar surfactant in the immature lungs. Surfactant lowers surface tension in the alveoli, which stabilizes the expanded state and prevents collapse of the alveoli on expiration. Without surfactant the alveoli tend to collapse and respiratory distress develops. The premature infant cannot maintain body heat due to the undeveloped neural thermal regulatory centers, and normal temperature maintenance becomes a problem. The premature infant is more prone to the development of kernicterus due to a greater than normal amount of bilirubin in the blood.

The effects of postmaturity on the infant are quite variable. Growth may continue, or it may stop, and the infant may actually have a reduced birth weight at the time of delivery. The increased incidence of stillbirths as pregnancy advances beyond term is now generally recognized.

The physical changes that typically appear in the postmature infant are thought to be related to placental insufficiency. The mildest changes include an abundance of scalp hair, long nails, reduced vernix, and loose skin with desquamated epithelium. Meconium staining of the fluid, skin, and vernix may indicate more severe fetal distress, and mortality during labor and delivery is likely to be higher in these infants than in those in whom only mild changes have occurred. Hypoglycemia is common in the postmature infant and must be treated. In the infant who has continued to grow, delivery may be difficult due to the large body size, and this infant will be more prone to sustain a birth injury; cesarean section should be considered.

Abnormal parturition

The main characteristic of normal labor is its steady progress.

Dystocia is abnormal or difficult labor characterized by lack of progress. Labor can become extremely difficult if any of the following conditions exist either singly or in combination:

1. Weak or uncoordinated uterine forces
2. Faulty presentation due to fetal position or abnormal development
3. Obstruction of the birth canal

Other factors that can adversely affect the course of labor include excessive analgesic or anesthetic administered to the mother especially during the latent phase, primigravidity, and premature rupture of the membranes while the cervix is closed and uneffaced. Psychologic factors such as excessive fear and anxiety can also prolong labor. These factors can act alone or in concert.

Most prolonged labor represents extension of the first stage, and any extension of either the first or second stage of labor results in an increased risk of perinatal death. Other potential dangers to the fetus as a result of prolonged labor include asphyxia and hypoxia due to the long labor itself and an increased incidence of traumatic birth injuries such as cerebral damage due to pressure on the head of the neonate and injury from the use of instruments in difficult rotation and extraction maneuvers. Premature rupture of the membranes also increases the infant's chances of an infection.

Another complication the infant may suffer is that of meconium aspiration. Aspiration of normal amniotic fluid is most likely a physiologic event. Fetal distress, a likely event in prolonged labor, may cause a defecation reaction and the subsequent contamination of amniotic fluid with meconium. The contaminated fluid may be quite thick, and aspiration of this fluid may create a mechanical obstruction of the airway, as well as a chemical pneumonitis that may develop in the lung tissue. The resulting respiratory distress may be quite severe. To minimize the extent of the damage due to aspiration, the neonate's mouth and nares should be suctioned prior to the delivery of the shoulders. Suctioning of the entire airway and endotracheal intubation to allow suctioning of the trachea and bronchia should be carried out as soon as possible after birth.

Prolonged labor represents a danger to the

mother as well. The incidence of traumatic injury to the birth canal, lacerations, hemorrhage, infection, and shock is sharply increased in the mother who experiences prolonged labor. Maternal exhaustion, which depletes energy stores and lengthens convalescence, is also a complication of prolonged labor.

Lack of neonatal adaptation to extrauterine life

Neonatal adaptation from intrauterine life to extrauterine life requires many complex physiologic adjustments: respiration must begin and be maintained, pulmonary circulation must increase, and the cardiovascular system must begin to meet the oxygen and nutritional needs of the neonate's tissues. When placental blood flow ceases, the foramen ovale and ductus arteriosus must close to ensure efficient cardiovascular function. Pathophysiologic mechanisms that prevent this adaptation include a failure to breathe at birth, immaturity of the respiratory system, which prevents normal respiratory activity from being maintained, and failure of the cardiovascular transport system. A syndrome that may indicate an infant's inability to adapt to extrauterine life is the sudden infant death syndrome (SIDS). This occurs between the ages of 3 weeks and 7 months rather than in the immediate postnatal period.

Respiratory distress. Pulmonary problems are the most frequent cause of neonatal death. Respiratory distress may be caused by factors external or internal to the neonate. Maternal sedation and anesthesia are external factors that may seriously depress the neonate's respiratory center. Prolonged hypoxia during a long and difficult labor may also make the neonate less responsive to normal respiratory stimuli. The factors with which this discussion is primarily concerned are those internal to the neonate. These factors include congenital defects and immaturity of the central nervous system regulatory centers and of the respiratory system.

The clinical manifestations of respiratory distress in the infant include intercostal retractions with inspiration, flaring of the nares, a "grunting" type of respiration, and an increase in apical pulse rate. As respiratory distress increases there will be a progressive increase in the number of apneic episodes. The baby's color will be extremely cyanotic.

Premature infants, infants of diabetic mothers, second born of twins, and perhaps infants delivered by cesarean section without prior labor appear to be most susceptible to the development of idiopathic respiratory distress syndrome (IRDS), or hyaline membrane disease. It is believed that a central factor in making the transition from intrauterine maternal dependence for oxygen to the initiation of stable respiratory function is an intact and fully developed surfactant system. A deficiency of surfactant predisposes to alveolar collapse, and the infant with surfactant deficiency must generate maximal ventilatory pressure to reexpand the lungs and maintain respiratory function.

IRDS is characterized by atelectasis, which results in hypoxemia and acidosis. Pathologic changes found in the lungs of infants with IRDS include degeneration of epithelial and endothelial cells of the alveolocapillary membrane and development of hyaline membranes, which line the alveolar sacs. Increasing end expiratory pressure by external ventilation is the recommended form of treatment to promote reexpansion of collapsed alveoli and to prevent the collapse of others.

Hyperbilirubinemia. Hyperbilirubinemia, or an increased amount of unconjugated bilirubin in the blood, may also complicate the neonatal period. Prior to birth, unconjugated bilirubin freely transfers across the placenta to the maternal circulation. Normally the liver conjugates bilirubin with glucuronic acid, which is synthesized from uridine diphosphoglucuronic acid in a reaction catalyzed by the enzyme glucuronyl transferase. Some studies have demonstrated a deficiency in both the enzyme and uridine diphosphoglucuronic acid in fetal livers of some mammals. Other substances are also conjugated with glucuronic acid and may compete with bilirubin for conjugation, leading to increased amounts of bilirubin in the blood.

Hyperbilirubinemia may be the result of increased destruction of red blood cells due to a hemolytic disorder or of increased bleeding due to difficult deliveries associated with oxytocin administration. The most common form of hyperbilirubinemia is *physiologic jaundice.* In fully mature, normal infants, jaundice increases for 3 to 4 days after birth due to the following factors: an increased rate of red cell destruction, which is normal, a reduction in hepatic uptake of free bilirubin, a decreased rate of conjugation, and decreased bacteria-mediated conversion of bilirubin to urobilinogen in the intestine, which allows more excreted bilirubin to be absorbed from the gut.

Unconjugated bilirubin can cause pathologic changes and degeneration of the basal ganglia in the brain, a condition referred to as *kernicterus.* The basal ganglia acquire a yellowish discoloration. Infants who survive demonstrate spasticity and incoordination.

There is a greater incidence of kernicterus among premature infants. Physiologic jaundice is usually more severe and prolonged in the premature infant, which partially accounts for the greater incidence of kernicterus. The premature infant is also more susceptible to disorders (other than hyperbilirubinemia) that may further contribute to hyperbilirubinemia and thus to the development of kernicterus. Hypoxia and acidosis reduce the protein-bound bilirubin, while hypothermia and hypoglycemia increase elements that compete with bilirubin for binding sites. Both these mechanisms increase bilirubin toxicity and are more likely to be present in the premature infant.

Phototherapy, or exposure to light, is used in the treatment of hyperbilirubinemia. Light increases peripheral blood flow, promotes excretion of bilirubin by the liver, and reduces absorption from the intestine due to shortened intestinal transit time. The exact mechanisms by which these effects occur are not completely clear.

Sudden infant death syndrome. The sudden infant death syndrome (SIDS) is presently the subject of much research regarding its etiology, pathogenesis, and the mechanisms by which it causes death. Based on intensive research conducted since 1972, it is now believed that SIDS babies have anatomic and physiologic defects not apparent at birth and that no one single mechanism is responsible for death as was previously believed. Current research is focusing on seven major areas regarding SIDS:

1. The anatomic pathology of SIDS
2. Developmental neurophysiology with emphasis on abnormal sleep patterns associated with disrupted autonomic activity
3. Cardiorespiratory and vagal responses to stimuli
4. Immunologic incompetence
5. Metabolic and endocrine factors
6. Epidemiology and genetics
7. Behavior and psychologic processes in those persons associated with a sudden, unexplained infant death

SIDS, called also *crib death* or *cot death,* has been acknowledged since biblical times; however, it is only relatively recently that it has been recognized as a specific disease entity. It is the leading cause of death in infants after 1 week of life. The characteristic picture is that of a healthy child, put to bed, who when checked on is found to be dead with no apparent signs of a struggle. The infant may have had a slight upper respiratory tract infection, but this is not always the case. Autopsy reveals no lesion of enough significance to have caused death. At this time there is no way of identifying those infants most susceptible. No genetic or hereditary patterns have been demonstrated, nor is there any known way of preventing SIDS.

SUMMARY

This chapter presented an overview of the normal reproductive process and the manifestations of disruption of that process. The mechanisms of reproductive dysfunction that were discussed in this chapter included lack of maternal adaptation to pregnancy, disruption of normal fetal growth and development, difficult parturition and its effect on the mother and neonate, and inability of the neonate to adapt to extrauterine life.

SUGGESTED READINGS

Altshuler, G., Russell P., and Ermocilla, R.: The placental pathology of small gestational infants, Am. J. Obstet. Gynecol. **121**:351, 1975.

Butts, P.: Magnesium sulfate in the treatment of toxemia, Am. J. Nurs. **77**(8):1294-1298, 1977.

Driscoll, J., and Mellins, R.: Idiopathic respiratory distress syndrome of infancy (hyaline membrane disease), Basics R. D. vol. 1, no. 5, June 1973.

Dwyer, J.: Human reproduction: the female system and the neonate, Philadelphia, 1976, F. A. Davis Co.

Farrell, P. M., and Avery, M. E.: Hyaline membrane disease, Am. Rev. Respir. Dis. **111:**657, 1975.

Givens, J., editor: Gynecologic endocrinology (based on proceedings of First Annual Symposium on Reproductive Medicine held at University of Tennessee, Memphis), Chicago, 1977, Year Book Medical Publishers.

Jewett, J. F.: Committee on maternal welfare, N. Engl. J. Med. **297**(18):1009-1011, 1977.

Novak, E., et al.: Novak's textbook of gynecology, ed. 9, Baltimore, 1975, The Williams & Wilkins Co.

Pitkin, R., and Scott, J., editors: The year book of obstetrics and gynecology, Chicago, 1978, Year Book Medical Publishers.

Pritchard, J., and MacDonald, P.: William's obstetrics, ed. 15, New York, 1976, Appleton-Century-Crofts.

Sell, E., and Harris, T. R.: The influence of ruptured membranes on fetal outcome, Pediatr. Res. **10:**432, 1976.

Tejani, N., Mann, L. I., and Weiss, R. R.: Antenatal diagnosis and management of the small-for-gestational-age fetus, Obstet. Gynecol. **47:**31, 1976.

U.S. Dept. of Health, Education and Welfare: The Sudden Infant Death Program of the National Institute of Child Health and Human Development, (NIH) 78-1436, Public Health Service, National Institutes of Health, 1978.

PART SEVEN

Pathophysiology of the body's structural and motor integrity

CHAPTER 16

Neuromuscular system: mechanisms and disorders

Kenneth J. Kant, Ph.D.

AT THE COMPLETION OF THIS CHAPTER THE STUDENT WILL BE ABLE TO:

- Differentiate between lower and upper motor neuron diseases.
- Predict sensorimotor deficits based on localized spinal cord trauma.
- Describe sensorimotor deficits resulting from a cerebrovascular accident.
- Describe the mechanisms of synaptic transmission difficulties and the resulting clinical manifestations.
- Describe the mechanisms and clinical manifestations of demyelination.
- Describe the visual system and pathologic conditions related to its function.
- Describe the auditory system and pathologic conditions related to its function.

Any change in central nervous function normally produces a complex alteration in a person's existence. A person may experience not only sensory or motor loss, depending on severity and duration of the malfunction, but also perceptual problems and behavioral changes resulting from the losses. In today's society a person who has experienced a heart attack, for instance, can modify his behavior appropriately and pursue a fairly normal existence. However, a person afflicted with a neuromuscular problem that does not permit normal-appearing behavior has the added psychologic stress of how to cope with his handicap.

NORMAL ANATOMY AND PHYSIOLOGY

Only a minimal review is supplied here. The student is referred to standard texts in anatomy and physiology for any necessary details.

Spinal cord

The spinal cord is contained by the vertebrae. It is encased in the three meninges: dura mater, arachnoid, and pia mater. The cord extends from the first cervical vertebra to the first or second lumbar vertebra (Fig. 16-1). The vertebral canal from L_3 caudally contains the spinal nerves that course down from the cord on their way to their appropriate exit points, for example, at the sacral level. These lower spinal nerves form the cauda equina. Spinal taps are done in this lower area below the termination of the cord because of the decreased risk of damaging nervous tissue there.

Each spinal nerve is composed of both sensory and motor axons, the sensory axons entering the cord through the posterior roots and the motor axons exiting the cord through the anterior roots on their way to skeletal muscles (Fig. 16-2). The cell bodies of the motor neu-

421

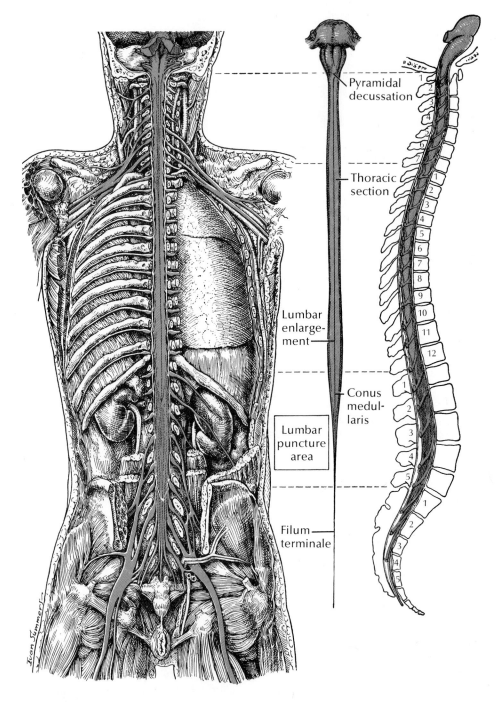

Fig. 16-1. Relation of spinal cord, part of brain, and some of spinal nerves to surrounding structures. (From Mettler, F. A.: Neuroanatomy, ed. 2, St. Louis, 1948, The C. V. Mosby Co.)

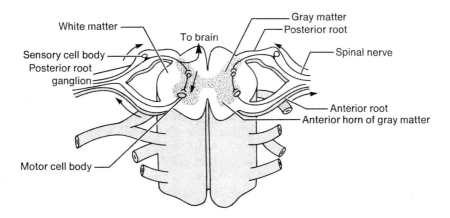

Fig. 16-2. Section of spinal cord (anterior view).

rons are in the anterior horn of the gray matter of the cord. The cell bodies of the sensory neurons are located in the posterior root ganglia lying adjacent to the cord. Connections between the sensory and motor neurons in the spinal cord are made by interneurons in the gray matter.

Sensory information is sent up to the brain through myelinated axons. If the ascending axon is part of the sensory (primary) neuron, it stays on the same side of the cord as its entry side until it gets to the medulla. Then it synapses with a second neuron, which crosses to the other side and ascends to the thalamus. From there, a third neuron carries the information to the sensory cortex. An example of such a pathway is the one for fine touch. For other sensory systems, such as pain and temperature, the first neuron synapses with the second neuron within a few segments in the gray matter of the cord. The second neuron crosses to the other side of the cord, enters the white matter, and ascends directly to the thalamus. There, as with the first example, the third neuron goes to the sensory cortex. Thus, some of the white matter of the spinal cord is used for specific sensory pathways to the brain. The remaining white matter is used for descending motor pathways. Each part of the brain affecting the motor neurons in the cord has its specific tract, for example, corticospinal and rubrospinal tracts.

Each spinal nerve serves one part of the body only, both for sensory information and motor control (Fig. 16-3). An awareness of these *der-matomes* can aid those caring for a patient with trauma to the cord. The areas of the body without sensation or voluntary muscle activity can be predicted if the damaged area is known, or vice versa, the traumatized area can be predicted according to the areas of the body showing a loss of sensation and voluntary control.

The *autonomic nervous system* employs the spinal cord and spinal nerves as well as a few cranial nerves in its role of modulating the involuntary motor activity of the body, for example, heart rate, intestinal motility, and sweating. The *sympathetic system* has its normally short preganglionic neurons exiting the cord from T_1 to L_3. These end in the sympathetic chain ganglia next to the cord or another sympathetic ganglion deeper in the body. From there, the normally long postganglionic neurons go to the organ being modulated. The *parasympathetic system* sends its normally long preganglionic neurons from the brain stem, that is, medulla, or the sacral region of the cord directly to the organ served. Within the organ are the normally quite short postganglionic neurons that are the effective modulators. Most organs are served by both systems (dual innervation), arterioles and sweat glands being two major exceptions. The sympathetic system is generally an activator, increasing heart rate, blood flow to skeletal muscle, bronchiolar diameter, and pupillary diameter while decreasing blood flow to skin and intestines and GI motility. The parasympathetic system is more concerned with regenerative functions. For instance, it facilitates

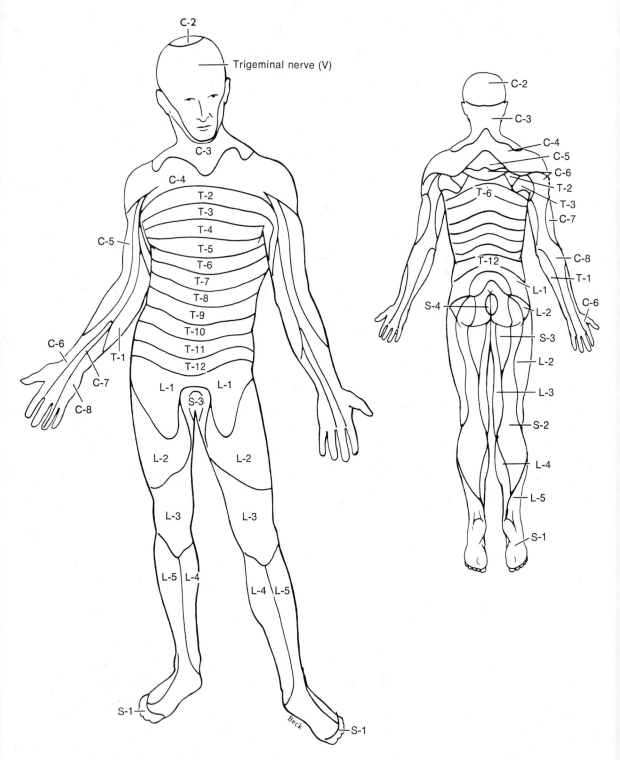

Fig. 16-3. Segmental innervation. (From Anthony, C. P., and Thibodeau, G. A.: Textbook of anatomy and physiology, ed. 9, St. Louis, 1975, The C. V. Mosby Co.)

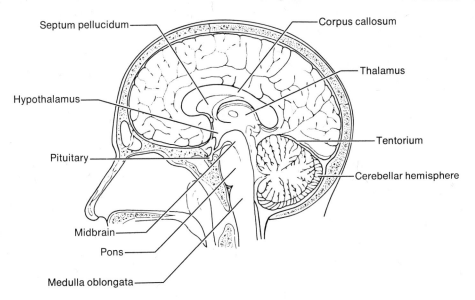

Septum pellucidum

Corpus callosum

Thalamus

Hypothalamus

Pituitary

Tentorium

Cerebellar hemisphere

Midbrain

Pons

Medulla oblongata

Fig. 16-4. Median sagittal section of brain and part of head.

GI motility, slows heart rate, and increases salivation.

Brain

The brain is contained by the cranium and, like the spinal cord, is surrounded by the meninges.

There are many ways in which to classify the various structures of the brain, but in essence it has two major divisions: the brain stem and the structures that grow out of the brain stem. The brain stem is a continuation of the spinal cord in the cephalad direction (Fig. 16-4). It starts at the point where the cord enters the cranial cavity. The characteristic cross-sectional appearance of the cord is lost as the brain stem begins, each division of the brain stem having its special grouping of neuronal cell bodies (gray matter or nuclei) and areas of myelinated axons (white matter or tracts). The first structure above the cord is the *medulla oblongata*. Above the medulla is the *pons.* The medulla and pons together are termed *hindbrain.* The pons and medulla, especially the latter, contain nuclei that have control of several vegetative functions. Cells that control inspiration and expiration are in these structures. Cells that modulate heart rate, arteriolar diameter, and the coughing and vomiting reflexes are in the medulla.

The next major portion of the brain stem is the *midbrain*. Various visual reflexes, such as eye blink and pupil diameter, are controlled in this area, as well as some "alerting" responses that occur to auditory stimulation.

The major forward structures of the brain stem are the *thalamus* and ventral to the thalamus, the *hypothalamus*. These form the diencephalic portion of the *forebrain*. The thalamus, as previously mentioned, is a relay (synaptic) point for the various sensory pathways going to the sensory cortex. It also has other functions. The hypothalamus can be divided structurally into several subunits, based on the nuclei within it. Although it is a relatively small structure, the hypothalamus has a large role in many body functions. There are cells that control temperature regulation by their influence on the medulla (heart rate, arteriolar diameter, and respiration). Other cells, in conjunction with cells in the cortex, activate or inhibit feeding and sexual behavior. Still other cells influence the activity of the pituitary and therefore several endocrine glands. Damage to the hypothalamus can have a vast effect on a person's vegetative, endocrine, and emotional behavior.

The telencephalic portion of the forebrain includes the many structures that develop from the brain stem (Fig. 16-5). These include the

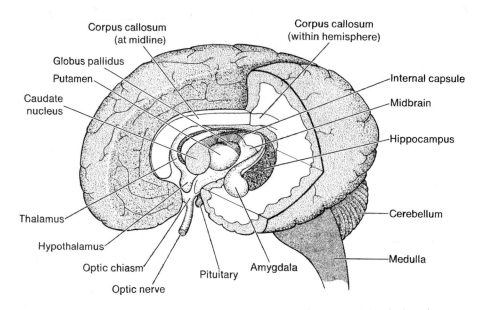

Fig. 16-5. Major subcortical structures; left hemisphere dissected, right hemisphere intact.

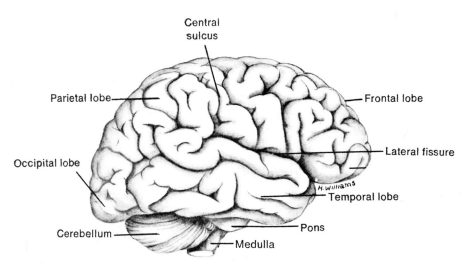

Fig. 16-6. Brain, lateral view. (Adapted from Francis, C. C., and Martin, A. H.: Introduction to human anatomy, ed. 7, St. Louis, 1975, The C. V. Mosby Co.)

basal ganglia (caudate nucleus, putamen, and globus pallidus), *limbic* structures (amygdala, hippocampus, septum, etc.), and the *neocortex*. The *cerebellum* also grows out of the brain stem; it is located posterior to the pons and is essentially part of the hindbrain.

Each cerebral hemisphere contains the outer neocortex (gray matter), the underlying, subcortical structures mentioned above, and connecting pathways between them. The cerebellum, of course, is a separate entity. The cerebral hemispheres are joined to each other largely through the *corpus callosum*, a thick band of white matter. Virtually any selected point on the neocortex of one cerebral hemisphere is joined to the corresponding point on the other side by the myelinated axons running through the corpus callosum. Another large band of white matter in each hemisphere is the *internal capsule*. Axons in this tract run from the thalamus to the cortex and from the cortex to several subcortical structures.

Each hemisphere is divided anatomically into four major lobes: frontal, parietal, occipital, and temporal (Fig. 16-6). Some portions of cortex in these lobes have specific functions, while the role of other sections is yet unknown. The sensory cortex, or more correctly the somatosensory cortex, is located in the anterior region of the parietal lobe, just behind the central sulcus. The visual cortex is in the occipital lobe at the posterior pole of the cerebrum. The auditory cortex is situated in the temporal lobe, on the superior surface of the lobe and virtually covered by the nearby parietal lobe. Sensory cortex gives us the ability to localize, identify, and discriminate the intensity of a stimulus. All sensory information except vision, hearing, and smell goes to the somatosensory cortex. Visual and auditory activity are directed to the appropriate cortex. Smell has no known sensory neocortex. Neural activity produced by odors is transferred to the amygdala, a limbic structure in the temporal lobe. From there, no known pathways have been found that carry smell information. Since we can localize, identify, and discriminate odors, some part of our neocortex must be used, but where it is has yet to be discovered.

Motor cortex is located in the frontal lobe, just in front of the central sulcus. This is the part of the brain that presumably is involved in the initiation of movement by the contraction of skeletal muscles. Two systems are mutually responsible for voluntary muscle movements: one quite simple, and the other considerably more complex. The simple one is the *pyramidal motor system*. The primary neurons have their cell bodies in the motor cortex, and their myelinated axons run through the internal capsule, through the brain stem and white matter of the spinal cord, finally ending in the anterior horns of the spinal cord on interneurons, which in turn synapse with the alpha motor neurons that go out to the muscles. All of the primary neurons cross to the side opposite their side of origin; 80% do so in the medulla, and the rest do so in the spinal cord before they reach their respective final segment. The axons of the primary neurons are obviously quite long. The role ascribed to the pyramidal motor system is initiation of finely controlled movements.

The more complex motor system is called the *extrapyramidal motor system*. The primary neurons are located in the motor cortex, mixed in with those of the pyramidal motor system. Their axons leave the cortex with most going to the basal ganglia, probably the caudate nucleus first. Some pass through to the midbrain. There are connections between the three structures of the basal ganglia, and these connections permit a great deal of integration and modification of the original neural activity. The basal ganglia also connect with a part of the thalamus so it has a role in modifying their output. From the basal ganglia, axons go to other nuclei in the midbrain and hindbrain. Finally the cells in these lower regions send their axons down the white matter of the spinal cord to end on interneurons in the anterior horns of the gray matter. These interneurons in turn synapse with the alpha motor neurons. The extrapyramidal motor system sends its influence down both sides of the cord about equally. The role of the extrapyramidal motor system is initiation of gross, postural movements. In reality, there is a large overlap in function between the two motor systems.

The cerebellum is intricately involved with motor function. Its role is one of modification; that is, it does not initiate movement but rather alters movements that are occurring. The cerebellum receives sensory information from the various sensory systems and also motor information from the two motor systems. Thus, in a sense, the cerebellum is told what is *supposed* to happen (motor system activity) and what *is* happening (sensory activity). The cerebellum "compares" the information and then, through its connections to the brain stem portions of the extrapyramidal motor system or directly to the spinal cord, alters the ongoing muscle activity, resulting in appropriate and accurate completion of the desired motor behavior.

The motor cortex and the sensory cortex are arranged in a specific fashion. Certain areas of the cortex represent certain body areas, for example, toe, leg, shoulder, and tongue. These cortical areas are arranged according to the order of the body area being served. The toes are represented at the midline deep in the longitudinal fissure, then the foot, ankle, leg, knee,

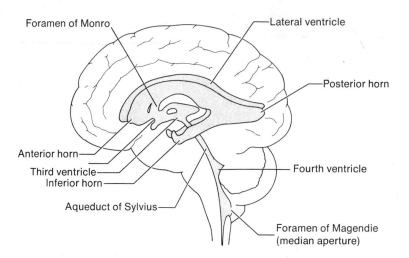

Foramen of Monro
Lateral ventricle
Posterior horn
Anterior horn
Third ventricle
Inferior horn
Aqueduct of Sylvius
Fourth ventricle
Foramen of Magendie
(median aperture)

Fig. 16-7. Ventricular system.

thigh, and so on, coming out of the longitudinal fissure and down the lateral surface of the brain. The lateral-most areas of sensory (or motor) cortex are devoted to the face, including large areas for tongue and lips. The actual size of the body area served is not a factor in the size of the cortical area representing it. What is important is the sensitivity of sensory discrimination of the area served or the degree of motor control. Thus, the tongue with its highly sensitive surface and finely controlled movements has a much larger area of cortex devoted to it than does the trunk, especially relative to their respective sizes. With this difference in mind it is understandable that a lesion in the cortex can have greater or lesser effects, depending on the area involved.

Many functions have been found for the various limbic structures, some functions shared and others apparently unique to one structure. A full discussion of all the limbic structures and each of their functions is not possible here. Basically these subcortical parts of the brain have both affective and vegetative roles, often shared with the hypothalamus. Rage, placidity, fear, and attack reactions are aspects of affective behavior apparently controlled by the septum and amygdala as well as by the neocortex and hypothalamus. The amygdala has some influence on sexual and feeding behavior as well as endocrine activity, most probably by its influencing activity in the hypothalamus. The

hippocampus, also in the temporal lobe, has a role in somehow consolidating short-term memory into long-term memory. Research on animals and humans frequently brings out new descriptions of functions of many of these limbic structures. By no means is the brain and the interrelated roles of its many parts deciphered.

Within the cerebrum are hollow areas called *ventricles* (Fig. 16-7). These ventricles are formed, at least in part, as a result of the telencephalic portion of the forebrain "folding over" as it grows out of the brain stem. The lateral ventricles, one in each cerebral hemisphere, run from the frontal pole to the occipital pole, with a large extension into the temporal lobe. The basal ganglia, amygdala, and hippocampus, as well as the overlying neocortex, are lateral to the lateral ventricles. The thalamus and septum are medial to them. At the midline, splitting most of the hypothalamus and thalamus, is the third ventricle. There is a fourth ventricle that forms a hollow area between the pons and cerebellum. The two lateral ventricles are connected to the third ventricle near its anterior end by short, relatively narrow channels (foramen of Monro). The third ventricle connects to the fourth by a longer, narrow tube (aqueduct of Sylvius). The fourth ventricle then connects to the subarachnoid space, between the arachnoid and pia mater through the foramen of Magendie. In this way the ventricles are connected to the "outside" of the brain and spinal cord.

Within each of the ventricles is a specialized structure called the *choroid plexus*. This choroid plexus is formed from pia mater that has "invaded" the ventricles from the outside and brain capillaries. It is the choroid plexuses that produce *cerebrospinal fluid* (CSF). This fluid, formed in the ventricles, normally flows out through the ventricles and their connections to the subarachnoid space. Here, through specialized projections of the arachnoid layer (villi), the cerebrospinal fluid is absorbed into venous blood. Approximately 750 ml of CSF is produced each day. The average volume of CSF in an adult is approximately 140 ml.

One other important brain area must be mentioned. Lying in the central region, or core, of the brain stem is a dense network of short-axoned, nonmyelinated neurons. There is very little recognizable structure, that is, clusters of cell bodies (nuclei) or bands of white matter (tracts). This region is called the *reticular formation*. It apparently receives sensory information through branches of the sensory pathways discussed earlier. It may provide a secondary, although much slower, route for sensory information to the cortex. A more important role for the reticular formation is determination of a person's level of consciousness (state of alertness). There appear to be pacemaker neurons in the lower brain stem that drive the activity of neurons in the nonspecific part of the thalamus (nonsensory, nonextrapyramidal part). These cells, in turn, project to all areas of the neocortex and activate the neocortex, or perhaps better stated, keep the cells of the neocortex in a more excitable state. This determines how reactive the neocortical cells are to other, more specific activation. The synaptic activity surrounding the ongoing effects of this system is reflected in the electroencephalogram (EEG). The more alert a person is, the faster, more irregular, and lower amplitude is the EEG. The less alert a person becomes, the slower, more regular, and larger amplitude is the EEG. The part of the reticular formation that presumably determines our state of alertness is termed the *reticular activating system*. What determines the circadian rhythm of sleep and wakefulness is a major area of research. One clue may be that the ratio of the concentrations of two synaptic transmitters, norepinephrine and serotonin, changes in the reticular formation as the level of sleep and wakefulness changes. Whether this is cause or effect is not certain.

DISORDERS IN TRANSMISSION
Cell damage

Damage along any part of the sensory pathways will lead to sensory loss. How localized (to body area) or discrete (to sense) the loss is depends on the location of the lesion.

Severe burns or other destruction of the skin will lead to loss of all sensation in that area. Sensation normally returns as the axons regenerate, but the presence of scar tissue prevents complete recovery to the pretrauma state. Pain normally is the first sensation to return.

Destruction of a spinal nerve results in a larger area of sensory loss (the dermatome) with all senses involved. In this instance, voluntary skeletal muscles served by the spinal nerve would also lose their function. The likelihood of recovery of function and the time for recovery to occur are determined by the effects of the trauma on the sensory cell bodies in the posterior root ganglia and the motor cell bodies in the anterior horn of the spinal cord. The closer the trauma is to these cell bodies, the less likely recovery will occur, and the longer regeneration of the axons will take if it does take place at all.

Damage to the spinal cord presents a different situation, depending on the extent of the lesion. Spinal cord trauma may result from a transection (complete or incomplete), compression (from a blunt trauma), or hyperextension and hyperflexion (whiplash). Complete transection or compression of the cord through its complete cross section results in total loss of all sensation on both sides of the body below the damaged area. Similarly, complete loss of voluntary muscle control occurs (spinal reflexes will likely be present after spinal shock wears off).

If the damage does not involve the entire cord, that is, it is more localized, then the loss of sensation and motor control may be considerably less. If the lesion were localized to a single tract, then only the sensory system (or motor influence) served by that tract would be lost below the lesion. The side of the body showing the sensory loss would reflect whether the sensory path affected was one of early cross-over in the cord, for example, pain and temperature, or of later crossover in the medulla, for example, fine touch or proprioception. If the lesion were in the pain pathway, then the loss would be contralateral to the lesion site. If the lesion were in the proprioceptive pathway, then the loss would be ipsilateral. Motor loss is always on the same side as the lesion.

The Brown-Séquard syndrome is an example of one-sided loss of function. It results from hemisection of the spinal cord or from a lesion involving one half of the cord. All sensory and motor pathways are destroyed in the area of the lesion on one side, while the other side is left intact (Fig. 16-8). Motor loss occurs only on the involved side. Proprioception and fine touch are lost below the trauma on the involved side. However, pain and temperature sensations are lost from the noninvolved side but are still present on the lesioned side. This difference results from the almost immediate crossover to the other side by the pain and warm and cold pathways. These senses on the lesioned side cross over to the nonlesioned side (below the lesion) and travel up the intact pathway, while those on the nonlesioned side cross below the lesion to the damaged side and cannot traverse the destroyed zone.

More commonly, damage to the spinal cord involves a compression of the posterior columns of white matter on both sides. Such a trauma interrupts the sensory pathways serving proprioception. Neither the cerebrum nor the cerebellum receives any information about limb position (position in space) or passive movements of the affected limbs. Pain, temperature, and fine touch can be sensed because the pathways for these senses travel up the anterior white matter and are not interrupted. Motor pathways are also intact, yet with the lack of proprioceptive information, the limbs remain flaccid. The exact cause of this phenomenon has not been determined. *Tabes dorsalis* is the name frequently applied to this loss, but originally the name referred to a stage in neurosyphilis when the posterior columns of white matter disappeared due to the death of sensory cell bodies in the posterior root ganglia. The motor loss is the same for either cause.

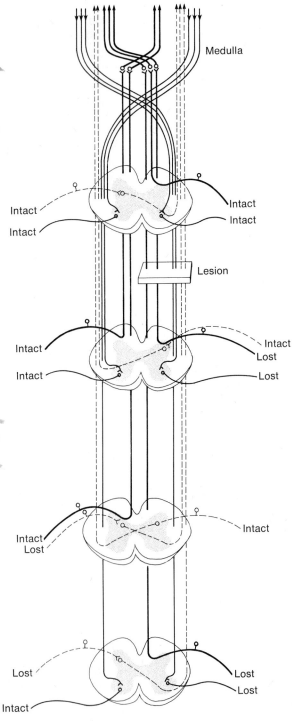

Fig. 16-8. Sensorimotor loss with hemisection.

When a person suffers a transection of the spinal cord he is often classed into one of two categories: paraplegic or quadriplegic. The classification is based on the level of the trauma and the resulting loss in function. The degree of loss is a consequence of the transection itself, whether it is complete or incomplete. Other traumas, such as compression, can have similar effects, and the individuals are classed according to the same criteria.

For a paraplegic the damage can occur anyplace from T_1 to L_2, with the most common site being T_{12}, L_1. This person normally has full use of the arms and shoulders but has lost sensation in and use of the legs. Frequently, back and abdominal muscle control are lost too. Voluntary bladder and bowel control may be lost. These responses can usually be trained reflexly if good nursing care is provided during the spinal shock period. The bladder must not be allowed to overdistend or become infected.

A quadriplegic patient is one with damage between C_4 and C_7. A transection at this high level leaves the person with no voluntary control of arms, trunk, or legs except perhaps for the shoulders. All sensation below the lesion is lost, as expected. Like the paraplegic person the quadriplegic loses voluntary control of the bladder and bowel. As already mentioned, good nursing care is essential to maintain a functional bladder and bowel in order to be able to retrain the functions after spinal shock is gone.

A paraplegic with damage in the area between T_4 and T_6 and a quadriplegic with a higher lesion both lose the normal reflexes that control blood pressure. This is because the sympathetic system with the controlling centers in the medulla exits the cord from T_1 to L_3. With a cut high in the cord the outflow from the medulla cannot get through. A quadriplegic patient, especially, can have orthostatic hypotension as a result. For the same reasons these individuals will have little if any temperature regulation. Another, potentially more serious result of such high damage is *autonomic hyperreflexia*. Any stimulus can cause a spinal reflex below the traumatized area. One rather easily elicited reflex is vasoconstriction. As more arterioles constrict, the arterial blood pressure rises. Even though the pressure receptors in the carotid sinus sense the hypertension and send the information to the medulla, the vasomotor centers there are not able to transmit through the damaged cord to produce a vasodilation, thus reducing the pressure. As the stimulation increases or persists, or the reflex becomes more easily obtained, the hypertension increases. Headache, facial flush, and sweating are all signs of autonomic hyperreflexia. If autonomic hyperreflexia is allowed to persist, the patient is likely to have a cerebrovascular accident (CVA, stroke). The simplest measure is to find the stimulus causing the response and remove it. The stimulus can be a pressure sore, a full bladder, a wrinkled bed sheet, or a nurse with strong hands or sharp nails.

Transection or compression causes a loss of transmission because the pathways are damaged. Another condition producing a similar effect is demyelination, in which the white matter degenerates. The myelin covering the axons produces the means for fast conduction of the action potentials (saltatory conduction). Any loss in myelin covering will slow or stop the action potential transmission. Thus, the white matter tracts affected would become afunctional with a resulting loss in sensory and motor information.

An example of a demyelinating disease is *multiple sclerosis* (MS). Portions of white matter in the cord and brain are affected. The sclerotic plaques are located randomly. The cause of multiple sclerosis is unknown. Research looking for viruses as causative agents has been unsuccessful. An altered immunologic system has been suggested (see Chapter 5), in which T cell immunity is decreased and B cell immunity is increased. Evidence for an antimyelin antibody, if it exists, has not been found. The mechanism that forms the MS plaques is unknown. There is a suggestion that a person's genetic makeup may determine the structures in which the plaques form (but not the development of the disease). The disappearance and reappearance of the symptoms may reflect physiologic and environmental factors that alter the ability of the poorly myelinated axons to conduct action potentials. A person with MS may have relief of symptoms when conditions are right to permit axonal conduction. Later, the symptoms may return when conditions are altered and no longer allow the axons to function.

Destruction in the sensory or motor pathways in the brain stem or neocortex can produce quite varied losses of function. After the sensory pathways merge in the thalamus and especially the neocortex, any loss resulting from damage in these higher areas is presented as a generalized sensory loss in a body area rather than a loss of a particular sensory system.

A lesion in the pyramidal motor system pathway can have extremely varied effects depending on its location. Damage to the neocortex would affect the corresponding body area. A lesion of similar size in the internal capsule would have a much larger body area affected due to the compacting of axons coming from the cortex in the internal capsule. Destruction in either area would show its effect primarily on the opposite side of the body. Lesions in the midbrain or lower brain stem may produce a small or large loss depending on their size, but, especially in the midbrain region, the loss is more likely to be bilateral because of the closeness of the two pyramidal pathways to each other.

Because of the complex nature of the extrapyramidal motor system, lesions in individual structures can have quite different results. In general, however, the motor deficits might be characterized as improper postural adjustments, either at the wrong time or to an improper degree. The effects are frequently bilateral but are not always in the same direction; that is, one side of the body may show a stronger flexor response, while the other side may have a stronger extensor response. The motor dysfunction may be one in which involuntary skeletal muscle movements occur only during voluntary movements or only during the period when no voluntary movements are taking place. Frequently, the different types of motor malfunction can be attributed to pathologic conditions within specific extrapyramidal structures, for example, athetosis and the caudate nucleus, and parkinsonism and the substantia nigra (in the midbrain).

Damage to the cerebellum leads to motor disturbances too. Muscle responses frequently are weaker and both slower to start and slower to stop. Without a properly functioning cerebellum it is much more difficult to rapidly and accurately execute a motor activity. Postural movement difficulties may be present, and even a normal static posture may be difficult to maintain. As with the two motor systems, localized damage to the cerebellum can have quite varied effects, depending on the locus of the lesion.

A cerebrovascular accident is another means by which transmission of information is seriously altered. A lack of oxygen through ischemia or the presence of whole blood through rupture of a vessel is deadly for neurons. Loss of function results from the number and location of neurons permanently destroyed. Those cells that are temporarily nonfunctional will with time return to normal activity so a patient may likely have recovery of some functions, at least in part, with time and training.

The location of the damage depends on the blood vessel involved. Blood to the brain is furnished by two arteries on each side, the internal carotid and vertebral arteries (Fig. 16-9). The vertebral arteries join as they move up under the hindbrain and form the basilar artery. The two internal carotids and the basilar artery are joined at the base of the hypothalamus by anterior and posterior communicating arteries. These vessels are of smaller diameter than the internal carotids and basilar artery but do provide a safety route for at least some blood to go to all parts of the brain should one of the supplying arteries be blocked. The communicating arteries form the circle of Willis. Arising from the circle of Willis are three arteries supplying blood to each cerebral hemisphere: anterior, middle, and posterior cerebral arteries. The anterior and middle cerebral arteries receive blood primarily from the internal carotid arteries, and the posterior cerebral arteries are supplied by the basilar artery. The anterior cerebral artery sends blood to the medial and superior surfaces of the frontal and parietal lobes. This area includes the lower extremity zone of the somatosensory and motor cortices. The middle cerebral artery serves the inferior surface of the frontal lobe and the entire lateral surface of the cerebrum. This area includes the major part of the somatosensory and motor cortices, the speech area in the left hemisphere, and

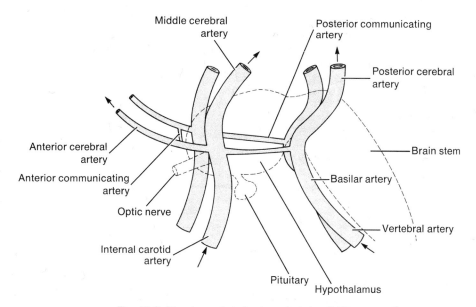

Fig. 16-9. Blood supply to brain and circle of Willis.

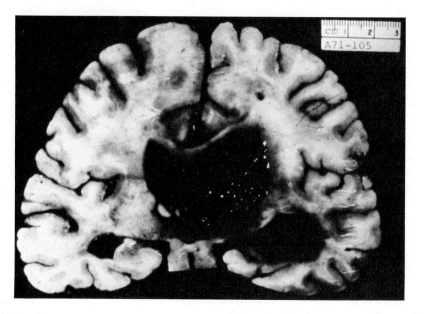

Fig. 16-10. Extensive rupture of cerebral vessel. (Courtesy Department of Pathology, University of Tennessee, Memphis.)

the auditory cortex. The posterior cerebral artery supplies blood to the medial and superior surfaces of the occipital lobe and the medial and inferior surfaces of the temporal lobe. These areas include the visual cortex and some of the limbic structures.

If blockage occurs in one of the internal carotids the effect is usually one sided, often lead-

ing to hemiplegia (and aphasia if the left side of the brain is involved). Obviously a major part of the cerebral hemisphere would be involved. If the basilar artery is blocked, the posterior areas of both hemispheres are damaged. Typical effects are double vision, difficulty in swallowing, and slurred speech.

If a blockage or rupture occurs in one of the

cerebral arteries, the effect can be less damaging, especially if the vessel involved is a small branch. The smaller the vessel, the less brain tissue being served, and the less brain tissue being damaged by ischemia or rupture. Fig. 16-10 shows an extensive rupture of a cerebral vessel.

When hemiplegia occurs, it does suggest that a large part of one hemisphere is involved, either directly or through damage to the internal capsule. The effect of damage on the right side is a left hemiplegia. Damage on the left side results in a right hemiplegia. This is because of the crossover by the motor and sensory systems. A person with right hemiplegia almost always will be aphasic too because the speech area is almost always located on the left side, regardless of preferred handedness. This person may have difficulty in comprehending speech. He also may appear cautious and anxious. A person with left hemiplegia can speak with little difficulty but may have other problems. For instance, he almost always is disoriented in space. He cannot find the midline of his body. Up and down and left and right become meaningless terms. He has virtually no money or number concept and cannot be trusted to take responsibility for taking his own medications. This person appears quite confident of his abilities and may attempt tasks for which he is not ready. Other differences exist between people with right and left hemiplegia, but there are similarities as well. Both will continue motor activity beyond its necessary use or continue to make certain sounds (perseveration). Both may have difficulty in performing simple tasks without some kind of clue being supplied (apraxia). Visual defects of various types may also occur in both types of hemiplegia. In both there is loss of sensation in the affected extremities. People who have suffered a CVA are very suggestible. Told they look tired, they usually will be. Told they are looking better, they will often act as if they feel better.

Cell hyperactivity

Up to this point all problems discussed are due to damage to cells or their axons, resulting in poor transmission of information. A group of motor problems, namely, the various types of epilepsy, exist that are the result of improper functioning of cells that are more active than they should be, resulting in improper transmission of neural activity.

Epilepsy can be caused by various factors, not all of them yet identified. Whatever the cause, the result is a population of neurons, usually in the cortex, that is anatomically and physiologically abnormal. Normally, cortical cells have a large number of axons from other cells ending on their dendrites and cell bodies. The abnormal cells have lost several of these synaptic connections. The result is a hyperexcitability.

Presumably the population of aberrant neurons is quite small at the onset, but with time and continued pathology more and more cells are included. In this way the focus, or malfunctioning area, increases in size and has greater effects. It is quite possible for a person to have several foci simultaneously, but presumably only the most active focus sets off the epileptic seizure. This phenomenon is analogous to the action of pacemakers in the heart and elsewhere.

What actually produces the epileptic attack is uncertain, but most likely the focus, being hyperexcitable, eventually causes those areas to which it connects to reach threshold and become active. These areas in turn activate the next in line and so on. Eventually an entire hemisphere or the entire cerebrum could be involved. Inclusion of the motor systems would result in localized muscle spasms or more generalized tonic or tonic-clonic behavior. Activation of the sensory cortex or sensory thalamus would yield appropriate sensations, including light flashes and sounds. Involvement of the higher brain stem structures might add "absence" and even unconsciousness. After the various brain structures are driven to hyperactivity, they may require a recuperative period, a time during which they cannot respond to stimulation. All of this would be quite variable, depending on the individual's neurologic state, that is, size and site of focus and degree of excitability of the focus and of the connecting structures.

There is good evidence to suggest that repeated activation of a brain structure, for example, by a focus, even on an infrequent schedule, leads to an easier excitement of that structure over time. This would result in more frequent or more easily activated epileptic seizures. This change in seizure threshold has been termed *kindling*.

Because of the wide variety of causes of epilepsy and the differing patterns of the seizures exhibited a standardized classification of seizures is difficult. Several classifications offered through the years have been found wanting for various reasons. The more traditional types of grand mal, petit mal, psychomotor, and focal (jacksonian) are far from sufficient yet still frequently used. Representatives of neurologic organizations from different countries developed a classification series that has been adopted by the World Health Organization. It is called the International Classification of Epileptic Seizures. A complete description here is not possible, but in essence the various types of epileptic seizures are broken down into (1) partial seizures, which begin locally and may or may not involve a larger mass of brain tissue, (2) generalized seizures, which are bilaterally symmetric and without local onset (these do not necessarily include the entire cerebrum), and (3) unilateral seizures, which largely involve only one side of the brain. A fourth classification is also offered and must be included until epilepsy is finally understood, namely unclassified epileptic seizures. The student is urged to seek out the various texts that describe the characteristic patterns of behavior presented during the different types of epileptic seizures.

Synaptic malfunction

Some diseases result from an intact system that is not functioning properly at the synaptic connections between the neurons or between the neurons and muscles. There are other diseases in which the synapses become afunctional due to cellular pathology.

Whenever an action potential reaches the end of an axon, a certain amount of chemical transmitter is released into the synaptic cleft. If enough transmitter makes contact with the receptors in the postsynaptic membrane, an appropriate depolarization (or hyperpolarization,

if transmitter and receptor dictate) takes place. If enough depolarizing (excitatory postsynaptic potentials [EPSP]) potentials occur, an action potential is produced in the axon of the postsynaptic cell. If a few hyperpolarizing (inhibitory postsynaptic potentials [IPSP]) potentials occur also, an action potential is likely prohibited from forming. In the special case of motor axon to skeletal muscle the depolarizing potential at the end-plate (end-plate potential [EPP]) is normally large enough on its own to produce an action potential in the muscle cell, thus leading to a contraction.

The transmitter is produced by biochemical processes in the neuron and is stored in vesicles at the axon terminal. The amount of transmitter released is a function of the size (amplitude) of the action potential. Calcium must be present at the axon terminal for the transmitter to be released. After release the transmitter is reabsorbed by the axon terminal or destroyed by enzymes at the synapse.

Any condition that alters the chemical nature of the transmitter, the quantity produced, the quantity stored, the quantity released, or the quantity remaining in the synaptic space will affect the synaptic activity produced by that transmitter. Similarly any condition that alters the quantity or responsiveness of the postsynaptic receptors will affect the synaptic activity of the related transmitter.

If too little chemical is released, its effectiveness is reduced. If the transmitter is not reabsorbed or destroyed, its effect is prolonged and possibly enhanced. If the receptor is bound by any chemical that prevents reaction with the transmitter, then the transmitter is ineffective. There are also other possible problem areas with a system as complex as the synapse.

Myasthenia gravis is a motor problem characterized by weakness of the skeletal muscles, especially those used frequently, such as the eye muscles and those controlling the lids. It is often found with a disorder of the immune system. It may be a result of an autoimmune reaction, but the actual cause is not defined yet. Whatever the initial cause, myasthenia gravis is evidenced as a neuromuscular problem because the receptors for acetylcholine in the synaptic end-plate of skeletal muscle cannot react with the transmitter. Therefore, no (or few) muscle action potentials are produced, and the muscles do not contract. There does seem to be a sufficient quality and quantity of acetylcholine released from the axon with each action potential, so the problem lies with the receptors in the postsynaptic muscle membrane.

Parkinsonism is an extrapyramidal motor problem in which the concentration of a synaptic transmitter decreases. The substantia nigra, in the midbrain, sends axons to the basal ganglia. The transmitter produced by these pigmented cells and stored in the axon terminals is dopamine. Presumably dopamine acts as an inhibitory transmitter in the basal ganglia. Its action is balanced by acetylcholine, coming from other areas, which presumably is an excitatory transmitter.

There are several causes of parkinsonism. Frequently there is degeneration of the pigmented cells in the substantia nigra. The result of such degeneration is a decrease in the amount of dopamine, both in the substantia nigra, where it is produced, and in the basal ganglia, where it is stored and released. As a result a chemical imbalance occurs between dopamine and acetylcholine because the cells producing acetylcholine and delivering it to the basal ganglia are still intact. Such an imbalance would produce more excitation of the cells than normal and may be the factor producing the parkinsonian tremor.

It is quite possible that further research into neuromuscular problems and even neuropsychiatric problems will reveal chemical imbalances between two or more transmitters as the basis for the difficulties. Some research on schizophrenia has already suggested this possibility.

LOWER AND UPPER MOTOR NEURON PROBLEMS

Any neuromuscular difficulty can be classified as either a lower motor neuron problem or an upper motor neuron problem. The distinction is based on the location of the pathology and the concomitant symptoms.

A lower motor neuron problem involves the motor neurons whose cell bodies are located in the anterior gray matter of the spinal cord or certain nuclei in the brain stem (cranial nerve nuclei). The axons of these lower motor neurons leave the cord or brain stem and go to skeletal muscle. A lower motor neuron is the only one that activates skeletal muscle directly. It is the only one that forms the neuromuscular junction, the synaptic end-plate. The lower motor neurons receive excitation and inhibition from the pyramidal and extrapyramidal systems, the cerebellum, and the sensory part of the cord. They are the cells that "decide" whether the muscles should contract. Damage to lower motor neurons prevents muscle contraction.

Upper motor neurons are the cells of the brain that influence the activity of the lower motor neurons. Upper motor neurons include the cells of the pyramidal and extrapyramidal motor systems and the cerebellum. The axons of these cells, whether they stay in the brain or continue into the cord, are still considered upper motor neurons. Damage to upper motor neurons alters muscle contraction but usually does not prevent it.

Symptoms of a lower motor neuron problem include (1) flaccid paralysis, weakness of voluntary movements, a decrease in muscle tone, and a loss of reflexes, (2) atrophy of the involved muscles if the motor axons are intact and degeneration of the muscles if the axons to them are cut, (3) fibrillation or fasciculation of the involved muscles, (4) a decreased response in the muscle from electrical stimulation of either muscle or nerve, (5) an increased responsiveness of the muscle to certain chemicals, especially acetylcholine, and (6) biochemical and histologic changes to the muscle.

The flaccid paralysis, weakness, and so on are due to the fact that damage to the motor axons or the motor cells in the anterior gray matter prevents appropriate activation of the motor neurons. Without activation of the motor neurons, the muscles cannot be activated. So the muscles do not contract.

Atrophy of the muscle is a result of disuse in which the muscle cells are not stimulated to produce sufficient contractile proteins. Degeneration is a result of much more than disuse. Presumably all neurons, wherever they are, have a stimulatory influence on the metabolism of the cells to which they go. Proper synaptic contact is apparently necessary for this trophic effect of one excitable cell on another. It is not necessary that action potentials occur with the normal resulting synaptic events. The close contact and presumably ongoing neurochemical stimulation is necessary. Without it, the postsynaptic cell would have an altered, abnormal metabolism that could result in its death. This is what apparently happens to muscle cells when the motor axons to them are cut and the axons themselves degenerate. The muscle cells lose the trophic influence from the motor neurons.

Fibrillation is the contraction of single muscle cells and is not visible through the skin. *Fasciculation* is the contraction of an entire motor unit (all the muscle cells activated by one motor neuron) and is visible. Both of these symptoms, when they occur, are the result of the hyperexcitability of the degenerating axons of the lower motor neurons or the degenerating membranes of the affected muscle cells. Action potentials are more easily produced, at least for a time, in degenerating membranes because of their "leakiness" to ions.

The decrease in response of the nerve and muscle to electrical stimulation reflects an alteration in the axonal and muscle membranes. The changes that occur lead to a depolarization of the membranes to the point that they can no longer generate action potentials in response to the electrical stimulation.

The increased responsiveness of the muscle membrane to circulating acetylcholine also reflects a change in the membrane. Where the acetylcholine receptors are normally only at the neuromuscular junction, they appear to be spread all over the membrane as a consequence of losing the trophic influence of the motor neuron. This widespread population of receptors makes the entire membrane sensitive to acetylcholine, whereas under normal conditions, only the synaptic area is responsive.

The biochemical and histologic changes in the muscle are related to each other and again are a consequence of the loss of trophic activity from the motor neuron. Some of the changes seen are in protein metabolism and the production and maintenance of the contractile elements of the muscle cell. The net result is a muscle cell that shows a decreased ability to function. Examples of lower motor neuron problems

include acute anterior poliomyelitis, which results from pathology of the motor cell bodies in the anterior horn of the gray matter in the cord, and peripheral nerve injury, which as the name implies is a problem stemming from damage to the spinal nerve.

A person with an upper motor neuron disease will show some of the following characteristics: (1) spastic paralysis, with increased resistance to passive movement of a limb, or paresis, an absence or weakness of voluntary movement, (2) no muscle atrophy, except from disuse, (3) hyperactive deep reflexes, such as the knee jerk and Achilles tendon tests, (4) decreased or absent superficial reflexes, such as the abdominal and cremasteric reflexes, and (5) positive pathologic signs, such as a positive Babinski test.

The spastic paralysis may be the result of an overactive stretch reflex causing a virtually constant contraction of the limb muscles. Those that normally oppose gravity are especially involved. The student should review the gamma motor neuron–muscle stretch receptor system. The mechanism involved in spasticity is most likely due to damage in extrapyramidal motor pathways that inhibit the gamma motor neurons. The gamma motor neurons become more active, resulting in an increased sensitivity to muscle stretch. Thus, the limb muscles develop a greatly exaggerated tone without any apparent stimulus. Passive movement of the involved limb elicits an exceptionally enhanced reflex opposing the motion. Overactive alpha motor neurons may also cause spasticity because of their direct influence on the muscles. The paresis, when it occurs, is a result of the motor pathways in the brain or cord not being able to sufficiently activate the alpha motor neurons.

The lack of any noteworthy muscle atrophy is due to the intact alpha motor neurons still having their neurotrophic influence on the muscle cells, even if there are no action potentials being produced. Atrophy from disuse may occur, as described earlier.

Hyperactive deep reflexes, as with spasticity, may be a result of overactive gamma motor neurons setting the reflex sensitivity to muscle stretch higher than normal. These responses suggest damage in the extrapyramidal motor system.

In the case of decreased or absent superficial reflexes the problem is more likely in the pyramidal motor system, but that is not yet definite. The decreased responsiveness (a negative sign) presumably results from a decreased influence on the alpha motor neurons by the upper motor neurons.

The positive pathologic signs may result from several possibilities: the absence of influence from a motor system, the presence of an increased expression from a motor system due to its no longer being inhibited by the damaged area, or a change in responsiveness of the two motor systems so one becomes more effective than normal. The positive Babinski reflex may be an example of the last possibility. It appears that all the muscles reflexly activated by stimulation of the plantar surface of the foot continue to respond in the abnormal state. The extension of the large toe is a result of the appropriate pathway responding with more activity than normal so the toe extends instead of flexing. A positive Babinski reflex is considered a sign of pyramidal motor system difficulties.

Examples of upper motor neuron problems include most of the diseases described earlier. Spinal cord trauma, involving the motor pathways, or a CVA, also involving motor pathways, are two examples. Other examples are multiple sclerosis, parkinsonism, cerebellar ataxia, and any other disease that alters the normal functioning of the cells in the pyramidal and extrapyramidal motor systems and the cerebellum.

DISORDERS IN MUSCLE FUNCTION

In order for muscle to contract, several physiologic steps must occur. The action potential must develop and progress along an intact, functional surface membrane. The bioelectrical effects of the action potential must be transferred to the deeper membranes of the sarcoplasmic reticulum, which must then release Ca^{++} to the sarcoplasm. The diffusing Ca^{++} must activate the ATPase system of the myofilaments, permitting the "sliding" of actin over myosin through the formation and consequent rupture of chemical bonds (bridges). In order to relax or return to the precontraction state, the Ca^{++} must be pumped back into the sarco-plasmic reticulum, and sufficient ATP must be generated.

As with all cells, the DNA within the many nuclei in a muscle cell are responsible for the coding of the many proteins, for example, filaments, enzymes, and membrane material, made in the cell. The mitochondria are responsible for many biochemical steps, including ATP production.

In a system as complicated as muscle contraction there are many steps that can go awry, each one alone being sufficient to seriously alter proper muscle function. If the membranes are improperly constructed, they may not be able to properly carry an action potential or hold (or release) Ca^{++}. If the DNA of a gene is incorrectly coded, a nonfunctional enzyme may be generated, and the entire cell may become nonfunctional. If the mitochrondia cannot produce sufficient ATP or other biochemicals, the entire cellular metabolism may be ruined. Any of the above conditions would result in a muscle that could not function in a normal fashion.

Muscular dystrophy includes many diseases under one general classification, each one having its own special characteristics. It is a disease of progressive muscle wasting with the motor nerves still intact. Thus, whatever trophic influence is presented by the nerves is not sufficient. Muscular dystrophy is apparently a genetically transmitted disease. The exact nature of the disease is still unknown. The source of the problem currently is thought to be the surface membrane of the cell. Most other subunits of the dystrophic muscle cell have been found to be functional, for example, filaments, sarcoplasmic reticulum, and several enzymes. The actual role the surface membrane might have in the development and progressive nature of the disease has not been worked out.

Another class of muscle diseases is called *myopathy*. Again the muscles progressively weaken. The causes of the different myopathies are apparently genetic, with the immediate problem of each usually being the absence of or improper construction of certain enzymes.

Generally the cause of the muscle-wasting diseases, where the nerves are intact, is genetic. The resultant incorrect production of or the lack of certain proteins is probably characteristic for each disease. Yet the connection between the missing or poorly produced proteins and the symptoms of the diseases has not been discovered. Obviously this area is one that still requires a great deal of research.

DISORDERS IN VISION AND AUDITION

For both vision and audition, as special senses, nervous pathways are utilized to relay information from the receptive area to the appropriate sensory cortex. For that reason these senses can be affected by the same pathologic changes discussed earlier for the nervous system in general. What makes them rather unique, in addition to the portion of our environment they "sample," is the biochemical or biophysical mechanisms employed to translate the stimulus to nervous energy (the action potential).

Vision

Light entering the eye first passes through the cornea, where a small amount of refraction occurs (Fig. 16-11). Next the light moves through the aqueous humor, which normally has little effect on its path. The next structure is the iris with its opening, the pupil. Varying amounts of light are allowed through, depending on the diameter of the pupil. The lens is next; it is the major element in the eye that controls the focusing of the light energy onto the retina. The shape of the lens, which determines its focusing point, is controlled by its own elasticity and by the tension on it from the ciliary muscles and suspensory fibers. When the ciliary muscles contract, they oppose the tension of the suspensory fibers, allowing the elasticity of the lens to have a greater effect. When the muscles are working, the lens takes on a thicker, shorter shape—a shape necessary for near vision. This process is known as *accommodation*. As people age, their lenses become less elastic. As a result, older people have more difficulty in clearly seeing a close object, for example, a book or newspaper.

The next area for light to pass through is the vitreous humor, a jellylike material that normally has little effect on the light. Finally the

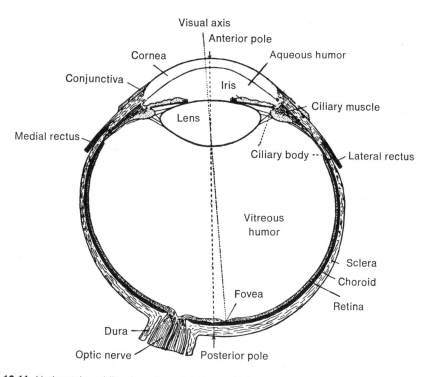

Fig. 16-11. Horizontal meridianal section of right eye. (Adapted from Bevelander, G., and Ramaley, J. A.: Essentials of histology, ed. 8, St. Louis, 1979, The C. V. Mosby Co.)

light reaches the retina, where, if conditions are right, the light energy is translated into action potentials in the optic nerve.

The retina lines a major portion of the inside of the eye. It lies in close association with the pigmented layer, the choroid. The outermost layer is the white of the eye, the sclera.

The retina is composed primarily of three layers of cells: the sensory cells (rod and cones), the bipolar cells, and the ganglion cells. The sensory cells are located closest to the pigmented layer. Light must travel through the ganglion and bipolar cell layers to reach the sensory cells. When light strikes the rods and cones, it is absorbed by the pigments in those cells. A chemical reaction then occurs that results in a change in the movement of ions through the cell membranes. Such ionic movement develops action potentials in the sensory cell axons, which may then, through normal synaptic activity, activate the bipolar cells. The bipolar cells combine the activity of several sensory cells. The ganglion cells similarly are activated by the bipolar cells and combine the results of bipolar cell activity. The ganglion cell axons leave the eye through the optic nerve and end in a special area of the thalamus reserved for vision. From there, axons of the thalamic cells end in the visual cortex. Some axon branches also go to the midbrain, where visually related reflexes are controlled.

All the ganglion cell axons leave the eye in the area called the *optic disc*. This is the entry and exit point respectively for the arteries and veins serving the vitreous side of the retina. The choroid contains blood vessels that supply the choroid side of the retina. No sensory cells exist in the optic disc. If part of an image falls on the optic disc, that part would not be seen. For this reason the optic disc is also called the *blind spot*. The rod and cone cells are fairly evenly distributed throughout the retina. There is a gradual change in relative numbers of each, however. There are more rods than cones in the anterior section of the retina, and there are more cones than rods in the more posterior part of the retina. The fovea is a special part of the retina that contains no rods, only cones. The fovea is in direct line with the cornea and lens and is the area that normally receives the focused image.

When we fixate, that is, fix our gaze on a particular object, our eyes move in such a way that the object's image is placed on the fovea.

The rods are sensitive to light at all frequencies of the visual spectrum. In essence they provide us with information on the intensity of light, or shades of gray. They require less light to become activated than do the cones. Thus, it is the rods that provide "night vision," and since there are more rods than cones at the anterior aspects of the retina, and no rods in the fovea, we can see an object at night better by fixing our gaze off to the side of the object. This puts the image onto an area where there are more rods.

There are three classes of cones, based on their particular sensitivity to light: red, green, and blue. Between the three classes, we are able to sense the various colors in our environment. The cones require more light energy than do the rods to become activated. Thus, as light intensity diminishes, the cones become less active and color vision disappears. The fovea, containing only cones, is the area of sharpest color vision.

The pigmented layer of the choroid has two important functions in addition to carrying blood vessels to that side of the retina. Any light not absorbed by the sensory cells is normally absorbed by the melanin in the pigmented layer. Such absorption prevents reflection of the light, with a resultant degradation of the focused image. The pigmented layer is also a storage site for vitamin A. Vitamin A is necessary for the re-formation of the visual pigments located in the sensory cells. These pigments absorb the light energy and as a result are broken down, initiating the biochemical events that result in the formation of the action potentials.

The optic nerves leaving each eye come together just anterior to the hypothalamus to form the optic chiasm. From the optic chiasm the axons continue as the optic tracts, one on each side of the hypothalamus, until they reach the visual portion of the thalamus. The optic chiasm is a crossover point for approximately half the axons in each optic nerve. The other half of the axons in each nerve do not cross but stay on the same side as the eye from which they came. Which axons cross over and which stay on the same side is determined by where they originate in the retina. Essentially the right half of each eye sends its axons to the right side of the brain, and the left half of each eye sends its axons to the left side of the brain. Using just one example, the temporal half of the right retina sends axons to the optic chiasm, where they then enter the right optic tract, staying on the right side. The nasal side of the left retina sends its axons to the optic chiasm, where they cross over and enter the right optic tract, joining the axons of the temporal half of the right retina. In this way an object on the left side of the visual field is perceived in the right side of the brain, because its image is formed on the right halves of both retinas. Similarly an object in the right visual field is perceived in the left side of the brain. Axons from the foveae apparently go to both halves of the brain, permitting depth perception, or stereoscopic vision.

Visual problems. Any alteration of the normal light path will necessarily result in a visual problem. Astigmatism is a condition in which lines of one orientation are in sharp focus while lines of different orientation are not; for example, vertical lines are clear while horizontal lines are fuzzy. The cause of astigmatism is a malshaped cornea. The small amount of refraction by the cornea is unequal for the different angles of light waves entering the eye. The lens cannot correct the difference, so the image cannot be completely in focus. Cataracts are cloudy lenses. Visual loss results because of the inability of light to pass through. The degree of loss necessarily depends on the degree of opacity of the lens. Cataracts may result from trauma to the eye, radiation on the lens, or elevated glucose in the aqueous humor (as with diabetes mellitus). A ruptured or detached retina obviously prevents proper image formation. If the condition is allowed to persist, the sensory cells will degenerate since they are not being supported by the choroidal blood supply. A possible cause of detached retina is physical trauma to the eye.

Anything that may affect the biochemical

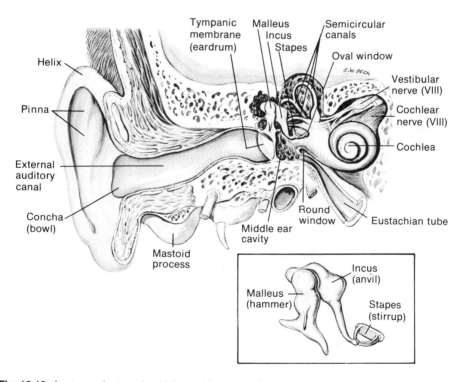

Fig. 16-12. Anatomy of external, middle, and inner ear. Auditory ossicles are shown enlarged in box. (From Schottelius, B. A., and Schottelius, D. D.: Textbook of physiology, ed. 18, St. Louis, 1978, The C. V. Mosby Co.)

events surrounding the translation of light stimulation to action potentials would also affect vision. Both hypovitaminosis A and hypervitaminosis A can affect the eyes. With too little or too much vitamin A stored in the pigmented layer, the normal process involving the regeneration of the visual pigments cannot occur.

The cells of the pigmented layer are constantly removing the ends of the sensory cells nearest the choroid. The portion of the sensory cells affected is called the *outer segment*. The sensory cells are also constantly renewing their outer segments. The visual pigments are located in these portions of the sensory cells. If something happens such that the choroid cells stop removing the ends of the outer segments, then cellular debris accumulates between the sensory cells and the choroid. This in turn prevents normal exchange between the capillaries of the choroid and the sensory cells. The final result is blindness due to a loss of function of the sensory cells. This disease in humans is called *retinitis pigmentosa*.

Once the image is translated into action potentials in the retina, any visual loss that might occur would be the result of nervous tissue malfunction. The possible causes for this have been discussed earlier in this chapter, for example, transection and demyelination.

If an optic nerve is affected, there is loss of vision in one eye. The loss is either partial or complete, depending on the extent of the damage.

If an optic tract is involved, the loss is half of the visual field for both eyes. The loss is for the visual field opposite to the affected optic tract. This is known as *hemianopia* and can occur as a result of a CVA or tumor.

If the optic chiasm is the trauma site, different types of losses occur, depending on the part of the chiasm lesioned. If a transection, for instance, is from side to side through the optic chiasm, all axons are cut, and total blindness occurs in both eyes. If the transection is from front to back, only the crossing axons are cut. As a result, each eye is half blind. The nasal area of each retina can no longer transmit information to the brain. Only the temporal halves of each retina would have an intact pathway.

Audition

Audition involves the translation of physical sound-wave energy into action potentials. This is done by the inner ear, aided by the external and middle ear structures (Fig. 16-12).

Sound waves enter the auditory meatus, or canal, and are directed to the tympanic membrane. This membrane separates the external and middle ear regions. The sound waves cause the eardrum to vibrate in synchrony. The eardrum functions to change the vibration of air into a vibration of a tissue. It changes the medium being vibrated. Attached to the eardrum is the first of the three ossicles, the malleus. The vibration of the eardrum is transferred to the malleus, then the incus, then the stapes, and finally another membrane, the oval window. The oval window separates the middle and inner ear regions. The function of the three ossicles is to transfer the vibration from the eardrum to the oval window and hence to the fluid in the inner ear, without loss of energy. There are small muscles attached to the ossicles. A reflex mechanism exists that contracts these muscles and thereby dampens the vibration of the ossicles. This dampening reduces the amplitude of the sound waves being transmitted. This reflex normally occurs after a loud sound. It is doubtful just how protective this reflex is when a person is exposed to intermittent loud noises, such as thunder and explosions. It is probably more important when a person is in an environment with a constant high level of noise, such as a foundry or a discotheque. In the conditions just mentioned the dampening effect is not enough to prevent some deafness.

In the inner ear are several bony chambers: the utricle, the saccule, the semicircular canals, and the cochlea. The first three structures are all involved with sensing head position in space, more specifically, acceleration, deceleration, and head rotation in all planes. The action potentials produced by the sensory cells in these chambers travel up the vestibular portion of the eighth cranial nerve. Their final destination is primarily the cerebellum. Some information also reaches the sensory cortex.

The cochlea is the one structure in the inner ear that is concerned with audition. It is shaped somewhat like the shell of a snail. It has three chambers that run the length of the coiled tube. Two of these, the upper and lower ones, are connected at the narrow end of the cochlea, the helicotrema. The middle chamber ends just before the helicotrema. The sensory cells for hearing are located in the middle chamber. All three chambers are filled with fluid. When the oval window is forced back and forth by the stapes, a physical wave is sent through the fluid in the upper and lower chambers. The round window at the large end of the lower chamber gives with each pressure wave, thereby reducing any dampening effect a more solid structure would have. Each frequency of sound produces an appropriate frequency of pressure waves in the cochlea. By mechanisms still unknown, the pressure waves for each frequency of sound activate a relatively small portion of sensory cells in one location of the middle chamber. In other words, each frequency of sound has a fairly specific group of sensory cells that is activated because of its location. The pressure waves corresponding to the highest frequency activate the sensory cells nearest to the oval and round windows. Those waves related to the lowest frequency activate the cells at the helicotrema. This is how the coding of frequency occurs. It is the sensory cells at the site of activation that code the stimulating frequency. The action potentials carrying the information of audition travel up axons in the cochlear portion of the eighth cranial nerve. There are several relay points in the auditory pathway, including the medulla, the auditory portion of the thalamus, and finally the auditory cortex in the temporal lobe. Auditory information from each ear goes to both auditory cortices.

Auditory problems. Any alteration in the sound transmission pathway would necessarily affect audition. Conditions as simple as wax in the auditory meatus, blocking the incoming sound waves, would produce partial deafness. Similarly a ruptured eardrum will reduce the transmission of sound waves to the ossicles. As a person ages, the ligaments of the ossicles stiffen. This causes a reduction in the transmitted energy to the inner ear and a partial deafness. The middle ear often fills with fluid during a middle ear infection. This condition limits action of the ossicles and the membranes, reducing hearing. Otosclerosis is a disease in which a bony growth attaches the stapes to the oval window, drastically reducing the transmission of energy to the cochlea.

Sensory cell damage in the inner ear is a major cause of deafness. Conditions leading to sensory cell death are varied, including genetic causes, some viral infections, and high-intensity stimulation such as in certain factories and rock bands. Many teenagers and young adults have hearing losses as a result of listening to loud music. Apparently the high-intensity stimulation sets up large pressure waves in the cochlea, in spite of the muscle reflex in the middle ear. The high-amplitude pressure waves over a sustained period damage the sensory cells. For factory workers the damage is often restricted to a narrow range of (usually high) frequencies. The frequency range affected by loud music is much larger.

Nervous system diseases can also affect the auditory system. The student should review the various causes and effects, such as trauma, demyelination, and CVA. Occasionally a person will show a loss of hearing as a result of antibiotic treatment, for example, streptomycin. Some antibiotics attack the eighth cranial nerve. The vestibular portion is affected more often than the cochlear portion, but both can be involved. Tinnitus, especially at higher frequencies, normally occurs first. Young children and older people are most susceptible to auditory nerve damage from these drugs.

ELECTROLYTE IMBALANCE AND THE NERVOUS SYSTEM

Any disease that influences the electrolyte concentrations of the extracellular space has an effect on all excitable tissue. The student should review those chapters that pertain to this topic.

A low potassium concentration (hypokalemia) results in hyperpolarized membranes, making it more difficult for excitable cells to reach threshold. Hyperkalemia has the opposite result. Only small changes either side of normal values are necessary to cause the heart to stop.

A low extracellular sodium concentration

(hyponatremia) mainly affects the amplitude of the action potential, reducing it. Less transmitter is released as a result, so the postsynaptic potentials are smaller in amplitude. Hypernatremia has the opposite effect. Many other physiologic functions are upset by changes in sodium concentration before the effects mentioned here are exhibited. Large changes in sodium concentration are possible before deleterious effects are shown.

Low calcium concentration in the extracellular space (hypocalcemia) reduces the amount of transmitter released at the synapse, increases the rate of potassium leaving the cardiac pacemaker cells, and leaves the membranes of excitable cells in general in an unstable, hyperexcitable state. Hypercalcemia generally has the opposite effect, especially on the cellular membranes. Only small changes in calcium concentration are possible before effects will be seen.

SUGGESTED READINGS

Brain, W. R., and Walton, J. N.: Brain's diseases of the nervous system, New York, 1969, Oxford University Press.

Drachman, D. B., editor: Trophic functions of the neuron, Ann. N.Y. Acad. Sci. **228:**1-423, 1974.

Eliasson, S. G., Prensky, A. L., and Hardin, W. B., Jr., editors: Neurological pathophysiology, New York, 1974, Oxford University Press.

Grob, D., editor: Myasthenia gravis, Ann. N.Y. Acad. Sci. **274:**1-682, 1976.

Gutmann, E.: Neurotrophic relations, Ann. Rev. Physiol. **38:**177-216, 1976.

Mountcastle, V. B., editor: Medical physiology, ed. 13, St. Louis, 1974, The C. V. Mosby Co., vol. 1.

Tower, D. B., editor: The nervous system, vol. 2: the clinical neurosciences, New York, 1975, Raven Press.

CHAPTER 17

Effects of immobility

AT THE COMPLETION OF THIS CHAPTER THE STUDENT WILL BE ABLE TO:

- Define the term *immobility* and discuss the relative nature and use of this term.
- State four qualitative measures used to estimate the degree of immobility present.
- Identify conditions in which the normal level of physical mobility is altered.
- Describe the systemic effects of immobility.
  Describe the clinical manifestations of these effects.
  Explain the pathophysiologic mechanisms by which these effects occur.
  Discuss the relationship between the severity and reversibility of these effects and the variables of the duration and the degree of immobility present.
- Describe and state the rationale for treatment measures used to minimize the effects of immobility.

Mobility is defined as the ability to move about freely. The term can be used to describe a state of free movement within all aspects of life: physical, psychosocial, political, economic, spiritual, geographic, and occupational. Mobility is highly valued in our transient society and is sometimes equated with freedom. Indeed, a certain sense of freedom does emanate from the ability to move about without restriction. Many individuals use their level of mobility to define their health status; that is, they view the inability to get out or perform their routine, daily activities as a manifestation of illness. Discussion of the concept of mobility within this chapter will be limited to the effect of altered levels of physical mobility upon the overall physiologic functioning of the human body.

Movement of the various parts or of the entire body is essential for the maintenance of both physiologic and psychologic well-being. Movement serves many purposes, such as providing the means for nonverbal communication and the expression of emotion in a socially acceptable way; for self-defense, as an individual can move away from harmful or noxious stimuli; and for satisfaction of basic and secondary needs, as the person participates in activities of daily living that are both life sustaining (eating, drinking, etc.) and life enhancing (recreation, work, etc.). The ability of any organism to interact with and react to the various forces and conditions operating within the internal and external environments is in itself considered a basic need, or a prerequisite to the occurrence of even minimal levels of function. Satisfaction of this need depends to a great extent on the organism's level of mobility.

In order for the level of physical mobility to be within normal limits, the nervous, muscular, and skeletal systems and the vestibular apparatus and proprioceptor organs must be intact and functioning. Trauma (accidental or surgical), disease, or altered levels of consciousness can result in impaired functioning of these organ systems with the result of altering the normal mobility level. Pathology of these organ systems is not the only condition from which an altered state of mobility may result, since restriction of movement can also be voluntary or prescribed. When any of these conditions are present and result in a departure from the normal level of physical mobility, a state of immobility exists.

This chapter will discuss the concept of immobility, conditions in which some degree of immobility may be expected, and the systemic effects of immobility. The treatment of the effects of immobility will be discussed in terms of a reversal of the pathophysiology that is present.

The term *immobility* can be defined as the inability to move about freely; it includes any condition in which movement is impaired or restricted. There is a wide spectrum over which the degree of immobility can occur; hence, use of the term is relative. The degree of immobility can be *absolute,* as in the comatose patient who is incapable of initiating any movement on his own. More frequently seen, however, is a lesser degree of immobility or immobility of one body part, as in a patient who is partially paralyzed or who has sustained a bone fracture and has a cast. The term takes on a relative meaning in these conditions.

The degree of immobility present can be assessed using four qualitative measures described by Spencer and associates (1965):

1. Physical inactivity, which is manifested by a reduction in body movement

2. Physical restriction or limitation of movement, which is manifested by an imposed reduction of movement

3. Constancy of body posture in relation to gravity, which results in a loss of the body's ability to adapt to changes in position and posture

4. Sensory deprivation, which causes a reduction in the stimulus to move and which is manifested by even greater physical inactivity A judgment regarding the degree of immobility can be made based on how many of the above conditions are present. The more conditions present, the greater will be the degree of immobility experienced by the patient. In the comatose patient all four conditions are present, and the degree of immobility is total. In comparison a patient with a fractured arm and a cast in place to restrict movement of the injured arm is able to continue to participate in activities

of daily living, making some minor adjustments to compensate for the temporary loss of use of the injured arm. The degree of immobility in this patient is considered minimal since only one condition, physical restriction of movement, is present.

The duration of the immobile state is another important variable to be considered in the clinical situation. Both the duration and degree of the immobility are determined by the primary cause of the disruption and by the individual's response to that disruption.

CAUSATIVE AND PREDISPOSING FACTORS

Alterations in the level of physical mobility can result from prescribed restriction of movement in the form of bed rest, physical restriction of movement through the use of external devices, voluntary restriction of movement, or impairment or loss of motor function. Prior to World War II, immobilization in the form of imposed bed rest was considered the treatment of choice for most medical and surgical conditions and was imposed during the period following childbirth as well. This form of treatment was begun in the mid nineteenth century (1860) under the influence of John Hilton of Guy's Hospital in London. His teachings regarding the benefits of bed rest as medical therapy were a drastic and radical departure from the accepted methods of treatment at that time. Prior to that time, confinement to bed was a sign of approaching death. Once bed rest became recognized as a therapeutic measure, it was prescribed as treatment for most disorders. Pathologic complications that occurred during convalescence were regarded as the inevitable results of the primary disease process rather than the results of the immobility caused by bed rest.

The observation that the incidence of complications seemed less in injured soldiers who were rapidly mobilized during World War II led to questions as to the real benefit of bed rest as a treatment measure. Research since that time has documented the negative effects of prolonged immobility and the positive effects of early mobilization following illness, injury, surgery, and childbirth. As a result of these studies the use of bed rest as acceptable treatment has been modified. Bed rest continues to be an acceptable therapeutic measure for the treatment of conditions such as ischemic coronary disease, in which the increased metabolic demands of increased activity cannot be met and attempts by the body to meet these demands would result in damage to the organ systems. Bed rest is also beneficial in conditions in which organ damage has been sustained, as the reduced work load promotes healing and repair of injured tissue; in conditions in which an anatomic abnormality is aggravated by the effects of gravity; and in conditions in which weight bearing by the muscles, joints, and bones is contraindicated.

Casts, splints, slings, and traction are means by which body parts are immobilized to allow the injured part to rest and heal. These are not the only means by which movement can be physically restricted, however. Sometimes, for safety reasons, a patient must be physically restrained, which creates an obvious impairment to normal mobility. Drainage devices, intravenous therapy, bulky dressings, and the necessity of being on a respirator or a monitoring device also physically restrict mobility.

Voluntary limitation of movement is often the first response to acute, temporary illness; a person just does not ''feel good'' and cuts down on his usual activities. The general achiness that often accompanies colds, flu, and fever makes the person even more reluctant to move about. The presence of pain or the fear that movement will cause pain also can cause a person to limit movement.

Impairment or loss of motor function usually occurs as a result of trauma or disease of the functional components of the motor system: brain, nerve pathways, motor end-plate, muscles, joints, or bones (see Chapter 16 for a discussion of the mechanisms by which nervous system disorders disrupt mobility and Chapter 4 for a discussion of inflammatory disorders that affect joint function and result in immobility).

A reduction in motor function may occur as a result of the loss of proprioceptive ability. A complete discussion of the effects of trauma is outside the scope of this book; however, immobility is a frequent sequela to trauma, either as a primary result of the injury sustained or as a secondary result of the treatment regimen.

In most diseases of the brain, nerves, joints, and bones the muscles are secondarily affected. Aside from inflammatory conditions, the most commonly seen muscular disorders of a primary nature are those known under the classification of *muscular dystrophy*. The muscular dystrophies are a group of hereditary diseases characterized by progressive pathologic changes in the skeletal muscles, which result in bilateral, symmetric wasting and weakness of the muscles. Each muscle fiber is affected individually, which leads to a mixture of normal and abnormal fibers. Change in size is most apparent in the abnormal fibers, some of which are atrophied and others hypertrophied. The large fibers are really pseudohypertrophic, as the increase in size is due to abnormal deposition of fat and connective tissue among the fibers. The basic defect causing these changes is unknown; however, evidence suggesting defective metabolism has been found. Current research in this area is focusing on the role of vitamin E in metabolism and its relationship to this group of diseases.

There are four types of muscular dystrophy, which differ from one another in the manner of genetic transmission, age at onset, progression of the symptoms, and the sites of the affected muscles. The signs and symptoms depend on the muscle groups affected. For instance, in the pseudohypertrophic type (Duchenne) the muscles of the calves and pelvis are especially affected, resulting in a waddling gait and lordosis, signs pathognomonic to this type. Onset is usually insidious in all types of muscular dystrophy. The nervous system is unaffected.

Bone fractures may occur as the result of external trauma or as the consequence of some deformity within the bone itself. Fractures that occur in the latter manner are called *pathologic* and are usually seen in disease states in which the bone matrix is decalcified or in which there is a general decrease in the total amount of bone tissue (reduction in mass), *osteoporosis*. Osteoporosis may have a variety of causes, among them immobility. *Osteomalacia* is a condition in which the bone matrix is not calcified. This term is also used to identify the disease process

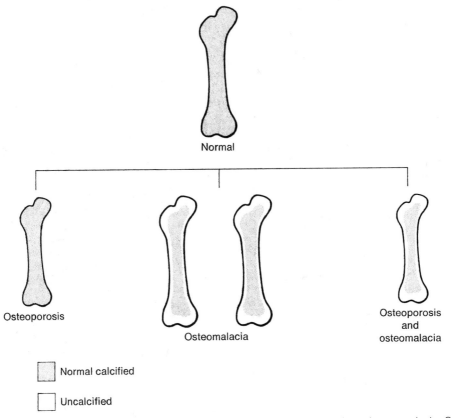

Normal

Osteoporosis

Osteomalacia

Osteoporosis
and
osteomalacia

▨ Normal calcified

▢ Uncalcified

Fig. 17-1. Differences in bone mass and mineralization in osteoporosis and osteomalacia. Osteoporosis results in a smaller but completely calcified bone. Osteomalacia results in normal-sized bones in which bone matrix is not calcified.

resulting from vitamin D deficiency in an adult, which is the same as rickets in children. Fig. 17-1 illustrates the differences between osteoporosis and osteomalacia that may also coexist.

Another disease state in which bone tissue becomes weaker than normal and subject to possible fractures is Paget's disease (osteitis deformans). Bone formation and resorption occur in an accelerated and random manner, mainly in the lumbar, sacral, and pelvic regions. The skull may also be involved. Other complications of Paget's disease include osteoarthritis (degeneration of the articular cartilage of the joint) due to the stress placed on the joints, high-output heart failure, and an increased incidence of bone tumors with metastasis. These last two complications are due to the increased vascularity of involved tissues. The etiology of this disorder is unknown at the present time. Other disorders of the bones that alter physical mobility include infectious processes, tumors, and congenital deformities. Various physiologic factors that influence bone deposition and resorption are summarized in Table 17-1.

Disease in organ systems not directly involved in motor function can also alter the level of mobility. A feature common to most diseases is a general reduction in physical activity. The more severe the disease, the more severe the reduction. This reduction in physical activity can be attributed to many factors: weakness, loss of endurance, decreased energy production, and reduction in normal organ function. In chronic, progressive disease this reduction in activity may be quite insidious. An example is

Table 17-1. Factors that influence bone deposition and resorption*

	Deposition	Resorption
Increase	Exercise, stress on bones Growth hormone (somatomedin) Fluoride†	Parathyroid hormone excess Vitamin D hormone [1,25 (OH) · D]‡ Adrenocortical steroid excess Calcium deficiency (dietary or malabsorption) Phosphorus deficiency (dietary, malabsorption, renal loss) Anabolic steroid deficiency (androgen, estrogen) Immobilization Acidosis Pregnancy and lactation Osteolytic neoplasms (including leukemia) Prostaglandins
Decrease	Immobilization, disuse, bed rest Growth hormone deficiency Adrenocortical steroid excess	Calcium Phosphorus Parathyroid hormone deficiency Calcitonin Magnesium deficiency Anabolic steroids Alkalosis Mithramycin Diphosphonates (P-O-P)

*From Pathophysiology. Altered regulatory mechanisms in disease, ed. 2. Edited by Edward Frohlich, J. B. Lippincott, Philadelphia, 1972.
†Fluoride in excess causes deposition of uncalcified osteoid and produces osteomalacia.
‡Osteolytic effect of parathyroid hormone requires presence of vitamin D hormone.

the emphysemic individual who leaves his second-floor walk-up apartment as little as possible because it ''just takes too much out of him'' to go out anymore.

Primary disease processes in organ systems outside the motor system may adversely affect its function and may even produce secondary pathologic changes within it. An example of this is sickle cell anemia. Degeneration of the heads of the femur and humerus may occur as a result of infarction due to arterial occlusion by the sickled cells. These bones are most susceptible to infarction because the arterioles supplying them are long and tortuous, collateral circulation is poor, and the rate of blood flow through the marrow is slow. In other words, hypoxia and acidosis, necessary prerequisites to sickling, will be present, especially in the distal portions of the bone. In addition, osteoporosis may occur in the vertebrae and may cause vertebral collapse. Another example is the *renal*

osteodystrophy that accompanies renal disease (see Chapter 11). Osteoporotic changes may accompany a number of pathologic conditions that occur outside of the motor system. Among these are hyperthyroidism, Cushing's syndrome, hepatic cirrhosis, hypogonadism, vitamin C deficiency, and gastrectomy.

Pregnancy, especially in the later stages, and obesity are physical conditions in which a voluntary reduction in physical activity often occurs. Obese individuals are more susceptible to the effects of immobility during convalescence and are often more difficult to mobilize. Alterations in the level of consciousness and severe catatonic states can also affect an individual's ability to move on his own in a safe manner.

The action of various drugs that may be ingested can alter the individual's level of mobility. One way in which this effect can occur is through drugs that affect the level of consciousness. Sedatives and some analgesics can make a person very lethargic and unwilling (even physically unable) to participate in any physical activity. Other drugs can have a more direct effect on motor function. Both steroid and heparin therapy can cause osteoporosis. Heparin promotes bone resorption by potentiating the action of parathyroid hormone and vitamins A and D and probably through some direct effect on bone as well. Steroid drugs cause osteoporosis through depression of osteoblastic (bone formation) activity, while osteoclastic (bone resorption) activity remains normal. Osteomalacia may result from the excessive intake of aluminum gels, which diminish intestinal phosphate absorption through the formation of insoluble aluminum phosphate. This mechanism serves as the basis for a type of therapy in conditions where serum phosphate levels are high. Osteomalacia may also result from the use of anticonvulsant drugs, which inactivate vitamin D. Ototoxic drugs, such as streptomycin, can impair an individual's sense of balance.

Sensory deprivation and overload can also affect an individual's mobility level. Studies in which sensory and motor stimuli were reduced or made monotonous have demonstrated that the subjects respond by consistently reducing the level of physical activity. This sets up a vicious cycle since immobility itself will cause a further reduction in sensory and motor input.

Another factor that may alter the level of mobility is age. As a consequence of the aging process, older persons generally reduce their physical activity, which is due to both reduced physical ability to move and lack of stimuli to move. This problem is compounded if a chronic disease accompanies the aging process. Retirement, lack of a substantial income, and loss of social contacts provide little motivation to go out. The physiologic processes involved in aging (see Chapter 18) result in a certain degree of motor function impairment. The osteoporosis of aging appears to be due to an imbalance between the bone formation and resorption processes. Women seem to be more susceptible to the development of osteoporosis than men, especially after menopause. This is most likely because of the loss of estrogen, which inhibits bone resorption to a certain degree, although the finding of increased numbers

of mast cells (which synthesize heparin) in the bone marrow of elderly, osteoporotic women indicates that other factors may also play a part.

It was stated earlier in this chapter that the duration and degree of immobility are related to both the cause of and the individual's response to the immobility. Depending on the cause, the immobility can be considered permanent or temporary and the degree either partial or absolute. No matter what the cause, immobility in itself has profound negative effects on all the body systems. The severity, that is, the scope and progression, of these effects is directly proportional to the duration and degree of the immobility. Additionally these effects themselves contribute further to the immobility. Fig. 17-2 illustrates this phenomenon; it is easy to see that the potential for development of a vicious cycle is present. A response to immobility that decreases the duration and the degree of the immobility will also have the result of minimizing the effects of the immobility and thus their potential for further altering the level of mobility to any great extent. Fig. 17-3 illustrates the interrelationship between immobility and a positive response to reduce the duration and degree of the immobility.

EFFECTS OF IMMOBILITY

The effects of immobility are both metabolic and functional and reflect a lack of use. Because of the dynamic interaction of all the body components, no system escapes the consequences of immobility. Interestingly enough, the manifestations of prolonged immobility seen in healthy individuals are identical to those seen in astronauts subjected to weightlessness and relative inactivity during space flight. In fact, studies conducted by the Air Force and the National Aerospace Administration are among those that have significantly increased the body of theoretic knowledge regarding the consequences and treatment of the effects of prolonged immobility.

It has already been mentioned that the treatment of injured soldiers during World War II was the impetus for questions regarding the effects of prolonged immobility. Prompted by the observation that the more rapidly mobilized soldiers seemed to experience fewer complica-

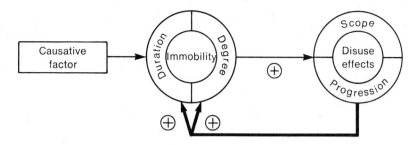

Fig. 17-2. Systems model of feedback relationship between immobility and its effects.

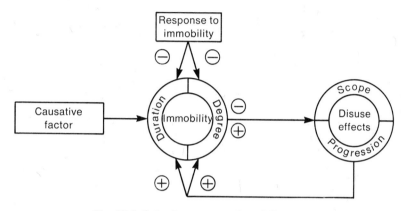

Fig. 17-3. Role of response to immobility.

tions, a group of researchers in the middle and late 1940s conducted what is now considered to be a classic study documenting the effects of prolonged immobility on healthy individuals (Deitrick et al., 1948). The subjects in this study were four young, healthy men. Physiologic parameters such as heart rate, muscle size and strength, response to position change, metabolic rate, and excretion of metabolic products were measured during three separate periods, each approximately 6 weeks in length: before immobilization, immobilization, and after immobilization. The data from each period was compared to determine the physiologic changes that had occurred and the length of time necessary for recovery from these changes. The results of this study have been consistently replicated in other studies involving normal subjects and in the experiences of astronauts on prolonged space missions.

The effects of immobility are a result of deconditioning, which is defined as loss of functional capacity secondary to lack of use (Spen-

cer et al., 1965). The effects produced in healthy subjects include the following:

1. Decreased basal metabolic rate
2. Decreased blood volume and red cell mass
3. Increased urinary excretion of calcium, phosphorus, and nitrogenous waste products
4. Decreased muscle mass
5. Decreased endurance for physical activity
6. Increased pulse rate
7. Inability to tolerate position change

In most clinical situations these effects occur with pathologic conditions, which compound the problem even further. Some of the effects of immobility seen in ill persons have not been observed in healthy subjects participating in immobility studies. The effects of immobility contribute to certain problems. These problem areas serve as the organizing element in the discussion of the effects of immobilization since they more accurately reflect the effect of immobility on the whole individual. The following problem areas can be expected to occur in the individual who is experiencing immobility in the presence of pathology:

1. Loss of endurance for physical activity
2. Decreased physical stability
3. Impaired oxygenation processes
4. Chemical disequilibrium
5. Disruption of normal elimination processes
6. Reduced integrity of the integument

Each problem area will be discussed separately in terms of the effects of immobility that contribute to the problem, the clinical manifestations, and the underlying pathophysiologic mechanisms.

Loss of endurance

Loss of endurance is primarily due to loss of the functional capacity of the muscles, which accompanies lack of use. The functional capacity is normally determined by the frequency, duration, and intensity of use. The functional capacity of a muscle that is used infrequently or only for short periods of time for nonstrenuous activity will be greatly diminished. This loss of functional capacity is characterized by loss of muscle mass, tone, and strength, which limits the amount of work that can be performed before the physiologic limit is reached.

The loss of muscle mass and strength due to decreased use is directly related to the principle that catabolic and anabolic processes balance each other: a reduction in catabolic processes leads to a reduction in anabolic processes and thus to a reduction in both cell size and available cellular energy. This reduction in cell size is referred to as *atrophy*. The loss of muscle mass due to disuse atrophy is both measurable and observable. In Deitrick's study, measurement of limb circumference and creatinine retention and x-ray examination documented a 4% to 10% loss in mass in the thighs and a 10% to 12.5% loss of mass in the calves. Such a loss can be seen in the obvious difference in size of two limbs following removal of a cast from one.

Loss of muscle strength in the immobilized legs measured between 13% to 20% in the Deitrick study. Deitrick also concluded that it took 4 to 6 weeks for recovery of preimmobility muscle mass and strength in healthy subjects.

The antigravity muscles of the lower limbs are those most affected, lending support to the theory that the normal stresses of gravity are important in maintaining function and development and therefore mobility. This is also true for muscle tone, a state of constant, partial contraction of the muscles. Standing upright requires a greater degree of muscle tone than does lying in bed. Muscle tone diminishes during the period of time an individual spends in bed or in a recumbent position. This loss of muscle tone further contributes to the loss of mass and strength because it represents a certain degree of disuse.

The problem of loss of endurance for physical activity can also be attributed in part to an increased cardiac work load. Cardiac function is most affected when the immobility involves assumption of the recumbent position and the inability to change position in relation to gravity. Upon assumption of the recumbent position with the head nearly flat, blood that normally pools in the lower extremities due to the effects of gravity is mobilized and thereby increases venous return to the heart. Because of the permissive nature of the heart's pumping function, cardiac stroke volume will be increased to accommodate the increased venous return, which results in an increased work load for the heart.

Inactive or immobilized individuals have a relative tachycardia when compared to active or athletic individuals of the same age and with the same physical characteristics. This is thought to be due to a dominance of vagal or parasympathetic effects in the active individual as compared to a dominance of sympathetic effects in the inactive individual. Both Deitrick's study and a study by Taylor and associates (1949) documented a progressive increase in the resting pulse rate over a prolonged period of immobility. Additionally the increase in the pulse rate of the immobilized subjects during exercise was greater in magnitude and required twice as long to return to preactivity levels than in the preimmobility period. These studies also determined that the pulse rate did not return to preimmobility levels for at least 6 to 8 weeks after resumption of activity.

Tachycardia contributes to the increased cardiac work load by increasing the amount of work performed per unit of time. Fatigue of the myocardium is a potential consequence of the increased energy expenditure in the presence of a reduced ability to supply energy to the myocardium since tachycardia reduces the diastolic period, which shortens both ventricular and coronary filling times. Tachycardia further contributes to the increased cardiac work load through this inefficient utilization of energy.

The problem of loss of endurance for physical activity can be attributed to both the diminished functional capacity of the muscles and an increased cardiac work load. Manifestations of this problem include weakness, easy fatigability, and an increased pulse rate, especially during exercise or activity. Loss of endurance will lead to a further reduction in physical activity since an individual will match his level of activity to his capacity or tolerance for such activity. Because of this, loss of endurance becomes a priority problem since it is a central feature in the cycle of immobility.

Decreased physical stability

Various definitions of the term *stability* can be applied to different aspects of normal physical movement; "the capacity to return to equilibrium after having been displaced" refers to a change in position, and "steadiness" refers to balance and coordination. To be "stable" means to be "not likely to give way" or "not easily thrown off balance." Certain results of immobility work together to disrupt stability and to reduce the potential for steady movement with the ability to change position readily and without danger of falling off balance or having the body "give way." The immobilized individual has difficulty in maintaining equilibrium while in motion in an upright, weight-bearing position due to the weakness, loss of joint mobility, osteoporosis, and postural hypotension that occur as direct consequences of the immobility being experienced.

Weakness is the result of both muscle atrophy, since the muscles lose strength as they atrophy, and a reduction in the general energy level due to slowing of the metabolic processes in the immobilized individual. Stability is severely affected by weakness because it is ex-

tremely difficult to attain or maintain an upright position or perform any activities requiring even minute amounts of energy when one feels weak. An ill individual may lack the necessary energy to maintain normal levels of mobility. When weakness is a manifestation of other problems an immobilized individual may experience, it can cause loss of stability.

Loss of joint mobility is a result of the pathologic changes that occur in the muscles and connective tissues in response to decreased activity. Because of these changes, the muscles and connective tissues become progressively more resistant to movement, and eventually the joint becomes fixed in one position. This condition is referred to as a *contracture*.

New connective tissue, which has a characteristic, loose appearance, is constantly being formed around the joints and muscles. This areolar nature of the connective tissue is maintained by its being stretched through normal movement. If movement becomes limited or absent, stretching of this tissue is concomitantly reduced or absent, and the connective tissue becomes denser, fixed, and less resilient, or fibrosed. This fibrosis hinders movement even more.

The muscles, because of decreased use and loss of tone, become either stretched, from being held in a lengthened position, or contracted, from being held in a shortened position. Fibrosis of the connective tissue around them will cause them to remain in these positions. An example of this is a deformity called *footdrop,* which is the result of the foot's not being supported while an individual remains in a non-weight-bearing position for any extended length of time. The foot becomes fixed in a position of plantar flexion since the tendon of the calf muscles will shorten while the anterior muscles of the leg tend to be stretched and will lengthen when the foot is allowed to remain in an unsupported position. Fig. 17-4 illustrates the normal position of the supported foot and the position that results when the foot is not supported, which becomes the position of footdrop. Normal use of the foot becomes impossible in the presence of footdrop.

Individuals who remain in bed for an extended period of time are particularly suscepti-

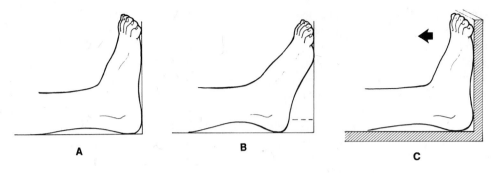

Fig. 17-4. Footdrop. **A,** Normal. **B,** Dropped. **C,** Corrected.

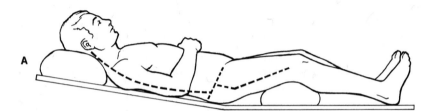

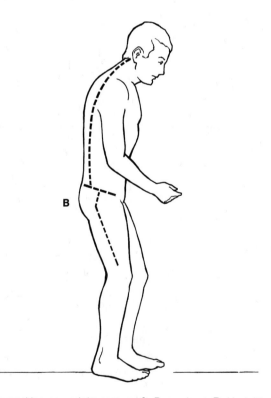

Fig. 17-5. Effects of bed-lying position on upright posture. **A,** Recumbent. **B,** Upright.

ble to the development of contractures. Flexion deformities are those most frequently seen as the use of flexion is one way of relieving discomfort, especially in the back, hips, and knees, and of maintaining body warmth. Flexion of the hips occurs whether the person is in a lying, semireclining, or sitting position in a soft bed. Flexion of the hips is increased when the knees are also flexed. Often the knees are flexed by means of a pillow, rolled blanket, or use of the knee Gatch to keep a person from slipping down in the bed. Fig. 17-5 illustrates this position. The head is positioned with the neck flexed. This position obviously discourages functional alignment of the bones and muscles for the weight-bearing position. Stiffness of the joints may be the first sign of loss of joint mobility.

It seems obvious that the presence of contractures will further impair the normal mobility of the individual and that a bedridden individual with a chronic, debilitating disease is especially at risk. Once contractures have begun to form, a greater than normal energy expenditure will be required to move since the added resistance at the joint must be overcome. Contractures may form in less than a week and may require months of steady therapy to reverse. In the meantime the individual is susceptible to all the other consequences of immobility as well. Table 17-2 lists the length of time required for recovery of full range of motion following immobilization for treatment of a shoulder dislocation.

A reduction in bone mass, or osteoporosis, is also a result of immobility that works to reduce physical stability. The processes of bone formation and resorption are normally in balance with one another; however, as a result of

Table 17-2. Mobility recovery rate for shoulder dislocation

Period of immobilization	Period of recovery
0 days	18 days
7 days	52 days
14 days	121 days
21 days	300 days

immobility this balance is disrupted to favor bone resorption, or destruction. The exact mechanism by which activity can stimulate bone growth is not completely understood at this time. It is a fact that the bones of athletic individuals are heavier than those of sedentary individuals. Activity and movement and the resultant mechanical stress on the bones is thought to stimulate bone growth through a *piezoelectric effect*, in which there is an electrical gradient and a flow of current that stimulates bone growth at the site of the stress where a negative potential is thought to exist. Lack of stress on the bones is thought to disrupt the electrical field and thus the stimulus for balanced bone growth and resorption.

There is also disagreement as to the exact effect of immobility on the balance between formation and resorption. Some authorities state that osteoclastic (destruction) activity increases while osteoblastic (formation) activity decreases, and others contend that both osteoblastic and osteoclastic activity increase but that the increase in osteoblastic activity is not as great as that of the osteoclastic cells. In any event, the result is the same: destruction of the matrix and release of the mineral constituents of the bone into the general circulation, with any excesses eventually excreted in the urine. Deitrick found that the level of calcium in the urine of his immobilized subjects rose on the second to third day after immobility began, indicating that bone resorption begins soon after the level of mobility is reduced. There was no radiologic evidence of osteoporosis in Deitrick's subjects; however, a loss of approximately 25% to 30% of the total body calcium must occur before x-ray changes are seen. The urinary loss of calcium may also lead to the development of other problems.

Weight bearing with stability in the osteoporotic individual cannot always be achieved since weight bearing can result in the body's "giving way." If osteoporosis is severe enough, pathologic fractures of the bones may occur. The neck of the femur, the ribs, and the lower end of the radius are most susceptible. Vertebral compression can also occur, resulting in back pain, which is a common complaint following long periods of immobility and which can become chronic. Individuals who are especially at risk for the development of severe osteoporosis are those in whom a pathologic process or some form of therapy that also causes osteoporosis is present concurrently with the immobility.

Postural hypotension refers to a fall in blood pressure during a change from the lying or sitting position to the standing position, which manifests itself as a feeling of dizziness or faintness upon rising. Under normal conditions the baroreceptor reflexes elicit an immediate sympathetic response to the reduction in arterial pressure that normally occurs as a person stands up. This sympathetic response causes the splanchnic and peripheral vessels to constrict, thus preventing pooling of blood in the lower extremities and maintaining arterial pressure. Failure of these vessels to constrict, as seen in immobilized individuals, results in rapid pooling of venous blood in the lower extremities, decreased venous return, decreased cardiac output, and reduced arterial pressure, causing dizziness and loss of consciousness. This effect has been consistently observed in all studies of immobilized individuals.

Studies have also demonstrated that postural hypotension occurs in the presence of intact sympathetic nervous system responses and that it occurs more frequently when the subjects are passively raised to an upright position. These observations have led to the conclusion that postural hypotension in response to immobility is the result of changes in the reaction of the vessels themselves rather than any change in sympathetic function. This change in the reactivity of the vessels is thought to be a result of disuse similar to the loss of tone in unused muscles; the vessels become acclimated to the lower blood pressure, higher flow, and the increased diameter of the supine position. Another conclusion is that the muscle tone and contraction in the lower extremities, which is necessary for actively assuming the upright position, aids in promoting vasoconstriction and inhibiting venous pooling. The muscles prohibit venous pooling by exerting a pumping action on the vessels as they contract. This effect is lost during periods of immobility, when the muscles are not used. Deitrick diminished the fainting response to passive placement in the upright position by wrapping his subjects' legs with elastic bandages, thus simulating the action of the muscles. Deitrick's subjects, whose legs were immobilized, began to faint in response to passive placement in the upright position after only 1 week of immobilization.

It seems apparent that the loss of physical stability would be detrimental to the maintenance or restoration of normal levels of mobility. Stability promotes and enhances normal mobility. Lack of physical stability further impairs it.

Impaired oxygenation processes

Several of the effects of immobility work together to impair oxygenation processes in the immobilized individual. Among these factors are a reduction in blood volume and red cell mass, decreased cardiac output, decreased expansion of the chest and lungs, increased work of breathing, stasis of the respiratory tract secretions with reduction of the diameter of the airways and development of hypostatic pneumonia, and thrombus and embolus formation. Not all these effects have been observed in healthy individuals who are immobilized; however, even in healthy individuals the effects of immobility will alter the oxygenation processes, although not to the same extent as in persons who are ill or debilitated.

A reduction in blood volume and red cell mass alters the oxygen-carrying capacity of the blood, and the decrease in cardiac output that is secondary to venous stasis alters the transport process by which oxygen is delivered to the body tissues. This has implications for periods during which the body's oxygen requirements may increase, requiring an immediate or greater than normal supply of oxygen. These effects of immobility are seen in healthy individuals but are potentially more dangerous in ill or debilitated individuals.

The reduction in chest and lung expansion and the increased work of breathing are interrelated. Respiratory activity is affected by the stimulus for respiration, the resistance against which the respiratory muscles have to work, and the strength of the muscles themselves.

With a reduction in activity there is also a reduction in the body's energy needs, which is reflected in a lowered BMR, indicating slowing of the metabolic processes. As a result of the slowing of the metabolic processes, less carbon dioxide is produced, removing the stimulus for respiration and causing the respiratory rate to drop. Additionally, tidal volume drops as a result of diminished chest expansion, which is caused by weakness of the muscles of respiration and by the pressure of the abdominal organs and the bed against the chest cavity, which create resistance to expansion. The combination of the weakness and the added resistance result in an increase in the work of breathing or the effort a person must put forth to breathe.

The effects described so far occur in anyone experiencing immobility. Stasis of respiratory tract secretions has not been a problem in the healthy subjects participating in immobility studies. Individuals who are prone to develop stasis of secretions during a period of immobility are those in whom ventilatory function is already impaired, the cough reflex is suppressed, and secretions are thicker than normal, or who are unable to move at all. Under normal conditions, mucus produced in the lungs is swept outward by the action of the cilia. When an individual is in the upright position, the bronchioles are in a vertical plane, and the mucus coats them in a fairly uniform manner. In the supine position, the bronchioles are predominantly in a horizontal plane, and the mucus tends to pool on the lower side as a result of the pull of gravity. The mucosa on the upper sides of the bronchioles tends to dry out, and the cilia are damaged by this drying. The cilia on the lower side are unable to move all the mucus that has become pooled. Thus several factors, namely, position, lack of ciliary action, and reduced respiratory excursion, contribute to statis of the respiratory secretions. The diameter of the bronchioles is reduced in the supine position, and this effect is intensified by the pooling of secretions within the bronchioles. Fig. 17-6 illustrates the effect of the pooled secretions on the size of the bronchiole.

The conditions just described predispose an individual to the development of hypostatic pneumonia or a mucous plug. Lack of deep

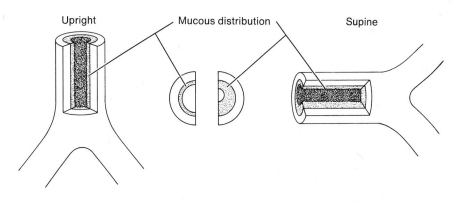

Effects on lumen diameter

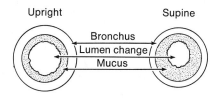

Fig. 17-6. Effect of recumbent position and gravity on distribution of respiratory tract secretions and diameter of bronchiolar lumen.

breathing can also result in atelectasis (see Chapter 8) due to "inspiratory failure." The pooled secretions provide a medium for bacterial growth, which may result in an inflammatory process, *pneumonia,* which is characterized by consolidation due to exudate filling the alveolar spaces. Hypoxemia occurs as a result of the shunting of pulmonary blood around a nonfunctional alveolus. Pneumonia can be caused by a variety of organisms, including the pneumococci, streptococci, staphylococci, various viruses, bacilli, and fungi, as well as by inspiration of food, vomit, or chemical agents. The signs and symptoms of pneumonia include dyspnea, fever, cough, pallor, malaise, and cyanosis if the hypoxemia is severe. In general they are the signs and symptoms of an acute inflammatory process in which the lung tissue is directly affected. Chest pain is often present and may indicate pleurisy. Inflammatory changes will be visible as hazy areas on the chest x-ray film. The color and consistency of the expectorated mucus will depend on the causative organism. Since the secretions pool in the dependent areas of the lung, it is in these areas that the infectious process will occur: namely, the lateral segment of the middle lobe, the apical segment of the lower lobe, and the axillary portions of the anterior and posterior segments.

As stated earlier, the persons most at risk are those who are totally unable to move or in whom ventilatory function is already impaired, mucus secretion is excessive, or the cough reflex is suppressed. Any combination of these factors would also predispose an individual to the development of respiratory problems. An example is the heavily sedated or anesthetized patient in whom the cough reflex is suppressed, respirations are depressed or rapid and shallow, the mucus is thick and tenacious, and the membranes of the upper respiratory tract are dry. These patients are prone to develop stasis of the respiratory tract secretions and hypostatic pneumonia. Poor posture in bed and the use of constrictive bandages or binders and clothing may also impair ventilatory function and cause these patients to be potentially more susceptible to the development of respiratory difficulties.

Venous thrombosis and pulmonary embolism. Venous thrombosis is another condition that the immobilized individual may develop and that contributes to the problem of impaired oxygenation processes. Basically the term *thrombosis* refers to a blood clot that has formed inside a blood vessel. The terms *thrombophlebitis* and *phlebothrombosis* are attempts to classify different types of venous thrombi by the initiating factor. Inflammation of the vein serves as the initiating factor in thrombophlebitis, while the thrombus itself serves as the initiating factor in phlebothrombosis, and an inflammatory response ensues. Clinically the effects are the same no matter what the sequence of events.

Because of the relatively slow flow of venous blood, veins are the most common site of thrombosis. A thrombus formed in slow moving blood is composed of layers of platelet aggregates (pale thrombus) alternating with a fibrin network containing leukocytes and red cells (red thrombus). This arrangement and the

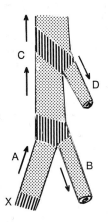

Fig. 17-7. Mode of extension of venous thrombosis. Thrombus occludes a small vein, *A,* at point *X,* and red thrombus (dotted areas) rapidly extends in stagnant column of blood up to entrance of next tributary, *B,* where platelet deposition forms a cap of pale thrombus (lined areas); when this occludes junction of *A* and *B,* red thrombus extends rapidly up to entrance of next tributary, *C,* and so on. Red thrombus also forms in each tributary as its entrance to major channel is occluded (arrows show direction of thrombosis). (From Muir's textbook of pathology, revised by J. R. Anderson, London, 1976, Edward Arnold [Publishers] Ltd.)

sequence of formation of a venous thrombus are illustrated in Fig. 17-7. It should also be noted that venous coagulation can spread the entire length of a vein.

Normally blood does not clot within the blood vessels; some abnormal condition or conditions must be present (see Chapter 5). Conditions that enhance the formation of thrombi include endothelial damage or changes in the vessel, venous stasis, and changes in the clotting tendency of the blood. Of these conditions, only venous stasis is directly influenced by immobility. Immobility contributes to venous stasis through loss of the pumping action of the muscles and by the very nature of the venous structure itself. Blood will pool in the direction of gravity; however, with activity and movement and the constant changing of body position, this pooling is reduced to a minimum. During inactivity it is enhanced in the dependent areas of the body. With a lack of muscular activity the pumping action that the muscles exert on the veins and that assists venous return is greatly diminished. The many bifurcations and valve pockets within the veins also contribute to localized areas of stasis during periods of immobility. This has been found to be even more pronounced in older people.

Venous stasis has not been found to be the sole cause of thrombus formation; however, stasis in combination with other factors may accelerate thrombus formation. Hypercoagulability due to an increase in the number and the adhesiveness of the platelets and a rise in the prothrombin time has been observed following trauma (accidental and surgical), childbirth, and myocardial infarction. These changes are maximal on the tenth day following the injury, which coincides with the time most thromboembolic episodes occur. Estimating the amount of endothelial damage in the veins that occurs as a result of immobility is extremely difficult if not impossible. Definitely some endothelial damage occurs when invasive treatment measures such as intravenous fluid therapy are used. These sites can serve as the point of initiation for thrombus formation. Whether endothelial damage occurs as a result of prolonged pressure on a vessel is a point of speculation.

Kinking of the vessel because of the position of the extremity may do more to create a disturbance of blood flow than to actually damage the intimal lining of the vessel. The turbulent flow that results may predispose to platelet deposition and hence thrombus formation.

The origin of thrombi in the immobilized, ill individual is probably multifactorial, with all the above mentioned conditons involved. Consider the postsurgical patient who is placed on his side with one leg on top of the other in the recovery room while still under the influence of an anesthetic agent. The fully alert, conscious patient would not tolerate the discomfort and would soon change position. The postsurgical patient cannot readily change position and may even be unaware of any discomfort from the position. Pressure points on the veins may cause venous stasis, and this situation in the presence of increased viscosity due to a postsurgical reduction in volume and hypercoagulability of the blood may accelerate thrombus formation in this patient.

Signs and symptoms of venous thrombosis depend on whether the pathologic changes occur in the superficial or deep veins. The clinical manifestations of a thrombus of a superficial vein include visible reddening of the affected vein and tenderness and hardness on palpation. A slight elevation in temperature and pulse rate occurs in response to the inflammatory process. Deep vein thrombosis following immobilization after surgery or during illness or bed rest usually occurs in the soleal veins of the calf. Local pain on compression of the calf may be the only symptom. If a major vein is involved and the thrombus is extensive, swelling of the leg because of the blocked venous return may occur. If the thrombus is not extensive, an increase in the circumference of the calf that is measurable but not necessarily visible may occur with redness, warmth, and tenderness in the affected area. The calf pain will be aggravated by movement, and *Homans' sign* (calf and popliteal pain upon dorsiflexion of the foot) is often present. There will also be the systemic manifestations of an inflammatory process: fever, leukocytosis, increased erythrocyte sedimentation rate, and an increased pulse rate.

Thrombus formation is a serious complication of immobility not just because of the disruption of venous circulation but also because of the potential danger of embolism. An embolism is the result of the thrombus or a portion of it detaching from the vein wall into the general circulation and becoming lodged in some other part of the circulation. The site of embolism secondary to thrombosis of the systemic veins is usually the pulmonary arteries and their branches, a condition referred to as *pulmonary embolism*, which can result in sudden death. Thrombosis of the veins of the lower extremities is the most common cause of pulmonary embolism.

The detachment of a thrombus from the wall of a vein may be the result of any number of activities that cause a sudden increase in venous return, for example, increased activity after a period of immobility, straining during a bowel movement, and isometric exercises. The straining associated with defecation, performance of isometric exercises, and even positioning oneself in bed cause what is called *Valsalva's ma-*

neuver, an attempt at forced expiration with the glottis closed. With closure of the glottis, intrathoracic pressure rises, causing a reduction in venous return and ventricular filling. During straining the cardiac output and arterial pressure fall, coronary filling is decreased, and the diameter of the femoral vein increases. With release of the glottis and the consequent drop in intrathoracic pressure, venous return will suddenly and maximally increase and arterial pressure will rise. This drastic change in the velocity of venous blood flow and the increased diameter of the femoral vein may facilitate a clot's becoming detached and passing into the circulation.

The clinical manifestations of pulmonary embolism depend on the size of the embolus and the portion of the pulmonary circulation that it occludes. A large embolus from the femoral or iliac trunk that occludes the pulmonary artery will cause sudden death preceded by a period of intense, severe dyspnea with cyanosis and gross neck vein distension. The effect is that of acute right-sided failure of the heart.

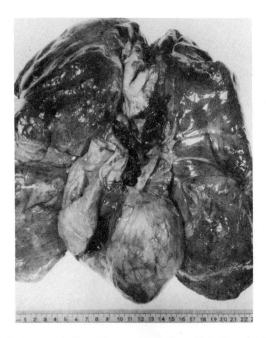

Fig. 17-8. Massive pulmonary embolism after postoperative phlebothrombosis in leg veins. Death occurred suddenly on sixth postoperative day. (From Anderson, W. A. D., and Kissane, J. M.: Pathology, ed. 7, St. Louis, 1977, The C. V. Mosby Co.)

Cardiac output and arterial pressure drop. Shock and loss of consciousness rapidly ensue as perfusion of the vital organs decreases. Death occurs within minutes to hours following the embolism (Fig. 17-8).

Smaller emboli can pass through the right side of the heart and pulmonary artery to become lodged in the branches of the pulmonary artery, which become progressively smaller. The patient may experience quite severe dyspnea of sudden onset. Chest pain may also be a complaint presenting in much the same way as that of a myocardial infarction. Other signs and symptoms will be the same as in right-sided heart failure because pulmonary vascular pressure and pulmonary resistance increase, and the right side of the heart can no longer pump out all the blood being returned to it. If the reduction in cardiac output is severe, signs of cerebral hypoxia may also appear: restlessness, confusion, or a change in the level of consciousness.

Infarction of pulmonary tissue may follow embolism, but because the bronchial arteries also supply the lungs, this rarely occurs. The clinical manifestations of infarction include tachycardia, tachypnea, chest pain, cough, hemoptysis, dyspnea, and a low-grade fever, and leukocytosis. Serum levels of the enzyme lactic dehydrogenase will be elevated, reflecting its loss from damaged tissue.

The treatment of pulmonary embolism is supportive since there is no cure for an embolism once it has occurred. Oxygen is administered to relieve hypoxemia and promote oxygenation of the tissues. Sedation may be used to relieve anxiety and promote rest, which in combination with absolute bed rest serves to reduce the work load of the heart and lungs. Vasopressor agents are used to restore normal arterial blood pressure if hypotension occurs since administration of large quantities of fluid is contraindicated due to the already existing state of heart failure. Anticoagulant therapy is initiated to prevent other thromboembolic episodes and extension of the already existing clot. Various surgical procedures can also be used for persons in whom anticoagulant therapy is contraindicated or who experience repeated episodes of embolization. Measures to prevent further thrombus formation in the lower extremities should be instituted to lessen the chances of recurrence.

• • •

It is apparent that delivery of oxygen to the tissues can be severely disrupted by several of the effects of immobility. The problem of impaired processes of oxygenation further retards restoration of normal levels of mobility since with less oxygen available, less energy will be available to meet the demands of increased activity.

Chemical disequilibrium

The effects of immobility that disrupt normal chemical equilibrium of the body include a negative calcium balance, a negative nitrogen balance, and a compartmental fluid shift in dependent areas. Calcium loss is promoted by the osteoporotic process induced by immobility. Calcium is released into the extracellular fluid as the bone is resorbed, and urinary excretion of calcium increases in order to maintain normal serum calcium concentrations during immobility. Hypercalcemia may result if immobility occurs in the presence of rapid bone turnover, that is, during growth periods or in the presence of Paget's disease. In these conditions the amount of calcium released due to the increased bone resorption of immobility exceeds the renal capacity for excretion. The renal excretion of calcium during periods of immobility has been found to be greater in men than in women. There is also impaired dietary absorption of calcium during immobility, causing increased fecal excretion. The combination of increased urinary and fecal excretion results in a negative calcium balance when the total amount excreted exceeds that taken in. Increasing the amount of calcium in the diet will have no effect on calcium balance since dietary absorption is impaired.

Deitrick's study demonstrated that urinary excretion of calcium began within the first week of immobility and reached a peak during the fourth to sixth weeks of immobility. The subjects in Deitrick's study lost between 1% and 2% of their body calcium during 6 weeks of immobility. It has been estimated that as much as 5% of the total body calcium may be lost in a young man who is immobilized for 3 months with a fractured femur. Urinary excretion of calcium is monitored not only because it is a sign of the degree of osteoporosis that occurs but also because this increased amount of calcium in the urine may negatively affect normal elimination processes.

The nitrogen balance provides a gross measure of protein utilization by the body. A *negative nitrogen balance* is said to exist when excretion of nitrogen due to the breakdown of protein exceeds intake. During periods of immobility urinary excretion of nitrogen increases to the extent that negative nitrogen balance results. Urinary excretion of nitrogen in healthy immobilized persons occurs on approximately the fifth or sixth day after immobilization. In certain disease states and as a result of trauma (surgical or accidental) and stress, protein is rapidly catabolized, and the potential for development of a negative nitrogen balance is great. Protein requirements will already be increased by these conditions, and immobility will compound this problem. Table 17-3 lists various pathologic conditions in which the protein requirements of the body are altered.

The loss of nitrogen is thought to reflect the depletion of muscle tissue as atrophy occurs. This is supported by the fact that the sulfur-nitrogen ratio of the urine remains unchanged during immobility, indicating that tissue rich in sulfur (e.g., skeletal muscle) is being broken down. Further contributing to the negative nitrogen balance that exists is the individual's decreased nutritional status. The decreased nutritional status and negative nitrogen balance also contribute to the loss of muscle mass and strength that occurs in immobility, and a vicious cycle ensues. Fig. 17-9 depicts the central role of anorexia in this vicious cycle.

The consequence of a state of negative nitrogen balance is a lack of adequate nitrogen for protein synthesis. With severe protein depletion the plasma protein concentration will decrease, although originally these proteins are spared.

Fluid shifts from the intravascular to the interstitial compartments in the dependent areas of the body as a result of the increased hydrostatic pressure secondary to venous stasis.

Table 17-3. Pathologic conditions altering protein requirements*

Condition	Increased	Decreased
Sepsis	X	
Fever	X	
Trauma—injury	X	
Fractures	X	
Burns	X	
Gastrointestinal disorders (ileostomy, colostomy, diarrhea and other malabsorption states, ulcerative colitis)	X	
Respiratory infections	X	
Parasitic infections	X	
Bacterial infections	X	
Viral infections	X	
Hepatic coma		X
Liver disease	X	
Massive hepatic necrosis		X
Proteinuria	X	
Renal disease (glomerulonephrosis)	X	
Renal failure, acute and chronic		X
Cancer	X	
Marasmus (protein-calorie malnutrition)	X	
Kwashiorkor (protein malnutrition)	X	
Pain	X	
Anxiety or other psychologic stress	X	
Profuse sweating	X	

*From Nutrition in clinical care by R. Howard and N. Herbold. Copyright 1978 McGraw-Hill Book Co. Used with permission of McGraw-Hill Book Co.

Blood will pool in the dependent areas of the body as a result of the cumulative effect of gravity, the reservoir nature of the veins, and the loss of pumping action of the muscles. As the volume of the pooled blood increases, the hydrostatic pressure of the blood at the venous end of the capillary bed will increase. An increase in the blood hydrostatic pressure will increase the hydrostatic pressure gradient, and when this gradient becomes higher than the osmotic pressure gradient, the Starling forces will be disrupted, favoring movement of fluid out of the intravascular compartment and preventing its return. Dependent edema results in any body parts on a level below that of the heart for any

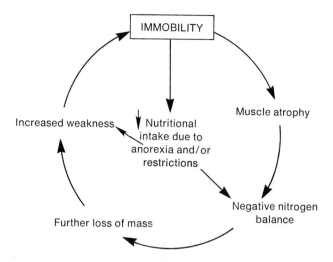

Fig. 17-9. Factors contributing to negative nitrogen balance of immobility and its contributory role, leading to further impairment of mobility.

period of time. Edematous tissue may be quite uncomfortable and is more easily injured. Edema of the lower extremities can make standing and walking extremely difficult, inhibiting mobility even more.

Disruption of normal elimination processes

Elimination from both the bladder and the bowel can be disrupted by the effects of immobility. Constipation is often seen in the ill person who is immobilized, but it is not a direct consequence of immobility per se. It is the result of weakened abdominal and perineal muscles and decreased gastric motility, which are the results of immobility. Decreased gastric motility also causes bloating and belching and may contribute to the feeling of anorexia that many immobilized individuals experience. Other factors probably also play a part in constipation. A change in diet, emotional stress, or some other change in activities of daily living can cause constipation in a well individual. The person experiencing illness and immobility is subject to any or all of these factors in addition to the effects of immobility. A person on bed rest in a hospital setting may experience difficulty using a bedpan since the anatomic position one must assume when using a bedpan does not allow maximal use of the muscles in the act of defecation. This person may be em-

barassed by the lack of privacy and may suppress the urge to defecate with the eventual result of constipation.

The supine position itself affects stimulation of the urge to defecate. Normally, as stool descends into the lower rectum, stimulation of the anorectal ring results in a desire to defecate. In the upright position this descent of fecal material is sudden, resulting in strong stimulation, whereas in the supine position, rectal filling is slow and stimulation is weak. Whether the urge to defecate is suppressed, weak, or nonexistent, the results are the same. The fecal material will continue to increase in size, and water will be reabsorbed, causing it to become hard. Defecation cannot occur at this point without a great deal of difficulty and discomfort. Straining at trying to pass a larger than normal, hardened mass of stool will cause a Valsalva maneuver, which is contraindicated in the immobilized individual for reasons already discussed.

Elimination from the bladder can be disrupted by renal calculi, retention of urine, and urinary tract infection. Like constipation these are not direct consequences of immobility per se but are the results of the high level of urinary calcium and the recumbent position seen in immobility. The formation of renal calculi or ''recumbency stones'' depends on several factors:

1. Urinary concentrations of calcium, citric acid, and phosphate
2. Ratio between the concentrations of calcium and citric acid in the urine
3. pH of the urine
4. Stasis of the urine
5. Presence of infection

Calcium is normally excreted in the urine and is kept in solution by the action of citric acid and the acidic condition of the urine. During periods of immobility, as a result of reduced metabolic activity, fewer acid products of metabolism are formed to be excreted, and the pH of the urine rises. Citric acid concentration remains the same as in the preimmobility period. The alkalinity of the urine and the altered ratio between citric acid and calcium concentrations favoring the calcium level enhances precipitation of calcium salts within the urine.

The recumbent position causes stasis of the urine in the renal pelvis as well as incomplete emptying of the bladder. In the supine position the effect of gravity causes urine to pool in the dependent calyces of the kidney. This is illustrated in Fig. 17-10. Stasis also favors precipitation of calcium salts out of solution in the urine. The effect of gravity in the upright position favors complete emptying of the bladder as well as the kidneys. Sometimes individuals are unable to void in a sitting or lying position, and retention of urine occurs. Retention can cause distension of the bladder to such a degree that small tears develop in the mucosa, providing a site for infection. Extreme fullness of the bladder can lead to dribbling of small amounts of urine; the bladder actually overflows. This is called retention with overflow. The presence of stagnant urine in the kidneys and bladder also increases the potential for infection. The presence of a urinary tract infection will even further enhance the conditions for renal stone formation; the urine becomes more alkaline, and the cellular debris from the inflammatory process provide nuclei for stone formation.

A reduction in the volume of the urine will also contribute to stone formation. When the individual first lies down, urinary volume will increase due to the increased blood flow to the kidneys. Urinary volume will decrease if fluid intake is reduced for any reason. This is an important point to remember for ill and bedridden persons. Often adequate amounts of fluid are not provided, and the person is unable to get his own. Sometimes there are stringent medical restrictions on the amount of fluid a person is allowed. In this case the quality of the fluid takes on special importance. Fluids and foods that will increase the acidity of the urine are recommended (acid-ash diet).

The signs and symptoms of renal calculi include hematuria, colicky flank pain, backache, and nausea and vomiting. Bloatedness, constipation, urinary retention or infection, and formation of renal calculi are very uncomfortable conditions that may lead to further reduction in the level of mobility.

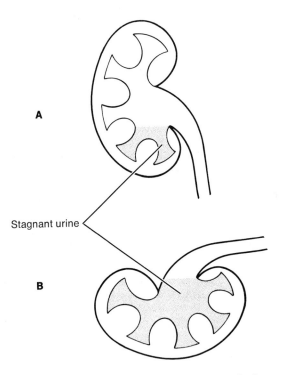

A

Stagnant urine

B

Fig. 17-10. Effect of position and gravity on distribution of urine in calyces of kidneys. **A,** Upright position. **B,** Recumbent (supine) position promotes stasis of urine in dependent calyces and inhibits complete emptying of urine.

Reduced integrity of integument

Reduced integrity of the integument is not seen in healthy immobilized individuals but is a serious and potentially devastating problem

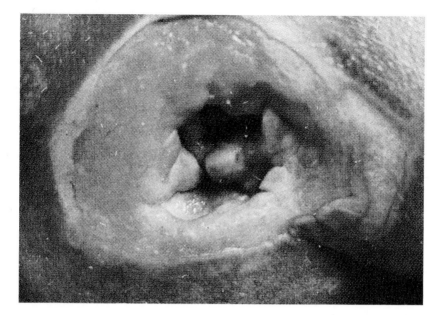

Fig. 17-11. Decubitus ulcer formation in debilitated patient. (From Beyers, M., and Dudas, S.: The clinical practice of medical surgical nursing, Boston, 1977, Little, Brown & Co.)

in the ill or debilitated individual. It is compounded by the presence of a negative nitrogen balance since tissue repair will be retarded as a result of it. Various terms are used to describe this problem: pressure sore, decubitus ulcer, or bedsore. These terms all refer to an open wound that results from prolonged pressure and friction on the skin and subcutaneous tissues due to immobility (Fig. 17-11).

The consequences of a pressure sore are increased susceptibility to infection, loss of body fluid, and further impairment of mobility. Any break in the skin will make an individual more susceptible to infection, since the skin constitutes the body's first line of defense. A pressure sore, especially a large one, may leak substantial quantities of body fluid containing protein and other constituents. A pressure sore may be extremely uncomfortable and may make turning and moving a person very difficult, thus contributing to further immobility.

Any person experiencing immobility in the presence of a pathologic process can be considered to be at risk for the development of a pressure sore, although in some persons the potential is greater than in others. Patients with impaired sensory input or motor function are

more predisposed to the develoment of pressure sores than are those who are on bed rest following surgery. Localized pressure areas can be created by external devices such as casts and traction apparatus and even catheters and tubing that exert a continuous pressure. Pressure is concentrated on the bony prominences of the body, and these areas are more likely to break down than others. There is less subcutaneous and fatty tissue in these areas, and the pressure becomes concentrated on these points rather than distributed and dissipated over larger areas of tissue; Fig. 17-12 illustrates the location of these points in various body positions. It is for this same reason that thin individuals are more susceptible to the development of pressure sores than are overweight individuals. Other factors that may be present and that can contribute to the formation of a pressure sore include edema, heat, negative nitrogen balance, lack of vitamin C, maceration (moistness and softening of the skin), anemia, circulatory disorders in which blood supply is reduced, and corticosteroid therapy (catabolism is increased). Age is another factor that must be considered. The incidence of pressure sores increases after age 65. Adolescent boys have

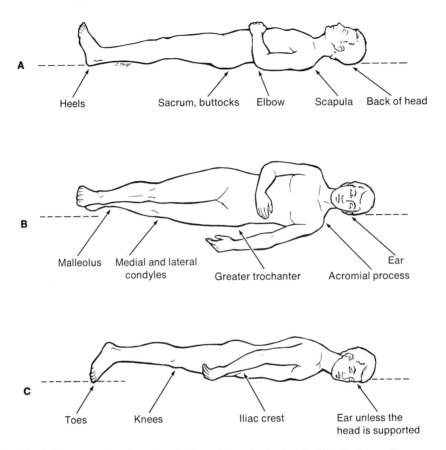

Fig. 17-12. Pressure points in various body positions. **A,** Supine. **B,** Side. **C,** Prone. These are positions at which pressure sores are most likely to form.

been found to be more susceptible to the development of pressure sores; this may be related to the intensity of the catabolic response to injury that they experience.

Another type of pressure that can contribute to pressure sore formation is *shearing force.* This kind of pressure is most frequently exerted when a patient is moved or repositioned in bed without being lifted or when he is allowed to slide down on the bed. The skin adheres to the exterior surface of the bed, and the various layers or subcutaneous tissue and even the bones slide with the direction of body movement. Blood vessels become kinked and damaged by this type of pressure.

Pressure prevents blood from being supplied to the tissues, which causes ischemic hypoxia. Waste materials will accumulate as the pressure prevents their removal also. The ischemic area

will initially appear as a white spot, which turns red as the pressure is relieved. A red spot that disappears quickly with relief of pressure and massage of the area to increase circulation indicates that no tissue damage has occurred. A red spot that does not disappear indicates hyperemia and the presence of tissue damage, that is, cell necrosis. When the superficial layer of skin becomes necrosed, the skin integrity will be broken.

The first sign of a deep pressure sore may be a small area of discoloration or tenderness or a hard lump. Development of deep-tissue pressure sores is often the result of shearing force because shearing force causes damage to the deeper tissues rather than the superficial tissues. A sinus tract may develop from the area of damage for the release of the products of tissue destruction. The first sign of damage in

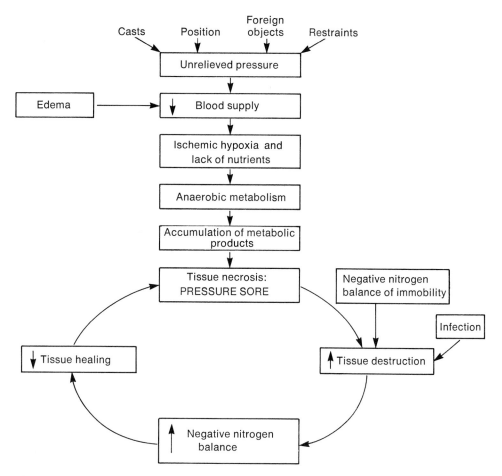

Fig. 17-13. Pathogenesis of pressure sore and resulting cycle once pressure sore has developed.

this case may be a small opening in the skin with the release of pus or serosanguineous drainage.

A pressure sore can form rapidly and once formed will continue to deteriorate rapidly. Since the cause of the damage is ischemia due to pressure, the duration of the pressure is an important variable. Obviously, the skin and subcutaneous tissue can tolerate some pressure before damage occurs, or sitting and lying would be impossible. The longer the pressure is exerted, the greater the degree of ischemia and the greater the chance that tissue damage will occur. Edematous tissue is more prone to pressure damage, since its blood supply is already impaired because of the disruption of pressures and forces in the capillary bed. For this reason the areas where dependent edema can occur in

the immobilized person must be closely observed. The presence of a negative nitrogen balance also contributes to the formation of a pressure sore. There are inadequate amounts of protein available to maintain the structural integrity of the tissues, thus facilitating the destruction of tissue, which in turn causes further reduction in the nitrogen balance.

The healing of a pressure sore occurs through second intention connective tissue repair because of the nature of the injury. This process is discussed in Chapter 4. Basically the site is filled with highly vascular granulation tissue over a matrix of fibrin. Eventually collagen fibrils are deposited, which serve as the basis for scar formation. Poor healing can be the result of many factors that may be at play due to the immobility. Lack of sufficient amounts

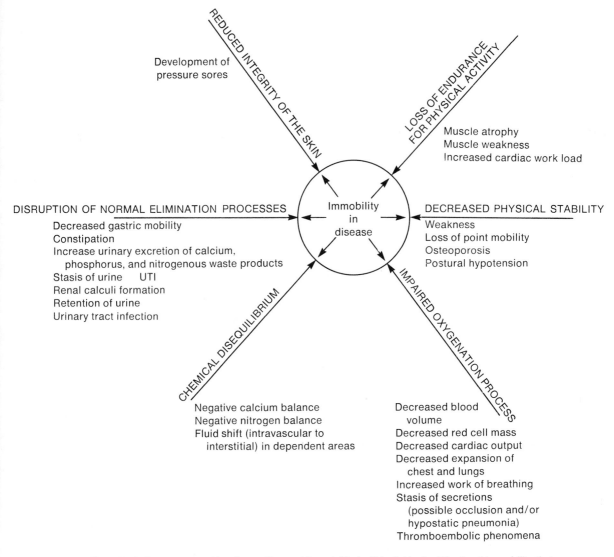

Fig. 17-14. Problems resulting from effects of immobility in ill individuals. Effects of immobility that contribute to each problem are listed. Arrows indicate reciprocal nature of immobility and problems.

of protein for tissue repair is a consequence of the negative nitrogen balance. Infection may occur, causing more tissue destruction and complicating the healing process. Continued pressure on the site will contribute to further damage. Lack of adequate amounts of vitamin C will impair collagen formation and slow healing. Fig. 17-13 illustrates the formation and perpetuation of a pressure sore. It is important to remember that once a pressure sore has formed, it is extremely difficult to treat. Prevention is the best treatment!

Summary

Each of the problems caused by the effects of immobility has the potential of reducing the level of mobility even further. The reciprocal relationship between the state of immobility and the problems it causes is illustrated in Fig. 17-14, which also summarizes the effects of immobility that contribute to each problem. It was stated earlier that no body system escapes the consequences of immobility. The effects of immobility as they affect the various systems of the body are summarized in Table 17-4.

Table 17-4. Systemic manifestations of immobility during convalescence

Circulatory	Gastrointestinal	Metabolic	Respiratory	Musculoskeletal	Genitourinary	Integument

↓Maximum cardiac output
↑Heart rate
Postural hypotension
Dependent edema
Thromboembolism
	Anorexia
	↓Gastric motility
	Belching
	Bloating
	Constipation (partially due to muscle weakness)
		↓BMR
		Negative nitrogen balance
			↓Excursion
			↓Diameter of airways
			Stasis of secretions → hypostatic pneumonia
			↑Work of breathing
				Muscles
				  Atrophy
				  Weakness
				  Shortening
				  ↓Elasticity of tendons and ligaments
				Joints
				  ↓Mobility
				  Contractures
				Skeletal
				  Osteoporosis
					↑Excretion of calcium (formation of urinary calculi)
					↑Urinary excretion of nitrogen
					↑Urinary excretion of phosphorus
					Stasis and retention of urine → urinary tract infection
						↑Susceptibility to breakdown (especially at pressure points and in edematous areas)

It must be remembered that, as an individual, each person will react to immobility in a different way. Not every individual who experiences immobility will experience all the potential problems just discussed or in the same way as others might. The extent of the problem depends on how long the immobility is left untreated. The severity of the effects is directly proportional to the duration and degree of the immobility; hence, a response to immobility in the form of treatment of both the duration and degree of the immobility is the limiting factor.

PHYSIOLOGY OF TREATMENT

Treatment of immobility must begin immediately if the degenerative changes that can occur are to be prevented. The effects of immobility are secondary to lack of use of the functional components of the motor system. The longer the immobility is left untreated, the more of these effects will occur, and some changes may become irreversible.

Lack of endurance and decreased physical stability can be prevented or at least minimized by range of motion exercises to all the joints while in bed, early ambulation and positional changes, and isotonic and isometric exercises. Weight-bearing activities will help decrease the amount of calcium lost by increasing bone deposition. The use of elastic stockings to prevent venous pooling in the extremities helps to prevent postural hypotension as well as thromboembolic phenomena. Deep-breathing exercises and change of position will prevent stasis of respiratory tract secretions and promote excursion of the respiratory muscles. Frequent position changes will also prevent stasis of urine and prolonged pressure on body parts. Use of a commode rather than a bedpan and provision of adequate amounts of fluid and roughage in the diet will promote normal elimination processes. The diet should also include high-protein food to improve the nitrogen balance and acid-ash foods to maintain the acidity of the urine. These are all relatively simple measures that can be taken to prevent the development of complications.

SUMMARY

Immobility is an important concept in the study of pathophysiology since some degree of immobility accompanies all illness and can have a significant effect on the progress and treatment of the disease entity. The effects of immobility may accelerate the pathophysiologic processes that are present. They may complicate the treatment of the disease and prolong the convalescent period. Certain consequences of immobility may even result in death.

An understanding of the effects of immobility and why they occur will lead to a greater understanding of how to prevent them. Even more important is the appreciation for the importance of preventing these effects that comes from this understanding.

SUGGESTED READINGS

Birkhead, H., Haupt, G., and Meyers, R.: Circulatory and metabolic effects of prolonged bed rest in healthy subjects, Fed. Proc. **22:**520, 1963.

Carnevali, D., and Brueckner, S.: Immobilization: reassessment of a concept, Am. J. Nurs. **70:**1502-1507, 1970.

Canda, K.: The hazards of bed rest, an unpublished paper, 1972.

Deitrick, J., Whedon, G., and Schorr, G.: Effects of immobilization upon various metabolic and physiologic functions of normal men, Am. J. Med. **4:**3-36, 1948.

Downs, F.: Bed rest and sensory disturbances, Am. J. Nurs. **74**(3):434-438, 1974.

Gosnell, D.: An assessment tool to identify pressure sores, Nurs. Res. **22:**55-59, Jan.-Feb. 1973.

Gruis, M., and Innes, B.: Assessment: essential to prevent pressure sores, Am. J. Nurs. **76**(11):1762-1764, 1976.

Kottke, F. J.: The effects of limitation of activity upon the human body, J.A.M.A. **196:**117-122, 1966.

Lerman, S., et al.: Parathyroid hormone and the hypercalcemia of immobilization, J. Clin. Endocrinol. Metab. **45**(3):425-428, 1977.

Lynch, T. N., Jensen, R. L., Stevens, P. M., et al.: Metabolic effects of prolonged bed rest: their modification by simulated attitude, Aerospace Med. **38:**10-20, 1967.

Mack, P., and LaChance, P.: Effects of recumbency and space flight on bone density, Am. J. Clin. Nutr. **20:** 1194-1205, 1967.

Reichel, J.: Pulmonary embolism, Med. Clin. North Am. **61**(6):1309-1318, Nov., 1977.

Ryback, R., Lewis, O., and Lessard, C.: Psychobiologic effects of prolonged bed rest (weightless) in young, healthy volunteers (study II), Aerospace Med. **42:**529-535, 1971.

Spencer, W., Vallbona, C., and Carter, R., Jr.: Physiologic concepts of immobilization, J. Phys. Med. Rehabil. **46:**89-100, 1965.

Taylor, H., Henschel, A., Brozek, J., and Keys, A.: Effects of bed rest on cardiovascular function and work performance, J. Appl. Physiol. **11:**223-239, 1949.

Verhonick, P., Lewis, D., and Goller, H.: Thermography in the study of decubitus ulcers, Nurs. Res. **21**(3):233-237, 1972.

Warren, R.: Osteoporosis, J. Oral Med. **32**(4):113-119, 1977.

William, A.: A study of factors contributing to skin breakdown, Nurs. Res. **21**(3):238-243, 1972.

Ziskind, M.: The acute bacterial pneumonias in the adult, Basics R.D. vol. 3, no. 2, 1974.

Zubek, J., Bayer, L., Mitstein, S., and Shepard, J.: Behavioral and physiologic changes during prolonged immobilization plus perceptual depravation, J. Abnorm. Psychol. **74:**230-236, 1969.

PART EIGHT

Pathophysiologic mechanisms in senescence

CHAPTER 18

Aging

AT THE COMPLETION OF THIS CHAPTER THE STUDENT WILL BE ABLE TO:

- Relate aging and death to energy, entropy, and the concept of humans as open systems in the steady state.
- Describe basic biologic characteristics of cells that make immortality unlikely.
- Discuss major theories of senescence and relate them to the physiologic changes observed in aging.
- Predict possible forms of future therapy for aging based on these theories.
- Describe factors that accelerate or delay aging and explain how these factors interfere with the normal pattern.
- Describe the general pattern of age-related changes that occur in all organ systems and discuss the various diseases of sensescence in relation to these general changes.
- Cite the abnormalities of function that occur during senescence and describe pathophysiologic patterns produced by these diseases.
- Describe progeria and list ways in which it resembles aging.
- Discuss the rationale for the current concepts of treatment of senescence and senescence-related problems.

It is perhaps appropriate that this textbook should close with a final chapter on the pathophysiology of aging, since this is the most universal pathophysiologic process. Yet it might have been equally appropriate to have begun this book with an aging chapter since aging is an ongoing development that begins as soon as or perhaps even before an ovum is fertilized. Aging is an irreversible, cumulative, predictable, universal process in all known multicellular living creatures. Senescence is part of the developmental process and must be viewed in that continuum. The rate at which it proceeds is species specific, and humans have the longest life span among the mammals. Within an individual, aging and death appear to be genetically programmed, at least according to the most popular theory of aging; that is, cellular DNA determines the rate and pattern of senescence that is unique to every person.

When systems theory is applied to the process of senescence and death, it can be seen that the elderly maintain a delicate steady state. Although many aged individuals claim to be well, over 30% of the people over 65 years of age have severe limitations on their function. Normal aging is accompanied by changes in such parameters as cardiac output, peripheral resistance, pulmonary function, and glomerular filtration rate, which in a young person would be considered signs of severe limiting disease. While the aged individual may maintain the steady state even in the presence of these functional impairments, a minor event such as a viral infection or a fall can set off a catastrophic chain of events that perpetuates positive feedbacks and pathophysiologic processes, leading to loss of the steady state and inability to restore equilibrium. Death occurs when entropy increases to such a degree that no new equilibrium can be reached.

Within the aging process are certain uniform

phenomena that characterize aging. Many other changes that can be associated with aging are symptomatic of disease in a younger person. Therefore, consideration of aging as both a normal and a disease process is valid. This leads to the question, "Is aging normal?" Is it intrinsic, or is it the result of exogenous factors that act on tissues and cells, causing them to undergo aging as we know it? To answer this question it is necessary to examine the normal pattern of senescence, both in general and in specific organs and tissues. We must also look to gerontologic research that is so active at the present time to answer basic questions about aging.

PATTERNS OF SENESCENCE

It will be recalled that cell death is a phenomenon that begins during embryogenesis and continues throughout the life of the organism. In no way can cell death per se be considered equivalent to the aging process. Cell death in many cell compartments results in cell renewal through differentiation of other cells. This has been well described in the gastrointestinal tract, epithelium, the hematopoietic series of cells, and the spermatozoa. Other compartments of cells do not renew at these rapid rates. Connective tissue, for example, has a slow turnover rate, and cell death in this compartment may lead to signs of aging, that is, a decrease in elasticity and increased cross-linkage of collagen fibrils. With aging there is a decrease not only in cell function but also in actual cell number, leading to atrophy of various tissues and organs. Connective tissue in general shows many more pathophysiologic signs of aging than does the epidermis of the skin, the lining of the gut, or the hematopoietic system, although all these systems are profoundly affected by senescence. Connective tissue also is ubiquitous, and therefore changes in this tissue will have far-reaching effects on organ function. The vasculature, for example, consists of tubes made patent by a lining of connective tissues, and therefore these vessels and the tissues they supply may be interfered with if the connective tissue becomes rigid and sclerosed.

The consideration that cell death is part of normal development and that rapid cell renewal systems are important in "saving" compartments of cells from senescence is verified by many studies. In terms of normal embryogenesis, cell necrosis is part of the normal development of organs and can be reversibly interfered with by transplantation of embryonic parts to other sites. This suggests that cell death is greatly influenced by environmental factors. Further support for this comes from research showing a hormonal reliance for cell death during embryogenesis, at least in some species. Environmental factors such as surrounding tissue, nervous supply, and hormones that have been shown to influence cell senescence and death are termed *epigenetic* factors. Much of the normal sequence of development both in the embryo and in the organism as it grows and matures appears to be genetically programmed. It is believed that there is tremendous redundancy in the genetic information contained in DNA and that only a small portion of the total DNA is switched on at any given time. The pattern of inactive and active DNA during embryogenesis, growth, and senescence makes up the program that ultimately determines both the quality and quantity of life. Epigenetic factors can influence the expression of this genetic program greatly by accelerating or slowing down senescence and death, such as by disease. Nevertheless, aging itself appears to be an irrevocable outcome of inherited genetic mechanisms. There is also evidence that the aging mechanism is extremely complex and subject to a time regulator or biological clock, which could be nervous, hormonal, or metabolic. For example, the hypothalamus has been suggested as the site that governs the aging rate of cells. Another possibility could be intrinsic to the aging cells themselves. As the cells age they accumulate mutations, which are not efficiently repaired. These mutations may themselves affect cell function, which then results in the changes associated with aging. Thus, the biological clock could be the irrevocable accumulation of mutations with time, which alters cells functions and causes deterioration.

In an attempt to determine whether genetic or epigenetic factors are most important in aging, cell cultures have been studied as model systems of aging. Maintenance of cell populations collected from animals at various stages in development has inevitably led to the same result. Cells in culture have a finite survival capability, and characteristic changes and declining reproductive capacity invariably occur. Another method of studying cell survival is by transplanting cells into young hosts and retransplanting the same cells into new young hosts when the original hosts age. These studies also show that there is a limitation on cell survival even in the most optimal environment. They indicate that there is a definite limit on the number of times a human cell can divide (about 50), and this limitation in turn determines the ultimate survival of the organism. It is interesting then to note that the number of population doublings of cultured normal embryo fibroblasts from the Galapagos tortoise is more than twice that of human fibroblasts under the same conditions. The Galapagos tortoise is the longest-lived organism, surviving for 175 years. This correlation would seem to indicate that there is a relationship between in vitro aging and in vivo aging, which is, of course, the central question in applying the results of laboratory studies to humans. Senescence is much more complex than aging of cells in vitro, with many interactions causing specific changes. Furthermore, different tissues age at different rates in the intact organism, and there is no question therefore that reduced division capability is only one part of the whole phenomenon of aging. It is interesting, however, to note that patients with *progeria* or *Werner's syndrome,* diseases perhaps associated with accelerated aging, have cells with reduced proliferative capacity.

With regard to the possibility of cellular immortality, it would appear that cells, particularly of a lymphoid line, that are grown in tissue culture and that appear not to age and die are cells that have undergone *carcinogenic transformation* (see Chapter 3). In other words, perhaps cell survival requires complete dedifferentiation and anaplasia, in a sense a return to an early evolutionary state. Indeed, the earliest cells in the course of evolution (and possibly modern unicellular organisms) must be considered ''immortal'' in that their reproduction was asexual, so no protoplasmic material was lost through cell necrosis. Death is the price that multicellular organisms pay for the pleasures of sexual reproduction.

One of the major cytopathologic changes observed in cells as they appear to age in cell culture is the accumulation of *lysosomes.* These cellular organelles are involved in inflammatory reactions and in autocatalysis, often being described as the digestive system or suicide bags of the cells. Not only do these structures increase in number, but their enzymatic contents change as well. Such changes are not observed in cell cultures that have been transformed and thus appear to be able to propagate indefinitely. Some of the normal lysosomal enzymes may be able to cause breaks in the chromosomes of cells, and the activity of these enzymes increases with the age of the cells. Thus, the lysosomal changes and accompanying enzymatic changes may share a cause-and-effect relationship with cellular senescence. Other observations regarding subcellular events that are associated with aging include an increase in the RNA accumulation with a decrease in RNA synthesis, an increase in the heterogeneity of the total cell population, and the striking capability of hydrocortisone to retard the aging process in tissue cultures.

Environmental factors in the cell culture situation can alter the pattern of senescence and death (e.g., hydrocortisone). Nutritional composition of the medium in which the cells are grown can affect the pattern of senescence, as can certain additives. However, characterizations of the additives, aged cell nutritional requirements, and effects of deprivation or excess are in a preliminary stage. The ultimate effect for diploid animal cells, regardless of their environment, is senescence and death. Thus, it would appear from many studies that at least in vitro cells are genetically programmed to age and die, and the environment can only act to alter the rate at which this inevitable process proceeds.

While cell cultures are relatively easy to maintain and study with regard to aging, the process of senescence in intact mammals is much more difficult to study. Such studies require that suitable experimental animals be studied throughout their life span in a single experimental design. Studies on rodents therefore last about 2 years, but larger animals such as monkeys and dogs require continual investigation, for as long as 12 years in dogs and 24 years in rhesus monkeys. The difficulty in maintaining large experimental and control groups is obvious. Therefore, most of the whole animal research in aging has been done with mice, rats, insects, and fish, and very little has been done with larger mammals with longer life spans. As always, the assumption that what is true for the rat must also be true for humans cannot be made with confidence.* Some studies of aging in humans have also been made, but they are not the longitudinal types of studies that are being done with laboratory animals. Nevertheless, such studies are extremely valuable, particularly when viewed in light of similar animal studies.

THEORIES OF AGING

Within the context of the approach of this chapter, which assumes that aging is a genetically determined rather than a solely environmentally determined process, several theories of aging are relevant.

Programmed theory

The programmed theory of aging implies that genes are turned on and off during the whole spectrum of development and that certain ''aging'' genes exist, which act to cause senescence. The mechanism of action for such genes is largely a matter for speculation, but possibly there could be errors in protein synthesis as the cell ages, with the eventual impairment of cell function. Such a situation would set up the classic positive-feedback pathophysiology that has been emphasized so often in this book. Accumulation of error-containing protein macromolecules themselves affects both intracellular and extracellular events in such a way as to further impair DNA transcription of RNA and RNA transcription of protein. Thus, the more errors that are made in the protein products of

the cell, the more enhanced and propagated is the initiating cause, namely, malfunctioning DNA. Of course, the inevitable result is death of the cell.

Another possibility supporting the programmed theory of aging is that DNA contains great redundancy of information and that mutations are continuously occurring in DNA. Furthermore, only a fraction of 1% of the DNA is active at any given time, the remainder being repressed. The redundant DNA information is called forth when changes or errors accumulate in the active genes. It is only when the mutations have caused such accumulated damage and no more reserve DNA is able to function that aging takes place. Such an accumulation is obviously time dependent and species specific, since the amount of linear sequencing and redundancy of DNA is characteristic of the species, with little variability among the species' members.

Further support for the programmed theory of aging comes from the suggestion that aging is the result of macromolecular effects due to repression of certain sequences of DNA, which code for certain sequences of ṘNA and then for certain proteins. Environmental accidents can be particularly damaging to such cells that have genetically programmed malfunctioning DNA codons, or errors in the transcription of DNA.

There is experimental support for all these hypotheses that support the programmed theory of aging. It is, nevertheless, difficult to explain why, in the evolutionary sense, DNA-directed, inevitable programmed aging came about. Presumably there must be some selective advantage for the species in the process of senescence and death. The most plausible explanation is that aging and death remove competition for food, sexual partners, and shelter for the young. This is, of course, epitomized by spawning salmon but is difficult to rationalize for other species, such as humans.

Stress theory

In contrast to the programmed theory of aging are other theories, such as the stress theory, which implicates epigenetic factors as most important in the pathogenesis of aging and death.

*George Sacher of Argonne National Laboratory has pointed out that if the data for carcinogenesis in rodents is applied unequivocally to humans, then humans should theoretically have 50 times the incidence of cancer than that which is observed.

Death is due then to the ultimate "wearing down" of the organism as a return to a thermodynamically more stable state. It is the result of accumulated wear and tear beyond the capacity of the organism to repair. Those compartments of cells that undergo rapid turnover and renewal are least affected by wear and tear, since the cells are short lived. Cells that do not turn over frequently or at all, such as connective tissue, muscle, and nerve, are most affected by stressors in the environment ultimately wearing down the organism. Thus, the stress theory of aging suggests that aging occurs in tissues with slow or no turnover and that these tissues indirectly damage other compartments of cells. The classic stages of the stress response were described in Chapter 6, namely, alarm, adaptation, and exhaustion. Thus, the stressed animal over the life span should enter the stage of exhaustion and decreased resistance to further stress.

Experimental evidence for this theory of aging is not convincing. The aged adrenal cortex can respond to stressors by secreting large amounts of corticosteroids, and the response is only slightly reduced as compared to young individuals. Furthermore, when the values are corrected for the decreased muscle mass in the aged one finds that the elderly can respond to stressors with great efficiency in terms of adrenocorticosteroid response. Of course, a physiologic decrease in corticosteroids in response to stress might occur if the target tissues of the hormones were unresponsive or refractory, regardless of the level of hormones in the blood. This has been suggested not only for the adrenocorticosteroids but also for thyroid hormone, insulin, epinephrine, vasopressin, ACTH, aldosterone, norepinephrine, gonadotropic hormone, and testosterone. Furthermore, in the rare syndrome of progeria, which is characterized by extraordinarily accelerated aging such that senescence and death occur in the early teens, there is a decreased tissue response to hormones generally. Of course, it is difficult to determine whether this tissue phenomenon is the cause or the effect of aging.

One important aspect of the stress theory is that exposure to stressors accelerates aging. This has been demonstrated for some but not all stressors and only when these stressors are continually applied. These include exposure to cold, repeated breeding, high altitude, radiation, and psychologic stress. Each individual, according to the theory, possesses a certain amount of *adaptation energy,* which is in part determined by his genetic makeup and in part by the degree of stress his body is subjected to. Certainly there is evidence that chronic stress plays a role in the pathogenesis of certain cardiovascular diseases, especially arteriosclerosis and myocardial infarctions, and the incidence of these conditions does increase with age. Whether this is due to decreased adaptation energy is not known, since, as mentioned earlier, the aged generally have a good adrenocorticosteroid response to stress. Thus, the role of stress in the aging process is not clear, but it would seem logical that the expression of genetically programmed sequential changes can be modified by the external environment, which includes many stressors that elicit the general adaptation syndrome. This in turn could ultimately lead to a stage of resistance and then exhaustion and act in positive-feedback pathophysiologic ways to enhance the expression of the genetic program.

Mutation theory

This theory correlates the aging process with irreparable mutations in the genetic material. Such mutations in somatic cells then lead to changes, which are characteristic of aging, in the cells and tissue. Mutations can lead to alterations in the structure, function, and absolute amount of enzymes produced by individual cells. There are many reports describing a loss in the enzymatic activity of cells as they age. Furthermore, the capacity to regulate enzymatic responses to hormonal stimulation is greatly depressed in the aged. Hormonal responsiveness has been particularly studied for insulin and corticosteroids. This changing ability to respond to hormones may reflect the biochemical pathology of the tissue resistance that has previously been mentioned with the stress theory of aging. Accumulated mutations could conceivably alter enzymatic responsiveness, but certainly other mechanisms are equally likely to do so. Radiation-induced life shortening is a phenomenon that may be correlated with mutations in critical tissues, which lead to secondary alterations in other tissues. Radiation senescence is not characteristic of normal aging, however, as the connective tissue does not appear to show an acceleration of the inelasticity and sclerosis normally found with age. While it is not questioned that humans, and all biologic organisms, accumulate genetic damage during their life spans and that gross chromosomal aberrations increase in frequency with age and may be associated with senile changes in behavior, it is still not clear if such changes are the actual cause of aging per se. Rather they could reflect inability to adequately repair damage, which in turn could be part of the intrinsic genetic program, which would dictate a loss in repair enzymes with age.

Free radical theory

Free radicals are reactive atoms or molecules with highly excited electrons. Such free radicals are therefore able to oxidatively attack certain molecules, such as lipids, which may undergo lipid peroxidation. Radiation certainly promotes the formation of peroxide free radicals, which are known to damage biologic membranes through oxidative attack of the membrane lipids. A decrease in enzymes that normally remove free radicals (e.g., peroxidase) may occur with age and may result in an increased concentration of these compounds. Free radicals can also be formed through the action of drugs and chemicals in the environment, and biologic systems can be protected from the attack of free radicals by chemicals known as *antioxidants*. Vitamin E and many food additives function this way. Vitamin E (α-tocopherol) is a normal constituent of most cells, where it appears to act as a scavenger for free radicals and thus to protect membranes and cytoplasmic organelles from peroxidation. Lipid peroxidation can lead to the formation of certain pigments, which have been identified with senescence. *Lipofuscin* is the most commonly deposited pigment in the nervous system, and its concentration there increases markedly with age. It has been suggested that an initial peroxidative event at cellular organelle membranes or enzymes occurs and is followed by cellular repair efforts. The cellular mechanism for repairing or removing the damaged structure is through the autophagocytic organelle, the lysosome. The lysosome is able to combine with cellular constituents, other membranes, and lipids and to form a structure that is then able to digest these structures. The great importance of lysosomes in brain physiology is apparent when one recalls that the neurons have no cell turnover at all and are therefore fixed and stable throughout the life span. Excellent reparative mechanisms must exist to ensure the functional and structural integrity of the nervous system. Lysosomes eventually become structures known as *residual bodies* when they have completed their hydrolytic autophagic digestion of whatever they originally combined with. Lipofuscin pigments, or age pigments, are in reality residual bodies formed from lysosomes that have reacted with peroxidated lipids, proteins, and other molecules. While there is no question that these pigments do accumulate in aging, it has not been conclusively established that they are harmful and that they in any way interfere with the cell function of the aged human neuron. Some investigators feel that the accumulation of lipofuscin pigments merely indicates that the neuronal reparative processes are functioning normally, and the innocent end product of this process is the lipofuscin residual body. It is certainly possible that the accumulation of these pigments with age aggravates pathologic damage caused by other agents of disease, and thus the aged's precarious steady state can be explained in light of such possible interactions. Much further research is required before the role of peroxidation and free radical formation, aging, lipofuscin pigment accumulation, and possible naturally occurring antioxidant defenses can be clearly described.

Slow virus infection theory

Since the advent of early electron microscopy the identification of viruses inside most cells has been considered evidence that many viruses may be present as passengers inside cells without causing pathologic damage. Further work has shown that some viruses present inside cells may be capable of remaining in either a latent state, which is subject to reactivation, or capable of producing a chronic subacute slow infection. Slow viruses have therefore been implicated as possible agents of aging. Their ubiquitous presence in all animals would lead to ultimate degeneration and disease of the infected cells, and thus senescence would be a viral infection with an ultimately fatal outcome. Another consideration that might be more meaningful would be that while not causative, slow viruses could nevertheless be involved in some of the degenerative changes that are associated with aging. Experimental backing for this possibility is found in the observations that certain slow virus infections of the central nervous system produce changes in the brain substance and vasculature that are extremely similar to the changes noted with normal senescence. The disease *kuru* is transmitted in primitive human tribes through the eating of infected nervous tissue of relatives as part of a mourning ritual. The agent is a slow virus that produces progressive brain degeneration. The symptoms develop insidiously, but once they are apparent, death usually occurs within 2 years. Another slow virus may be involved in Creutzfeldt-Jakob disease. These diseases have been transmitted experimentally from humans to chimpanzees and their viral nature proven. A number of other degenerative nervous system diseases have also been tentatively identified as caused by slow or latent viral infections. Some of these latent viruses have been successfully grown in tissue culture, and their cytopathic effects have been demonstrated in vitro. This may indicate that similar cellular damage occurs in their presence in vivo. It has been suggested that these latent viruses are normally present within human cells and that they are slowly activated with aging, resulting in chronic degenerative-tissue changes that characterize senescence. Silent viral infection is well described in humans for herpes simplex. Varicella (chickenpox) virus can cause herpes zoster lesions along sensory nerve roots in later life. Epstein-Barr virus, which has been implicated in the serious infectious response that occurs in some patients after open heart surgery with cardiac bypass or heart transplantation, is also considered to be silent or latent in many normal individuals. These viruses all can be reactivated under appropriate environmental conditions.

Herpes simplex can be reactivated by sunlight, radiation, trauma, and stress, causing the familiar coldsore, or fever blister. Herpes zoster causes the painful disease shingles, which also can be repeatedly reactivated by environmental stimuli. *Epstein-Barr virus,* the causative agent of infectious mononucleosis and Burkitt's lymphoma, is present in an apparently latent form in most human leukocytes but can be activated to pathogenicity by immune suppression. Rubella virus also can persist in human tissues without causing further apparent damage to the host, as observed in children with rubella syndrome. The same property has also been recently described for measles virus and for a papovavirus in a disease that is associated with immunosuppression, progressive multifocal leukoencephalitis. Thus, latent viruses do exist in human tissues and are capable of slow infection or reactivation. Their role in aging, however, remains to be discovered.

Autoimmune theory

Another theory of aging suggests that aging is an autoimmune disease, with the production of autoantibodies leading to cell damage and necrosis and producing the changes of senescence. There is evidence that autoantibodies increase with age, as does the incidence of known autoimmune disorders. Furthermore, the changes associated with autoimmune phenomena can be viewed as senescentlike changes. Also, if development, growth, and aging are all part of the same process, then the process of self-recognition that occurs in early life through poorly understood but probably ultimately genetic means could occur in reverse in senescence. Thymic involution occurs with age and may result in the organism's depending on IgM antibodies rather than IgG, with the result that autoimmune phenomena are more likely to occur in the absence of the more highly specific IgG. Both T cell–and B cell–mediated immunity decrease with age, and this is associated not only with autoimmune diseases but also with cancer and general susceptibility to infections. T suppressor cell function declines during senescence. There also appears to be a qualitative difference in the T cells between young and old animals. Implantation of old T cells into young mice results in a reversible state of immunodeficiency that is characteristic of the aged mice. This is perhaps one of the best pieces of evidence for cellular aging in vivo. It is thought that certain extrinsic factors may be involved in the development of autoimmunity with age. One such splenic factor is believed to cause the immune cells to respond less well to antigen. In light of this it is interesting to note that splenectomy has been one of the most effective life-lengthening measures in experimental animals.

Although certainly interesting and provocative, the autoimmune theory probably only will help explain some of the changes that are found in senescence, rather than identifying autoimmunity as the ultimate cause of aging.

EARLY CALORIC RESTRICTION AND DELAYED AGING

The most striking experimentally induced delay in aging and death in the laboratory rodent and in many other animals is caused by early restriction of food intake. This phenomenon was first demonstrated by McKay in 1939 and has been confirmed many times. The mode of action of early caloric restriction is obscure, but the absolute amount of food, the time of restriction, and the nature of the diet all appear to be important in determining the life-lengthening effect. The amount of protein, carbohydrate, and total calories varies in different studies and in different animals. Caloric restriction of about 60% of the normal intake in a diet relatively low in protein and high in carbohydrate fed ad libitum to rats in the postweaning period had the greatest effect. Calorie restriction to control the obesity that usually results in rats fed ad libitum was essential although not severe enough to interfere with sexual vigor and development. Absolute growth was decreased in these animals. They were generally more active, sleeker, and leaner and appeared much younger than control rats of the same age. The major effect of early caloric restriction on delayed senescence and death may be related to the absence of obesity in the animals, which acts to protect them from the diseases normally associated with advancing age in the rat. These include cardiovascular, muscular, renal, and

malignant diseases that appear to be similar to the diseases of old age in humans.

Another interesting possibility is that early caloric restriction inhibits potentially tumorogenic cells early in the growth period, so that ultimate carcinogenic transformation of these cells is delayed significantly. Rats (and people) do not die of old age per se but from the ravages of the many diseases that are associated with normal senescence. A major disease of the aged is cancer, and its incidence is increasing as the proportion of elderly individuals among the general population also increases. Malignancy in this population might well be correlated with obesity or accelerated growth during certain critical periods, either of which acts to promote or initiate carcinogenesis. In this regard it is interesting to note that calorie-restricted rats do not develop tumors with the same frequency as control rats. Furthermore, age and caloric intake in the rat are the two major determinants of ultimate tumor development during the rat's life span. The incidence of certain tumors can actually be predicted by the rat's weight at 70 days old.

The relationship of growth in the early stages of life to ultimate senescence and death are major areas of research at the present time. It does appear that rapid early growth is associated with a shorter life span. Among mammals, man has the longest growth and development period and the longest life span as well. Whether this relationship indicates a fundamental expression of the genetic sequencing and timing program is a matter for speculation. It is interesting to examine the theoretic life spans attainable for different species as measured in calories dissipated per gram of tissue. This would be in a sense a measure of the "living efficiency" of an organism. Data appear to indicate that caloric life span increases as the brain-body ratio increases, as well as with the length of the somatic growing period and brain maturation period.

It may be that early caloric restriction allows for ultimately more effective utilization of calories throughout the life span. The body in a sense "learns" to conserve energy very early during the critical growth periods. Critical periods for humans have not been defined, but the postweaning period in the laboratory animal seems to be the time at which restriction produces the greatest life lengthening. Prenatal restriction in all animals, including humans, sets up pathologic changes in the developing fetus (see Chapter 2). Immediate postnatal restriction as well is not effective. If it can be presumed that there is some degree of applicability of this work to humans it suggests that the prevention of childhood obesity carries with it the possibility of a healthier and longer life.

Other agents that have been shown to prolong life in experimental animals include immunosuppression, a germ-free environment, hypothermia, antioxidants, anti-cross-linking agents, prednisolone, and posterior pituitary extract. None of these agents are comparable or strikingly additive with the effects of early caloric restriction, however.

AGENTS THAT DECREASE LIFE SPAN
Radiation

Ionizing radiation has been reported to significantly shorten life span by accelerating aging. Part of this effect appears to be due to the carcinogenic effect of radiation, as tumors increase in incidence in irradiated populations of mice. Irradiation also causes increased body weight and fat deposition, conditions associated with premature onset of various diseases and early death. The types of pathologic lesions associated with irradiation include nephrosclerosis and infection. Single exposure of young mice to whole-body radiation produces essentially the same pattern as that produced by cumulative, spaced low doses. Whether these effects of radiation truly mimic natural aging or are the specific pathologic effects of radiation on cells and tissues is not known. As has been mentioned before, radiation does not cause certain characteristics of normal senescence such as connective tissue sclerosis and collagen cross-linking. It is doubtful that normal senescence can proceed without these phenomena, at least in humans.

Nutrition

It would seem logical that aging can be accelerated by a poor, unbalanced diet and retarded by a good diet. It has been difficult to verify this experimentally, however, no matter how logical it sounds. Certainly the relationship of obesity to various diseases associated with senescence (diabetes, cardiovascular disease) has been well demonstrated (see Chapter 12). The effects of early caloric restriction may in fact be due to the prevention of obesity. Even genetically obese rats, which have a very high incidence of disease and early senescence, can be made to live longer and are healthier when they are calorically restricted and their obesity prevented. Nevertheless, the composition of the diet itself in retarding aging appears to be dependent on the species and strains of animals, and no information is available for humans. The changes in dietary requirements throughout the life span are not well described, and essentially nothing is known about the changes that may occur in the requirements of the aged human. Table 18-1 shows the decrease in nutrient intake with age; only calcium is well below recommended allowances, but all nutrients decrease with age. Table 18-2 shows the recommended daily dietary allowances for older adults. Caloric allowance is decreased about 10% from that recommended for a mature adult. Other nutrients are not decreased, indicating that nutrient enrichment of diet per calories recommended should be carried out. Little experimental data exists on changing nutritional needs of the elderly.

It is believed that since general metabolism is decreased in the aged there is a need for fewer calories and vitamins. Certainly the aged eat less and at irregular intervals more than do the young or middle-aged adults. The social pressures associated with eating may change, however, with age and may account for these differences.

One concomitant of aging that essentially is universal over the age of 80 is *osteoporosis*. This process begins in middle adulthood and is most common in women. Some nutritionists believe that the osteoporotic process can be delayed by dietary factors before it has actually begun. According to a number of studies, bone density is significantly increased in vegetarians, but more work needs to be done to confirm these results. It is conceivable that a meat-rich diet can cause acid overloading, which is asso-

Table 18-1. Mean nutrient intake per day for men*

	Age in years			
	35-54	**55-64**	**65-74**	**75+**
Calories (kcal)	2,643	2,465	2,051	1,866
Protein (g)	107	99	82	72
Fat (g)	133	124	100	90
Carbohydrate (g)	244	228	204	191
Calcium (g)	0.77	0.70	0.67	0.60
Iron (mg)	16.9	16.2	13.4	1.3
Vitamin A (IU)	6,650	9,740	5,640	4,720
Thiamine (mg)	1.4	1.4	1.2	1.1
Ascorbic acid (mg)	75	78	67	54

*From U.S. Dept. of Agriculture, Household Food Consumption Survey, 1965-1966.

Table 18-2. Recommended dietary allowances for persons over 50 years*

	Women	Men
Calories (kcal)	1,800	2,400
Protein (g)	46	56
Vitamin A (IU)	4,000	5,000
Vitamin E (IU)	12	15
Ascorbic acid (mg)	45	45
Niacin (mg)	12	16
Riboflavin (mg)	1.1	1.5
Thiamine (mg)	1.0	1.2
Calcium (mg)	800	800
Iron (mg)	10	10

*From Recommended Dietary Allowances, 8th rev. ed., National Academy of Science, Washington, D.C., 1974.

ciated with a withdrawal of calcium from the bones. High-protein diets may also cause the same phenomenon. There is some evidence that osteoporosis can be partially prevented by water fluoridation, protein restriction, and increased calcium intake during childhood and early adulthood.

GENERAL CHANGES WITH AGE

Before the various changes that characterize senescence in the different organ systems are discussed, a general description of the structural and functional changes that occur with aging will be given.

Atrophy and involution

A general characteristic of aging is atrophy and involution of many structures. Accompanying these changes in size are also characteristic changes in function. The sexual organs involute markedly, particularly in women, a process that begins during the menopausal middle years. Accompanying the involution of these organs and glands is a decrease in the secondary sexual characteristics and a decline in sexual appetite. The body fat distribution changes in women, and the muscular bulk and strength decline markedly in men. One exception to the atrophy is the high incidence of prostatic hypertrophy that occurs in men as they age (see Chapter 3).

Other organ systems undergo involution as well. The incidence of obesity declines from its peak incidence during the middle years. Height diminishes on the average 2 inches due to kyphosis and thinning and softening of the cartilaginous intervertebral discs. Loss of pigmentation of the hair is a nearly universal characteristic, and the hair itself often becomes thin and sparse.

Sclerosis

Connective tissue throughout the body undergoes a process of hardening and loss of elasticity, leading to sclerosis. This may be marked in structures such as arteries, which are supported by connective tissue, and in the skin. The dermis rather than the epidermis is affected, giving the skin its characteristic wrinkled appearance. The sclerotic process appears to involve increased fibrous content of connective tissue as well as increased cross-linking of collagen molecules. As a result of this widespread process many organs and tissues can be affected. The contribution of this to the decline in function that accompanies senescence is difficult to measure but may be one of the major ways that secondary aging changes in tissues occur.

General organ function

While the aged person may be maintaining a steady state, it is done so in the presence of much functional decline. Thus, the steady state is precarious, and pathologic damage to one organ or organ system will therefore have far-reaching effects on other systems. Furthermore, the incidence of disease increases with age, and not only will this contribute to the senescent process, but in many cases it will also lead to death. The aged person thus is not able to cope effectively with environmental changes that induce loss of the steady state.

Some notable functional declines that occur with aging are in glomerular filtration rate, cardiac index, respiratory function, fluid and electrolyte balance, basal metabolic rate, nerve conduction, velocity, and memory. The aged person often has some sensory and motor deficits, and the special senses such as hearing and eyesight undergo diminution with age. There is an increased incidence of mental illness as well, much of which may go unreported and untreated due to the general tolerance of most cultures toward peculiar or deviant behavior in the elderly. Depression is extremely common, and the incidence of suicide among men is highest after age 75.

Common diseases of senescence

In senescence there is a tendency to develop infections more easily, and the immune system also is deficient and subject to pathologic alterations. The gastrointestinal tract is the most common area of complaint in the elderly, with constipation, diverticulosis, and gallstones extremely common. Diabetes mellitus increases with age (see Chapter 12). Cardiovascular disease is nearly universal, although its severity may vary among individuals. Malignancies increase in incidence in the aged population. Osteoarthritis and osteoporosis are considered normal pathologic changes that occur with age; they are nearly universal, causing severe disability. Chronic obstructive lung disease also is often present in the elderly.

Integumentary system

The skin is composed of a stratified epithelium separated by a basement membrane from a connective tissue dermis. The connective tissue is composed of fibroblasts, tissue cells, and fibers such as collagen, reticulin, and elastin.

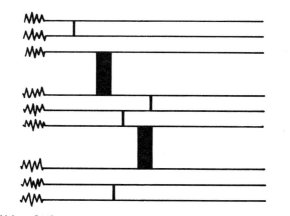

$$P-(CH_2)_3-CHO+NH_2-(CH_2)_4-P-P-(CH_2)_3-CH=N-(CH_2)_4-P$$

Fig. 18-1. Collagen cross-linkage. Collagen may be cross-linked intramolecularly as indicated by thin bands connecting protein strands or intermolecularly as shown by thick bands holding molecules of collagen together. This cross-linkage causes a rigidity of structure, leading to eventual sclerosis of all connective tissues. Nature of molecular bond formed by a common type of cross-linkage is indicated at bottom.

Collagen and elastin are proteins elaborated by the connective tissue cells and found in all connective tissues. The functions of connective tissues are related to transport, deposition of materials, and support. The nature of collagen is such that a variety of possible cross-linkages between collagen molecules can occur, thus altering the nature of the connective tissue. The collagen molecule is diagrammed in Fig. 18-1, and the nature of possible cross-linkage is indicated. Cross-linkage is not a pathologic process in all circumstances. It occurs in healthy human collagen under the influence of the tissue environment and various hormones. Thus, it is a phenomenon that can be regulated in response to the needs of the organism. One type of cross-linkage of collagen might facilitate transport of substances through the tissue matrix, whereas another might give the connective tissue more tensile strength and facilitate the supportive function.

Senescence is accompanied by an increase in the cross-linking of collagen molecules within the connective tissue throughout the body. Thus, molecular changes occur with aging of the organism. The collagenous fibers do not turn over very much and are of course not renewed by cell division. Therefore, they can accumulate errors with age, and repair of these errors obviously is not efficient. The types of cross-linkage that occur when collagen ages are conversion of intramolecular adol cross-links into stable cross-links of both an intramolecular and an intermolecular nature. The second type of linkage is that of the Schiff base type, which is formed as covalent bonding of the aldimine type. Cross-linkage of collagen confers more rigidity upon the connective tissue in which the collagen is found. Such cross-linked collagen is less soluble than normal collagen and physically stronger. It would appear that the association of collagen molecules in this manner is the most entropic and therefore most probable form, indicating a return of the connective tissue with age to the most thermodynamically stable state. The increase in collagen fiber formation is accompanied by an increase in elastin fiber formation as compared to the relative amount of connective tissue matrix. The hexosamine:collagen ratio is high-

est in the newborn and declines with age. It is also low in the chronically ill. Thus, with advancing age the amount of connective tissue ground substance and the number of cells decrease, while the collagen fiber formation, strength, and insolubility all increase. Calcium salts are also deposited in connective tissue with age, causing calcification. These changes cause the dermis of the skin to fold and buckle; the overlying epidermis also folds mechanically as the dermis changes. The epidermis itself undergoes very little change with age, being composed of a rapid turnover compartment of epithelial cells, which constantly desquamate and are replaced. It is believed that the epithelium has the potential to far outlive the organism itself. The skin does wrinkle with age, but this effect is entirely due to the dermal changes that have been described rather than to any properties of the epidermis.

The pigmentation of the skin changes with aging, and age spots (senile lentigo) are commonly found. The source of pigmentation in the human skin is melanocytes, which are under the influence of hormonal and environmental factors. Skin turgor is nearly universally lost to some degree, and the skin often has a lax appearance. The most common skin lesions associated with senescence are seborrheic keratosis characterized by irregular round or oval lesions that are brown and often warty, comedones (blackheads), dermatophytosis (a fungal infection), and dry, scaly skin. Nevi also occur often in the aged group. Cherry angiomas are commonly present, increasing in incidence after the third decade.

Musculoskeletal system

Bone and joints. Profound changes occur in the musculature and the skeleton, some of which have been alluded to previously. Bone is an extremely active and dynamic tissue. It is constantly undergoing remodeling according to the stresses put on it so as to serve its major function, *support*. The microstructure of bone consists of cells and mineralized matrix, which form a complex array of haversian canals and osteons. The matrix of the bone is mainly composed of calcium hydroxyapatite crystals, which form a latticelike structure. A portion of the calcium in bone is exchangeable with the blood; this is influenced by the activity of calcitonin and parathyroid hormone. This exchangeable pool of calcium diminishes with age, and thus the bone becomes demineralized, or less dense. The bone becomes brittle and is subject to fracture when stressed. Demineralized bone does not provide adequate support for musculature and viscera. Fibrous and fatty infiltration of the haversian canals contributes to the instability of the demineralized bone. The microvasculature of the bone also may be compromised by arteriosclerotic changes that occur with age, and this plays a role in the difficulty of bone healing that is common following fractures in the aged. Minute foci of necrosis and microfractures characterize the increasingly porous bone of old age.

Osteoclasts, which are giant resorptive bone cells that break down bone in preparation for new bone formation or growth and healing, are thought to be increased in number with senescence. Osteoclastic activity is also influenced by parathyroid hormone and is one mechanism by which calcium is removed from bone.

The initiating factors in osteoporosis are not known, although osteoporosis seems to be an intrinsic part of the aging program. There are several ways in which the rate of its development can be altered, some of which have been described. It has been suggested that somatotropin, gonadal insufficiency, and hyperactivity of the adrenal cortex all increase the rate of osteoporosis. The osteoporotic process appears to begin at the age of 40 and occasionally, especially in females, at the age of 30. Osteoporosis and bone atrophy and softening are all signs of senile changes.

Cartilage also changes with age, as evidenced by softening of the fibrocartilaginous intervertebral discs, which then may invade the bodies of the vertebrae, contributing to kyphosis and decrease in stature. The cartilage in general, like other connective tissues, becomes calcified with age, and bone may actually form in the cartilage of very old persons. Degeneration of the cartilage also accompanies calcification and therefore contributes to the decreased general elasticity of the skeleton. The articular cartilage is not spared these changes, and the joint capsules erode with age. As cartilage degenerates it appears that reparative efforts ensue, which result in bony overgrowth, causing "lipping" of the bone around the joint or the formation of bone spurs, which may project into the joint. Osteoarthritis is one of the most common disabling afflictions that occur normally with senescence. The joints themselves are hypertrophied, and there is a decreased flexibility, which leads to stiffness, pain, and limitations of motion. Crepitus, or noise in the joints upon movement, is common, and loose bodies (joint mice) may also be present.

Muscle. As do most structures, muscles atrophy with age. There is associated with this a loss of muscular strength and decreased capacity for muscular work. It should be recalled that muscle is a tissue with very slow or no turnover and thus may reflect aging changes more markedly than other tissue. The microstructure of the muscle changes with age, accumulating collagen and elastin fibers. The cells themselves lose nuclei, the myofibrils lose their striations, and cellular degeneration results in atrophy and replacement of muscle fibers with adipose and connective tissue. These changes may be prevented to some degree by exercise, nutrition, and genetic factors. The changes observed in muscle with age may be caused by a lack of activity and use of the muscles, as well as by the skeletal changes that also occur. A primary aging process in muscle seems likely as well, as hand grip strength declines markedly with age, although the use of the hand does not decrease with age.

Cardiovascular system

The myocardium, a muscle, is subject to the aging changes that have been described. Furthermore, it is composed of excitable cells capable of automaticity. Some studies indicate that ionic movement across the cardiac cell membrane is disrupted with aging of the myocardium. Fatty and connective tissue infiltration, degeneration and atrophy of individual fibers, and accumulation of lipofuscin pigments in the heart all occur with aging. These changes in the heart muscle are accompanied by senile changes in the epicardium and valves of the heart and in the conduction system. The endocardium thickens diffusely in the left atrium, causing left atrial hypertrophy. The other chambers of the heart undergo some hypertrophy, fatty infiltration, and sclerosis. The valves become thickened and fibrotic with advancing age, and the mitral valve in particular is subject to some degree of calcification. There are increases in the elastic fiber content and fat in the nodes and conduction system of the heart. It can be seen then that there are macroscopic and microscopic changes in the heart that must cause some derangement of function and also increase the susceptibility of the heart to injury under circumstances such as hypoxia or infarction. Furthermore, it has been demonstrated that coronary flow is decreased significantly in the aged, and the older animal does not appear as able to increase oxygen extraction during hypoxia as does the younger animal.

Other physiologic parameters of cardiac function decrease with age. The length-tension relationship, which is the basis of the Frank-Starling mechanism and by which stroke volume is determined through end diastolic volume, is disturbed in the elderly. The stiffer ventricle has a higher filling pressure, or left ventricular end diastolic pressure, than does the younger ventricle. Therefore, sudden stress in the older animal, which would require operation of the Frank-Starling mechanism, results in the maintenance of a higher left ventricular pressure for a longer period of time, thus contributing to an elevated end diastolic pressure. This in turn can contribute to congestive heart failure and pulmonary edema.

Another parameter that changes with age is the duration of isometric relaxation and contraction in the older heart. These alterations may reflect intrinsic changes in contractile properties with age or may be due to catecholamine depletion or decreased calcium removal from the actin and myosin of the myofibrils. When the heart rate increases for various reasons, the effects of prolonged relaxation and contraction could compromise ventricular filling such that incomplete relaxation occurs between contractions, causing higher left ventricular end diastolic pressure and higher pulmonary venous pressure, contributing again to the development of pulmonary edema and congestive heart failure.

Cardiac output may decline to half of normal by age 80; if this is expressed as cardiac index (liter/min./m^2), total cardiac function declines with declining cardiac output.

The vascular system is also profoundly affected by the aging process. Thus, the heart must pump blood through sclerotic vessels, and the total peripheral resistance increases as a function of age so that some degree of hypertension is considered a normal concomitant of senescence. There have been many studies done on the incidence of atherosclerosis with age and the influence of factors such as obesity, diet, activity, and habits. These have been discussed elsewhere in this book as also has the basic process of atherosclerosis. Atherosclerosis is the most important cause of arteriosclerosis, and although atherosclerosis is multifactorial in its determination, age appears to be the most common cause.

While many authorities consider atherosclerosis to be a multifactorial group of diseases, the pathophysiologic changes that occur with age in various arteries in the body must be examined in terms of senescent changes, since the process of atherosclerosis appears to be directly influenced by life span. The atherosclerotic process appears to preferentially involve certain parts of the arterial tree more frequently than others (e.g., coronary arteries, arterial branches, and the distal abdominal aorta). It appears that there are intrinsic properties of these vessel walls that predispose them to atherosclerotic plaque formation. It is conceivable that senescent changes in the arterial walls themselves may lead to plaque formation. It has been suggested that an initial lesion must occur before the atherosclerotic plaque formation ensues, namely, a myointimal cellular proliferation. This cellular proliferation may occur as the result of a number of possible processes, including endothelial injury and platelet factors, neoplastic changes in the arterial wall, and clonal senescence. Clonal senescence might occur as part of normal aging in which a clone of intimal smooth muscle cells has a limited life span and therefore undergoes an irreversible aging process, leading to decreased replicative ability.

Some experiments have been described in which cell cultures of various segments of the arterial tree were shown to have a diminished capacity for replication with age of the donor animal. This indicates that intrinsic aging of the smooth muscle cells of the arterial walls may occur. When the differentiated cells are not replaced adequately, the feedback regulation of cellular division is interrupted. This causes a compensatory proliferation at sites where the cells have aged and have not been replaced by differentiated cells from the intimal, smooth-muscle, stem-cell compartment. Cells stimulated to replace the aged differentiated cells are atypical and produce the early myointimal lesions that are the forerunners of atherosclerotic plaque formation.

Other explanations for intimal proliferation are possible, an important one being the effects of endothelial injury and platelet activation on the development of early lesions. Certainly it is conceivable that both processes can contribute to the development of atherosclerosis with aging.

There are other changes in vessels that commonly occur with senescence. Connective tissue aging leads to hardening and loss of elasticity of the tissue. Blood vessels have a fibrous wall of connective tissue, containing ground substance, collagen and elastic fibers, and fibroblasts. With aging this tissue is subject to sclerosis, which leads to narrowing of the vessel lumen and increased rigidity and resistance to blood flow. The increase in collagen fiber deposition and cross-linkage as well as calcium deposition that occurs in the dermis may also be observed in the blood vessels. It is a change that is noninflammatory and not necessarily associated with atherosclerotic plaque formation. Obviously these connective tissue changes that occur with senescence can lead to a number of pathophysiologic processes, a prime one being tissue hypoxia, the effects of which may be quite profound. The brain function depends greatly on oxygenation, and senile vascular changes can lead to microfoci of tissue ischemia, or in the case of large vessel atherosclerosis, large areas of infarction with brain tissue necrosis. Thus, the effects of hypoxia with age-related vessel changes may be minor, such as memory lapses, or profound, such as paralysis, coma, and death. Other tissues are subject to hypoxia, most particularly the renal, hepatic,

and splanchnic beds. Indeed, when the decreasing cardiac output distribution of the aged is examined, it is apparent that the cerebral, coronary, and muscular blood flow are all maximally maintained at the expense of the visceral circulation. In fact, with advancing age it may be that the cerebral circulation receives a proportionately greater percentage of the cardiac output than in the younger person.

There is abundant evidence that cardiovascular decline with age is associated with intellectual impairment. The effects of cardiovascular disease appear to act together with the intrinsic aging changes in the nervous system.

Another pathophysiologic consequence of the age-related vascular changes is the development of some degree of hypertension (blood pressure greater than 140/90 mm Hg) with age. Thus, with each year of aging the peripheral resistance has been reported to increase 1%. Blood pressure elevation with age occurs in men in response to the rising peripheral resistance. Both systolic and diastolic pressures increase up to the age of 60, at which point the systolic pressure increases and the diastolic pressure actually may decrease. Women generally have both higher systolic and diastolic pressures than men by the age of 70. The possible pathophysiologic consequences of hypertension have been described in Chapter 9.

Respiratory system

The bronchial tree and lungs undergo changes with age that result not only in decreased respiratory function but also in chronic obstructive lung disease (COLD) such as emphysema. The connective tissue of the bronchial tree undergoes characteristic age-related changes, and the lungs themselves also develop changes that are emphysematous in nature but that may not be correlated with the clinical signs and symptoms of COLD. The alveoli are often enlarged and the bronchial ducts dilated. The enlargement of the alveoli appears to be due to weakening and stretching of the alveolar septal membranes, which have the tendency to rupture. When this occurs the membranes of the ruptured alveolus immediately fuse to an adjacent alveolus, thus preventing the escape of air into the intrapleural space. Furthermore, the adjacent alveolar membrane may also be stretched and may rupture. The two fused alveoli then form a new alveolar sac. This dilation, rupture, and fusion are processes that can be considered emphysematous. Corresponding to the alveolar changes are capillary defects. The acinar capillary network may become crowded and disorganized. Thus, not only is the integrity of the alveoli decreased by the aging process, but the gas exchange capabilities of the alveolocapillary membrane may be severely limited. Such changes would contribute to the decreased vital capacity, Pa_{O_2}, and maximum breathing capacity, and to the increased residual volume that are all associated with old age. Also important in the pathophysiology of these phenomena are the changes in the thoracic cage that occur with senescence. There is a reduction in thoracic cage volume due to kyphosis and osteoporotic changes in the vertebral column and ribs.

The respiratory alterations that are normal in old age increase the elderly's susceptibility to severe pathophysiology when infections, stresses, and cardiac problems develop. The steady state is precarious at best in old age, and a minor pulmonary infection may set off a variety of responses that can lead to eventual pulmonary hypertension, respiratory failure, and cardiac decompensation.

Genitourinary system

As explained previously, the renal circulatory perfusion is decreased during the aging process, and glomerular filtration rate and kidney function both decline. There is a steady loss of nephrons from the kidneys, which begins at the age of 40, such that by 75 years of age only 60% of the nephrons are left. This may predispose the kidney to development of disease, which does occur with increased incidence in the aged. The aged kidney is not able to concentrate urine as effectively and is also less sensitive to the action of ADH. The kidney is able to maintain acid-base and fluid-electrolyte balance under normal circumstances, but these functions may be impaired in the aged kidney during stress. The kidney changes during senescence may be caused by infection or vascular disease. Many elderly people have significant pyuria in the absence of any clinical signs of

pyelitis. Furthermore, the vascular changes in aging result in decreased renal plasma flow, decreased kidney perfusion, and often afferent arteriolar atrophy. It is possible also that renal senescence is intrinsic to the kidney cells, being accelerated or retarded by environmental factors. The process of renal senescence is difficult to evaluate as it does not occur in germ-free rats. Therefore, the relative contribution of latent infection and arteriosclerosis in the aged must be further assessed.

The kidneys may also be implicated in the pathogenesis of hypertension (see Chapter 9), and both nephrosclerosis and hypertension are increased in incidence during senescence. The loss of nephrons with age and the declining kidney function are situations in which environmental factors may again act as a threat to the steady state in that the kidney's normal excretory, acidification, and base conservation processes are inadequate when the organism is severely stressed. Thus, if heart failure and compensatory vasoconstriction occurred, resultant renal ischemia could have a more profound effect in the older person, and renal failure would be the more likely 'sequela in the aged.

The reproductive systems of both the male and female undergo involution. It appears that the ovaries and the testes are affected by hormones, but whether their aging process is through intrinsic primary degeneration or by refractoriness to the hormones that stimulate them is not known.

Male reproductive system. Although atrophic changes occur throughout the male reproductive system and are often accompanied by degeneration, pigment deposition, and fibrosis, the capacity to produce viable sperm is retained in many men over the age of 60.

Nevertheless, many men do gradually lose sexual drive and capacity to produce viable sperm. Hormonal influences on male reproductive tract senescence have not been studied in detail, but it has been suggested that the senile hypothalamus in both men and women may play the most important role in determining the aging process, through the hypothalamic-hypophyseal-gonadotropic hormones. Testosterone levels decline progressively after the age of 50.

The cause of prostatic hypertrophy is not known other than that it is definitely linked to the aging process. It appears that the connective tissue component of the prostate is affected primarily, and this in turn causes the glandular epithelium to undergo morphologic changes.

Female reproductive system. The remarkable changes that occur in the structures of the female reproductive system throughout the life span have been the subject of much research. The cyclic 28-day cycle of the uterus occurs in most women for about 30 years and then becomes irregular, finally ceasing during the female climacteric or menopause. The ovarian hormones no longer are produced in sufficient quantities, and women at menopause begin to show signs of senescent pathology such as atherosclerosis and osteoporosis. It ap-

pears that estrogen protects women from these processes in the premenopausal period.

It had previously been thought that the determining factor in the timing of the menopause was the final loss of all ova from the ovaries through the repeated cyclic ovulation of the menstrual period. Thus, the ovary was considered to age by primary means, having an inherent biological clock, the timekeeper for which was the total number of viable ova. There are still many proponents of this theory. Others, however, believe that the ovary itself is theoretically capable of function long after the time of menopause but that hormonal factors influence its activity and result in its aging. The hypothalamus has been implicated as the major regulator of all endocrine activities and the site of the human biological aging clock

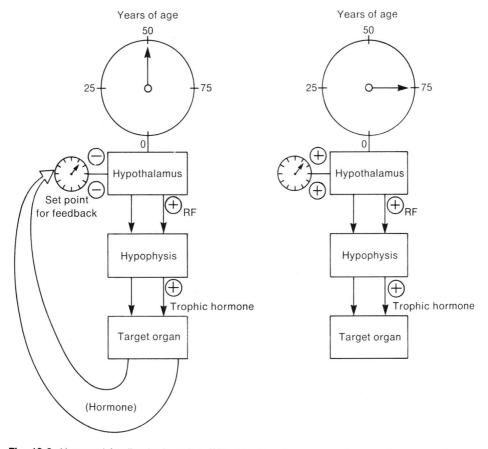

Fig. 18-2. Hormonal feedbacks in aging. With age, target organs such as ovaries can no longer produce hormones when stimulated. This leads to loss of negative-feedback inhibition on tropic hormone source, resulting in continuous outpouring of tropin, which has no effect on target gland. RF = releasing factor.

through its own intrinsic senescence. Its mode of action might be the development of decreased sensitivity to circulating steroids with aging, such that its regulatory functions on hormonal production become progressively disturbed.

A further effect would be glandular hyperactivity, since the negative-feedback system is operating at a higher set point or threshold to the gland product. While the steady state is thus maintained, an imbalanced internal environment can easily be provoked by secondary factors that set up pathophysiologic mechanisms, which result in age-associated changes in many organ systems.

Whatever mechanism is responsible, at about the age of 50 the ovaries begin to atrophy, produce less and less estrogen, and the uterus also involutes, with the cessation of menstruation and loss of fertility. Corresponding to the fall in estrogen secretion is a rise in pituitary gonadotropin release. This is seen as the result of the loss of negative-feedback inhibition of estrogens on pituitary gonadotropin production and release. Both FSH and LH are elevated throughout the postmenopausal period. With regard to the theory of hypothalamic elevation of threshold to feedback inhibition, the female menopause would occur by the following mechanism. The hypothalamus becomes less sensitive to the negative-feedback inhibition of estrogen on releasing factor for FSH and LH. This is determined by some sort of genetic program in the cells of the hypothalamus. As a result the hypothalamus produces FSH and LH, which act to stimulate the ovaries. The hypersecretion process eventually results in exhaustion of ovarian capacity to produce estrogen and permit ovulation. This is diagramed in Fig. 18-2.

When the menopause becomes established, a variety of changes occur, most of which are partially preventable by the administration of estrogen preparations. The estrogens do not, however, retard the basic aging process. Furthermore, the use of these hormones in postmenopausal women is controversial in the light of new evidence that they may be carcinogenic at this period of life.

The atrophic changes that occur after meno-pause in the female reproductive tract may cause problems. Thinning of the vaginal membrane appears to predispose elderly woman to chronic infection, and the vulva and vagina may be extremely irritable. Estrogen administration may result in alleviation of these problems through promotion of vaginal wall hypertrophy.

Endocrine system

The interaction of the hypothalamic-hypophyseal-hormonal circuit has previously been alluded to, and it has been speculated that the same type of mechanism, that of elevated threshold to feedback inhibition, may operate at all levels of endocrine function and cause the secondary changes of senescence in target organs.

Metabolism is intimately regulated by hormonal influences. It can be generally said that anabolic processes predominate during the growth and developmental periods and that catabolic processes predominate during the maturation and senescent periods. The environment in which a tissue functions is also closely correlated to hormonal influences, and it is reasonable to therefore suggest that the endocrine system, by altering the tissue environment and the net catabolism of the organism, may serve as the ultimate timekeeper or biological clock, determining the rate of senescence of the various tissues. It is also reasonable to suggest that certain critical tissues are most affected by these endocrine mechanisms and thus show senescence as a primary phenomenon. These tissues then can exert a great variety of effects on other tissues, causing them to undergo a secondary or induced senescence.

Adrenocorticosteroids. No consistent changes in plasma cortisol occur with aging, and in fact the aged appear to have an adequate adrenocorticosteroid response to stress. However, it has been suggested that target organs of the steroids are less sensitive to the actions of these hormones.

According to Selye's stress-adaptation theory, chronic stress in an individual eventually leads to a stage of exhaustion, in which further stress cannot be tolerated due to ultimate depletion of the adrenocorticosteroid reserves. This has been considered equivalent to a process in which "adaptation energy" is decreased by constant stress. The life process is accompanied by many stresses, and theoretically aging may occur as the adaptation energy stores are depleted. Primarily implicated in the loss of "adaptation energy" are the catatoxic steroids (see Chapter 6), which may normally function in a protective manner and which may become deranged in senescence.

Thyroid hormone. Thyroxin, triiodothyronine, and thyrocalcitonin are hormones released by the thyroid. The first two act to stimulate metabolism, and the third acts on calcium and phosphate metabolism. The thyroid gland atrophies during senescence as do many organs and glands. Thyroid function also declines with age, which may be due to a decreased need for the hormone by the aged tissues. Basal metabolic rate (BMR) is decreased in the elderly, and some of the normal senescent changes in a sense mimic hypothyroidism, although a cause and effect relationship between these signs and hypothyroidism in the aged has not been shown. In fact, myxedema in the aged can be successfully treated with thyroid hormones. It would appear, however, that in times of stress such as with an acute febrile illness the thyroid gland is able to respond equally well in the old individual as in the young. Thus, the gland itself does not appear to be functionally impaired in senescence, but rather the peripheral utilization of the hormone by target tissues is depressed in the aging process.

Pituitary hormones. The pituitary gland undergoes atrophy and senile degenerative changes with age. It appears that some depression of function is likely. It has been suggested that growth hormone secretion decreases during senescence. Administration of growth hormone to young animals may result in prolongation of life, but this effect is not observed in older animals. It will be recalled that this hormone increases anabolic pathways of metabolism in many tissues, including bone, muscle, and liver. Excess growth hormone results in giantism in humans, and many pathologic growth processes appear to be accelerated by excess growth hormone in the laboratory animals. These include nephrosclerosis, periarteritis

nodosa and hypertension, and various malignancies, all diseases associated with senescence.

ACTH release from the hypophysis does not appear to decrease with age, and TSH release as well appears to remain normal or actually increase with age. Gonadotropin output is increased after menopause, and this also occurs to a slight degree in men. The pituitary gland itself then appears capable of producing hormones throughout the life span. In general the pituitary production of hormones does not seem to be a major cause or accompaniment of aging.

Tissue sensitivity. Target tissues of hormones may become less and less sensitive to the hormones with advancing age. The hormone production occurs therefore at a high rate, and the target tissue begins to show signs of pathologic changes due to the relative lack of the hormone, which may be manifested as age-related diseases or as merely normal senescent processes. Much experimental research has indicated the validity of this concept, but conclusive evidence for most tissues is still lacking.

One intriguing theory related to tissue unresponsiveness to hormonal stimulation with age is related to the increasing calcification of many soft tissues with senescence. Calcium also appears to accumulate in the cell membranes and might interfere in many ways with membrane function and membrane receptors, such as those that are believed to exist for hormone interactions. Increased membrane calcium may interfere with the adenyl cyclase system, which is involved in producing cyclic AMP, the second messenger for many hormone-mediated responses. Calcium in the membrane may inhibit the rate of turnover of membrane lipoproteins and thus favor the accumulation of alterations in the membrane such that the membrane "ages" and the tissue is also adversely affected.

Another possible mechanism for tissue unresponsiveness might be the actual effect of the hormones that act on the tissue over a period of many years. Thus, repeated stimulation of the target tissue by the hormone produces changes that accumulate with age and cause signs of senescence.

Digestive system

The digestive system above all others appears to cause disturbing problems in the elderly. Splanchnic bed hypoxia may occur in the arteriosclerotic process that accompanies aging, as it does in the kidney. Therefore, the gut, like the kidney, is a common site for age-related pathology. By far the most common complaint of the elderly is constipation, but it is difficult to ascertain if this results from primary GI tract atony, from the decreased mobility of the aged, or from the repetitive utilization of laxatives, which ultimately damage the bowel's capability to perform the defecation reflex.

The salivary glands' activity is decreased in the elderly, accounting for the dryness of the mouth and mucous membranes. The muscular atrophy of the chewing and swallowing muscles and the usual lack of teeth impair the elderly's ability to eat, and this of course may contribute significantly to the poor nutrition that is characteristic of the elderly population in general.

The esophagus and stomach both may have a thinning of the mucous membrane lining; atrophic gastritis is common and may be associated with vitamin B_{12} deficiency and pernicious anemia. There is also an associated risk of gastric carcinoma.

The small and large intestines also change with age and may show degenerative changes, pigment deposition, and calcification. Furthermore, in the large intestinal wall the increased incidence of diverticulosis indicates that the muscular lining may become weakened with age.

The pancreas has also been reported to show senile changes histologically. The liver, on the other hand, rarely shows fibrosis and the other degenerative changes of senescence. The individual parenchymal cells may show signs of aging such as large and unusual nuclei and cytoplasmic organelle variation. Other studies on aged human livers have shown no gross morphologic or functional alterations in the liver with aging. Enzymatic activities of the liver have been reported to remain at a normal level throughout the life span.

Nervous system

Changes in the brain, spinal cord, and peripheral nerves can occur through hypoxic changes due to age-related vascular disease or through intrinsic properties of these tissues. The nervous system consists of highly differentiated cells that do not divide after approximately the first 18 months of life in the human infant. Thus, damage in these cells cannot be compensated for by cell replacement. Damage is either repaired or it accumulates. Thus, aging of the nervous tissue has far-reaching effects on normal physiology and behavior and may lead to pathology. While there is no question that neuronal cells are lost with aging, recent research has shown that neurons are capable of repair and in fact are constantly turning over components of the cell membrane as well as most of the cellular organelles. The chromosomes are not as well repaired as other cytoplasmic and nuclear components due perhaps to a repressing protein, which has been found in neurons and spermatozoa.

Many theories of aging have ascribed a central role to the brain, in which the brain functions as the timekeeper or biological clock for the entire organism. Certainly it is obvious that changes in the brain would effect the functioning of many organs. Whether this implies a biological clock control function of the brain is debatable, however.

The rate of senescence is related to various factors that have previously been described. Positive correlations include brain size, neuron: glia ratio, and perhaps early environmental factors that tend to increase the size and connections of neurons and glial cells. Environmental factors include sensory stimulation and an enriched social and learning environment. It would also appear that neuronal circuits, which are very active, are more likely to be retained and have a longer life span. Of course, all these factors are dependent on the integrity of the vascular perfusion and microvasculature of the brain, and it is conceivable that the function of the brain in old age is intimately connected to blood supply rather than to intrinsic properties of neurons. Characteristically it appears that those neuronal structures that develop first during brain formation and maturation are the last to be affected by senility. These later areas are primarily in the association cortex, with loss greater in the left than in the right hemisphere.

Changes in brain with age. The EEG (electroencephalogram) changes slightly with age in the human. These changes have an earlier onset and a slower decline than other waning physiologic functions such as renal or respiratory function. They are possibly due to age-related cellular impairments of neurons in the brain. The role of lipofuscin pigments, which accumulate so strikingly in brain tissue with age, is still not clear. Possible changes in the normal neurotransmitters may be implicated, and some alterations have been reported to occur with aging. These include acetylcholine, dopamine, norepinephrine, serotonin, γ-aminobutyric acid, and glutamine. These declines in certain parts of the brain of various neurotransmitters may be associated with changes in the enzymes that normally regulate their concentration.

Neurofibrils also appear to become tangled and disoriented in the aged neurons. These structures are believed to transport neurotransmitter substance down the axon to the synapse.

Plaques may form, which consist of amyloid surrounded by degenerated nervous tissue cells. Amyloid is believed to be antigen-antibody complexes that have been degraded by neuronal phagocytes. This may implicate a role for the immune system in senile brain changes.

The brain weight declines, and calcification of the meninges may occur. The lateral ventricles may be enlarged, and the cerebral cortex atrophies. These changes are usually most striking in individuals with senile dementia (chronic brain syndrome), a disorder of old age associated with mental detorioration, cerebral cortex and basal ganglia atrophy, and accelerated senescence. The syndrome may appear in individuals as young as 45 years old, in which case it is usually correlated with cerebral arteriosclerosis and is known as Alzheimer's dementia. Changes in the brain vessels rarely occur alone, and systemic pathology therefore is often present. The onset of the acute disease, which then develops into a chronic process, often follows a severe stress such as a cerebrovascular accident, a drug reaction, cardiac failure, or renal disease. This disorder progresses and ultimately ends in death within from 1 year to occasionally over 10 years after the onset of symptoms. The signs and symptoms of senile dementia include loss of memory, confusion, delirium, impaired intellectual function, and lack of judgment. While the neurologic status of the elderly does change with age, these alterations appear to be greatly exaggerated in senile dementia. Changes in the sensorium, gait, muscular tremors, reflexes, and special senses (taste, olfaction, pain) are all frequently found in the aged.

Signs of impaired short-term memory are often found in the aged, while long-term memory appears often unaffected. The permanence of long-term memory appears to be correlated to the DNA of the neuronal cells involved in the memory circuits. It is speculated that the aged suffer a loss of ability to learn and remember due to the accumulation of defects in the brain system that processes and stores memory and that involves DNA changes. Short-term memory can be influenced by such factors as electroshock therapy, direct electrical stimulation of the brain, and drugs, while long-term memory is not affected by these factors. Thus, it would appear that each learning experience must go through a process of becoming a permanent tracing in the brain, and this process may be interfered with in the aged brain. Memory processing involves mediation by hormonal and neurochemical substances, and these may be affected by aging.

Brain lipid content and turnover both decrease with age and may be related to declining enzymatic activity of the brain. The enzymes produced in the brain tissue may be altered in form and thus inactive. Another possibility is that the DNA of the aged brain cell is subject to inactivation by cross-linkage. The association of DNA with histone proteins may be involved in the cross-linking property. Cross-linkage of essential segments of DNA would act to functionally remove information from the organism.

As has been discussed, pigment accumulates strikingly in the brain as it ages. This is a nonspecific sign of aging, as pigment accumulation occurs throughout the body during senescence. The accumulation is most marked in fully differentiated cells, which are not believed to divide during adult and senescent life. Whether the accumulation of these pigments results *in* aging or is the result *of* aging is unknown. However, certain clinical syndromes known as the *neuronal ceroid-lipofuscinoses* are associated with the accumulation of lipopigments in brain cells and to some degree in body cells. Lipopigments accumulate in these rare genetic conditions and cannot be removed by any known cellular mechanism. It appears that they are cross-linked polymers of biologic molecules with dialdehydes. Dialdehydes are produced by lipid peroxidation in many cells and thus are available to cross-link with molecules and in a sense to serve as a physiologic fixative. Patients with these syndromes show signs of diffuse neuropathy, but cells containing large amounts of the pigment appear to be able to function normally. It is theoretically possible that age pigments may not chemically interfere with the functioning of the cells, as the residual bodies act to sequester the pigments inside a membrane-limited compartment. However, the effect of accumulation may ultimately be distension and mechanical impairment of the cell; in the neuronal ceroid-lipofuscinoses the rate of pigment accumulation appears to be greatly accelerated above that of the normal individual, such that the pigment accumulation approximates that of an aged person during the first years of life. The neurologic effects of pigment may be manifested in both the diseased child and the elderly individual when normal biosynthetic pathways are not able to compensate for the increased pigment production. The cells in this case undergo morphologic changes and eventually die.

Since there are about 10 to 12 billion neurons in the human brain and about five times as many supporting glial cells, the effects of aging on these latter cells cannot be ignored. Furthermore, the complex array of interacting fibers from myriads of different nerve cells in the brain forms a suprastructure on the brain matrix, which also may be altered by the aging process. Additionally astrocytes are interposed between the nervous tissue and capillaries of the vascular system, forming the blood-brain barrier. Also the Schwann cells and oligodendrocytes that form the myelin layers of the nerves are intimately involved in providing the normal structural integrity of the brain and may be affected by the senescent process. Therefore, it is not only the tremendous complexity of the brain function that must be dealt with in aging research but also the topographic diversity.

Nerves. The motor nerve must always be viewed in relationship to the muscle it innervates and thus forms a motor unit with. It has been found that the conduction velocity and neurotransmitter substance release is decreased in the motor nerves of the aged. This is not associated with degeneration of the nerve per se, but the effects of these alterations on the muscle are profound, resulting in or contributing to the atrophy that is common in senescence. It is of interest that physical training of muscles in the young may retard the basic process of muscular atrophy, in that the nerves are kept in a tonically active state. This has great implications for the care of the elderly, who have a need for preservation of mobility for as long as possible.

The sensory nerves are also affected by senescence, and a decline in special sensory acuity is nearly universal. It has been noted that the aged, like the very young, are likely to develop sensory deprivation, a phenomenon that is associated with a wide variety of physiologic and psychologic abnormalities. The deficits that occur in vision and hearing have been studied in regard to the aging process, but other special sensory changes are not well researched. These include vestibular, olfactory, taste, somesthetic and kinesthetic, pain, and touch sensitivities.

DISEASE MODEL: PROGERIA

The rare and impressive disorder of *progeria* (Fig. 18-3) has been implicated as a disease of accelerated aging. In this condition there is a cessation of growth and appearance of many signs suggestive of senescent pathology. The

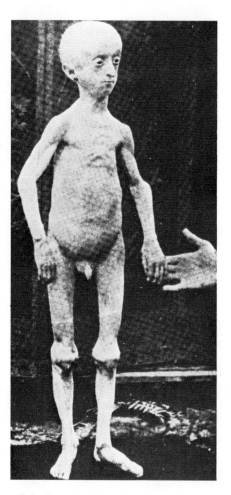

Fig. 18-3. Progeria. Teenaged boy with progeria. Similarities between changes observed here and those associated with normal aging are obvious. (From Burgess, J., and Everett, A., editors: Hypothalamus, pituitary, and aging, 1976, Courtesy Charles C Thomas, Publisher, Springfield, Ill.)

hair becomes gray, the skin wrinkled, generalized fibrosis and atrophy develop, premature atherosclerosis and connective tissue tumors are common, and death occurs early in life. Adult progeria develops in later life and is known as *Werner's syndrome*. It is characterized by processes similar to those in the juvenile form, which is also known as *Hutchinson-Gilford syndrome*. The people afflicted with these conditions have a bizarre senile appearance, which may coexist in the juvenile form with features of childhood. The primary teeth, for example, are often retained. Only

52 cases of the juvenile progeria syndrome have been described in the literature. Thus, it has been difficult to study the pathologic changes in progeria in an attempt to understand if the condition is in reality accelerated aging. Some observations have been made on cells from patients affected with progeria that indicate that the cells are antigenically and biochemically abnormal and in some respects similar to cells from aged people. Pathologic examination of progeria tissue indicates that collagen cross-linking, fibrosis, and lipofuscin accumulation occur, as in senescence. Ninety percent of the cases examined appear to have coronary or aortic atherosclerosis. Serum cholesterol and lipoprotein levels are also often elevated. Patients with Werner's syndrome show many of these changes even more markedly, and the disease is known to be hereditary. An endocrine cause has been investigated in progeria, and the incidence of diabetes is reported to be very high. However, the pituitary gland appears to be normal in these conditions.

Good evidence would indicate that the processes of accelerated senescence, or progeria, bear a superficial relationship to those of normal aging, but important differences appear to exist, and progeria as a disease model of aging cannot be presently accepted.

PHYSIOLOGY OF TREATMENT

The goal of gerontologic research is not only to gain an understanding of the basic cellular processes that occur in aging but also to ultimately delay or prevent aging and death and to improve the quality of life by the prevention of age-related diseases. Thus, many therapeutic approaches to senescence have been suggested. Many are based on various theories of aging. For example, antioxidant therapy might prevent the cross-linking of biologic molecules and thus retard the aging process. Infusions of RNA have been attempted in the elderly to restore learning capabilities and memory. A drug known as *Gerovital H₃* has been used, mostly in Europe, for the treatment of senescent pathology. This drug is a monoamine oxidase inhibitor that has proved to be clinically effective in the treatment of depression, hypertension, arthritis, and angina pectoris. It has been shown that mono-amine oxidase, an enzyme involved in the breakdown of catecholamines, is markedly elevated in humans after the age of 50. Other treatment modalities that have been used for senescent changes include procaine, stimulants such as amphetamines, vasodilators, hyperbaric oxygen, huge doses of vitamins, and hormones. The general effectiveness of these forms of treatment is difficult to measure, although most treatment has resulted in short-term therapeutic benefits.

The modern gerontologic approach to the treatment of senescent deterioration is based on three major phenomena: (1) free radical formation, (2) tissue hypoxia, and (3) macromolecular disorders, particularly of the polyribosomes, upon which protein synthesis proceeds.

Therapy for free radical formation

The approach to the treatment of free radical–related pathology is based on the supposition that these highly reactive compounds damage biologic membranes and molecules through such processes as lipid peroxidation and cross-linking of large biologic molecules with each other. Free radical formation is a prominent result of radiation and is further enhanced in the presence of oxygen. It can be partially prevented by certain antioxidant free radical "scavenger" drugs such as vitamin E and butylated hydroxytoluene (BHT). Addition of these agents to the diet of mice increases their life span, while feeding of polyunsaturated fats, which are most capable of free radical formations, shortens life span. The addition of antioxidants to the diet may eventually be shown to significantly increase longevity in humans.

Therapy for hypoxia

Hypoxia as a result of age-related vascular disease may be a major agent in promoting pathophysiologic changes that occur in aging. Cerebral hypoxia in particular is suspected of inducing most if not all of the neurologic manifestations of senility. Cellular hypoxia leads to abnormal function and structure, and necrosis is ultimately inevitable. Therefore, therapy aimed at reducing the effects of cerebral hypoxia in the aged has been done through the use of hyper-baric oxygen chambers. Significant improvement in many of these patients has been reported. Of course, as previously mentioned, oxygen increases the possibility of free radical formation, which may limit the efficacy of oxygen therapy. It has been found that the improvement in function, such as in learning and memory, is retained long after the period of maximum hyperoxygenation, so it is believed that the period of increased oxygen tension of the tissues results in some changes that are therapeutic and maintained. A possibility is that RNA and protein synthesis occurring during the period of oxygenation results in long-lived proteins that are involved with intellectual function.

Therapy for molecular disorder

It is generally believed that long-term memory requires the synthesis of specific RNA and protein. The actual changes in DNA, RNA, and protein during learning are probably extraordinarily complex. Thus, disturbances in this macromolecular system may impair memory and learning. The polyribosomes of aged human cells are abnormal both structurally and functionally. These cytoplasmic organelles may be the site of action of many drugs that are therapeutic in senility, including phenytoin, procainamide, pemoline, and amphetamines. Procaine has been used for many years, as has Gerovital H_3, which is a derivative of procaine. The latter drug is now being tested extensively in the United States.

Another form of therapy: prevention

While it is obvious that death cannot be prevented, certainly it appears that many of the changes that occur with senescence may be delayed by diet, exercise, drugs, and life-style. Identification of the actual pathophysiologic mechanisms that perpetuate the aging process is in the preliminary stage, yet this research has resulted in several concepts that can be applied to the prevention of age-related pathology and the treatment of such conditions. It is likely that research will provide us with information that can be used to significantly increase longevity and health. Certainly humans are capable of living to well over 100 years, as evidenced by certain populations of individuals in Russia and South America. Attainment of this life span is conceivable for all humans once the basic pathophysiology is well defined.

CONCLUSION

The study of pathophysiology ultimately may not only eliminate the disorders that afflict us but also result in the lengthening of productive lives. Death has been viewed in this book as a return to the most thermodynamically probable state. Pathophysiology is the process by which this return to entropy and loss of the steady state are effected. Physiology then is the constant interaction of processes to produce the thermodynamically unlikely phenomenon of living matter in the steady state. The interfaces between physiology, pathophysiology, and life and death are complex and tightly woven. It is impossible to study and understand one without the other. The student of pathophysiology comes to appreciate the significance of this statement only when he comes in contact with patients who suffer and die due to the frustrating lack of knowledge that still exists in all areas of pathophysiology or when he sees the therapeutic result of medical and nursing intervention based on a sound understanding of and respect for the findings of investigations into pathophysiologic mechanisms.

SUGGESTED READINGS

Andrew, W.: The anatomy of aging in man and animals, New York, 1971, Grune & Stratton.

Bakerman, S., editor: Aging life processes, Springfield, Ill., 1969, Charles C Thomas, Publisher.

Comfort, A.: The position of aging studies, Mech. Ageing Dev. **3:**1-31, 1974.

Cristofalo, V., Roberts, J., and Adelman, R., editors: Explorations in aging, New York, 1974, Plenum Press.

Edge, J., Pump, K., Arias-Stella, J., et al.: The aging lung: normal function, New York, 1974, MSS Information Corporation.

Elias, M., Eleftheriou, B., and Elias, P.: Special review of experimental aging research, Bar Harbor, Me., 1976, EAR.

Everitt, A., and Burgess, J., editors: Hypothalamus, pituitary, and aging, Springfield, Ill., 1976, Charles C Thomas, Publisher.

Garn, S.: The earlir gain and later loss of cortical bone, Springfield, Ill., 1970, Charles C Thomas, Publisher.

Nandy, K., and Sherwin, I., editors: The aging brain and senile dementia, New York, 1977, Plenum Press.

Ordy, J., and Brizee, K., editors: Neurobiology of aging, New York, 1975, Plenum Press.

Palmore, E., editor: Normal aging, Durham, N.C., 1970, Duke University Press.

Pryor, W.: Free radical pathology, C & EN, June 7, 1971.

Rockstein, M., and Chesky, J.: Theoretical aspects of aging, New York, 1974, Academic Press.

Sacher, G., editor: Aging in relation to development and reproduction. Sixth Annual AUA-ANL Biology Symposium, Argonne National Laboratory, October 1971.

Smith, D., and Berwin, E., editors: The biologic ages of man, Philadelphia, 1973, W. B. Saunders Co.

Strehler, B., editor: Advances in gerontological research, vol. 3, New York, 1971, Academic Press.

Strehler, B., editor: Advances in gerontological research, vol. 4, New York, 1972, Academic Press.

Thorbecke, J., editor: Biology of aging and development, New York, 1975, Plenum Press.

Glossary

acanthocyte an abnormal erythrocyte characterized by spiny projections that give it a thorny appearance.

aerobic oxygen dependent.

anabolism metabolic chemical reactions involved in the synthesis of body components; the process by which nutrients are taken up by the cell and converted into complex cellular constituents.

anaerobic not dependent on oxygen.

anasarca severe generalized edema.

ankylosing spondylitis a chronic disease involving the spine, which produces changes similar to those seen in rheumatoid arthritis; it is characterized by inflammation of the sacroiliac, costovertebral, and intervertebral joints with ossification and fixation of the spinal joints, which may result in complete immobilization of the spine and thorax.

antichalones agents that reverse the action of chalones.

antitrypsin substance that inhibits trypsin.

arteriosclerosis thickening, hardening, and loss of elasticity of the walls of the blood vessels; these changes may occur in either the intima or media.

arthropathy joint disease.

Arthus reaction the development of a severe localized inflammatory reaction soon after interdermal injection of an antigenic substance; it is thought to be an immediate hypersensitivity reaction.

asterixis flapping tremor characterized by involuntary jerking movements, especially in the hands; best elicited by having patient extend his arms, dorsiflex his wrists, and spread his fingers. It is also called *liver flap* because of its frequent occurrence in patients with impending hepatic coma, although it may be seen in other forms of encephalopathy.

atheroma fatty degeneration or thickening of the arterial wall.

atherosclerosis a form of arteriosclerosis in which there are localized accumulations of lipid-containing material (atheroma) within or beneath the intimal surfaces of blood vessels; a common cause of arterial occlusion.

autocatalysis progressive catalysis of a reaction by its own products.

autosomes any ordinary paired chromosome other than the sex chromosomes.

azotemia excess of urea or other nitrogenous compounds in the blood.

bradycardia slow heart rate, below 60 per minute in adult and 70 per minute in child.

carotenemia carotene in the blood; characterized by yellowing of the skin.

catabolism reactions of metabolism by which complex cellular substances are broken down into smaller simpler compounds.

cataract clouding of the lens or capsule of the eye, which obstructs vision; this condition can be caused by aging, injury, or infection.

centromere clear region of the chromosome, which marks the junction of two chromatids and location of attachment to the spindle during cell division.

chalone substance that regulates specific intracellular activity, including cell proliferation.

chelating agent chemical agents known as ligands, which form a ring structure surrounding a metallic ion by firmly binding it with coordinate bonds; the entire complex is termed *chelate, metal complex,* or *coordination compound.*

chronotropic affecting the rate of rhythmic movements such as the heart beat.

Chvostek's sign contraction of muscles around the mouth in response to tapping the facial nerve in front of the ear.

chyme semiliquid partially digested food found in the stomach and small intestine during digestion.

cleavage mitotic divisions of the fertilized egg cell.

clone a strain of cells descended from a single cell in tissue culture; this cell population is not only genetically identical but also genetically distinct from similar cells.

conjunctivitis inflammation of the mucous membrane that lines the eyelid.

cor pulmonale chronic: hypertrophy of the right ventricle due to disease of the lungs; acute: dilation and failure of the right side of the heart.

Cori cycle pathway in carbohydrate metabolism; the breakdown of muscle glycogen with the formation of lactic acid, which is reconverted to glycogen in the liver, catabolized to glucose, carried back to the muscles, and again converted into muscle glycogen.

cystic mastitis inflammation of the breast characterized by stromal and epithelial hyperplasia and cystic dilation of the ducts; the affected breast has a diffuse nodular texture.

deamination removal of an amino group, —NH$_2$, from amino compounds.

dermatoglyphics a study of the surface markings of the skin of palms, fingers, toes, and soles; utilized in law enforcement for identification and in medicine as a genetic indicator.

dialdehydes chemical compounds containing two aldehyde groups.

differentiation the process of acquiring functionally specific characteristics through the cellular diversification of embryologic development.

diploid having one complete set of homologous chromosomes or twice the haploid number, as seen in normal somatic cells of higher organisms.

diurnal cyclic events of a 24-hour nature.

dystocia diffiult labor or childbirth.

endergonic reaction that requires energy.

endotracheal intubation insertion of a tube into the trachea, which bypasses the upper airways and allows direct ventilation of bronchi and smaller airways.

entropy a measure of the randomness or disorder in a system; a state of maximum probability.

equifinality the phenomenon by which a final state may be reached through many different pathways.

exergonic reaction that liberates energy.

exophthalmos abnormal protrusion of the eyeball.

exudate substances such as cells, protein, cellular debris, and fluid, which escape from blood vessels into surrounding tissue, usually as result of inflammation.

falciparum malaria infection caused by the organism *Plasmodium falciparum,* one of the most virulent malaria parasites; transmitted only by the bite of the female anopheline mosquito, the disease is characterized by high fever, chills, convulsions, shock, and death.

fibroblast flat, elongated cell with cytoplasmic processes at each end, from which connective tissue is developed.

free radical atom or group of atoms having at least one unpaired electron; their existence is brief due to their extreme reactivity.

gamete basic reproductive cell whose union in sexual reproduction intiates a new individual; a mature female or male reproductive cell: the ovum or spermatozoon.

genotype collection of genes that make up the genetic apparatus of an organism.

glia the supporting structure of the brain and nervous tissue; also used to denote a gluelike tissue.

glucose-6-phosphate dehydrogenase specific enzyme that catalyzes the release of two hydrogen ions from glucose-6-phosphate.

glycogenolysis catabolism of glycogen in body tissue to glucose.

glycoproteins conjugated proteins in which the nonprotein groups are carbohydrates; for example, the mucins, mucoids, and the chondroproteins.

haploid possessing one complete set of nonhomologous chromosomes or half the number of chromosomes in somatic cells of higher organisms; normal state of gamete cells after reduction division of gametogenesis; the haploid number in humans is 23.

haversian canal central unit of haversian system, which is surrounded by concentrically arranged layers of matrix and cells; it carries blood vessels, which transmit nutrient material to the bone.

hemosiderin iron-containing pigment derived from the hemoglobin of red cell breakdown; functions as a storage form of iron.

hepatoma a tumor of the liver; also transition stage between adenoma and carcinoma of the liver.

hepatomegaly enlargement of the liver.

heterozygous having corresponding genes on two different genomes.

homozygous having corresponding genes on two identical genomes.

hyaline crystalline and nearly transparent.

hypercapnia increased concentration of carbon dioxide in the blood; syn. hypercarbia.

hyperphagia abnormally increased consumption of food; sometimes symptomatic of hypothalamus injury.

hyperplasia increase in mass due to increased number of cells in a tissue or organ.

hypertrophy overgrowth; generally an increase in bulk; use may be restricted to denote increase in mass through increase in size but not in number of individual tissue elements.

hypocapnia decreased concentration of carbon dioxide in the blood; syn. hypocarbia.

hypolipoproteinemia deficiency of lipoproteins in the serum; seen in hypobetalipoproteinemia and Tangier disease.

hypophysectomy removal of the pituitary gland.

hyposthenuria excretion of urine of low specific gravity, indicative of loss of concentrating ability.

hypoxemia insufficient oxygenation of the blood; a lower than normal concentration of oxygen in the arterial blood.

hypoxia inadequate cellular oxygenation, which can result from deficiency in either the delivery or utilization of oxygen at the cellular level.

iatrogenic induced by treatment; literally, "doctor caused."

immunization process of gaining protection from a specific pathogenic entity through exposure to antigenic substance while infected by disease or by injection of a vaccine that stimulates antibody production.

inotropic influencing the contractility of the muscular tissue, especially myocardium.

intermittent claudication pain, tenderness, and weakness of the calf, which occurs with exercise and subsides after a period of rest; may be due to occlusion of the arterial blood supply, arteriosclerosis, or atherosclerosis.

karyolysis destruction of the cell nucleus.

karyorrhexis fragmentation of the chromatin in cellular nuclear disintegration.

kernicterus deposition of bile pigments in the nuclear masses of the brain, which results in pathologic changes in the tissue.

kinins biologically active small polypeptides generated in plasma during the first phase of the inflammatory response; their effects include vasodilation, increased permeability to proteins, and attraction of neutrophils.

lactase intestinal enzyme that hydrolyzes lactose and other β-galactosides.

micelle 1. ultramicroscopic colloid particle; 2. living unit made up of one or more molecules and capable of growth and division.

microsome ultramicroscopic granular particle of the endoplasmic reticulum observed after cells are broken by centrifugation.

microvilli microscopic hairlike projections from the free surface of a cell, which greatly increase its surface area.

myelogenous originating in the bone marrow.

oligodendrocyte cell that forms part of the neuroglia of the central nervous system; processes from these cells form a partial investment for some myelin sheaths.

omphalomesenteric duct narrow tube, which, in the embryo, connects the umbilical vesicle (yolk sac) with the mid gut of the embryo.

oogenesis formation and development of female gametes (ova).

operon gene in genetics, a portion of a chromosome consisting of an operator region (at the initial end of the gene where the synthesis of mRNA is indicated) and closely linked structural genes or clusters; the cluster is controlled by the operator through the action of inducer and repressor proteins.

osseous relating to or having the properties of bone.

osteoblast bone cell that is responsible for the formation of one tissue.

osteoclast bone cell that is responsible for resorption (tearing down) of bone.

osteomalacia condition in which the bone matrix is not calcified.

oxidative phosphorylation electron transfer from donor to acceptor with resultant phosphorylation of ADP to form ATP; occurs in the mitochondrion of the cell via the respiratory pigments of the electron transport chain.

papilledema edema and inflammation (swelling) of the optic nerve at its point of entrance into the eyeball.

parabiotic 1. anatomic and physiologic union of two organisms as of joined twins or experimental union of laboratory animals; 2. reversible suspension of conduction through a nerve fiber.

paresthesia abnormal cutaneous sensation such as numbness, tingling, or prickling: heightened sensitivity.

penetrance in genetics, the frequency or phenotypic manifestation of a trait present in the genotype of an individual.

phenotype observable characteristics of an organism; the expression of a given genotype.

photophobia unusual intolerance or sensitivity to light.

piezoelectric effect stimulation of bone growth by an electrical gradient and flow of current, with growth occurring at the site of compressional stress due to the negative potential caused by compressional stress.

pinocytosis cellular process of actively engulfing liquid; a phenomenon in which minute incuppings or invaginations are formed in the surface of the cell membrane and close to form fluid-filled vesicles.

plasmid a group of genetic elements that never become integrated into the host chromosome but remain as independent, self-replicating units, including bioblasts, plasmagenes, plastids and viruses; some plasmids are responsible for the resistance transfer factors, which confer resistance to antibiotics.

pneumothorax collection of air in the pleural cavity, which causes pressure changes that collapse the lung tissue.

polar body cell that separates from an oocyte during

the first or second meiotic division; contains little cytoplasm and consists mostly of nuclear material.

polycythemia excessive number of red cells in the blood.

postprandial occurring after a meal.

postural hypotension a fall in blood pressure that occurs during a change from a lying or sitting position.

progeny descendants of animals; offspring of plants.

progressive multifocal leukoencephalitis rare disease present usually in patients with another underlying disorder or who have been given immunosuppressive drugs; characterized by multifocal demyelination of the white matter of the brain with loss of oligodendroglia, cells that elaborate and support myelin sheath.

proprioception awareness of posture, movement, changes in equilibrium and the knowledge of position, weight, and resistance of objects in relation to the body.

prostaglandins a group of chemically related, long-chain hydroxy fatty acids present in most body tissue; their specific actions are not fully established, but they do affect smooth muscle, nerves, liver, adipose tissue, circulation, and the reproductive organs.

protease protein-splitting enzyme.

pruritus severe itching.

pyruvate kinase enzyme that catalyzes the reaction of phosphopyruvic acid with ADP to form ATP and pyruvic acid, which completes glycolysis.

repressor gene regulatory gene, that contains the coded information for the synthesis of repressor protein; combines with an operator gene to prevent RNA synthesis, which inhibits enzyme synthesis.

retrolental fibroplasia formation of an opaque fibrous membrane behind the lens of the eye; usually occurs in premature infants exposed to high oxygen concentration for a long period of time.

Schwann cells cells around certain nerve fibers; they deposit lipid insulator sheath (myelin).

sclerosis hardening of an organ or tissue; especially a hardening due to excessive fibrous tissue formation from inflammation or disease of the interstitial tissue.

sebaceous producing or pertaining to sebum, an oily, fatty secretion.

secretagogue agent that stimulates secretion.

shearing force pressure that results from subcutaneous tissue and bone sliding with movement while the skin remains stationery.

spermatogenesis formation and development of male gametes (spermatozoa).

splenomegaly enlargement of the spleen.

steatorrhea excess of fat in the stools, seen in malabsorption syndromes.

steroid hormone secreted from the adrenal cortex, which is derived from cholesterol via similar synthetic pathways.

stratification an ordered, layered system.

synovial membrane membrane lining the capsule of a joint, which secretes synovia, a clear lubricating fluid.

tachycardia rapid heart rate; heart rate over 100 per minute in adult and 120 per minute in child.

Tangier disease familial disease characterized by a deficit of serum lipoprotein and abnormal cholesterol storage.

tetany condition characterized by intermittent tonic spasms, which are usually paroxysmal and involve the extremities.

thermoregulation maintenance of a body at a specific temperature regardless of fluctuations in its environmental temperature.

tracheostomy or tracheotomy incision of trachea with insertion of a tube to permit ventilation past an obstruction.

transamination reversible transfer of an amino group, $-NH_2$, from one compound to another or transposition of an amino group within a compound.

Trousseau's sign muscular spasms of the hands and wrist as a result of compression of the brachial artery for 1 to 5 minutes.

uremia the accumulation of toxic nitrogenous wastes in the blood due to renal dysfunction.

vagotomy break in the continuity of the impulses carried by the vagus nerve.

Valsalva's maneuver an attempt at forced expiration with the glottis closed, which causes increased intrathoracic pressure.

vasculitis inflammation of a blood vessel.

xanthoma rounded yellowish lipid plaque found usually on the eyelids.

Index